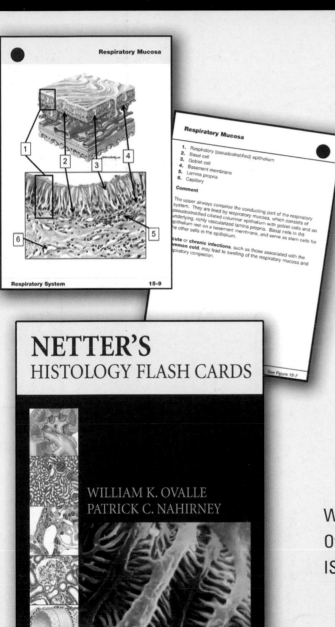

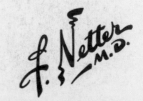

NETTER'S ESSENTIAL HISTOLOGY

William K. Ovalle, PhD
Patrick C. Nahirney, PhD

Illustrations by
Frank H. Netter, MD

Contributing Illustrators
Joe Chovan
John A. Craig, MD
Carlos A.G. Machado, MD
James A. Perkins, MS, MFA

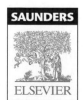

SAUNDERS
ELSEVIER

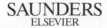

1600 John F. Kennedy Blvd.
Ste 1800
Philadelphia, PA 19103-2899

Netter's Essential Histology　　　　　　　　　　　　　　ISBN: 978-1-929007-86-8

Library of Congress Cataloging-in-Publication Data
Ovalle, William K.
　Netter's essential histology / William K. Ovalle, Patrick C. Nahirney; illustrations by Frank H. Netter; contributing illustrators, John A. Craig, Carlos A.G. Machado, James A. Perkins.—1st ed.
　　p.　;　cm.
　Includes bibliographical references and index.
　ISBN 978-1-929007-86-8
　1. Histology.　2. Histology–Atlases.　I. Nahirney, Patrick C.　II. Netter, Frank H. (Frank Henry), 1906–1991.　III. Title.　IV. Title: Essential histology.
　[DNLM:　1. Histology–Atlases. QS 517 O96n 2008]
　QM551.O94 2008
　611′.018–dc22　　　　　　　　　　　　　　　　　　　　2007003957

Acquisitions Editor: Elyse O'Grady
Developmental Editor: Marybeth Thiel
Publishing Services Manager: Linda Van Pelt
Project Manager: Priscilla Crater
Design Direction: Lou Forgione
Cover Designer: Patrick C. Nahirney

Printed in China

Last digit is the print number:　9　8　7　6　5　4　3　2　1

To the memory of my father—who, on my 10th birthday, gave me my first microscope and showed me how to use it. He was always the consummate teacher, who instilled in me a lifelong interest in serving others.

And to my partner—Robert Wilson Peck—who puts everything in perspective and continues to remind me of what is important.

William K. Ovalle

PREFACE

Histology is fundamental to many branches of medicine, applied science, and allied health professions. A visual science, it deals with microscopic structure as it relates to function. *Netter's Essential Histology* provides a contemporary and visual overview of normal histology by incorporating classic Netter illustrations and new drawings in the Netter style, original light and electron micrographs, and succinct explanatory text. As a pictorial guide, it highlights salient microscopic features of cells, tissues, and organs of the body. Its user-friendly and logical format is especially relevant in today's revised, problem-based, integrated curricula for students in medicine, dentistry, and undergraduate science programs. Allied health care professionals, clinical residents, medical laboratory technologists, teachers, and researchers will also benefit from its use.

Rapid advances in biomedical sciences and new curricula have required more efficient information presentation. To meet these challenges, *Netter's Essential Histology* concentrates on essentials of histologic organization and core concepts. The book draws attention to the morphologic continuum and integrates gross anatomy, embryology, histology, cell biology, and ultrastructure in a concise fashion. It also provides information with special clinical relevance.

Each chapter begins with an overview and then leads in logical sequence from low- to high-magnification micrographs with brief captions. Summaries of embryonic development are included when appropriate for better understanding. Concise, up-to-date, comprehensive text accompanies the illustrations and micrographs on the same page. To encourage self-directed learning, understanding of fundamentals rather than excessive detail is stressed, with emphasis on correlation of structure to function related to contemporary medicine. Many clinical boxes in the text give insight into pathology and aid appreciation of the importance of comprehending normal structure to understand abnormality and disease.

Light micrographs prepared with staining methods commonly used in histology and pathology utilize human tissues taken from biopsy, autopsy, and cadaveric specimens. High-resolution electron micrographs are mostly of freshly fixed rodent specimens and, in some cases, human materials. Electron micrographs are used selectively to enrich knowledge of fundamental cellular constituents as related to function.

Netter's Essential Histology serves multiple purposes. It is a visual guideline of histologic information essential for prospective physicians and other health care professionals. It aids students and specialists studying slides under a microscope and examining digitized images on a computer screen. It facilitates recognition and interpretation of microscopic sections and provides relevant frames of reference for understanding basic histologic principles. It helps clarify lectures, supplements standard textbooks, and provides a comprehensive review for course examinations. It also assists students in preparing for National Board and Licensing Examinations. Finally, the book is intended to awaken readers to both the intricacies of the human body and the sheer beauty of its cells, tissues, and organ systems.

William K. Ovalle
Patrick C. Nahirney

ACKNOWLEDGMENTS

When first approached by Mr. Paul Kelly with the possibility of writing a histology book incorporating Netter illustrations, I was not only deeply thrilled with the opportunity but also enormously honored and humbled. During my early student days in Anatomy at Temple University School of Medicine in Philadelphia, one of my gross anatomy professors—a dear friend and colleague of Dr. Frank Netter—knew how much I cherished Dr. Netter's lifelike and detailed drawings of the human body. Fortunately, I was then given the opportunity to meet and visit the infamous Dr. Netter one day at his studio in New York. On that memorable morning, Dr. Netter graciously showed me some new pencil sketches and beautiful watercolors with overlays he had just created. He carefully explained the process of gouache—a watercolor technique—he had been using, and shared his thoughts about how the artwork must lead the observer's eye to essentials of the topic at hand. His trademark and exquisite drawings—like those of no one else—not only brought anatomy "alive" for me, but continue to contribute greatly to medical education around the world.

Shortly after I agreed to take on the task of writing this book—combining my own histology micrographs with Netter drawings—I asked my former doctoral student, Dr. Patrick C. Nahirney, to be co-author. I owe an enormous debt of gratitude to him for eagerly participating in this endeavor with me. He is an indefatigable worker who has contributed the majority of original, high-quality electron micrographs. In addition, he was always available at a moment's notice to provide the most cogent and up-to-date scientific points related to the text. He is a talented and accomplished scientist with a distinctive ability to effectively bridge the gap between light and electron microscopy.

I am extremely grateful to the remarkable medical artist—Dr. Carlos Machado—who contributed many new and splendid plates to the book. His ability to accurately and forcefully translate conceptual ideas or tarnished copies of my old blackboard drawings into brilliant, three-dimensional art pieces is admirable. His contributions to the book are exceptional, contemporary pieces. They are a noteworthy testament to the Netter legacy. I also appreciate the artistic contributions of Dr. John Craig, Mr. Jim Perkins, and Mr. Joe Chovan.

In addition to Paul Kelly, whose idea it was to first embark on the project, I am especially indebted to three key individuals at Elsevier. Their guidance, critical input, and support were absolutely invaluable throughout the process of producing the book. Ms. Marybeth Thiel, Developmental Editor, patiently provided much needed direction, and kept us on track with necessary deadlines. Her expert knowledge, keen sense of professionalism, and overall capability were exceptional as she carefully coached us along—every step of the way. I profoundly thank Ms. Judith Gandy, Editor, whose extraordinary insight and unwavering attention to detail were invaluable. She not only aptly transformed the original manuscript into succinct and intelligible text, but also gave invaluable advice on artwork, clinical points, and scientific details. Ms. Elyse O'Grady, Editor of Netter Products, was incredibly helpful with web-related issues, design, and the production of flashcards. Her steadfast support was very much appreciated.

I am grateful for the generosity of several colleagues, friends, and authors, who permitted me to reproduce some of their original micrographs. Dr. Pierre R. Dow—with whom I have worked closely in research and teaching for over three decades—deserves special credit, especially for his inspiration, enthusiasm, and advice. Drs. Bruce J. Crawford, A. Wayne Vogl, Martin J. Hollenberg, and R. Michael Patten—members of my department—were especially generous in providing their beautiful electron micrographs. I also thank Dr. John Hansen from the University of Rochester, and Dr. William C. Gibson from the University of Victoria. In addition, two other departmental colleagues deserve special mention. The late Drs. William A. Webber and Vladimir Palaty contributed greatly, not only in providing their original micrographs, but also to the overall development of my professional career.

I thank other members of my staff—Ms. Monika Fejtek, Mr. Ian M. Patton, and Mr. George Spurr—who were very helpful with the preparation of histologic specimens, compilation of computerized graphics, and provision of expert technical advice. Their contributions have been a great asset to the book.

I gratefully acknowledge the "anonymous" external reviewers who gave generously of their time, and shared their expertise in carefully and critically reviewing each chapter. I thank: Brian R. MacPherson, Ph.D., Vice-Chair and Holsinger Endowed Professor of Anatomy in the Department of Anatomy and Neurobiology at the University of Kentucky College of Medicine; Jeffrey D. Green, Ph.D., Professor, Cell Biology and Anatomy, Louisiana State University School of Medicine; Larry J. Ream, Ph.D., Associate Professor of Anatomy, Vice Chair, Department of Neuroscience, Cell Biology and Physiology, Director, Graduate Programs in Anatomy and in Physiology & Biophysics, Boonshoft School of Medicine, Wright State University.

No words can express my gratitude to the long line of medical, dental and graduate students who I have been privileged to know over the years, and who continue to teach me. In the words of Sir William Osler—the renowned Canadian physician: "in the bewildering complexity of modern medicine. . . . no one can teach successfully who is not at the same time a student."

Finally, I thank the many teachers and role models who truly have molded my professional career. I am particularly grateful to Dr. Steven J. Phillips, my graduate advisor and histology professor at Temple University School of Medicine. In my early student days, he solemnly sat me down on countless Saturday mornings in front of the electron microscope, and instilled an excitement of cell structure and fascination of the unknown. I also owe a special debt of gratitude to Drs. Sydney M. and Constance L. Friedman, who offered me my first professorial position in the Faculty of Medicine at the University of British Columbia. By example, they led our wonderful department for over 30 years, and warmly provided me a "home" in the Department of Anatomy, now a Division in Cellular and Physiological Sciences at UBC. Their unwavering guidance and support throughout my career, and in the writing of this book, have been immeasurable.

William K. Ovalle

First of all, it's truly an honor to coauthor a textbook with the Dr. Frank H. Netter legacy. I wish to thank Dr. William K. Ovalle for his gracious invitation to coauthor *Netter's Essential Histology*. As my mentor in graduate studies, it is he who inspired my appreciation of histology and the anatomical sciences. His compassion and extraordinary dedication to medical education have set a high standard for me to follow.

A special thanks to the Elsevier production staff who worked closely with us, Marybeth Thiel, Elyse O'Grady, and Priscilla Crater, and our editor, Judith Gandy, who were always quick with a helping hand and highly focused on our goals.

There are many other people to whom I owe my gratitude, but I would especially like to acknowledge Dr. Pierre R. Dow, Professor Emeritus of Anatomy, a good friend and a character who first introduced me to Dr. Ovalle. As well, my former colleagues at the University of British Columbia, Drs. A. Wayne Vogl and Bruce J. Crawford, and the late Drs. William A. Webber and Vladimir Palaty, all truly masters of their discipline, deserve a special round of thank yous. And I would like to acknowledge Drs. Donald A. Fischman and Kuan Wang, inspiring, knowledgeable, and helpful mentors in my academic career.

Finally, I express my deepest thanks and appreciation to my parents, Denise and William Nahirney, who have always been so exceptionally supportive of all my endeavors in life.

Patrick C. Nahirney

ABOUT THE AUTHORS

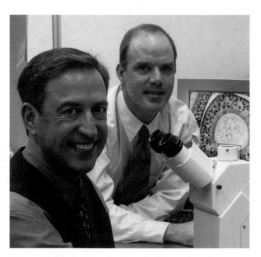

William K. Ovalle (left) and Patrick C. Nahirney (right)

WILLIAM K. OVALLE was born in Panama, and graduated from St. Joseph's University in Philadelphia, Pennsylvania with a B.S in Biology. He went on to receive his doctoral degree from Temple University School of Medicine, in Philadelphia. He was awarded a Predoctoral Traineeship in Anatomy from the National Institutes of Health and was elected to membership in Sigma Xi. He later became a Muscular Dystrophy Association Postdoctoral Fellow, and trained for two years in the Department of Surgery at the University of Alberta in Edmonton, Canada. In 1972, Dr. Ovalle joined the Department of Anatomy, Faculty of Medicine at the University of British Columbia in Vancouver, rapidly ascending the ranks to full professor in 1984. He has taught gross human anatomy, histology, and neuroanatomy to medical/dental students and surgical residents. In addition, he has been Director of Medical/Dental Histology at UBC since 1977. Over the years, he has published extensively on aspects of normal and diseased muscle, including the muscle spindle. During his tenure at UBC, he has served as Head of the Department of Anatomy (now Cellular and Physiological Sciences), subsequently returning full time to his scholarly interests in human histology. He has served as Councilor for the Canadian Association of Anatomists, as Chairman of Science Policy for the Canadian Federation of Biological Societies, as member of the Scientific Advisory Board for the Muscular Dystrophy Association, and as a member of Educational Affairs for the American Association of Anatomists. In 1992, he was awarded Certificate of Merit by the Panamerican Association of Anatomists. Over a long and rich history as a histologist and educator, he has responded to the changing needs of his discipline—moving from a microscope focus to pioneering the development of a virtual histology website for use in the expanded and distributed medical curriculum in British Columbia. This educational innovation has been the focus of other curricula around the world. Dr. Ovalle has been recognized repeatedly for teaching and educational leadership with several notable awards, including the Killam University Teaching Prize (the highest teaching award at UBC), several Medical Undergraduate Society Awards for Teaching Excellence, the Faculty of Medicine 50th Anniversary Gold Medal, and Honorary UBC Medical Alumnus.

PATRICK C. NAHIRNEY was born in 1967 in Winnipeg, Manitoba, Canada. He received a B.Sc. degree in Biology (cum laude) from Washington State University in 1990 and obtained his M.Sc.(1993) and Ph.D. (2000) degrees under the mentorship of Dr. Ovalle in the Department of Anatomy, Faculty of Medicine, at the University of British Columbia, Vancouver, Canada. He then went on as a Postdoctoral Fellow in Cell and Developmental Biology at Cornell Medical College. He has trained in and taught the three core medical and dental anatomy courses (gross anatomy, histology, neuroanatomy) and performed research in various aspects of muscle structure and disease, as well as coronary blood vessel formation. Dr. Nahirney has been a member of the American Association of Anatomists since 1991, has served on their Board of Directors for four years, and has received numerous awards for his research activities. His dedication to morphological detail and motto of 'seeing is believing' remain constant in his research and academic pursuits.

Frank H. Netter, MD

FRANK H. NETTER was born in 1906, in New York City. He studied art at the Art Student's League and the National Academy of Design before entering medical school at New York University, where he received his MD degree in 1931. During his student years, Dr. Netter's notebook sketches attracted the attention of the medical faculty and other physicians, allowing him to augment his income by illustrating articles and textbooks. He continued illustrating as a sideline after establishing a surgical practice in 1933, but he ultimately opted to give up his practice in favor of a full-time commitment to art. After service in the United States Army during World War II, Dr. Netter began his long collaboration with the CIBA Pharmaceutical Company (now Novartis Pharmaceuticals). This 45-year partnership resulted in the production of the extraordinary collection of medical art so familiar to physicians and other medical professionals worldwide.

Icon Learning Systems acquired the Netter Collection in July 2000 and continued to update Dr. Netter's original paintings and to add newly commissioned paintings by artists trained in the style of Dr. Netter. In 2005, Elsevier, Inc. purchased the Netter Collection and all publications from Icon Learning Systems. There are now over 50 publications featuring the art of Dr. Netter available through Elsevier, Inc.

Dr. Netter's works are among the finest examples of the use of illustration in the teaching of medical concepts. The 13 book *Netter Collection of Medical Illustrations*, which includes the greater part of the more than 20,000 paintings created by Dr. Netter, became and remains one of the most famous medical works ever published. *The Netter Atlas of Human Anatomy*, first published in 1989, presents the anatomical paintings from the Netter Collection. Now translated into 16 languages, it is the anatomy atlas of choice among medical and health professions students the world over.

The Netter illustrations are appreciated not only for their aesthetic qualities, but, more important, for their intellectual content. As Dr. Netter wrote in 1949, ". . . clarification of a subject is the aim and goal of illustration. No matter how beautifully painted, how delicately and subtly rendered a subject may be, it is of little value as a *medical illustration* if it does not serve to make clear some medical point." Dr. Netter's planning, conception, point of view, and approach are what inform his paintings and what make them so intellectually valuable.

Frank H. Netter, MD, physician and artist, died in 1991.

CONTENTS

I: CELLS AND TISSUES

1

THE CELL

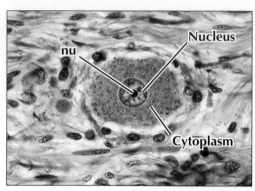

▲ **Light micrograph (LM) of part of the dorsal root ganglion.** A large nerve cell contrasts with smaller cells around it. The nerve cell has a rounded nucleus with a small, dark nucleolus (**nu**). Its cytoplasm is speckled with a bluish meshwork— the ribosomes and rough endoplasmic reticulum. 500×. *H&E.*

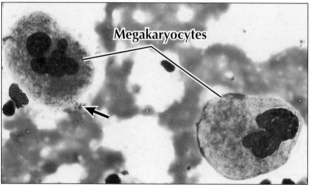

▲ **LM of megakaryocytes in a bone marrow smear.** These large cells have frothy, finely granular cytoplasm. Each cell has one large multilobulated nucleus that is polyploid and intensely basophilic. These cells produce platelets (**arrow**)—small cytoplasmic fragments—that are released into peripheral blood. Surrounding closely packed cells, many of which are erythrocytes, are small. Mature erythrocytes lack nuclei. 530×. *Wright's.*

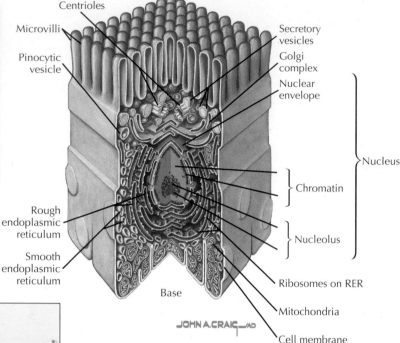

▲ **A composite cell cut open to show organization of its main components, as seen via electron microscopy.** A plasma membrane surrounds the cell, which is polarized, with basal, lateral, and apical domains. Its cytoplasm contains various organelles and inclusions, which surround a nucleus. Some organelles are membrane bound, but some are not. The apical cell border has many finger-like projections called microvilli. Lateral cell borders are areas with intercellular junctions.

1.1 OVERVIEW

The human body is organized into four **basic tissues (epithelial, muscle, nervous,** and **connective)** that consist of cells and associated *extracellular matrix.* The **cell** is the fundamental structural and functional unit of all living organisms. The body contains about 60×10^{12} cells—some 200 different types whose size and shape vary widely—but all have a common structural plan. The *eukaryotic cell* is a mass of **protoplasm** surrounded by an external **plasma (limiting) membrane.** The two components of the protoplasm are the **nucleus,** which holds the *genome* consisting of *chromosomes,* and the **cytoplasm,** a complex aqueous gel made of water (about 70%), proteins, lipids, carbohydrates, and organic and inorganic molecules. **Organelles** (specialized structures with functional capability) and **inclusions** (relatively inert, transitory structures) are in the cytoplasm. Except for mature erythrocytes, without a nucleus, most cells have one nucleus that conforms to the cell's shape. A few cells, such as osteoclasts and skeletal muscle cells, may be multinucleated. A **nuclear envelope** invests the nucleus, whose substance, called **chromatin,** contains one or more **nucleoli.** Internal cell structure is modified to reflect function: muscle cells, for example, are modified for contraction; nerve cells (or neurons), for conduction; connective tissue cells such as fibroblasts, for support; and glandular epithelial cells, for secretion.

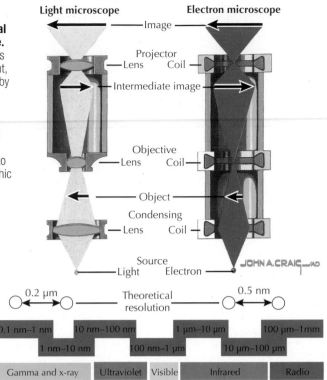

▶ Optical parts of a conventional light (or bright-field) microscope. This compound microscope transmits light through three glass lenses. Light, first focused on a stained specimen by a substage condenser lens, passes through the specimen and then an objective lens, which magnifies and projects the illuminated image to the ocular lens. The ocular lens further magnifies the image and projects it to the eye of the viewer or a photographic plate. Most tissues are colorless, so color dyes serve as stains that differentially absorb light so that structures in specimens may be distinguished.

◀ Optical parts of a transmission electron microscope (TEM). A TEM transmits a beam of electrons through an ultrathin section of tissue that has been cut via an ultramicrotome. Several coiled electromagnetic lenses deflect electrons and use the same principle as that of light microscope lenses to condense, focus, and magnify images. Electrons from a heated tungsten filament (or cathode) are drawn toward an anode within a vacuum column. Electrons are not visible to the naked eye, so a fluorescent screen or photographic plate records the image as a black and white electron micrograph (EM). The advantage of the TEM is great resolving power.

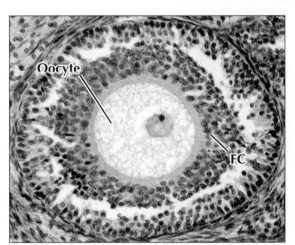

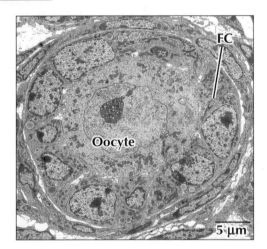

◀ ▶ Comparative views of the ovary as seen with light (Left) and electron (Right) microscopes. Images show a large oocyte surrounded by smaller follicular cells (**FC**). The LM is a paraffin section stained with hematoxylin and eosin (H&E). Hematoxylin, a blue cationic stain, binds to anionic (negatively charged) basophilic sites in tissue sections. Eosin, a pink anionic stain, binds to acidophilic (positively charged) tissue components. The EM is a thin plastic section stained with heavy metals (lead citrate and uranyl acetate). **Left:** 200×; **Right:** 1800×.

1.2 MICROSCOPES AND TECHNIQUES

Histology is the study of body **tissues** and **cells,** their constituents. Cells cannot be seen with the naked eye, so the primary tool used to study them is the **microscope.** It produces enlarged images of cells and enhances contrast for resolving details. Of several kinds of microscopes, two major ones are **light** and **electron microscopes.** They have different lenses and sources of illumination and provide complementary information at different levels of *resolution* and *magnification.* The ability to discriminate two points that are close together is the *resolving power* of a microscope. It is related to the light wavelength. A conventional light microscope uses bright-field illumination, with a resolving power of about 0.2 μm. Study specimens absorb visible light; glass lenses focus and magnify specimens. Most cells absorb very little light, so **staining** is needed to increase light absorption. Cells and tissues first undergo sequen-

tial processing steps. **Fixation** in aldehydes and **dehydration** in alcohols are followed by **embedding** in paraffin or plastic. Specimen **sections** (or slices) are made with a **microtome,** followed by staining with color dyes. The illumination source of the *transmission electron microscope* (TEM) is a beam of electrons, which has a smaller wavelength. The resolving power of the TEM, 0.2-0.5 nm, is about 10^3 greater than that of the light microscope. For the TEM, ultrathin sections are cut after specimens have been fixed and embedded in plastic. Sections are then stained with heavy metals to enhance contrast, and black-and-white, not color, images result. A *scanning electron microscope* (SEM) is used for thick specimens or whole cells that have been fixed, dried, and coated with a thin metal film. It provides three-dimensional surface views. A *high-resolution SEM* (HRSEM) allows internal morphology of cells and organelles to be discerned with great depth of focus.

▶ **LM of chondrocytes in hyaline cartilage.** The main function of these principal cells of cartilage is to synthesize and secrete surrounding extracellular matrix (**ECM**). Each cell has one round to ellipsoid nucleus and pale-stained cytoplasm. The ECM, which is also stained, contains proteins and carbohydrates secreted by the cells. 400×. *H&E.*

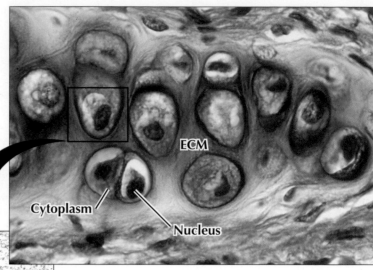

◀ **EM of a chondrocyte with its nucleus and cytoplasm.** Heavy metal stains combine with different parts of the cell to render them dark or light. Areas that appear dark, such as cell membranes and organelles, are electron dense—they scatter electrons that have passed through the section. Conversely, areas that do not scatter electrons are lighter (electron lucent). Note that assorted organelles pack the cytoplasm. 2000×. *(Courtesy of Dr. B. J. Crawford)*

▶ **High-resolution scanning EM (HRSEM) of a chondrocyte.** This image shows internal surface contours of a cell in three dimensions. Cells are frozen, fractured open, and coated with a thin metal film, and then surfaces are scanned. The resolving power of the SEM is not as great as that of the TEM, but tissue sections need not be cut for an SEM. Complementary information is obtained from the two microscopes. 2000×. *(Courtesy of Dr. M. J. Hollenberg)*

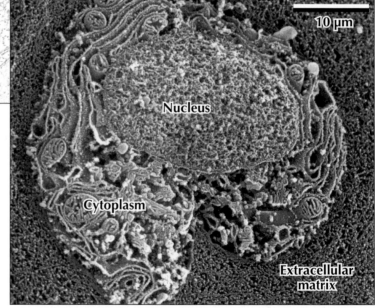

1.3 DIFFERENT APPEARANCES OF CELLS ACCORDING TO TECHNIQUE

Histologic techniques provide different but complementary views of cells and thus a useful morphologic base, which can aid understanding of cell function in health and disease. Paraffin sections are routinely stained with **hematoxylin and eosin (H&E)** and examined with a light microscope. Cell **nuclei** (which are rich in nucleic acids such as DNA and RNA) have an affinity for hematoxylin (a basic dye), stain blue, and are termed **basophilic.** In contrast, the **cytoplasm** of cells and **extracellular matrix** typically have an affinity for eosin (an anionic dye), stain pink, and are **eosinophilic** (or *acidophilic*). With superior resolving power, a **TEM** provides better elucidation of cell details, such as membranes and organelles, than a light microscope. Different parts of cells have distinct affinities for metal stains used on thin sections, so resulting two-dimensional images show variations in electron density, recorded in black and white. **HRSEM** images of freeze-fractured cells show three-dimensional spatial relationships of organelles and inclusions.

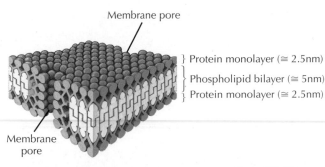

Membrane pore

} Protein monolayer (≅ 2.5nm)
} Phospholipid bilayer (≅ 5nm)
} Protein monolayer (≅ 2.5nm)

Membrane pore

▲ **Classic trilaminar model (after Davson and Danielli).** This 1935 model proposed that the plasma membrane is a bimolecular lipid sandwich with protein absorbed on each side of the lipid.

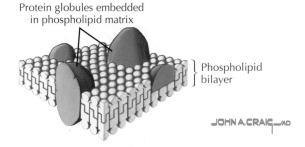

Protein globules embedded in phospholipid matrix

} Phospholipid bilayer

JOHN A. CRAIG—AD

▲ **Fluid mosaic model (after Singer and Nicholson).** This 1972 model proposed that the plasma membrane is a fluid lipid bilayer in which proteins are partly or completely embedded.

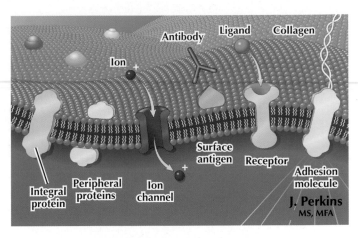

Antibody   Ligand   Collagen
Ion
Integral protein   Peripheral proteins   Ion channel   Surface antigen   Receptor   Adhesion molecule

J. Perkins
MS, MFA

▲ **Current rendition of the plasma membrane.** The phospholipid bilayer is associated with integral and extrinsic proteins, which serve many functions—tissue organization via adhesion molecules, bidirectional transport of substances via ion channels, cell recognition by surface antigens, and intercellular communication via neurotransmitter and hormone receptors.

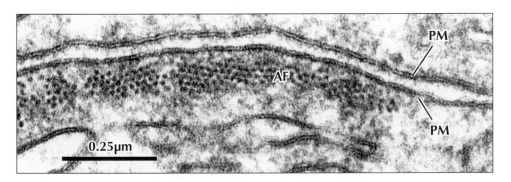

PM
AF
PM
0.25μm

▲ **EM of cell membranes.** Each plasma membrane (**PM**) of two adjacent cells has a trilaminar appearance. Actin filaments (**AF**) close to the cell surface are seen in transverse section. 100,000×.
(Courtesy of Dr. A. W. Vogl)

1.4 ULTRASTRUCTURE AND FUNCTION OF CELL MEMBRANES

Membranes—semipermeable barriers that selectively regulate movement of ions, water, and macromolecules—are ubiquitous in cells. They vary in composition depending on cell type and location, but all consist of about 35% lipids, 60% proteins, and 5% carbohydrates. The **cell** (or **plasma**) **membrane** forms an external boundary. Intracellular membranes surround nuclei and membrane-bound organelles. Membranes are beyond the limit of resolution of a light microscope and are thus difficult to visualize without special techniques. By high-magnification electron microscopy, membranes have a trilaminar appearance: two dark lines separated by a thin electron-lucent zone. The entire **trilaminar membrane,** or **unit membrane,** is 5-8 nm thick. Membranes are made of a lipid bilayer, with a structure consistent with a highly dynamic **fluid mosaic model:** two hydrophilic phospholipid leaflets with polar phosphate heads that point outward. The hydrophobic fatty acid tail regions form the internal membrane framework. Cholesterol molecules, dispersed throughout the membrane, impart fluidity to it. **Intrinsic (integral) globular proteins** lie in the lipid bilayer and span the membrane thickness. **Extrinsic (peripheral) proteins** are also anchored to the membrane and associate with outside or inside surfaces of the bilayer. Carbohydrates often form a fuzzy coat called the *glycocalyx* on the outside of membranes. Membranes contain **channels** and *ion pumps* made of proteins that regulate the cell's internal milieu by creating electrical charge differences. Membranes also contain **receptors** for hormones and growth factors, such as receptors for neurotransmitters in plasma membranes of neurons and muscle cells.

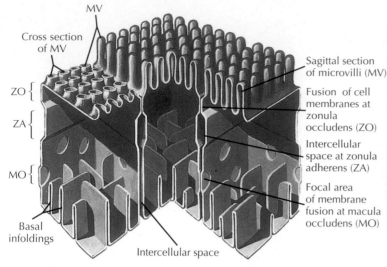

ZO
ZA
MO

Cross section of MV
MV

Sagittal section of microvilli (MV)

Fusion of cell membranes at zonula occludens (ZO)

Intercellular space at zonula adherens (ZA)

Focal area of membrane fusion at macula occludens (MO)

Basal infoldings

Intercellular space

▲ **Parts of three cells with microvilli on apical surfaces and junctional complexes at lateral borders.** A typical junctional complex comprises several types of intercellular junctions, such as tight junctions (zonula and macula occludens) and zonula adherens, seen here.

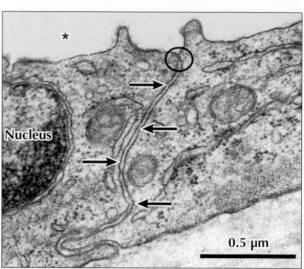

▲ **EM of a tight junction between two epithelial cells in the wall of a renal tubule.** Plasma membranes (**arrows**) of two adjacent cells interdigitate with each other. A tight junction (**circle**) is close to the tubule lumen (∗). Part of the nucleus of one cell is at the left. 50,000×. *(Courtesy of Dr. W. A. Webber)*

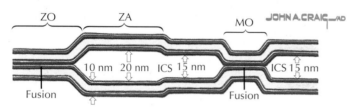

ZO ZA MO

JOHN A. CRAIG—AD

10 nm 20 nm ICS 15 nm   ICS 15 nm

Fusion   Fusion

▲ **Part of opposing plasma membranes of two cells.** The relative thickness of the intercellular space (**ICS**) at the junctions is seen. Fusion of adjacent cell membranes with occlusion of the ICS occurs at tight junctions. The macula occludens is a variant of this type of junction.

▼ **EM of tight junctions between two epithelial cells in the retina.** The trilaminar appearance of opposing plasma membranes (**PM**) of the cells is obvious. Several focal tight junctions (**circles**) are seen. 100,000×. *(Courtesy of Dr. B. J. Crawford)*

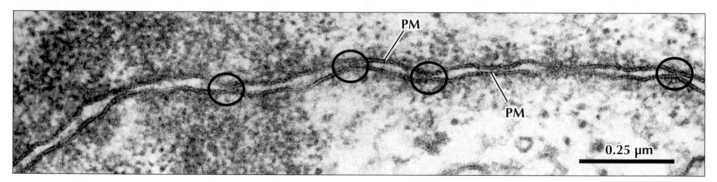

1.5 INTERCELLULAR JUNCTIONS: ULTRASTRUCTURE AND FUNCTION OF TIGHT JUNCTIONS

To increase adhesiveness, most adjacent cells have simple interdigitations between them. Cell membranes interact with extracellular matrix by adhesive contacts consisting of cell adhesion molecules. Cells also show more specialized modifications of **plasma membranes**—intercellular junctions of different kinds. There are three major types: **tight** (**zonula** and **macula occludens**), **anchoring** (**macula** and **zonula adherens**), and **gap** (or **communicating**) **junctions.** Tight junctions are common between epithelial cells and are closest to the luminal surface, where they form an occluding, belt-like seal between cells. At different sites, they form permeability barriers to prevent indiscriminate passage of material. The

tightness and permeability features of these junctions depend on cell type and location. In endothelia of specialized capillaries, they are the basis for the *blood-brain, blood-ocular,* and *blood-testis* barriers. In other sites, they define a boundary between apical and basolateral domains of plasma membrane. In high-magnification electron micrographs (EMs), plasma membranes of adjacent cells appear fused at one or more focal contact sites that eliminate intervening **extracellular spaces.** Each contact site contains *transmembrane proteins,* such as occludin, and different classes of *claudins.* Other cytoplasmic proteins, as well as *cadherin* proteins, reinforce the sites. A freeze-fracture EM shows tight junctions with a network of ridges and opposing grooves, which correspond to transmembrane proteins. *Actin filaments* of the *cytoskeleton* also associate with cytoplasmic sides of tight junctions.

▼ **Parts of three cells.**

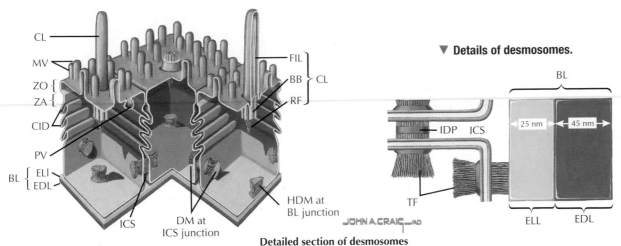

▼ **Details of desmosomes.**

JOHN A.CRAIG—AD

Detailed section of desmosomes

BB = Basal body	EDL = Electron-dense lamina	IDP = Intermediate dense plaque	ZA = Zonula adherens
BL = Basal lamina	ELL = Electron-lucent lamina	MV = Microvilli	ZO = Zonula occludens
CID = Cellular interdigitations	FIL = Filaments	PV = Pinocytic vesicle	
CL = Cilia	HDM = Hemidesmosomes	RF = Root fibrils	
DM = Desmosomes	ICS = Intercellular space	TF = Tonofibrils	

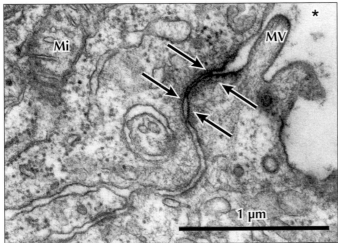

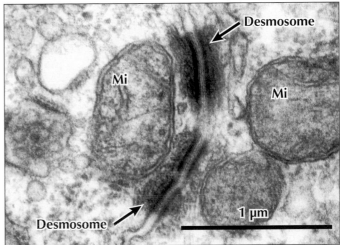

▲ **EM of a zonula adherens between adjacent epithelial cells in the kidney.** Interdigitating lateral cell borders show a zonula adherens (**arrows**) close to the lumen (∗). Cytoplasmic densities under the plasma membranes contain actin filaments, some of which are entering a microvillus (**MV**). Part of a mitochondrion (**Mi**) is seen. 40,000×. *(Courtesy of Dr. W. A. Webber)*

▲ **EM of desmosomes between adjacent epithelial cells in the kidney.** Dense cytoplasmic plaques on both sides of each junction correspond to accumulated intermediate filaments. An electron-dense line extends along the center of the intercellular space of the desmosomes. Mitochondria (**Mi**) are also in the cytoplasm. 40,000×. *(Courtesy of Dr. W. A. Webber)*

1.6   INTERCELLULAR JUNCTIONS: ULTRASTRUCTURE AND FUNCTION OF ANCHORING JUNCTIONS

Two kinds of anchoring junctions, **zonula adherens** and **macula adherens (desmosome),** hold cells together. They usually occur between lateral borders of adjacent epithelial cells. They resist mechanical stress and prevent lateral disruption by stabilizing the epithelium. Cytoplasmic **actin filaments** anchor zonulae adherentes; **intermediate filaments (tonofilaments)** anchor desmosomes. In most epithelia, a zonula adherens usually encircles the apical part of the whole cell just below the tight junction. Transmembrane proteins, consisting mostly of *cadherin* molecules, are on both sides of the junction. Their extracellular domains span the narrow gap (20 nm) between adjacent cells; their intracellular domains interact with other cytoplasmic proteins (*vinculin* and *α-actinin*) to anchor actin filaments of the cytoskeleton. Desmosomes are more complex, plaque-like junctions in epithelial cells, as well as in cardiac and smooth muscle cells, that resemble spot welds and strongly hold cells together at focal points. Dense cytoplasmic plaques are on the cytoplasmic sides of opposing plasma membranes. The intercellular space (20-25 nm wide) often shows a dense line in the center that parallels opposing cell membranes. This space contains transmembrane cadherins (*desmogelins* and *desmocollins*) that span it and link adjacent plasma membranes. Accessory proteins in the dense plaques (*desmoplakin* and *plakoglobin*) anchor intermediate filaments. Depending on location, desmosomes may have different types of intermediate filaments, such as *keratins,* associated with epithelial cells, and *desmin,* in cardiac muscle cells.

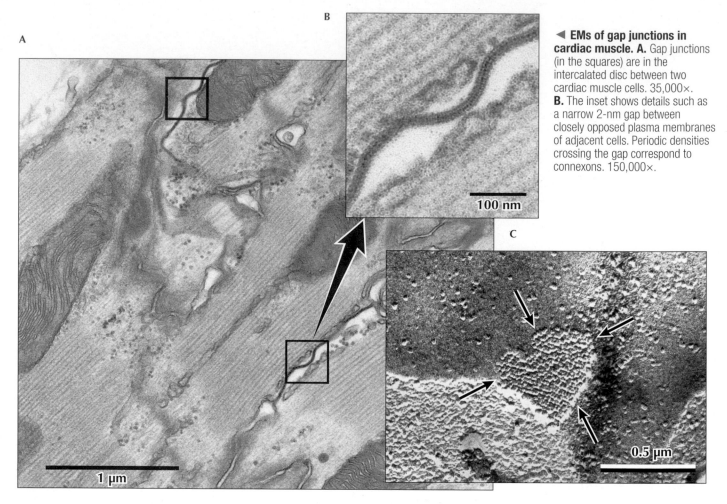

◀ **EMs of gap junctions in cardiac muscle. A.** Gap junctions (in the squares) are in the intercalated disc between two cardiac muscle cells. 35,000×. **B.** The inset shows details such as a narrow 2-nm gap between closely opposed plasma membranes of adjacent cells. Periodic densities crossing the gap correspond to connexons. 150,000×.

▶ **Freeze-fracture EM replica of a gap junction. C.** This technique allows interior and surface topography of membranes to be seen without fixation. A specimen is rapidly frozen in liquid nitrogen and then fractured with a metal knife under high vacuum. The fracture usually splits membranes along a plane in the center of the lipid bilayer. A replica of exposed surfaces is made by coating with a thin film of heavy metal, such as platinum. Here, the gap junction (**arrows**) is a plaque-like area containing a cluster of tightly packed intramembrane particles. 50,000×. *(Courtesy of Dr. B. J. Crawford)*

1.7 INTERCELLULAR JUNCTIONS: ULTRASTRUCTURE AND FUNCTION OF GAP JUNCTIONS

Metabolic, ionic, and low-resistance electrical communication occurs between adjacent cells via gap junctions, in which a narrow gap of about 2 nm separates opposing cell membranes. Gap junctions are difficult to discern in routine EMs; elucidation of structural details requires *freeze-fracture methods* or other techniques that use *immunocytochemistry* with antibody probes. Gap junctions are specialized sites composed of large, tightly packed **intercellular channels,** which connect cytoplasm of adjacent cells. Each cylindrical channel, 10-12 nm long and 2.8-3.0 nm in diameter, consists of a pair of half-channels, termed **connexons,** which are embedded in the cell membranes. Each connexon comprises six symmetric protein subunits, called **connexins,** that are **transmembrane proteins** surrounding a small central aqueous **pore** (diameter: 1.5-2.0 nm). Across the narrow gap, a connexon of one cell is aligned with that of the adjacent cell so that the central pores form one continuous conduit, thereby allowing direct communication. No leakage of ions or fluid out of cells and into the extracellular space occurs. Each of about 20 different connexin proteins has a separate gene encoding it. Connexons, like other *voltage-gated channels* in membranes, can undergo reversible conformational changes to open or close gap junction channels.

CLINICAL POINT

Several diseases result from mutations in genes encoding connexins, which are named according to molecular size. Recessive mutations in connexin-26, with a molecular size of 26 kD, lead to the most common cause of **inherited human deafness,** which often affects the elderly. Connexin-26 is usually involved in K^+ transport in cells that support cochlear hair cells. An X-linked form of **Charcot-Marie-Tooth disease** is due to mutations in connexin-32 and causes degeneration of myelin sheaths in central and peripheral nervous systems. A mutation in connexin-50 leads to **cataracts** in the lens of the eye.

▼ Nuclear components.

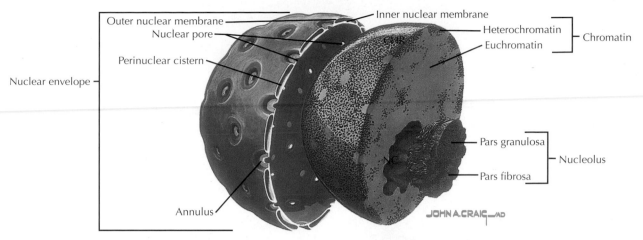

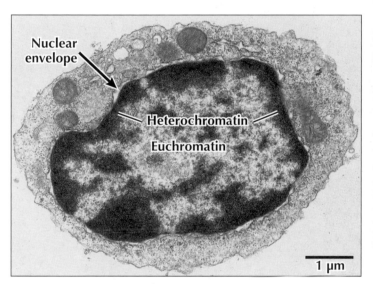

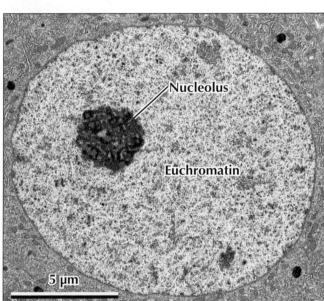

▲ **EM of a lymphocyte.** Its nucleus shows euchromatin in the center and darker stained heterochromatin, which appears as dense patches, around the periphery. A discernible nuclear envelope separates nucleus from cytoplasm. 12,750×.

▲ **EM of the perikaryon of a nerve cell in a spinal ganglion.** This cell is active in protein synthesis, so its nucleus is mainly euchromatic with almost no heterochromatin. A spherical nucleolus, also in the plane of section, is eccentrically placed and electron dense; it lacks a membrane. 5600×.

1.8 ULTRASTRUCTURE AND FUNCTION OF THE NUCLEUS AND NUCLEOLUS

The nucleus—the largest, most conspicuous structure in the cell—contains genetic material. Size and shape may depend on cell type: usually spherical or ellipsoidal, a nucleus may also be elongated (as in columnar epithelial cells) or lobulated (as in polymorphonuclear leukocytes and megakaryocytes). Most cells have one nucleus; some (e.g., hepatocytes) may be *binucleated,* others (e.g., osteoclasts, skeletal muscle fibers), *multinucleated.* The nucleus consists of **nucleolus, chromatin, nuclear matrix,** and **nuclear envelope.** The nucleolus, the most conspicuous part of the nucleus, is a dense, ovoid, discrete area (up to 1 μm in diameter) with no membrane around it. Its size, number, and location may depend on a cell's functional activity. The nucleolus is the site of *ribosomal RNA* (rRNA) transcription and production of *ribosomes.* It has a high content of RNA, so it is intensely basophilic by light microscopy. In EMs, the nucleolus shows two areas, the **pars granulosa** and **pars fibrosa,** that have no clear boundary between them. The pars granulosa, in peripheral nucleolar regions, is the main site of preribosome assembly. It consists of densely packed clusters of preribosomal particles (diameter: 15-20 nm) that are rich in ribonucleoprotein. The more central pars fibrosa contains a dense, irregular network of fine filaments (5 nm in diameter), rRNA genes, and transcription factors. The nucleolus disassembles in the prophase of mitosis but then reorganizes in daughter cells when cell division is complete.

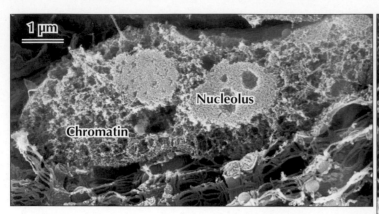

▲ **HRSEM of the interphase nucleus of a skeletal muscle fiber.** The chromatin is a network of slender filamentous threads. More densely packed spherical areas are two nucleoli. 11,000×.

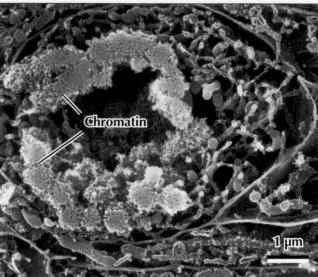

▲ **HRSEM of the nucleus of a dividing cell at anaphase.** At this stage of mitosis, chromosomes are seen as condensed chromatin strands, with an internal appearance of a loosely organized mass of looped fibers. 11,000×. *(Courtesy of Dr. M. J. Hollenberg)*

◄ **EM of a satellite cell in skeletal muscle in the prophase stage of mitosis.** Chromatin is condensed and forms thickened thread-like structures. Here, the nucleolus and nuclear envelope have disassembled. Satellite cells are stem cells on surfaces of skeletal muscle fibers. During growth and regeneration, these cells are activated and undergo mitosis to form new skeletal muscle fibers. 8000×.

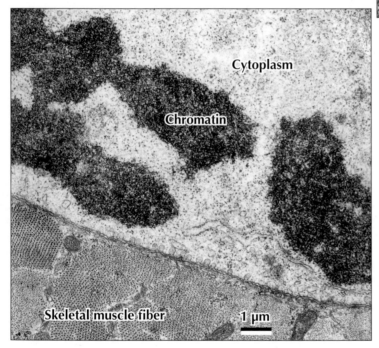

1.9 ULTRASTRUCTURE AND FUNCTION OF THE NUCLEUS: CHROMATIN AND MATRIX

Intensely stained substance of the nucleus is chromatin, which appears as irregular clumps. It consists chiefly of highly folded **DNA,** a nucleic acid, combined with structural proteins, mostly histones. It also contains nonhistone proteins and **RNA** that has been transcribed from DNA. Chromatin has a strong affinity for basic dyes, such as hematoxylin, used in light microscopy. Nuclear chromatin usually exists in two forms: **euchromatin** and **heterochromatin.** The pale or lightly stained euchromatin, which is dispersed regions of uncoiled **chromosomes,** is transcriptionally active and is prominent in protein-synthesizing cells. The condensed heterochromatin is transcriptionally inactive. It stains darker with basic dyes and in EMs looks more electron-dense compared with euchromatin. A typical nucleus has different amounts of the two forms. Heterochromatin is usually near the *nuclear envelope.* Intervening sponge-like areas between chromatin and nucleoli make up the **nuclear matrix.** It is rich in nonhistone proteins such as *condensins.* It also contains a meshwork of 10-nm intermediate filaments, called *nuclear lamins,* most of which adhere to the inner aspect of the nuclear envelope. The matrix, best seen via special techniques used with EMs, is a structural scaffold that organizes chromosomes during *meiosis* and *mitosis.* It also helps regulate gene transcription.

CLINICAL POINT

Chromosomes are thread-like structures of DNA and other proteins. Human cells have 23 pairs of chromosomes, the smallest being chromosome 21. Improper segregation of chromosomes during cell division may lead to a chromosomal abnormality. The most common inborn autosomal chromosome disorder is **Down syndrome (trisomy 21).** It usually occurs at fertilization via nondisjunction of chromosome 21 during meiosis and results in three (not two) copies of chromosome 21. Mental retardation, hypotonia in infancy, and specific facial features characterize the syndrome. Its frequency is about 0.1% of the total number of births; the risk increases with advancing age of the mother.

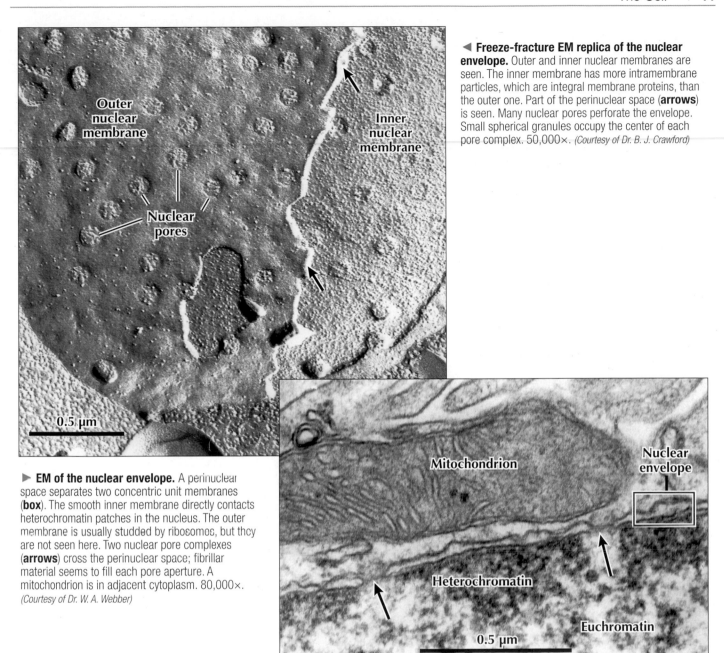

Outer nuclear membrane

Nuclear pores

Inner nuclear membrane

0.5 µm

◄ **Freeze-fracture EM replica of the nuclear envelope.** Outer and inner nuclear membranes are seen. The inner membrane has more intramembrane particles, which are integral membrane proteins, than the outer one. Part of the perinuclear space (**arrows**) is seen. Many nuclear pores perforate the envelope. Small spherical granules occupy the center of each pore complex. 50,000×. *(Courtesy of Dr. B. J. Crawford)*

► **EM of the nuclear envelope.** A perinuclear space separates two concentric unit membranes (**box**). The smooth inner membrane directly contacts heterochromatin patches in the nucleus. The outer membrane is usually studded by ribosomes, but they are not seen here. Two nuclear pore complexes (**arrows**) cross the perinuclear space; fibrillar material seems to fill each pore aperture. A mitochondrion is in adjacent cytoplasm. 80,000×. *(Courtesy of Dr. W. A. Webber)*

Mitochondrion

Nuclear envelope

Heterochromatin

Euchromatin

0.5 µm

1.10 ULTRASTRUCTURE AND FUNCTION OF THE NUCLEAR ENVELOPE

A nuclear envelope encloses the nucleus of interphase cells and separates nucleus from cytoplasm. It consists of two parallel **unit membranes** separated by a narrow space (10-70 nm wide) termed the **perinuclear space (cisterna).** The **outer membrane** is studded externally by **ribosomes** and is continuous with cytoplasmic *rough endoplasmic reticulum* (RER). Thus, the perinuclear space is continuous with the RER lumen. The **inner membrane** lacks ribosomes, and its innermost surface is in contact with clumps of **heterochromatin** in the nucleus. Many small octagonal apertures, called **nuclear pores,** perforate the envelope. About 10 nm in diameter, they permit selective, bidirectional exchange of small molecules, ribosomal subunits, and other substances between

nucleus and cytoplasm. Their number and distribution vary widely according to activity and type of cell; they are especially numerous in metabolically active cells. The outer rim of each pore forms by fusion of outer and inner nuclear membranes. A **nuclear pore complex** spanning the opening of each pore consists of eight proteins, or *nucleoporins,* around a central plug or granule. This complex is a molecular sieve and allows passive diffusion of molecules smaller than 10 nm but requires larger molecules to be transported by an energy-dependent mechanism that opens the pore. A meshwork of **intermediate filaments** associated with the nuclear side of the envelope consists of *lamins,* proteins that make up the *nuclear lamina.* These lamins maintain nuclear shape, help reinforce the nuclear envelope, and anchor ends of chromosomes.

▼ **Mitochondria with shelf-like and tubular cristae.**

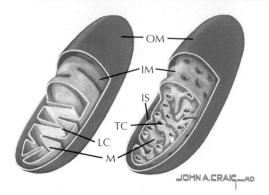

IM = Inner membrane
IS = Intracristal space
LC = Lamellar cristae

M = Matrix
OM = Outer membrane
TC = Tubular cristae

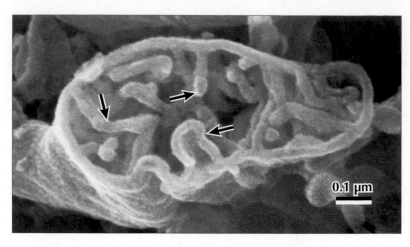

▲ **HRSEM of a mitochondrion.** A fractured open view reveals internal cristae (**arrows**). 100,000×.

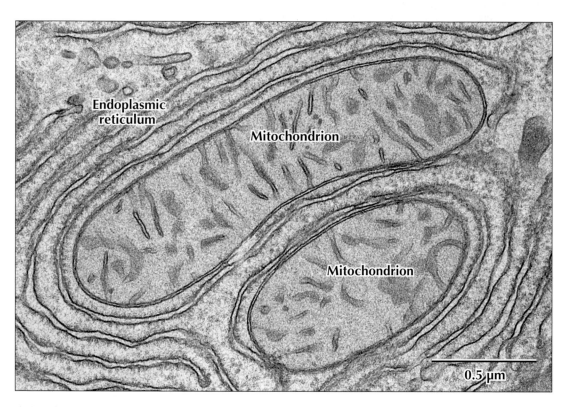

▲ **EM of mitochondria in a hepatocyte.** Their shape varies with plane of section and type of cell. Here, one is elongated; the other, more ovoid. Each has thin, shelf-like cristae that project into the mitochondrial matrix. Endoplasmic reticulum cisternae are in the cytoplasm. 54,000×.

1.11   ULTRASTRUCTURE AND FUNCTION OF MITOCHONDRIA

Mitochondria are the most recognizable membrane-bound organelle. They are usually scattered throughout the cytoplasm of most cells, but they often concentrate in specific areas where high energy utilization, in the form of ATP, occurs. Such areas include apical regions of ciliated cells, basal areas of ion-transporting cells, and subsarcolemmal areas of skeletal and cardiac muscle cells. Their number and size vary with metabolic activity and type of cell: mature erythrocytes have none; a hepatocyte has up to 2500. They are 1-10 μm in size and may be elongated, spherical, or pleomor-

phic. These very dynamic organelles show constant motion, fusion, and division in cells. EMs reveal that two membranes separated by an intermembrane space of 8-10 nm invest them. The outer mitochondrial membrane has a smooth contour, which corresponds to the organelle's shape. The membrane consists mostly of a large channel-forming protein, porin, which increases membrane permeability for passage of molecules and metabolites for ATP synthesis. The inner mitochondrial membrane, however, shows transverse shelf-like or tubular folds—the cristae. They project into the inner chamber of the organelle, called the mitochondrial matrix, which has a finely granular increased electron density.

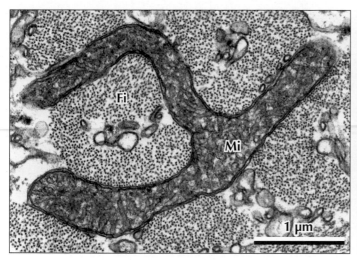
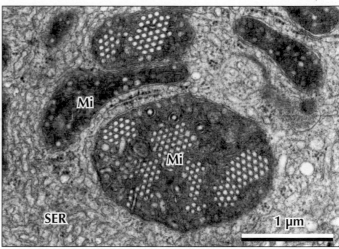

▲ **EMs of mitochondria in two different cells. Left.** This mitochondrion (**Mi**) in a skeletal muscle fiber is branched and has a high density of tightly packed cristae. Contractile filaments (**Fi**) are in the cytoplasm. **Right.** The mitochondria in a steroid-secreting cell have tubular, not shelf-like, cristae and a dense mitochondrial matrix. Abundant smooth endoplasmic reticulum (**SER**) is in the cytoplasm. 24,000×. *(B Courtesy of Dr. D. M. Pfeiffer)*

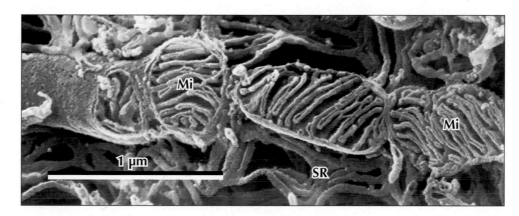

▲ **HRSEM of mitochondria in a diaphragm muscle fiber.** This highly aerobic, skeletal muscle fiber has many large mitochondria (**Mi**). Prominent shelf-like cristae extend across the entire breadth of each organelle and markedly increase surface area for oxidative metabolism. Sarcoplasmic reticulum (**SR**), a form of SER, is also seen. 46,000×.

1.12 ULTRASTRUCTURE AND FUNCTION OF MITOCHONDRIAL CRISTAE AND MATRIX

Mitochondrial **cristae** vary greatly in size, shape, and number depending on cell type and metabolic activity. Cristae greatly increase surface area for ATP synthesis and reactions related to *electron transport, Krebs citric acid cycle,* and *oxidative phosphorylation.* The **matrix** contains many enzymes needed for oxidation reactions of the Krebs cycle. Cristae usually, but not always, extend across the interior of a mitochondrion. Most cells have flattened, lamellar cristae, which are usually perpendicular to the longitudinal axis of the mitochondrion. Tubular and tubulovesicular cristae are most common in **steroid-secreting cells,** where cristae also contain enzymes for *steroidogenesis.* Unlike other organelles, mitochondria have a degree of autonomy in a cell. They have their own closed-loop *DNA, RNA,* and *ribosomes* in the matrix. Like bacteria, mitochondria are thought to be symbiotic organisms that infected a primitive cell millions of years ago and then remained in a useful relationship. Mitochondria sequester calcium and other divalent cations that are stored as small **matrix granules** (diameter: 30-50 nm). They can respond to a cell's functional demands. They are especially prominent in osteoblasts that form bone matrix and in ion-transporting cells, such as those of the kidney and small intestine.

CLINICAL POINT

Diseases that affect mitochondria, resulting mainly in muscle weakness and dysfunction, are known as **mitochondrial myopathies.** More than 50 harmful mutations in mitochondrial DNA can cause the typically inherited disorders. They vary from mild to life-threatening, the most common symptoms being severe muscle weakness, cramps, and spasm and cardiac involvement. **Chronic progressive external ophthalmoplegia,** the most common form, affects extraocular muscles; **Leber's hereditary optic neuropathy** affects vision. Brain involvement may lead to neurologic seizures in **mitochondrial encephalomyopathies.** Prognoses vary, and treatments depend on specific causes.

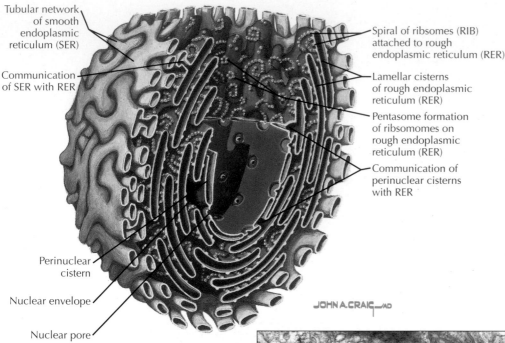

Tubular network of smooth endoplasmic reticulum (SER)

Communication of SER with RER

Spiral of ribsomes (RIB) attached to rough endoplasmic reticulum (RER)

Lamellar cisterns of rough endoplasmic reticulum (RER)

Pentasome formation of ribsomomes on rough endoplasmic reticulum (RER)

Communication of perinuclear cisterns with RER

Perinuclear cistern

Nuclear envelope

Nuclear pore

JOHN A. CRAIG—AD

◄ **Three-dimensional schematic of the ER.** This organelle is a continuous array of membrane-bound tubules, vesicles, and cisternae. A smooth-surfaced membrane encloses a central lumen, which is separated from the cytoplasm. Tubules often have flattened expansions called cisternae. Communications exist between RER and SER. The perinuclear space of the nuclear envelope is also continuous with the RER.

► **EM of part of a hepatocyte showing sagittal and cross-sectional SER.** Abundant in hepatocytes, SER exists as small, branching tubules and multiple stacks of flattened cisternae. Here, the SER is closely associated with lipid droplets. A pleomorphic mitochondrion and a few profiles of **RER** also occupy the cytoplasm. 20,000×.

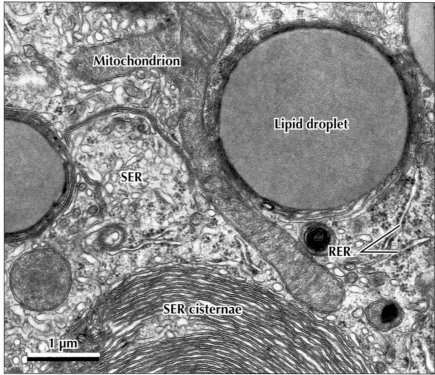

Mitochondrion

Lipid droplet

SER

RER

SER cisternae

1 μm

1.13 ULTRASTRUCTURE AND FUNCTION OF SMOOTH ENDOPLASMIC RETICULUM

The **endoplasmic reticulum** (ER) is a tortuous, communicating network of slender **tubules,** small circular **vesicles,** and flattened membranous **sacs (cisternae).** Its amount, distribution, and complexity vary widely depending on cell type and function. The anastomosing tubules may be scattered singly in the cytoplasm, but they often occur as stacks of multiple, parallel cisternae. The central cavity of the ER is separated from the cytoplasm by a closed membrane that is thinner but looks like the cell's plasma membrane. The two major forms of this delicate organelle are **smooth (SER)** and **rough (RER).** The RER, studded externally with ribosomes, looks granular, but the SER consists of smooth-surfaced

membranes lacking ribosomes and thus appears agranular in EMs. The many functions of the SER depend on location. In hepatocytes, SER participates in carbohydrate metabolism. It uses enzymes (such as glucose-6-phosphatase) in its membranes to convert *glycogen* to *glucose.* Hepatocytes have abundant SER that routinely degrades lipid-soluble drugs (such as barbiturates) and alcohol, via various *drug-metabolizing enzymes* (such as cytochrome P450) on its surface. Steroid-secreting cells (such as those in ovary, testis, and adrenal gland) that store cholesterol have large amounts of SER, which functions in lipid and lipoprotein synthesis. In muscle cells, SER, called **sarcoplasmic reticulum,** engages in calcium ion regulation, which is critical for contraction to start.

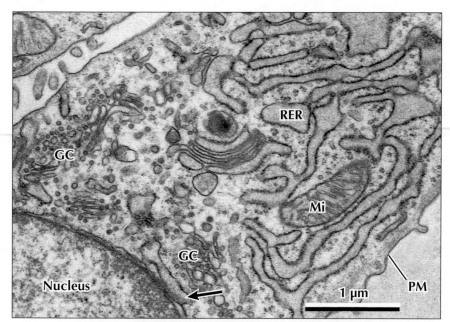

◀ **EM of part of a fibroblast in a growing tendon.** The **RER** consists of an extensive network of branching membrane-bound tubules, studded externally with ribosomes. Its luminal contents are moderately electron dense and amorphous. Note the continuity of the RER and perinuclear space (**arrow**). Many free ribosomes are in the cytoplasm. In cells secreting protein for export, abundant RER is usually associated with one or more supranuclear Golgi complexes (**GC**). A mitochondrion (**Mi**) and plasma membrane (**PM**) are also seen. 25,000×.

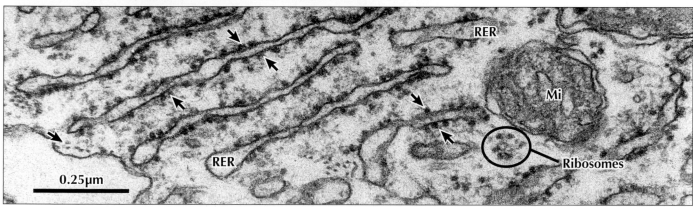

▲ **Higher magnification EM showing details of the RER.** Association of ribosomes (**arrows**) with RER membranes is clear in this protein-synthesizing fibroblast. Polypeptide chains synthesized on ribosomes are discharged into the RER lumen. The cytoplasm holds several elongated RER cisternae (**RER**), many free ribosomes (**circle**), and a mitochondrion (**Mi**). Many cell types that secrete proteins have this RER arrangement: fibroblasts of connective tissue (secrete collagen), nerve cells (in which RER plus ribosomes are named Nissl substance), pancreatic acinar cells (produce digestive enzymes), pancreatic islet cells (produce the hormone insulin), and plasma cells (produce antibodies called immunoglobulins). 100,000×. *(Courtesy of Dr. B. J. Crawford)*

1.14   ULTRASTRUCTURE AND FUNCTION OF ROUGH ENDOPLASMIC RETICULUM

External **ribosomes** on the RER produce a rough or granular appearance in EMs, like small beads or coarse sandpaper—thus the term *rough*. RER consists of an interconnecting network of membrane-enclosed **cisternae** and **vesicles**. Its membranes are continuous with the outer membrane of the *nuclear envelope*. Ribosomes sit on the outer (cytoplasmic) surfaces of RER cisternae and form rosettes or a linear pattern. **Polyribosomes,** which are ribosomes connected by messenger **RNA** (mRNA) strands, also bind to external RER surfaces. RER engages in synthesis and export of *proteins* and *glycoproteins*. It is the site of translation,

folding, and transport of newly formed proteins that become part of the cell membrane as *integral membrane proteins* and *transmembrane receptors* or that are proteins secreted by *exocytosis*. Ribosomes assemble **polypeptides** that are threaded into cisternae lumina. Newly formed protein is then folded into its native configuration. Once proteins are synthesized, most travel to the **Golgi complex** in *transfer vesicles*. The RER membrane has a receptor to bind the larger ribosome subunit and an adjacent pore to permit newly formed protein to enter and be sequestered in the RER lumen. Many different cell types that synthesize and secrete proteins contain an extensive, well-developed RER.

▼ Section of a single ribosome.

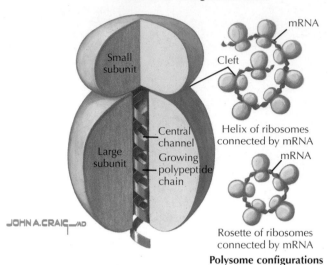

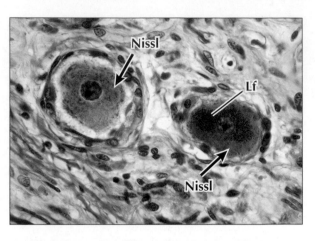

▲ **LM of nerve cells with cytoplasmic basophilia.** Nissl substance, which stains blue, occupies the cytoplasm. It indicates abundant ribosomes and RER, and thus protein synthesis. Lipofuscin (**Lf**)—a wear-and-tear pigment—is also seen in one cell. 440×. *H&E.*

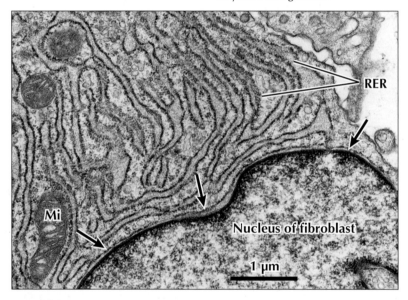

▲ **EM of part of an active fibroblast.** This cell secretes protein for internal use and export. Its cytoplasm contains abundant free ribosomes and ribosomes attached to cisternae of **RER**. Note the outer nuclear envelope (**arrows**) studded with ribosomes around the nucleus. Mitochondria (**Mi**) are also in the cytoplasm. 17,000×.

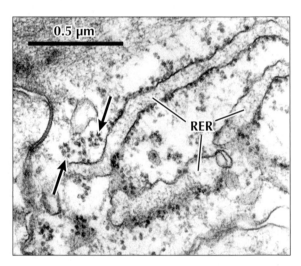

▲ **Higher magnification EM of part of a protein-synthesizing cell.** Several RER cisternae (**RER**) with attached ribosomes are seen. The cytoplasm also shows free ribosomes, many of which are rosettes (**arrows**) attached by thin strands of mRNA. 50,000×. *(Courtesy of Dr. B. J. Crawford)*

1.15   ULTRASTRUCTURE AND FUNCTION OF RIBOSOMES

Ribosomes are small, spherical, electron-dense particles that synthesize proteins. Of uniform size, their diameter is 15-20 nm. They consist mostly of **RNA** and associated proteins. **Free ribosomes** in the cytoplasm occur as single particles or rosette-like clusters, termed **polyribosomes,** which consist of several ribosomes arranged along a thread of mRNA. Single ribosomes are inactive; polyribosomes actively synthesize protein by assembling amino acids into polypeptides. Ribosomes may also be attached to membranes of RER and to the **outer nuclear membrane.** Free ribosomes synthesize proteins for internal use by the cell, but ribosomes attached to RER synthesize proteins for export from cells or proteins destined for lysosomes. Ribosomes are small and thus below the limit of resolution of the light microscope, but their polyanionic nature makes them strongly basophilic because

they have an affinity for basic dyes such as hematoxylin. In H&E-stained sections, they impart **cytoplasmic basophilia** to cells actively synthesizing protein. A high-resolution EM reveals that each ribosome consists of two unequal-size subunits that bind together during mRNA translation. The **large subunit** contains two RNA molecules and about 49 proteins; the **small subunit,** one RNA molecule and about 33 small proteins. Ribosomal subunits and their associated proteins are synthesized in the *nucleolus* and reach the cytoplasm via *nuclear pores*. Ribosomes, with binding sites for both mRNA and transfer RNA *(tRNA)*, translate a coded genetic message from mRNA that is first transcribed in the nucleus. Translation involves movement of a ribosome along the mRNA chain, and the two subunits perform different functions in translation. tRNA transports amino acids to ribosomes for polymerization and polypeptide synthesis. mRNA decoding and polypeptide synthesis occur in a cavity between the subunits.

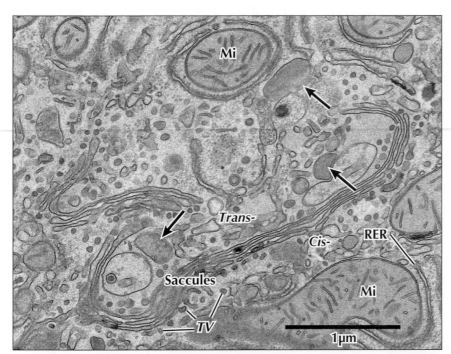

◄ **EM of the Golgi complex in a hepatocyte.** The *cis*–face on the convex side is associated with many small transfer vesicles (**TV**) and RER. Several flattened saccules are in the medial compartment. Many vesicles and vacuoles (**arrows**) are at the *trans*–face on the concave side. Mitochondria (**Mi**) are seen. 30,000×.

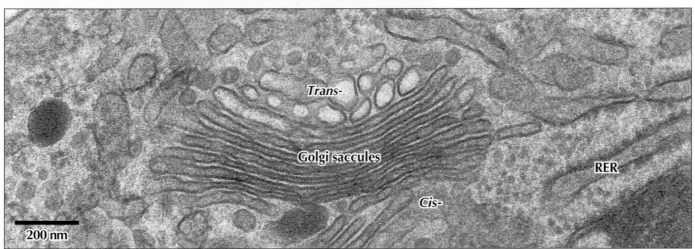

▲ **High-magnification EM of the Golgi complex showing its functional compartments.** All components of the complex are smooth-surfaced membranes without ribosomes. The *cis*–face (convex side) is close to the RER. The parallel saccules of the medial compartment are slightly curved, some with slightly dilated ends. The *trans*–face (outer, concave side) shows many vesicles and vacuoles. The smallest ones closest to the *trans*–face have a clear lumen; those farther away are larger and more moderately electron dense. 76,000×.

1.16 ULTRASTRUCTURE OF THE GOLGI COMPLEX

The Golgi complex (or apparatus) was first discovered in neurons by the neurohistologist Camillo Golgi in 1898. He used the light microscope with silver stains, which he developed to study and describe the Golgi. He called it the *apparato reticolare interno*, and it now bears his name. The ultrastructural complexity of this dynamic organelle was not fully understood until the use of electron microscopy in the mid-1950s. Located in the center of the cell, the *cytocentrum*, the Golgi is close to the nucleus and centrosome. It is a complex array of flattened, slightly curved, closely packed **membrane-bound sacs (cisternae)** with associated **vesi-cles** and larger **vacuoles.** This highly polarized, compartmentalized organelle has convex and concave sides and three functionally distinct compartments: a **cis-Golgi network** of vesicles on the convex side, a **medial compartment** of stacks of flattened **saccules,** and on the concave side a **trans-Golgi network** of vesicles and vacuoles for distribution and sorting of secretory products. Some cells have one Golgi complex; others, which actively synthesize proteins and polysaccharides, have many. The Golgi complex adds proteins to sugars to form glycoproteins, assembles polysaccharides, elaborates membrane lipids, and produces **lysosomes** that are kept by cells.

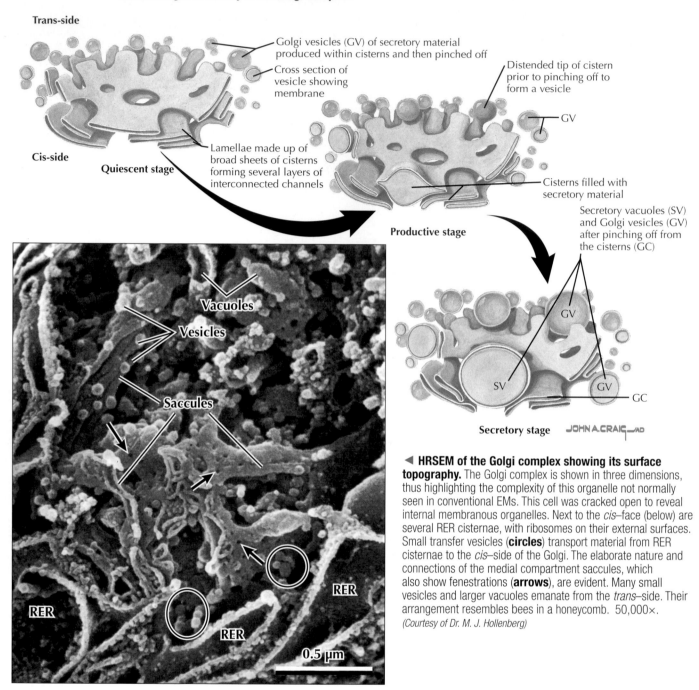

▼ **Various stages of activity of the Golgi complex.**

Trans-side

Golgi vesicles (GV) of secretory material produced within cisterns and then pinched off

Cross section of vesicle showing membrane

Cis-side

Quiescent stage

Lamellae made up of broad sheets of cisterns forming several layers of interconnected channels

Distended tip of cistern prior to pinching off to form a vesicle

GV

Cisterns filled with secretory material

Productive stage

Secretory vacuoles (SV) and Golgi vesicles (GV) after pinching off from the cisterns (GC)

GV

SV

GV

GC

Secretory stage

JOHN A. CRAIG—AD

Vacuoles

Vesicles

Saccules

RER

RER

RER

0.5 µm

◄ **HRSEM of the Golgi complex showing its surface topography.** The Golgi complex is shown in three dimensions, thus highlighting the complexity of this organelle not normally seen in conventional EMs. This cell was cracked open to reveal internal membranous organelles. Next to the *cis*–face (below) are several RER cisternae, with ribosomes on their external surfaces. Small transfer vesicles (**circles**) transport material from RER cisternae to the *cis*–side of the Golgi. The elaborate nature and connections of the medial compartment saccules, which also show fenestrations (**arrows**), are evident. Many small vesicles and larger vacuoles emanate from the *trans*–side. Their arrangement resembles bees in a honeycomb. 50,000×.
(Courtesy of Dr. M. J. Hollenberg)

1.17 FUNCTIONS OF THE GOLGI COMPLEX

A major role of the Golgi complex is to sort and package secretory proteins that are produced in the RER. By budding and fusing of **vesicles,** newly synthesized secretory material in the lumen passes from the proximal *(cis)* to the distal *(trans)* side of the organelle. **Transfer vesicles** from the RER fuse with the *cis*-Golgi complex to then deliver newly formed protein into flattened **saccules,** where protein is chemically modified. Each medial compartment saccule contains a different group of processing enzymes in its membranes—the *integral membrane proteins.* These chemical reactions, termed *posttranslational modifications,* include proteo-

lytic processing of protein precursors, glycosylation, phosphorylation, hydroxylation, and sulfation. The endoplasmic reticulum and Golgi complex also produce most lipids, especially those associated with membranes, which are kept by cells and organelles. Cytoplasmic *microtubules* closely associated with the Golgi complex help move and transfer vesicles and **vacuoles** to different parts of a cell. Vesicles associated with the *trans*-**Golgi network** have one of three purposes. They may form **secretory vesicles** that release contents by exocytosis to the cell exterior; they may fuse with the *plasma membrane* for insertion of proteins and lipids into it; or they may become *lysosomes.*

▼ Various stages in activity of lysosomes.

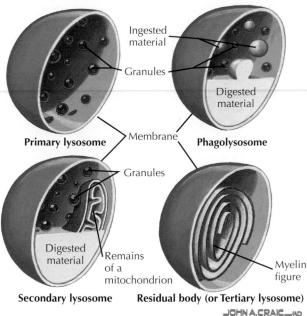

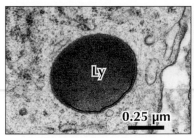 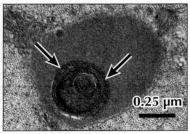

▲ **EMs of lysosomes. Left.** A primary lysosome (**Ly**) is enclosed by one membrane and has homogeneous, electron-dense granularity in its lumen. **Right.** In contrast, a larger secondary lysosome has partly digested material (**arrows**) in its lumen. 40,000×.

▶ **EM of a tertiary lysosome.** Also called a residual body (**RB**), it is much more variable in shape and appearance than primary and secondary lysosomes. Note both electron-dense and electron-lucent areas in its lumen. Lysosomes arise from the *trans*–face of the Golgi complex, so they are often seen nearby. Several mitochondria (**Mi**) are in the cytoplasm; the cell's plasma membrane (**PM**) is indicated. 40,000×.

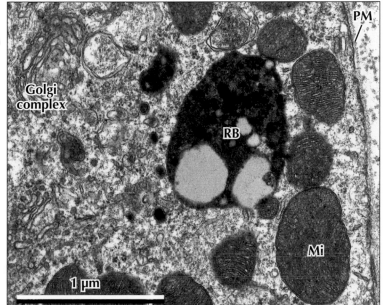

1.18 ULTRASTRUCTURE AND FUNCTION OF LYSOSOMES

Lysosomes are a heterogeneous collection of membrane-bound vesicles and vacuoles that derive from **Golgi complex** vesicles. They contain 50 or more *hydrolytic enzymes,* most being glycoproteins that are active at acid pH, and they stain cytochemically for *acid phosphatase.* Lysosomes are spherical or irregular in shape, with diameters of 0.25 0.8 μm. Present in most cells, they are especially abundant in cells engaged in *phagocytosis.* They serve in defense against infection by engulfing viruses, bacteria, and other pathogens. They are an intracellular digestive system for normal turnover and removal of worn-out organelles in cells. Also, in response to cell injury, they aid *autolysis* of cells—a self-destructive role, which leads to cell death when packaged lysosomal enzymes are released. Newly formed electron-dense **primary lysosomes** have a homogeneous, granular content with no digested material inside. They become **secondary lysosomes,** which are normally larger and more heterogeneous in appearance and electron density. They usually contain remnants of digested material. **Tertiary lysosomes (residual bodies),** the oldest lysosomes, have completed digestive functions and are prominent in long-lived cells such as nerve and cardiac muscle cells. They often have bizarre shapes and are almost entirely filled with debris, including concentric lamellae, indigestible material, and crystalline deposits. They often accumulate *lipofuscin,* a wear-and-tear pigment. Lysosomal membranes contain a unique phospholipid resistant to degradation by lysosomal enzymes, so other cell components are separated from them.

CLINICAL POINT

Tay-Sachs disease, a *lysosomal storage disease,* is an often rapidly fatal genetic disorder in which harmful amounts of the ganglioside GM2 accumulate in nerve cells because of a deficient lysosomal enzyme, hexosaminidase A (hex A). Progressive, abnormal increases in residual bodies in nerve cells of the brain result and cause severe brain damage, deafness, and blindness. Both *infantile* and *late-onset* forms are due to mutations in the hex A gene on chromosome 15. Diagnosis can be by a simple test that measures blood hex A or by a prenatal test, such as *amniocentesis,* to reveal the absence of hex A.

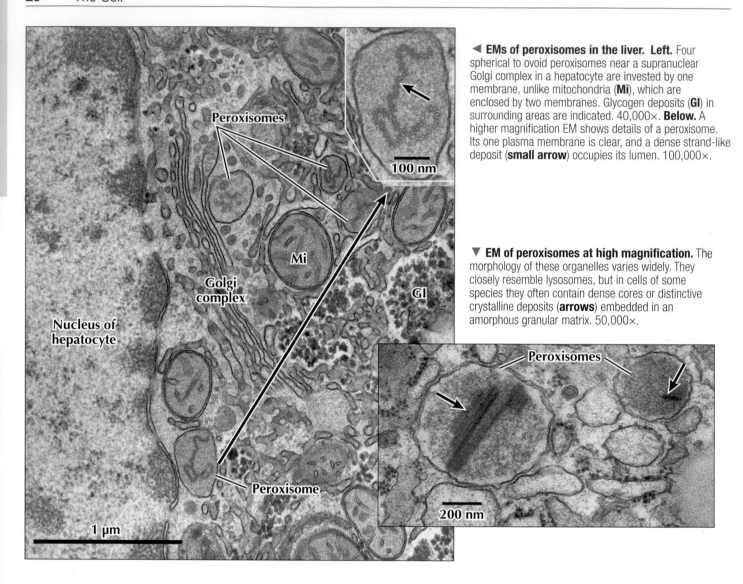

◀ **EMs of peroxisomes in the liver. Left.** Four spherical to ovoid peroxisomes near a supranuclear Golgi complex in a hepatocyte are invested by one membrane, unlike mitochondria (**Mi**), which are enclosed by two membranes. Glycogen deposits (**Gl**) in surrounding areas are indicated. 40,000×. **Below.** A higher magnification EM shows details of a peroxisome. Its one plasma membrane is clear, and a dense strand-like deposit (**small arrow**) occupies its lumen. 100,000×.

▼ **EM of peroxisomes at high magnification.** The morphology of these organelles varies widely. They closely resemble lysosomes, but in cells of some species they often contain dense cores or distinctive crystalline deposits (**arrows**) embedded in an amorphous granular matrix. 50,000×.

1.19 ULTRASTRUCTURE AND FUNCTION OF PEROXISOMES

Peroxisomes are ubiquitous, membrane-bound organelles that are spherical to ovoid and are 0.1-0.5 μm in diameter. Belgian scientist Christian de Duve originally named lysosomes in the 1950s; in the 1960s, he recognized peroxisomes as discrete organelles and also named them. He was awarded the Nobel Prize in Physiology or Medicine in 1974 for pioneering work on organelle structure and function. Found in almost all cells, peroxisomes are especially prominent in **hepatocytes** and in **proximal tubule cells** of the kidney. Peroxisomes perform various anabolic and catabolic functions depending on cell type and environmental conditions. They mainly engage in oxidative reactions that use molecular oxygen; they contain *oxidative enzymes* such as *catalase* and *uric oxidase*. In many species, they may have a dense crystalline core of *urate oxidase*. Functions include cell respiration, fatty acid metabolism, alcohol degradation, transamination, regulation of H_2O_2, and bile acid metabolism. Peroxisomes also synthesize specialized *phospholipids*, such as *plasmalogen*, which is needed for

myelination of nerve cells. Like lysosomes, they have one **plasma membrane,** but it is thinner and more permeable than that of lysosomes. Like mitochondria, they are self-replicating organelles. However, they do not have their own DNA or ribosomes and need to import proteins from the cytoplasm. They are often closely associated with **endoplasmic reticulum.** An internal **matrix** looks finely granular in EMs.

CLINICAL POINT

Several rare inherited diseases are caused by peroxisomal impairment. The most common and severe, **Zellweger,** or **cerebrohepatorenal, syndrome,** leads to abnormalities in brain, kidneys, and liver. Affected infants die soon after birth, which is most likely due to faulty neural cell myelination in utero. The primary defect is an inability to import newly formed proteins across peroxisomal membranes. Plasmalogens, which are produced in peroxisomes, are the most abundant phospholipid in myelin sheaths of nervous tissue. Thus, peroxisomal disorders usually lead to serious neurologic defects, including abnormal myelin caused by deficient plasmalogen.

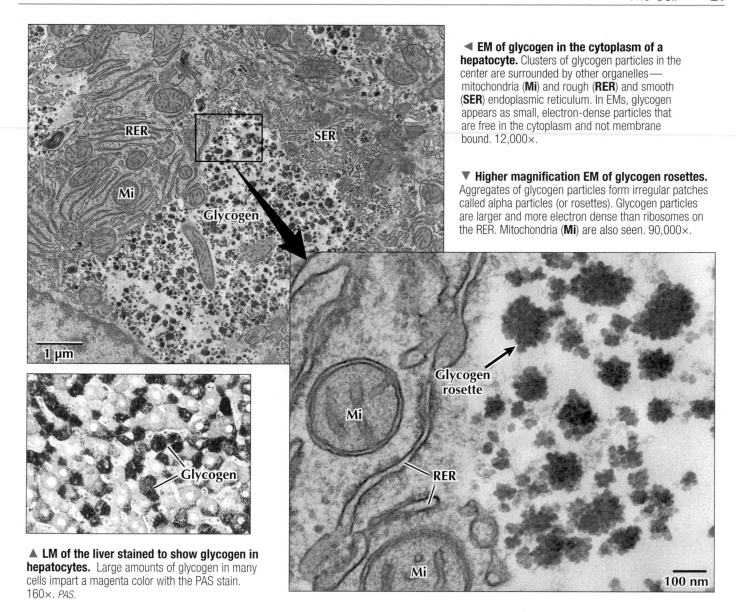

◀ **EM of glycogen in the cytoplasm of a hepatocyte.** Clusters of glycogen particles in the center are surrounded by other organelles—mitochondria (**Mi**) and rough (**RER**) and smooth (**SER**) endoplasmic reticulum. In EMs, glycogen appears as small, electron-dense particles that are free in the cytoplasm and not membrane bound. 12,000×.

▼ **Higher magnification EM of glycogen rosettes.** Aggregates of glycogen particles form irregular patches called alpha particles (or rosettes). Glycogen particles are larger and more electron dense than ribosomes on the RER. Mitochondria (**Mi**) are also seen. 90,000×.

▲ **LM of the liver stained to show glycogen in hepatocytes.** Large amounts of glycogen in many cells impart a magenta color with the PAS stain. 160×. *PAS.*

1.20 ULTRASTRUCTURE AND FUNCTION OF INCLUSIONS: GLYCOGEN

In contrast to organelles—the functionally active parts of cells—**inclusions** are relatively inert, dispensable, transitory components that vary in type and distribution. Usually metabolic byproducts or stored nutrients, they include glycogen, lipid droplets, and pigment granules. Glycogen is a D-glucose polymer, which is mostly stored in cytoplasm of hepatocytes and in skeletal muscle cells. Smaller amounts also occur in cells of other tissues. Synthesis, storage, and breakdown of glycogen occur rapidly according to need. Glycogen is not usually seen in routine sections and appears washed out unless special techniques, such as light microscopic histochemistry with *periodic acid-Schiff* stain, are used to preserve and stain it. In EMs, glycogen appears as non-membrane-bound, electron-dense **granules** with an irregular shape. At 20-40 nm in diameter, they are usually larger and denser than ribosomes. In liver cells, isolated glycogen granules are called **beta particles.** They often form larger, **rosette-like aggregates** termed **alpha particles,** with diameters of 90-95 nm. Glycogen is often close to SER, where there is a rapid conversion to glucose. Once SER enzymes break down glycogen, glucose leaves cells and goes via circulation to other tissues as a major energy source.

CLINICAL POINT

The more than 10 inherited inborn errors of metabolism that affect synthesis or breakdown of glycogen are called **glycogen storage diseases** (GSDs). These *autosomal recessive disorders* usually occur in childhood. Symptoms vary, but some are life threatening. One form, **von Gierke disease (type 1 GSD),** is a deficiency of the enzyme glucose-6-phosphatase. It leads to an abnormal accumulation of glycogen in muscle and liver cells, which causes clinically important end-organ disease and morbidity. Diagnosis is made by biochemical assay and physical examination. A muscle or liver biopsy may be needed for confirmation.

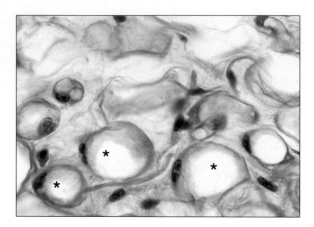

▲ **LM of fat cells in adipose tissue.** Lipid is not well preserved in routine sections and looks washed out. Here, several fat cells (adipocytes) contain lipid (*), which pushes nuclei to the periphery. Cells thus have a signet ring appearance in transverse section. 480×. *H&E.*

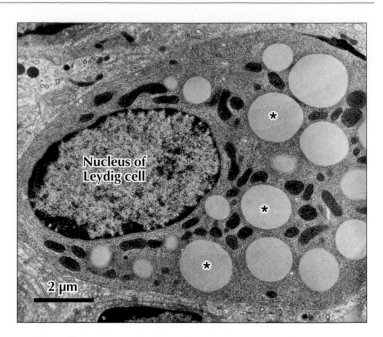

▲ **EM of lipid droplets in a steroid-secreting cell.** Several spherical lipid droplets (*) occupy the cytoplasm. This interstitial cell of Leydig produces testosterone, a steroid hormone. Precursors to the hormone are stored as cholesterol in lipid droplets. 7500×. *(Courtesy of Dr. A. W. Vogl)*

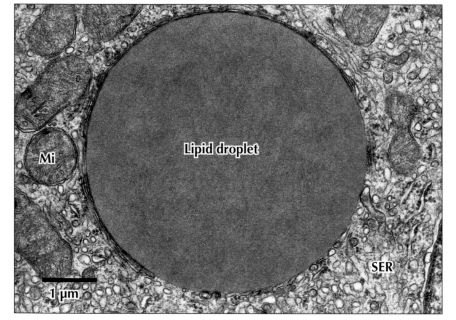

◄ **Higher magnification EM of a lipid droplet.** A large spherical lipid droplet is moderately electron dense. **SER** surrounds the droplet, which has no membrane. The close association of lipid to SER is functionally important: SER is the site of production of lipid, lipoproteins, and cholesterol derivatives. Several mitochondria (**Mi**) occupy the cytoplasm. 15,000×.

1.21   ULTRASTRUCTURE AND FUNCTION OF INCLUSIONS: LIPID DROPLETS

Lipid (or fat) is stored in the cytoplasm of many cells. Fats are insoluble in water, so they form spherical lipid droplets that vary widely in size. These **inclusions** are storage sites for energy used in cell metabolism. **Adipocytes** (fat cells) are the main storage sites for lipid in the body, with functions of thermal insulation, physical padding, and shock absorption. In these cells, droplets often coalesce to from one large droplet (up to 90 μm in diameter) that fills the cytoplasm and pushes other organelles to the cell periphery. Lipid is released from cells into the bloodstream for other cells to use as needed. Cells also use lipid for normal turnover of membranes. Lipid droplets normally lack a plasma membrane and consist of *triglycerides* and esters of *cholesterol.* Hepatocytes,

the main sites of cholesterol synthesis, contain variable numbers of lipid droplets. These inclusions are often closely associated with SER, where synthesis of lipid, cholesterol, and lipoproteins occurs. Cholesterol is a precursor to *steroid hormones,* so steroid-secreting cells (such as those in adrenal cortex, testis, and ovary) also contain many small lipid droplets. Adrenal cortex cells typically look spongy because of lipid content and are thus called *spongiocytes.* Organic solvents used for histologic specimen preparation commonly extract lipid unless special methods are used, so in routine sections, lipid-containing areas are usually clear, vacuolated spaces. The use of glutaraldehyde and osmium fixation for EMs preserves lipid as distinct, round droplets. Depending on chemical composition, some droplets in EMs may appear *electron-dense,* but others may be more *electron-lucent.*

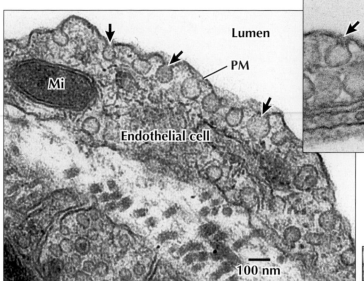

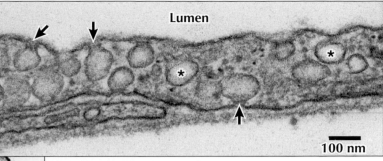

▲ **EM of caveolae and vesicles at high magnification.** Details of caveolae (**arrows**) and cytoplasmic vesicles (∗) are seen in this capillary endothelial cell. In life, blood would usually be in the capillary lumen. 80,000×.

▲ **EM of caveolae and vesicles in an endothelial cell.** Several flask-shaped invaginations of luminal plasma membrane (**PM**) form caveolae (**arrows**). In transcytosis, they pinch off from the surface to form vesicles, which enter the cytoplasm, travel across the cell, and discharge contents to the opposite surface. 50,000×.

▶ **EM of synaptic vesicles at a neuromuscular junction.** The terminal end of a nerve cell contains many small, smooth-surfaced synaptic vesicles (**arrows**). They hold the neurotransmitter acetylcholine, which is discharged by exocytosis into the synaptic cleft. Mitochondria (**Mi**), which supply energy, are in the cytoplasm of both the nerve cell and muscle cell. 60,000×.

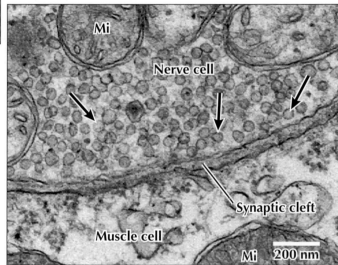

1.22 ULTRASTRUCTURE AND FUNCTION OF CYTOPLASMIC VESICLES: ENDOCYTOSIS, TRANSCYTOSIS, AND EXOCYTOSIS

Cells have several kinds of membrane-bound vesicles that form by invaginations of **plasma membrane.** They then enter the cytoplasm by pinching off from the surface and are transported to other parts of the cell. **Endocytosis** uses vesicles for cell uptake of extracellular fluid, macromolecules, and solutes. A nonselective form, called *fluid-phase endocytosis* (*pinocytosis,* meaning cell drinking), involves smooth-surfaced vesicles (diameter: 50-80 nm) that pinch off from cell membranes to enter cells. *Receptor-mediated endocytosis* is highly selective uptake of macromolecules such as hormones and growth factors. Shallow surface depressions, named *coated pits,* give rise to *clathrin-coated vesicles* (diameter: about 200 nm). Specific macromolecules bind with more than 20 distinct types of *transmembrane receptors.* Clathrin disassembles soon after a vesicle enters the cytoplasm. This pathway is used in metabolism of *cholesterol,* which most cells need for their membranes. Cholesterol is synthesized in the liver, travels in the bloodstream as *low-density lipoproteins* (LDLs), and is transported into cells by receptor-mediated endocytosis. Selective endocytosis is also mediated by small flask-like invaginations of plasma membrane termed **caveolae,** with diameters of 50-100 nm. They are coated by the protein *caveolin.* Many caveolae in endothelial cells mediate **transcytosis,** whereby vesicles derived from caveolae are taken across a cell and release their contents at another surface. Caveolae function in signal transduction, uptake of pathogenic bacteria, and oncogenesis. Other kinds of cytoplasmic vesicles, most derived from the Golgi complex, engage in **exocytosis.** In this pathway, vesicles move to the cell surface, fuse with plasma membrane, and discharge contents to the cell exterior. **Synaptic vesicles** of neurons and **secretory vesicles** of most secretory cells release products in this way.

CLINICAL POINT

Familial hypercholesterolemia is an autosomal dominant disorder caused by a mutation in the gene on chromosome 19 that encodes LDL receptors. Defective receptors lose an affinity for coated pits, so cell uptake of cholesterol is blocked. Greatly elevated serum cholesterol may lead to premature *atherosclerotic lesions* in walls of blood vessels such as coronary arteries. An untreated disorder may result in *myocardial infarction, stroke,* and death in midlife. Treatments include low-saturated-fat diets, aerobic exercise, and cholesterol-lowering drugs.

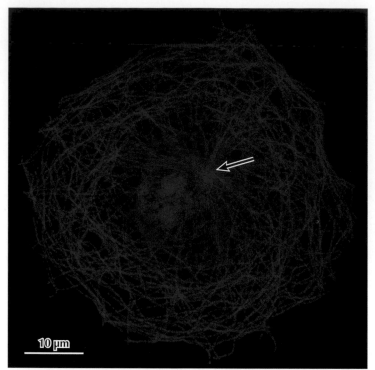

◀ **LM of a cell showing the microtubular organization of its cytoskeleton.** This cultured fibroblast from monkey kidney was treated immunocytochemically to reveal microtubules. The fluorescent immunolabel—an antibody to tubulin—shows the extensive network of microtubules in the cytoplasm. Microtubules originate from the microtubule-organizing center (**arrow**), which is named the centrosome. The nucleus is stained blue with a DNA-intercalating dye. 1800×. *Anti-β tubulin and DAPI (4',6-Diamidino-2-phenylindole).*

▶ **EM of microtubules in a cultured cell.** The cytoplasm contains microtubules (**arrows**), seen in longitudinal section. Microtubules resemble railroad tracks, on which other organelles such as mitochondria are transported from one part of a cell to another. Mitochondria (**Mi**) and plasma membrane (**PM**) are indicated. 42,500×. *(Courtesy of Dr. A. W. Vogl)*

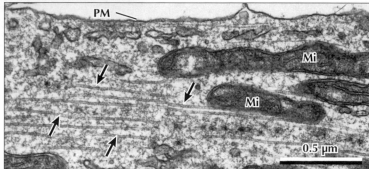

1.23 ULTRASTRUCTURE AND FUNCTION OF MICROTUBULES

Microtubules are hollow, semirigid cylindrical **organelles** that resemble drinking straws in EMs. Of uniform diameter (25 nm), they are unbranched and extremely variable in length. They are found in most cells but are especially abundant in neurons, platelets, leukocytes, and dividing cells. They are the main constituent of *cilia, flagella,* and *centrioles.* They also help provide mechanical strength and establish cell shape as a major part of the **cytoskeleton.** They engage in *intracellular transport* of organelles (such as **mitochondria** and **cytoplasmic vesicles**), ciliary and flagellar motility, and cytokinesis during cell division. They have no membrane; their walls are composed of linear polymers (**protofilaments**) of the globular protein *tubulin.* The 13 protofilaments in each microtubule are formed by alternating *alpha* and *beta subunits* in a staggered assembly, which gives rise to a helical design of tubulin heterodimers in the cylinder wall. Microtubules undergo continuous turnover in cells. They are intrinsically unstable and constantly elongate by polymerization and shorten by depolymerization. They also exhibit structural polarity, with a *plus end* (with exposed beta subunits) and a *minus end* (with exposed alpha units). Microtubule growth usually occurs at the plus end, where

tubulin is added in the presence of guanosine triphosphate. The minus end grows relatively slowly and is often anchored to another organelle or structure. Microtubules interact with *microtubule-associated proteins* that modulate their stability in assembly and disassembly. Two microtubule motor proteins, *kinesin* and *dynein,* move along microtubules, kinesin toward the plus end and dynein toward the minus end.

TECHNICAL POINT

Immunocytochemistry is a powerful research and diagnostic labeling technique using antibodies to show proteins and other molecules, called antigens, in cells. Antibodies to cell components are generated by injection of purified antigen (e.g., protein) into a host. Host immune cells that recognize a specific amino acid sequence in the protein produce antibodies. Antibodies are purified and used on tissue sections or cultured cells to show the protein of interest. Monoclonal and polyclonal antibodies may be used, but the former are more specific. Several systems may detect an antibody-antigen complex, the most common in light microscopy being a fluorescent tag that emits light at a certain wavelength when excited. Other systems use enzymes such as horseradish peroxidase and alkaline phosphatase to convert substrates into a visible precipitate.

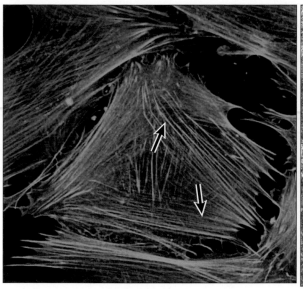

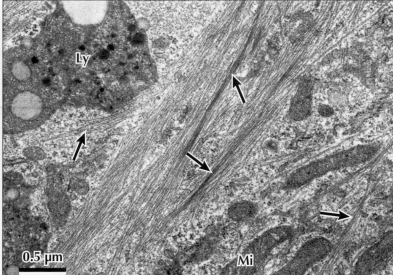

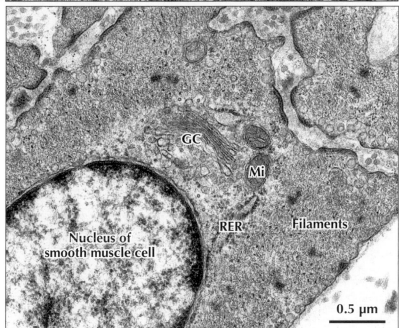

▲ **LM of mammary epithelial cells showing the distribution of actin filaments.** In this confocal microscopic image, the fluorescently label phalloidin demonstrates F-actin in actin filament bundles (**arrows**). Filaments crisscross the cell in the center of the field. 400×. *Phalloidin–Fluorescein Isothiocyanate (FITC). (Courtesy of Dr. J. G. Goetz)*

◀ **EM of intermediate filaments in a cultured cell.** A dense, interweaving network of intermediate filament bundles (**arrows**) makes up the cytoskeleton. Mitochondria (**Mi**) and a tertiary lysosome (**Ly**) are in the cytoplasm. 25,000×. *(Courtesy of Dr. A. W. Vogl)*

▶ **EM of actin and intermediate filaments in part of a smooth muscle cell.** In this transverse section, many closely packed filaments—the small, dense punctate profiles—predominate in the cytoplasm. Their diameters identify them as thin (or actin) and intermediate filaments. A supranuclear Golgi complex (**GC**), a few mitochondria (**Mi**), and rough endoplasmic reticulum (**RER**) are also indicated. 25,000×.

1.24 ULTRASTRUCTURE AND FUNCTION OF CYTOPLASMIC FILAMENTS

The **cytoskeleton** of most cells consists of two kinds of slender rod-like filaments, termed **intermediate** and **actin filaments,** as well as microtubules. These non-membrane-bound organelles vary in diameter, protein content, distribution, and mechanical properties. Intermediate filaments, 8-12 nm in diameter, form wavy bundles in a three-dimensional branching network. They mainly provide mechanical support to cells, are flexible but prevent excessive stretching, and interact with microtubules and actin filaments. Made of a heterogeneous family of *intermediate filament proteins,* they have a rope-like molecular structure. Six distinct classes of intermediate filaments exist, with 50 genes encoding them. Different cell types express specific kinds of intermediate filaments. *Nuclear lamins,* the most widespread, reinforce the inner nuclear envelope and help organize chromosomal archi-

tecture in interphase. Other intermediate filaments transmit mechanical forces between cells via *desmosomes,* and to the extracellular matrix via *hemidesmosomes. Keratin* is found only in epithelial cells and provides mechanical integrity to the epidermis of skin. *Desmin* is in muscle cells; *vimentin,* in mesenchymal cells; **neurofilaments,** in nerve cells; and **glial filaments,** in glial cells. Actin filaments, also called **thin filaments** or **microfilaments,** have cytoskeletal and motility functions. With diameters of 6-8 nm, they are made of the fibrous protein *actin.* They are flexible but resist deformation and transmit forces. They also contribute to cell movement and interact with **thick (myosin) filaments** in muscle cells during contraction. They are dispersed throughout the cytoplasm of nonmuscle cells or are arranged as linear bundles. They are found in *microvilli* or just beneath the plasma membrane, determine the shape of the cell surface, and contribute to cell locomotion, cytokinesis, and phagocytosis.

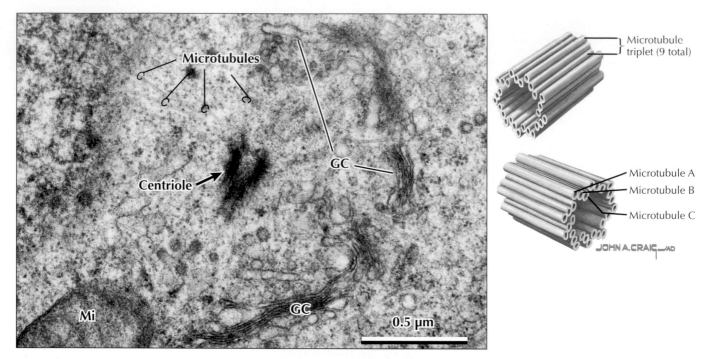

Microtubules

Centriole

GC

GC

Mi

0.5 μm

Microtubule triplet (9 total)

Microtubule A
Microtubule B
Microtubule C

JOHN A.CRAIG—AD

▲ **EM of part of a centriole in oblique section.** This small, cylindrical non-membrane-bound organelle is about 0.5 μm long and 0.15 μm wide. The self-replicating organelle is made of nine peripheral microtubular triplets, which are best seen in transverse section. Note that the centriole is near vesicles and saccules of the Golgi complex (**GC**). The area next to the centriole also contains many microtubules and a mitochondrion (**Mi**). 55,000×.

▶ **EM of microtubules in the cytocentrum.** This part of the cytoplasm next to the nucleus contains many microtubules (**arrows**) radiating in different directions. Mitochondria (**Mi**) and other organelles occupy other areas. Nuclear pores are seen in this grazing (tangential) section of the nucleus. 25,000×. *(Courtesy of Dr. A.W. Vogl.)*

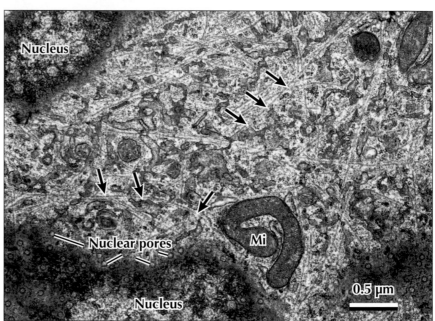

Nucleus

Nuclear pores

Mi

Nucleus

0.5 μm

1.25 ULTRASTRUCTURE AND FUNCTION OF THE CENTROSOME AND CENTRIOLES

The centrosome is the major microtubule-organizing center of a cell and the site for generation of new cytoplasmic **microtubules** and the **mitotic spindle.** This non-membrane-bound organelle is usually near the nucleus and often partly surrounded by a **Golgi complex.** The centrosome is made of a pair of centrioles—the **diplosome**—oriented at right angles or obliquely to each other. Each centriole is a short cylinder about 200 nm in diameter and 500-700 nm long. Each consists of a ring of nine sets of fused **microtubule triplets** that, in transverse section, resemble vanes of a turbine. In many cells, microtubules radiate from the centrosome in a star-like astral design and contribute to cell shape. Centriolar microtubules contain different forms of *tubulin,* plus isoforms of

the calcium-binding protein *centrin.* These microtubules are more stable than most cytoplasmic microtubules. Around the centrioles is a **pericentriolar matrix** containing proteins, which initiate polymerization of cytoplasmic microtubules and anchor them. The matrix also interacts with the Golgi complex and helps target Golgi-derived vesicles to different parts of a cell. Centrosomes are prominent in dividing cells: In mitosis, they induce development of the mitotic spindle by migrating to opposite poles, dividing, and serving as foci for microtubules needed for chromosomal movement. Under the cell surface, they induce development of *basal bodies,* which closely resemble centrioles and are organizing centers for microtubules of *cilia* and *flagella.* Centrosome abnormalities are often seen in malignant tumor cells, which suggests a close relation between such defects and *carcinogenesis.*

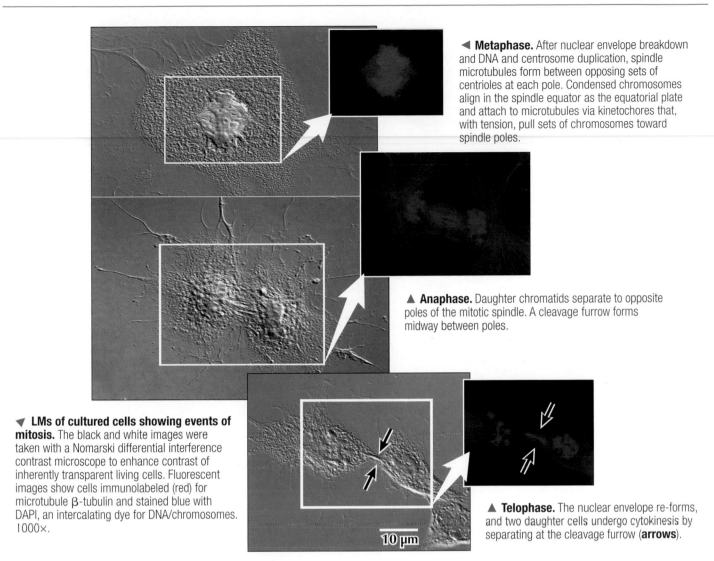

◀ **Metaphase.** After nuclear envelope breakdown and DNA and centrosome duplication, spindle microtubules form between opposing sets of centrioles at each pole. Condensed chromosomes align in the spindle equator as the equatorial plate and attach to microtubules via kinetochores that, with tension, pull sets of chromosomes toward spindle poles.

▲ **Anaphase.** Daughter chromatids separate to opposite poles of the mitotic spindle. A cleavage furrow forms midway between poles.

▼ **LMs of cultured cells showing events of mitosis.** The black and white images were taken with a Nomarski differential interference contrast microscope to enhance contrast of inherently transparent living cells. Fluorescent images show cells immunolabeled (red) for microtubule β-tubulin and stained blue with DAPI, an intercalating dye for DNA/chromosomes. 1000×.

▲ **Telophase.** The nuclear envelope re-forms, and two daughter cells undergo cytokinesis by separating at the cleavage furrow (**arrows**).

1.26 THE CELL CYCLE, MITOSIS, AND OTHER CELLULAR PROCESSES

The time between two successive divisions of a cell, called the cell cycle, consists of an orderly sequence of events that produce two daughter cells with identical copies of the *genome* of the parent cell. Its two major phases are **interphase** and **mitosis**. A time of continuous cell growth, interphase comprises a G_0 phase (quiescence), G_1 **phase** (initial cell growth), **S phase** (DNA synthesis, duplication of chromosomes and centrioles), and G_2 **phase** (preparation for cell division). These lead to mitosis (**M phase**). At interphase, **chromosomes** are not clearly seen in the nucleus, but clumps of condensed **chromatin**, named *heterochromatin*, and a *nucleolus* are seen. The cytoplasm also contains a pair of **centrioles,** the organizational sites for **microtubules**. Mitosis is also divided into phases. In **prophase,** the nuclear envelope disassembles, chromatin condenses, and the nucleolus disappears. Chromosomes, each made of a pair of parallel strands termed **chromatids** joined at a **centromere,** can be seen. Centrioles migrate to opposite poles of the nucleus. In **metaphase,** the **mitotic spindle** forms together with the **equatorial plate,** where chromosomes align in the middle of the cell. The spindle is made of microtubules that extend to both poles or connect centrioles to chromosomes. In **anaphase,** sister chromatids separate and begin migration to opposite poles of the mitotic spindle. A **cleavage furrow** forms by infolding of the cell equator. At **telophase,** chromatids complete movement to opposite poles of the spindle, chromatid DNA disperses, and nucleolus and nuclear envelope re-form. A constriction of cytoplasm, the *contractile ring,* forms, which leads to **cytokinesis** and separation of daughter cells. Two other important events affect cell life. **Apoptosis** is a normal process in certain tissues: programmed to die, cells become rounded, with nuclear pyknosis and plasma membrane blebbing, and are phagocytosed by macrophages. **Meiosis** is division of nuclear material from diploid to haploid in gametogenesis, which allows recombination and assortment of genotypes.

CLINICAL POINT

Tumor cells divide more rapidly than do normal cells and are thus more susceptible to chemotherapeutic **mitosis inhibitors** such as the vinca alkaloids **vinblastine** and **vincristine.** These naturally occurring extracts of the periwinkle *Catharanthus roseus* are clinically useful because they halt mitosis by arresting cells in metaphase. They prevent spindle formation in dividing cells by blocking tubulin polymerization (no microtubules form) and by inducing depolymerization of already formed microtubules. Vinblastine is mainly useful for treating *Hodgkin disease, advanced testicular carcinoma,* and *breast cancer;* vincristine, for *acute leukemia* and other *lymphomas.*

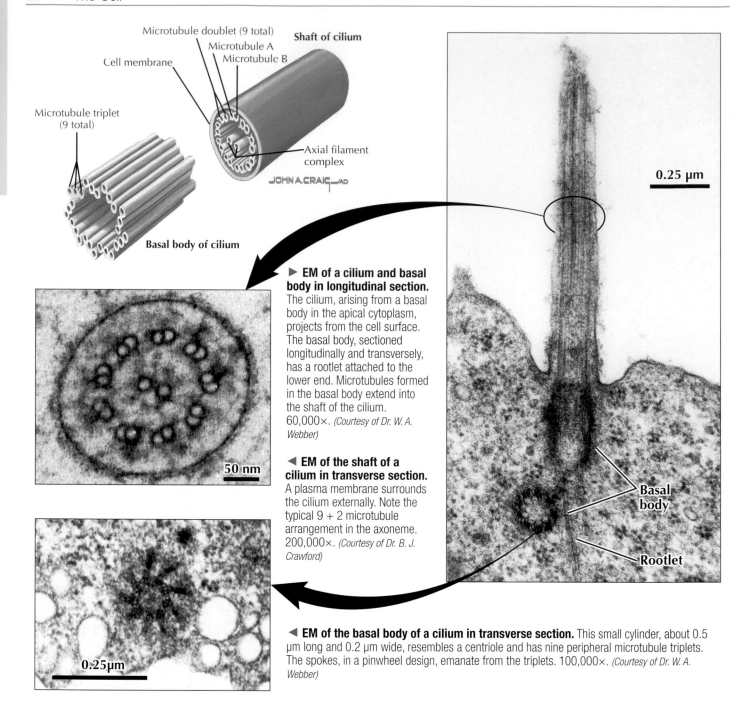

Microtubule doublet (9 total)
Cell membrane
Microtubule A
Microtubule B
Shaft of cilium
Microtubule triplet (9 total)
Axial filament complex
JOHN A. CRAIG—AD
Basal body of cilium

▶ **EM of a cilium and basal body in longitudinal section.** The cilium, arising from a basal body in the apical cytoplasm, projects from the cell surface. The basal body, sectioned longitudinally and transversely, has a rootlet attached to the lower end. Microtubules formed in the basal body extend into the shaft of the cilium. 60,000×. *(Courtesy of Dr. W. A. Webber)*

◀ **EM of the shaft of a cilium in transverse section.** A plasma membrane surrounds the cilium externally. Note the typical 9 + 2 microtubule arrangement in the axoneme. 200,000×. *(Courtesy of Dr. B. J. Crawford)*

◀ **EM of the basal body of a cilium in transverse section.** This small cylinder, about 0.5 μm long and 0.2 μm wide, resembles a centriole and has nine peripheral microtubule triplets. The spokes, in a pinwheel design, emanate from the triplets. 100,000×. *(Courtesy of Dr. W. A. Webber)*

0.25 μm

50 nm

0.25μm

Basal body

Rootlet

1.27 SPECIALIZATIONS OF THE CELL SURFACE: CILIA AND BASAL BODIES

Cells have different kinds of surface specializations—*microvilli, stereocilia,* **cilia,** and *flagella*—that are associated with specific functions. Microvilli are simple, finger-like projections of cell surface that are found on epithelial cells in several sites, such as small intestine and kidney. Their major role is to increase surface area for absorption. Unbranched and 1 μm long or shorter, they contain a core of *actin filaments.* Stereocilia are unusually long, branched microvilli that are on free surfaces of epithelial cells lining parts of the male reproductive tract and inner ear. Cilia, with the most complex internal structure, are mobile extensions of the cell surface and are typically 10-12 μm long and about 0.2 μm in diameter. Their structure is similar that of flagella, but their beating patterns are different. Cilia are found in parts of the respiratory and female reproductive tracts. Flagella, found in sperm cells, are longer than cilia. Some cells may bear one cilium, but most have many cilia that beat in synchrony. They originate from **basal bodies,** which are identical to **centrioles.** Basal bodies, in the apical cytoplasm at the cilium base, are hollow cylinders made of nine triplets of **microtubules,** with no central microtubule pair. Cilia are surrounded by a **plasma membrane** and consist of an **axoneme** with a 9 + 2 microtubule arrangement. Two *dynein side arms,* consisting of a motor protein and ATPase to generate force for movement, are bound to the outer microtubule doublets. Dynein arms of one doublet interact with the microtubule of the next doublet to cause sliding of microtubules past each other and bending of the cilium, thus producing ciliary movement.

2

EPITHELIUM AND EXOCRINE GLANDS

▼ Classification of epithelia.

▲ **Schematic of nonkeratinized stratified squamous epithelium as seen with the light microscope.** The epithelium acts as a protective barrier and is typical of wet surfaces—linings of the oral cavity, esophagus, anal canal, part of the urethra, and vagina. It also covers the cornea.

2.1 OVERVIEW

Epithelium is one of the four **basic tissues,** with a wide distribution and many functions. It consists of continuous sheets of **cells** that cover exposed body surfaces. It also lines internal cavities, such as those of the *digestive, respiratory, cardiovascular,* and *genitourinary* systems. During embryonic development, epithelium invaginates into underlying tissues to proliferate and form secretory *glands.* Its two classes are thus **covering and lining** and **glandular.** A **selective barrier** that protects other tissues, it transports material along its surface uni- or bidirectionally. Other functions include *synthesis, secretion, absorption,* and, because cells are exposed on free surfaces, *sensory reception.* Epithelium is made almost entirely of contiguous and adhesive cells bound together by *intercellular junctions* and a small amount of *extracellular matrix.* Epithelium has tissue polarity and an apical (or free) surface, lateral surfaces between adjacent cells, and a basal surface in contact with an underlying *basement membrane.* Epithelia lack a direct blood supply and are fed via diffusion from underlying tissues. Unlike other basic tissues, epithelia have a high *mitotic index* with constant cell renewal—an advantage because cells undergo mechanical stress and trauma. However, they are suscep-

tible to formation of **malignant tumors** called **carcinomas.** Epithelia have diverse embryonic origins and may come from *ectoderm, mesoderm,* or *endoderm.* Covering and lining epithelium is classed histologically according to the shape of the surface cells—**squamous, cuboidal, columnar, pseudostratified,** or **transitional**—and the number of cell layers—**simple** or **stratified.**

CLINICAL POINT

Epithelial cells have a high mitotic index and are exposed to the surface, which gives pathogens and carcinogens free access to them. The most common types of **cancerous** (or **malignant**) **tumors** (or **neoplasms**) in adults originate from epithelial cells; these tumors invade or metastasize to distant tissues and organs. Neoplasms that grow slowly are **benign** tumors and include papillomas, which arise from surface epithelium, and adenomas, which originate from glandular epithelium. Malignant neoplasms of surface epithelium are carcinomas, and those originating from glandular epithelium are adenocarcinomas. Knowing a tumor's histologic characteristics often helps determine diagnosis, staging, and treatment.

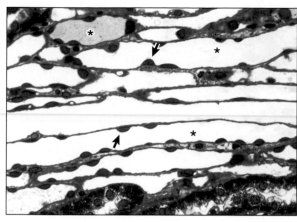

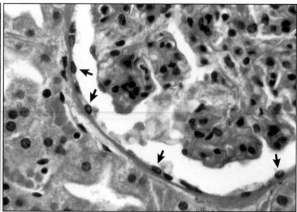

▲ **Light micrograph (LM) of part of the renal medulla.**
Simple squamous epithelial cells line loops of Henle (✶). Nuclei
(**arrows**) of the cells bulge into tubule lumina. 340×. *Toluidine
blue, plastic section.*

▲ **LM of the cortex of the kidney showing part of a renal
corpuscle.** Simple squamous epithelial cells (**arrows**) form the
parietal layer of Bowman's capsule. These attenuated cells have
oval to flat nuclei. 445×. *H&E.*

▼ **Simple squamous epithelium**

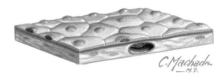

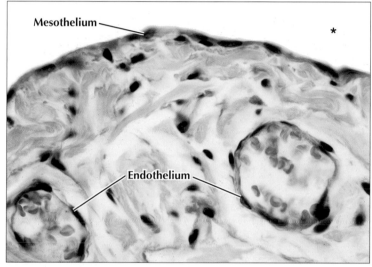

▲ **LM of the serosa of the urinary bladder.** Simple squamous epithelial cells
make up a mesothelium that covers the bladder and lines the peritoneal cavity (✶).
Compare the simple squamous epithelium of venules in underlying connective
tissue, called endothelium. 680×. *H&E.*

2.2   STRUCTURE AND FUNCTION OF SIMPLE SQUAMOUS EPITHELIUM

Simple squamous epithelium consists of a single layer of flattened
cells usually joined by **intercellular junctions** and resting on a
basement membrane whose thickness depends on location. The
cells, shaped like scales (Latin *squama*), are best seen in a surface
view and have irregular, serrated outlines that fit together like
pieces of a jigsaw puzzle. One nucleus is in the widest part of each
cell, so a local bulge protrudes into the free surface. In a plane
perpendicular to the surface, cells look like spindles with tapering
ends on both sides of the nucleus. Cell borders are hard to see in
hematoxylin and eosin (H&E) sections, but special techniques
and electron microscopy can elucidate them. This type of epithelium is typical at sites that make up **blood-tissue barriers.** Thinness of the epithelium also permits diffusion and bidirectional
movement of gases, fluids, and nutrients from the free surface to
underlying tissues. Names of this epithelium depend on location:
simple squamous epithelium of the lining of the heart, blood
vessels, and lymphatic channels is an **endothelium; mesothelium**

consists of simple squamous cells forming **serous membranes**
lining internal body cavities. This distinction is important to
pathologists because cells behave differently in inflammation and
tumor formation. Simple squamous epithelium in the kidney
constitutes the parietal layer of **Bowman's capsule** and thin **loops
of Henle;** it is also found in the middle and inner ear, and in lungs
where it lines pulmonary alveoli.

CLINICAL POINT

Rare, aggressive tumors called **malignant mesotheliomas** may arise
from parietal and visceral serous membranes of pleural, peritoneal,
and pericardial cavities. **Pleural mesothelioma**—the most common—
is usually caused by occupational exposure to asbestos. It has a long
latency time (25-40 years) from first contact to onset of symptoms,
which include shortness of breath, chest pain, and pleural fluid accumulation. Magnetic resonance imaging, positron emission tomography, needle biopsy, and electron microscopy are useful for diagnosis.
The often poor prognosis is due to a tendency to metastasize to lymph
nodes and other organs. Surgery, radiation, and chemotherapy can
help in some cases.

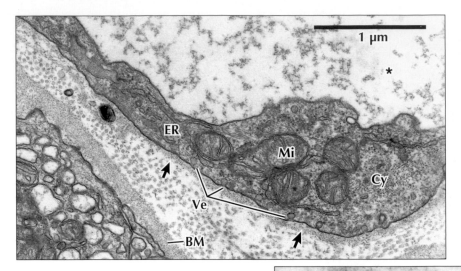

◀ **Electron micrograph (EM) of part of an endothelial cell of a capillary.** The basal part of the cell rests on a thin basement membrane (**arrows**); the apical surface faces the lumen (∗). The cytoplasm shows mitochondria (**Mi**), an extensive cytoskeleton (**Cy**), transcytotic vesicles (**Ve**), and scattered profiles of endoplasmic reticulum (**ER**). A thicker basement membrane (**BM**) of an adjacent epithelial cell is seen. 30,000×.

▲ **EM of a tight junction between the ends of two simple squamous epithelial cells.** A large area of plasma membrane fusion (**arrows**)—between overlapping cell processes where they touch and interdigitate—forms a tight junction. A mitochondrion (**Mi**) and rough endoplasmic reticulum (**RER**) occupy the cytoplasm. 80,000×.

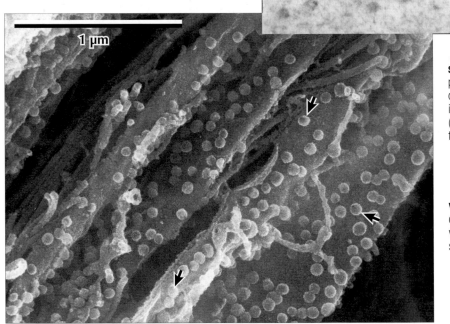

◀ **High-resolution scanning EM of cytoplasmic vesicles in squamous epithelial cells.** The cytoplasm, fractured open, shows many transcytotic vesicles (**arrows**). The spherical vesicles, of uniform size, indicate active transport across cells. 44,000×.

2.3 ULTRASTRUCTURE AND FUNCTION OF SIMPLE SQUAMOUS EPITHELIUM

Ultrastructure of simple squamous epithelial cells reflects their functional diversity. The rich, varied organelle content of the cytoplasm indicates high metabolic activity, active synthesis and secretion, and selective permeability. Cells usually have a complex **cytoskeleton** to maintain shape and provide internal scaffolding to resist pressure changes and wear and tear. The cytoskeleton consists of a network of *intermediate filaments (tonofilaments),* which are interwoven in each cell. Prominent actin-containing *thin filaments (microfilaments)* and motor proteins allow changes in cell shape and provide pliability. This epithelium is a metabolically active diffusion barrier at many sites, with striking features: smooth-surfaced **transcytotic vesicles** (first termed pinocytotic vesicles) and clathrin-coated *endocytotic vesicles,* which participate in transepithelial transport. The many **intercellular junctions** include *desmosomes* and *intermediate junctions,* which anchor cells together, and **tight junctions,** which act as a permeability barrier to indiscriminate passage of material. *Gap junctions* also allow ionic and metabolic communication between cells.

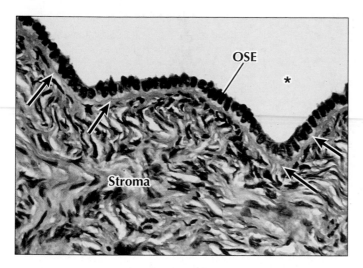

▲ **LM of the ovarian surface epithelium (OSE).** Simple cuboidal epithelial cells, with cuboidal nuclei, cover the ovary's surface. The free epithelial surface abuts the peritoneal cavity (∗). A thin amorphous layer under the epithelium is the basement membrane (**arrows**). Connective tissue, which makes up the stroma, is at bottom. 400×. *H&E.*

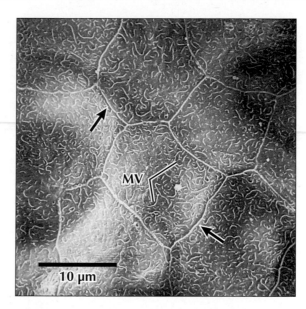

▲ **Scanning EM of simple cuboidal epithelial cells.** On surface view, cells are polygonal. Cell borders (**arrows**) are white linear densities; short surface projections, or microvilli (**MV**), extend from cell surfaces. 2000×.

▼ **Simple cuboidal epithelium**

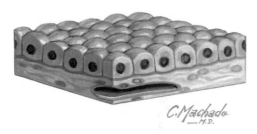

▶ **LM of a portal triad in the liver.** Simple cuboidal epithelium lines a small bile duct. Compare the simple squamous epithelium (endothelium) that lines a venule, arteriole, and lymphatic channel. 790×. *H&E.*

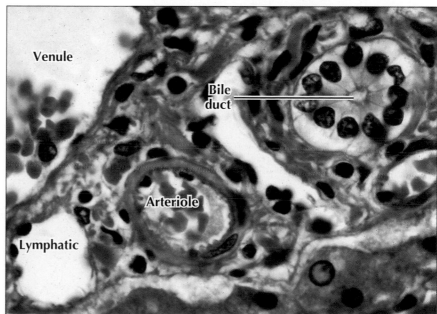

2.4 STRUCTURE AND FUNCTION OF SIMPLE CUBOIDAL EPITHELIUM

Simple cuboidal epithelium consists of one layer of cells whose height roughly equals their width, so in sections perpendicular to the surface, cells resemble small box-like cubes. Cells in horizontal section appear to be a mosaic of polygonal tiles. As in other epithelia, cells rest on a **basement membrane** that firmly attaches to underlying connective tissue. Each cell has one spherical, centrally placed nucleus. This epithelium provides protection, forms conduits for gland ducts, and may be specialized for active secretion and absorption. On the surface of the ovary, it is **ovarian surface epithelium.** It also lines renal tubules and small collecting ducts of the kidney, which engage in ion transport. The thyroid—an endocrine gland—contains spherical follicles of these cuboidal cells. The parenchyma of most *exocrine glands,* such as salivary glands and pancreas, consists of cuboidal to columnar epithelial cells in grape-like clusters called *acini.* In the eye, cells of pigmented epithelium of the retina and epithelium of the ciliary body are simple cuboidal and specialized for ion transport and secretion. Free surfaces of these cuboidal cells often have **microvilli,** which are best seen by electron microscopy. Their cytoplasm has more organelles than that of simple squamous epithelial cells, with more mitochondria and endoplasmic reticulum, which are evidence of high metabolic and functional activities.

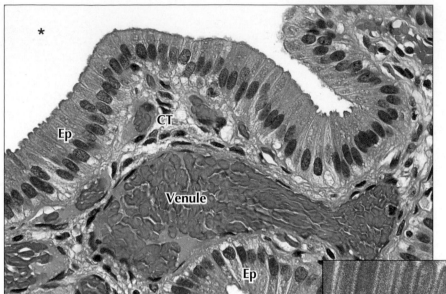

◀ **LM of the inner lining of the gallbladder.**
Simple columnar epithelium (**Ep**) lines the lumen (∗).
One row of regularly arranged, elongated nuclei lies
at the bases of these cells. Apical cell surfaces bear
a fringe-like border of microvilli, which is better shown
by electron microscopy. Compare the simple
squamous epithelium (endothelium) that lines the
lumen of a venule in the connective tissue (**CT**).
625×. *H&E.*

▼ **Simple columnar epithelium**

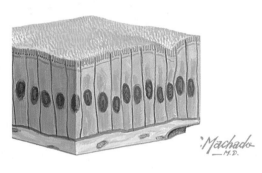

Machado M.D.

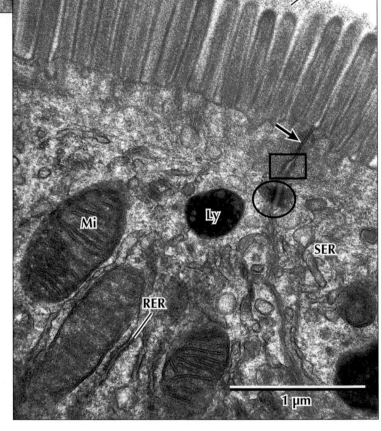

▶ **EM of a striated border in intestinal epithelium.** At the
lumen (∗), apical surfaces of two simple columnar epithelial cells
are studded by uniform, closely packed microvilli (**MV**) covered by a
fuzzy glycocalyx (**Gl**). Many densely packed cytoplasmic organelles
include mitochondria (**Mi**), rough (**RER**) and smooth (**SER**) endoplasmic reticulum, and lysosomes (**Ly**). A junctional complex—tight
junction (**arrow**), intermediate junction (**rectangle**), and desmosome (**circle**)—attaches lateral cell borders. 36,000×.

2.5 STRUCTURE AND FUNCTION OF SIMPLE COLUMNAR EPITHELIUM

Simple columnar epithelium consists of one layer of cells that are
taller than they are wide and look like closely packed, slender
columns. Bases of cells rest on a *basement membrane;* apical
surfaces contact a lumen. The ovoid nucleus is centrally or basally
placed. This epithelium, widely distributed in the body, is mainly
found in sites engaged in protection of wet surfaces, nutrient
absorption, and secretion. It forms major ducts of glands, convoluted tubules of the kidney, and inner lining of the stomach, small
and large intestines, gallbladder, small bronchi of the lungs, and

parts of the male and female (oviducts and uterus) reproductive
tracts. Free surfaces of cells often bear **microvilli**—thin, finger-
like cellular projections—for increased surface area. When microvilli are large (1-2 μm high), uniform in size, and closely packed,
they form a **striated border.** Lateral cell borders have **junctional
complexes,** which include an apical **tight junction, intermediate (adherens) junction,** and **desmosome.** The cytoplasm is
packed with many **organelles.** At certain sites, the epithelium
may consist of more than one type of cell, with mucus-secreting
goblet cells being common. In some areas, the epithelium may
have cilia.

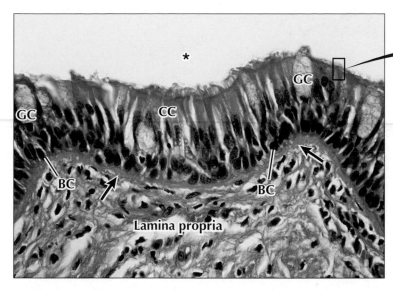

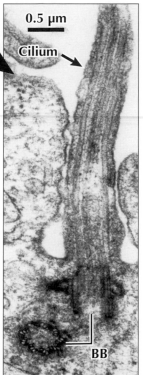

▲ **LM of pseudostratified ciliated columnar (respiratory) epithelium with goblet cells.** The airway lumen (∗) is indicated. Two or three layers of nuclei are visible. Tall columnar cells (**CC**) with elongated nuclei and apical cilia intermingle with pale-stained goblet cells (**GC**) whose washed-out appearance is due to mucus. One row of small basal cells (**BC**) rests on a basement membrane (**arrows**). The connective tissue at bottom is the lamina propria. 565×. *H&E.*

▶ **EM of one cilium in longitudinal section.** This surface specialization is a feature of cells in respiratory epithelium. It consists of a typical 9 + 2 arrangement of microtubule doublets, which make up the axoneme. A basal body (**BB**), at the base, has nine microtubule triplets, normally in a 9 + 0 configuration. 20,000×. *(Courtesy of Dr. W. A. Webber)*

▼ **Pseudostratified epithelium**

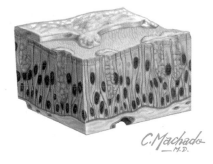

▶ **LM of pseudostratified epithelium in the epididymis.** Two layers of nuclei are typical. Note the row of small basal cells (**BC**) and columnar cells (**CC**) with apical stereocilia (**arrows**) that abut the lumen (∗). The lamina propria contains a venule. 665×. *H&E.*

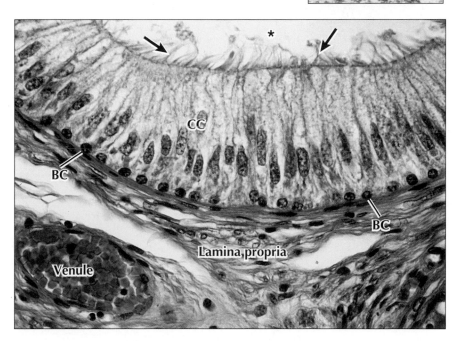

2.6 STRUCTURE AND FUNCTION OF PSEUDOSTRATIFIED EPITHELIUM

Pseudostratified epithelium consists of more than one type of epithelial cell, of varied size and shape. In sections perpendicular to the surface, the **nuclei** usually appear at different levels, so two or three layers of crowded nuclei are seen. A basal layer belongs to replacement (stem) cells with mitotic potential for regeneration. More apical layers contain elongated nuclei of tall columnar cells, many of which may have **cilia** on their free surfaces. All cells contact an underlying **basement membrane,** but only some reach the free surface and do not penetrate the whole thickness of the epithelium. These features give the epithelium a false impression of stratification—thus, its name. More aptly a type of simple epithelium, it lines many parts of the upper **respiratory tract** (nasal cavities, auditory tube, nasopharynx, larynx, trachea, and large bronchi). **Mucous goblet cells** usually occur in this epithelium, and where they mingle with **ciliated columnar cells,** the tissue is called **respiratory epithelium.** It acts as a mucociliary escalator to entrap and rid airways of foreign particles by sweeping, coordinated ciliary motion. Pseudostratified epithelium lacking goblet cells is also found in parts of the **male reproductive tract,** where some cells have apical nonmotile **stereocilia** and mainly lining, secretory, and absorptive roles are performed.

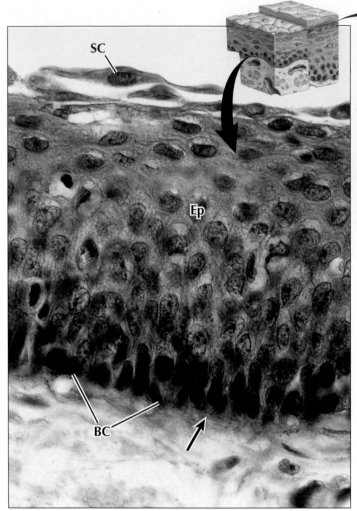

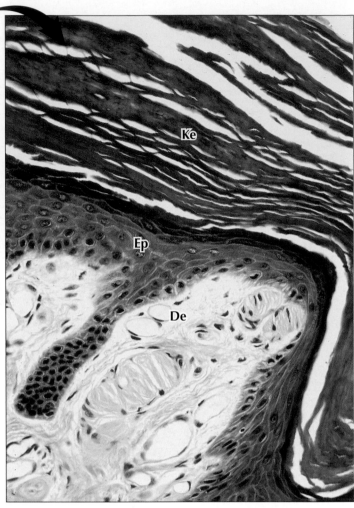

▲ **LM of nonkeratinized stratified squamous epithelium in the oral cavity.** Small basal cells (**BC**) form one layer that contacts a thin basement membrane (**arrow**). Intermediate areas of epithelium (**Ep**) contain polygonal cells; surface squamous cells (**SC**) undergo desquamation. 1030×. *H&E.*

▲ **LM of keratinized stratified squamous epithelium of skin.** Keratinocytes in this multilayer epithelium (**Ep**) change shape from basal to superficial layers, where cells are flatter and filled with keratin (**Ke**). Papillae of underlying dermis (**De**) are made of loose connective tissue. 240×. *H&E.*

2.7   STRUCTURE AND FUNCTION OF STRATIFIED SQUAMOUS EPITHELIUM

Stratified squamous epithelium is a tough, resilient multilayered epithelium that mainly protects against abrasion and dehydration. It also prevents invasion of pathogens, bacteria, and other infectious agents. Its name derives from the shape of the outer layer of flattened cells. Two types exist—**keratinized** and **nonkeratinized.** In areas exposed to air and subject to abrasion, such as **epidermis** of **skin,** the surface layer consists of dead cells lacking nuclei and containing plates of the protein **keratin,** which strengthens and waterproofs the tissue. This keratinized stratified squamous epithelium, with a dry, scale-like surface, also lines the outer surface of the tympanic membrane, parts of the **oral cavity** (gingiva and hard palate), and some mucocutaneous junctions (lips and distal anal canal). In other areas covered with fluid and with a moist surface, superficial **squamous cells** retain nuclei and lack keratin. This nonkeratinized stratified squamous epithelium lines most of the oral cavity, pharynx, epiglottis, vocal cords, esophagus, anal canal, vagina, parts of the male and female urethra, and cornea. Secretions from closely associated glands lubricate the surface of this epithelium.

CLINICAL POINT

After injury by trauma or infection to skin and other soft tissues, the capacity of epithelial cells to undergo mitosis and regenerate is clinically important. Complex reparative events known as **wound healing** include an inflammatory phase followed by proliferative and remodeling stages. Epithelial cells from nearby areas replicate, change shape, and migrate across the defect to cover the wound. Cells secrete various growth factors and activators that enhance repair. Angiogenesis, whereby new capillaries grow from endothelial cells, also occurs. The basement membrane is critical for rapid recovery; if it is destroyed, healing is relatively slow.

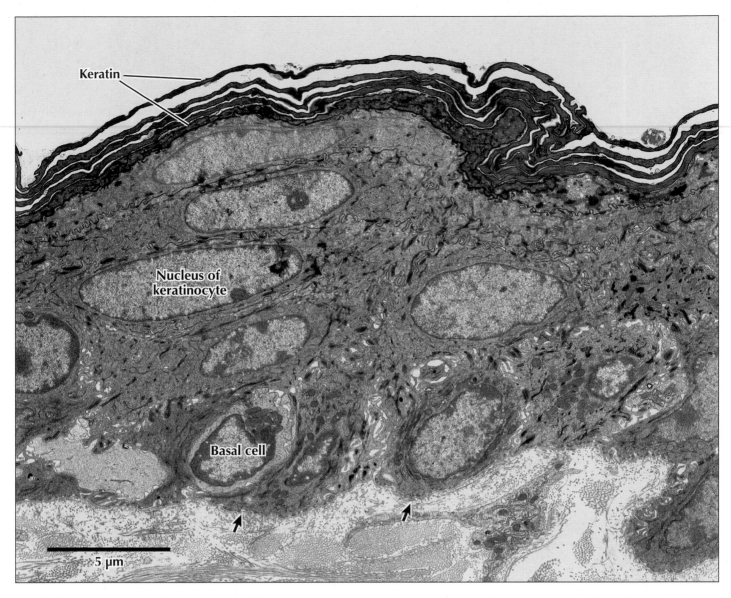

▲ **EM of keratinized stratified squamous epithelium in thin skin**. The basal round cells next to the basement membrane (**arrows**) are reserve stem cells. Just above them, keratinocytes differentiate, migrate upward, and transform into squamous cells toward the surface. An outer layer consists of flat keratin-filled scale-like dead cells. 6400×.

2.8 ULTRASTRUCTURE AND FUNCTION OF STRATIFIED SQUAMOUS EPITHELIUM

Electron microscopy provides ultrastructural details of this epithelium. It has many cell layers, whose numbers depend on location. In both types of stratified squamous epithelium, proliferation of basal germinative cells is critical to replace cells lost at the surface. **Basal cells** are mitotically active and continuously divide into daughter cells that mature and are pushed toward the surface to die and slough off. This process is called *desquamation*. **Keratinized epithelium** that makes up the epidermis of **skin** is renewed every 15-30 days; nonkeratinized epithelium of the oral cavity has a much more rapid turnover rate. Cells of both epithelia—**keratinocytes**—have many *intercellular junctions*, which are mostly *desmosomes* that connect cells to counteract

external forces of friction. For added strength, an extensive internal cytoskeleton, made mostly of keratin *intermediate filaments*, internally reinforces cells.

CLINICAL POINT

Epithelial **dysplasia** is a premalignant change in epithelium—an alteration in cell structure encoded in the genome plus an abnormal appearance of the tissue. **Cervical dysplasia**, a precancerous lesion in epithelium of the cervix, is caused by *human papilloma virus (HPV)* and is usually found via a screening test called the *PAP smear*. **Oral dysplasia** involves increased mitotic activity of oral epithelium with cell shape changes and loss of stratification of epithelial cells. Mutations in *tumor suppressor genes*, which normally act as negative regulators of cell proliferation, characterize many dysplasias and may be studied by immunohistochemical assays.

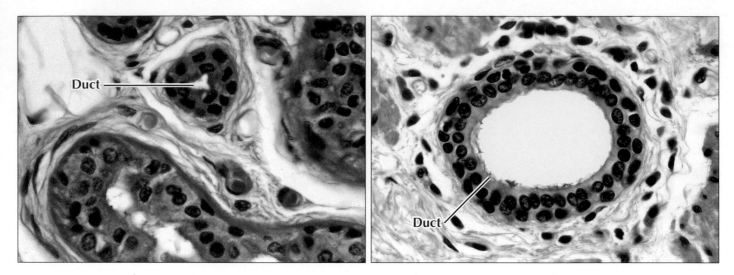

▲ **LMs of stratified cuboidal epithelia.** This epithelium forms ducts of a sweat gland (**Left**) and an esophageal mucous gland (**Right**). It typically consists of a double layer of cells. **Left**: 520×; **Right**: 625×. *H&E.*

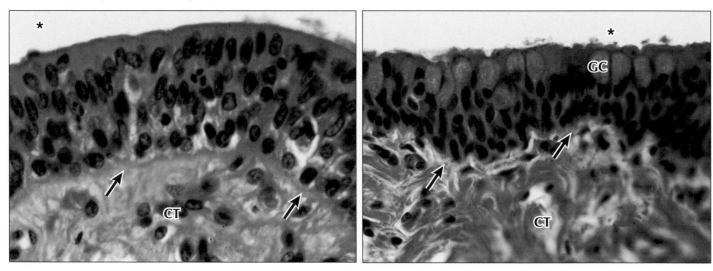

▲ **LMs of stratified columnar epithelia.** Both have a surface layer of columnar cells in contact with free space (∗). This multilayered epithelium occurs in the male urethra (**Left**) and palpebral conjunctiva (**Right**). The conjunctiva also has goblet cells (**GC**). The epithelia rest on a thin basement membrane (**arrows**) and cover loose connective tissue (**CT**). 680x. *H&E.*

2.9 STRUCTURE AND FUNCTION OF STRATIFIED CUBOIDAL AND COLUMNAR EPITHELIA

Stratified cuboidal and stratified columnar epithelia have limited distribution in the adult; they are more common in the embryo and fetus. Both contain two or more layers of cells, and because they are stratified, they are mainly protective and better suited than simple epithelia to withstand wear and tear. Stratified cuboidal epithelium, usually two layers of cells, lines **ducts of sweat glands** and other **exocrine glands.** Stratified columnar epithelium is in the pharynx and larynx, **conjunctiva** of the **eyelids,** major ducts of **exocrine glands,** and parts of the **male urethra.** It also occurs at sites of epithelial transition, interposed between two other types of epithelia. Such abrupt epithelial interfaces occur in the epiglottis and rectoanal junction. These sites are unstable and thus may undergo malignant change. This epithelium usually consists of basal cells (cuboidal), intermediate cells (more polyhe-

dral), and superficial cells (columnar). In the urethra and conjunctiva, two to five layers of cells make up the epithelium. It may often be confused with pseudostratified epithelium. This epithelium has **mucus-secreting goblet cells** that provide lubrication to the surface.

CLINICAL POINT

Pink eye, or **conjunctivitis** (inflammation of the conjunctiva), is the most common acute eye infection in children. It is usually caused by bacteria or viruses, allergy, or irritation from contact lens use. The normally seasonal **allergic conjunctivitis** leads to ocular redness and itching, crusting of eyelids, and photophobia. **Bacterial conjunctivitis** occurs more often than the viral form, the most common causative agents being *Haemophilus influenzae* and *Streptococcus pneumoniae.* Outbreaks of **adenovirus conjunctivitis** have been linked to contaminated equipment and swimming pools.

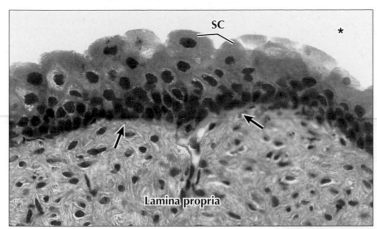

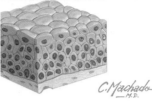

◀ **LM of transitional epithelium in a distended bladder.** Two or three layers of nucleated epithelial cells are typical of the bladder filled with urine. The largest, most superficial cells (**SC**) are round and bulge into the lumen (∗). Cells more intermediate in position are cuboidal. Basal cells, the smallest and most closely packed, abut a thin basement membrane (**arrows**). The lamina propria is made of loose connective tissue. 375×. *H&E.*

▶ **LM of transitional epithelium in a contracted bladder.** Many more layers of cells are seen here than in an expanded bladder. Dome-shaped surface cells (**SC**) in contact with the lumen (∗) have pale nuclei with prominent nucleoli. Polyhedral intermediate cells (**IC**) have well-defined cell borders and washed-out cytoplasm that reflects abundant glycogen. Tightly crowded basal cells (**BC**) abut an indiscernible basement membrane, under which is lamina propria. 600×. *H&E.*

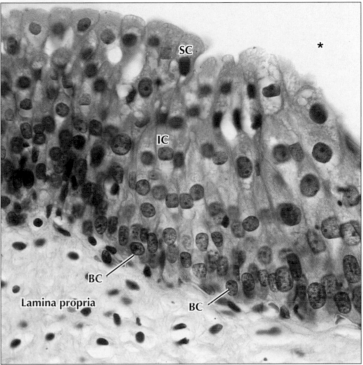

2.10 STRUCTURE AND FUNCTION OF TRANSITIONAL EPITHELIUM (UROTHELIUM)

Multilayered transitional epithelium is more aptly termed a *urothelium*, in that it is restricted to lower parts of the *urinary tract*, where it lines the renal pelvis, ureters, **urinary bladder,** and part of the urethra. The original term—transitional—is a misnomer; this epithelium was erroneously thought to be intermediate between stratified squamous and stratified columnar epithelium. Its appearance is not static. It rapidly adapts to contraction and distention; it changes from a tall epithelium with five to seven cell layers (empty state) to a thinner epithelium with only two or three cell layers (distended state). The **basal layer** of small cuboidal to columnar cells contacts a thin **basement membrane.** They serve as precursor stem cells and have a turnover rate of 12-24 weeks. The most **superficial layer** in contact with the lumen consists of relatively large, often binucleate cells. Their free surfaces are convex and they span several cells underneath, so they are called **umbrella cells.** Their apical cell membranes may show densely stained crust-like plaques in H&E

sections. Polyhedral **intermediate cells** are between the two layers. Electron microscopy shows all cells of this epithelium in contact with the basement membrane via long cytoplasmic processes, not unlike cells of pseudostratified epithelium. Urothelium acts as a *permeability barrier* and protects tissues from noxious effects of urine, but it can also stretch to accommodate urine volume.

CLINICAL POINT

A common *malignant neoplasm* of the urinary tract is **transitional cell carcinoma.** It arises from the urothelium of the renal pelvis, ureter, or bladder and is often fatal unless treated. *Hematuria* (blood in urine) and pain from gradual obstruction to urination are usual presenting symptoms. Its cause is unknown, but risk factors include cigarette smoking and occupational exposure to organic compounds such as benzidine and asbestos. Computed tomography, magnetic resonance imaging, and ureteroscopy are useful for diagnosis, and biopsy should be performed for histologic staging to determine treatment.

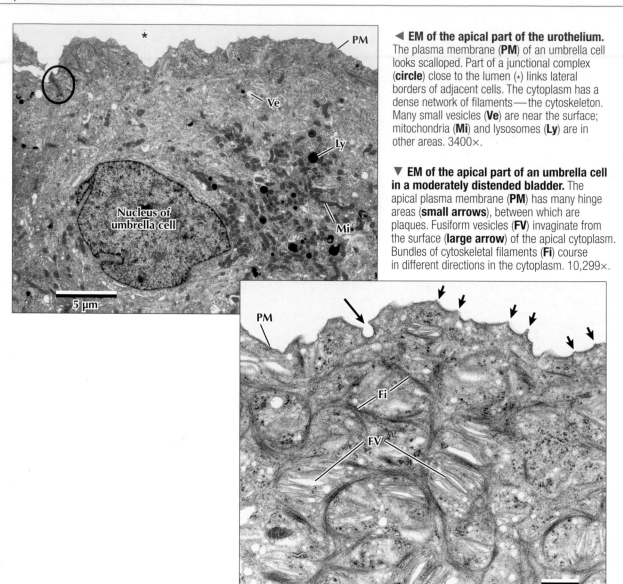

◀ **EM of the apical part of the urothelium.** The plasma membrane (**PM**) of an umbrella cell looks scalloped. Part of a junctional complex (**circle**) close to the lumen (✱) links lateral borders of adjacent cells. The cytoplasm has a dense network of filaments—the cytoskeleton. Many small vesicles (**Ve**) are near the surface; mitochondria (**Mi**) and lysosomes (**Ly**) are in other areas. 3400×.

▼ **EM of the apical part of an umbrella cell in a moderately distended bladder.** The apical plasma membrane (**PM**) has many hinge areas (**small arrows**), between which are plaques. Fusiform vesicles (**FV**) invaginate from the surface (**large arrow**) of the apical cytoplasm. Bundles of cytoskeletal filaments (**Fi**) course in different directions in the cytoplasm. 10,299×.

2.11 ULTRASTRUCTURE AND FUNCTION OF THE UROTHELIUM

Highly pliable urothelium has direct contact with urine, so surface **umbrella cells** have unique ultrastructural features to maintain a watertight permeability barrier. Intercellular **junctional complexes** contain many *tight junctions,* which reduce movement of water, ions, and solutes between cells. The apical **plasma membrane** is unusually thick and, like myelin of nervous tissue, has a high lipid content. These thick membranes usually have a scalloped appearance because of many stiff, concave **plaques** mixed with interplaque regions called **hinges** (or **microplicae**). Plaques, containing asymmetric membrane particles and unique proteins called *uroplakins,* cover 70%-90% of the umbrella cell surface. Membrane-bound **fusiform vesicles** are also abundant in apical cytoplasm. Originating in the *Golgi complex,* they become closely associated with the apical cell membrane. The apical cytoplasm contains a network of **cytoskeletal filaments** made of *actin* and *cytokeratins* that are involved in cell-cell adhesion and also provide mechanical strength to cells during bladder distention and contraction. To accommodate constant changes in luminal urine content, plaques provide a dynamic mechanism that promotes cyclic folding and unfolding of apical plasma membranes of umbrella cells. Fusiform vesicles alter the surface area of the apical membrane by pinching off from the plasma membrane when the bladder empties and fusing with it when the organ fills with urine.

CLINICAL POINT

Epithelial **metaplasia** occurs when a mature differentiated epithelium changes into another adult-type epithelial tissue. Usually an adaptive response to chronic irritation or exposure to a pathogen, it is reversible. The fate of precursor cells changes, but existing differentiated cells do not. **Squamous metaplasia** is found in the urinary bladder, uterine cervix, and respiratory tract. In the cervix, normal simple columnar epithelium may be replaced by nonkeratinized stratified epithelium. Cigarette smoking may cause squamous metaplasia in airways where normal respiratory epithelium becomes a more protective nonkeratinized stratified squamous epithelium.

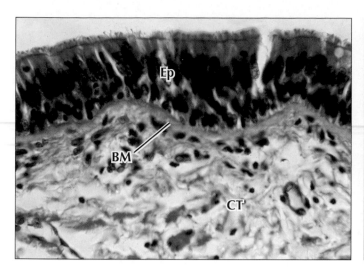

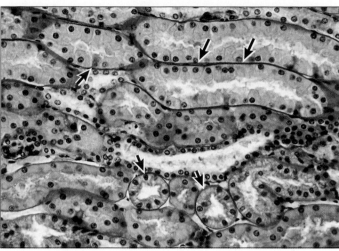

▲ **LM of the basement membrane in a trachea.** At the boundary between respiratory epithelium (**Ep**) and connective tissue (**CT**) is the highly flexible basement membrane (**BM**). Its contour follows that of the epithelium. 600×. *H&E.*

▲ **LM of basement membranes in the cortex of a kidney.** Thin linear densities (**arrows**) that are PAS positive (magenta) surround renal tubules. PAS has an affinity for carbohydrates in these membranes. 320×. *PAS.*

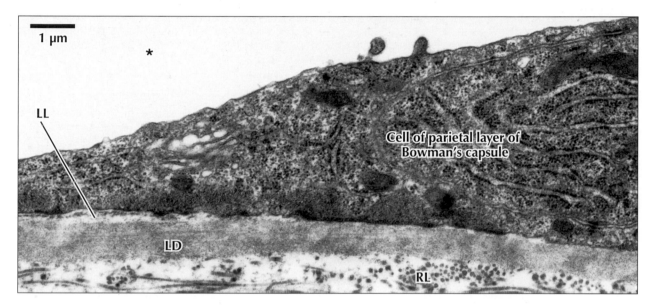

▲ **EM of Bowman's capsule in a kidney.** A prominent basement membrane under the parietal layer of Bowman's capsule has three layers: thin lamina lucida (**LL**), thicker lamina densa (**LD**), and outer reticular lamina (**RL**). The lamina densa is commonly thick at this site but much thinner in most other parts of the body. The reticular lamina contains a delicate interweaving network of reticular fibers. The lumen of the renal corpuscle (∗) is called Bowman's space. 12,000×.

2.12 STRUCTURE AND FUNCTION OF BASEMENT MEMBRANES

Most epithelia rest on an amorphous extracellular layer—the basement membrane—at the boundary between epithelium and underlying connective tissue. Where it surrounds other types of cells such as muscle cells, adipocytes, and Schwann cells, it is called an **external lamina.** It is usually poorly visualized by H&E but stains intensely with *periodic acid-Schiff* (PAS) and silver. With the advent of electron microscopy, the basement membrane has also been called the **basal lamina.** The two terms are often used interchangeably, which may cause some confusion, but the basal lamina is just lamina lucida and lamina densa. A basement membrane supports and cushions epithelia, is a semipermeable sieve or selective filtration barrier, and controls epithelial cell differen-

tiation in growth and tissue repair. These membranes vary in thickness and contain *glycosaminoglycans* and *proteoglycans* (heparan sulfate; perlecan), *glycoproteins* (laminin, entactin, and fibronectin), and *collagen.* By electron microscopy, this membrane has three layers. The **lamina lucida** is a pale zone (10-50 nm wide) of low density, just next to basal **plasma membranes** of epithelial cells. An intermediate zone, wider and more electron dense, is the **lamina densa.** Its thickness (20-300 nm) depends on location. *Type IV collagen* in both layers is a fine meshwork embedded in an amorphous matrix. The outer layer, the **reticular lamina (lamina fibroreticularis),** consists mostly of a delicate network of **reticular fibers** *(type III collagen).* Epithelium produces the lamina densa, but fibroblasts in connective tissue elaborate the reticular lamina.

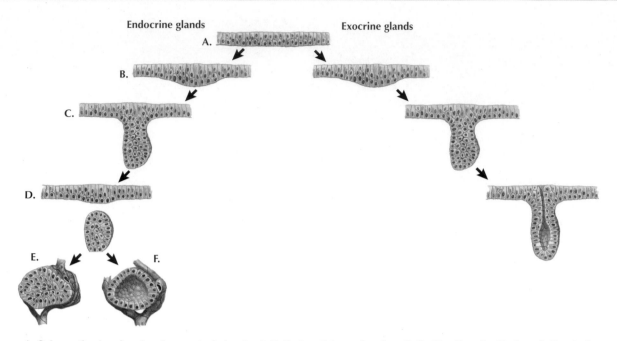

▲ **Schematic showing development of glands. A.** Epithelium lining and surface. **B.** Proliferation of epithelium. **C.** Penetration into underlying connective tissue. **D.** Formation of lumen, which opens on a free surface, and thus an exocrine gland. **E.** Some cells separate from surface epithelium to form endocrine glands. Capillaries are in close contact with cords of epithelial cells. **F.** In some glands (e.g., thyroid), lumina form in follicles but without surface connections.

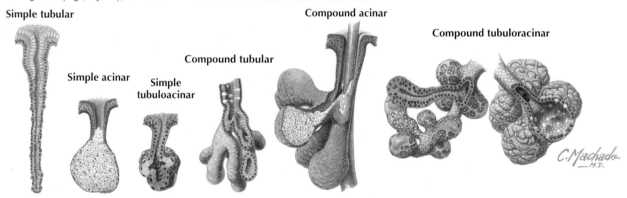

▲ **Different types of exocrine glands.** A simple unbranched duct corresponds to a simple gland; a branched duct, to a compound gland.

2.13 OVERVIEW OF EXOCRINE GLANDS

All glands, classified as either exocrine or endocrine, develop embryonically from **surface epithelium;** groups of surface cells differentiate, proliferate, and penetrate underlying connective tissue. Their main function is to synthesize and secrete extracellular products. **Endocrine glands** are ductless and release products, called *hormones,* directly into the bloodstream. These glands are arranged in cords or clumps of cells, close to a complex network of **capillaries,** for hormone transport. **Exocrine glands** connect to the surface by ducts, which take the secretions to the surface or lumen. The epithelial, or functional, component of all glands is **parenchyma;** the mainly supportive connective tissue part is **stroma.** The parenchyma of most exocrine glands consists of **secretory units,** made of groups of epithelial (secretory) cells around a lumen that are continuous with an **excretory duct system** (also lined by epithelial cells). Ducts serve as passive conduits or modify the composition of secretions produced by cells in secretory units. Exocrine glands are classified in several ways. They may be **multicellular** (most common) and have secretory units and ducts. They may be **unicellular:** one secretory cell (e.g., **goblet cell**) lies between other cells in an epithelium. Glands may be classified by shape and arrangement of secretory units as **tubular** (like a test tube), **alveolar** (Latin, for hollow sac or cavity), **acinar** (Latin, for grape or berry), or mixed (**tubuloacinar** or **tubuloalveolar**). They may be grouped by structure of the duct system: **simple** or **unbranched,** as in sweat glands, or **compound** or **branched,** as in most organs (e.g., pancreas and liver). They may be classified by the type of secretions: **mucous,** when secretions are a viscous glycoprotein called *mucus;* **serous,** when secretions are watery and enzyme-rich; or mixed **seromucous,** when one gland secretes both types. Glands may also be organized by mode of secretion; the most common, *merocrine,* involves release (or exocytosis) of secretory vesicles from cells by fusion with plasma membranes. *Apocrine secretion,* as in mammary glands, involves release of apical cytoplasm of cells. *Holocrine secretion* in sebaceous glands of skin involves disintegration and release of whole cells.

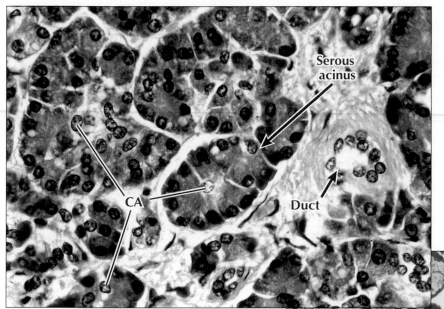

◀ **LM of part of the exocrine pancreas.** The exocrine part of the gland consists of closely packed spherical or pear-shaped serous acini. Several columnar to pyramidal acinar cells, with round basal nuclei, face a small central lumen in each **serous acinus**. Basal cytoplasm is basophilic; apical cytoplasm is more eosinophilic. Small clear centroacinar cells (**CA**) in acini centers help distinguish this purely serous gland from others, such as the parotid salivary gland. A small **duct**, in the connective tissue stroma, conveys secretions from acini to larger pancreatic ducts. 385×. *H&E.*

▶ **LM of part of a mixed salivary gland.** Several pale **mucous acini** surround two round **serous acini**. Serous cells have conspicuous, dark-stained secretory vesicles; mucous cells look vacuolated and washed out. EM in 2.15 shows the area in the square in detail. 600×. *Toluidine blue, plastic section.*

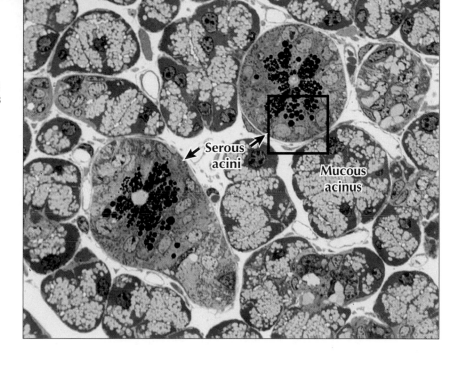

2.14 STRUCTURE AND FUNCTION OF SEROUS CELLS

Serous cells produce a watery, proteinaceous secretion, which usually contains enzymes, so their histologic appearance reflects protein synthesis and secretion. Cells occur in secretory units of pure **serous glands,** such as **parotid, lacrimal gland,** and **exocrine pancreas,** and in **mixed seromucous glands,** such as major and minor salivary glands and in walls of upper respiratory airways. These cuboidal, columnar, or pyramidal cells are seen in groups of grape-like clusters called secretory **acini.** Tightly packed cells with dark-stained cytoplasm surround a small lumen in the acinus. Serous cells are polarized and have basal, apical, and lateral domains and a basal spherical nucleus. They rest on an inconspicuous basement membrane, which encloses the whole acinus.

In some glands, small stellate cells share the basement membrane with serous cells. Not seen well in routine H&E sections but better resolved by electron microscopy, these myoepithelial cells lie in contact with basal aspects of serous cells. They serve a contractile role by promoting release of secretory product into lumina of **excretory ducts. Secretory granules** dominate the apical cytoplasm of serous cells, so it is relatively eosinophilic. The basal half of the cells contains fine granular cytoplasm that is intensely basophilic because of abundant rough endoplasmic reticulum. Vertically oriented mitochondria, which are best seen by electron microscopy, are often associated with basal striations in the cells. Lateral boundaries of cells are not well shown by light microscopy. Excretory ducts that come from acini are initially lined by *simple cuboidal epithelium.*

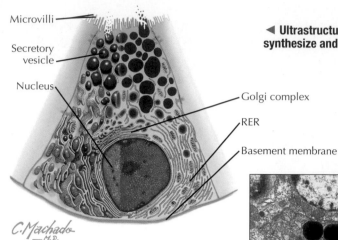

Microvilli

Secretory vesicle

Nucleus

Golgi complex

RER

Basement membrane

C. Machado
_M.D._

◀ **Ultrastructural features of a typical epithelial cell —a serous cell—specialized to synthesize and secrete protein for export.**

▶ **EM of part of a serous acinus in a parotid gland.** A cluster of serous cells with basal nuclei is oriented around the acinus lumen (∗). Lateral borders of these pyramidal cells closely interdigitate. Mitochondria (**Mi**) and cisternae of rough endoplasmic reticulum (**RER**) are in basal cytoplasm. Conspicuous electron-dense secretory vesicles (**SV**), of varied size and shape, dominate apical cytoplasm. They contain precursors of secretory product that is released into the lumen by exocytosis. At the acinus base, the thin process of a myoepithelial cell (**ME**) shares the thin basement membrane with the serous cells. 4600×.

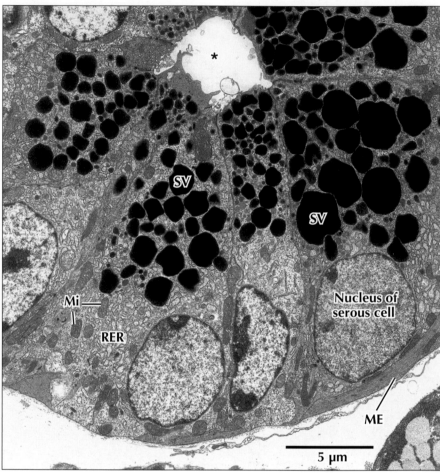

2.15 ULTRASTRUCTURE AND FUNCTION OF SEROUS CELLS

Ultrastructural features of serous cells are consistent with synthesis, storage, and release of secretory product into a lumen. All serous cells, at any site, are polarized **secretory cells** with the same basic plan, plus minor variations. **Organelle** content and disposition are typical of those in cells producing protein for export. The basal half of a cell holds one **euchromatic nucleus** with one or two **nucleoli;** the basal cytoplasm contains many *free ribosomes, polyribosomes* attached to messenger RNA (mRNA) strands, and parallel flattened **cisternae** of **rough endoplasmic reticulum** (RER). Amino acids taken up by cells at the base are first incorporated into ribosomes attached to RER membranes. Newly synthesized polypeptides are then released into the RER lumen and

delivered by transfer vesicles to the formative (cis-) face of the *Golgi complex.* Interspersed among RER cisternae are many **mitochondria,** which produce energy, as ATP, for active protein synthesis. Contents of transfer vesicles are released into Golgi saccules for macromolecular processing and addition of carbohydrate moieties to secretory product. Condensing vesicles from the maturing (trans-) face of the Golgi concentrate secretory product and become electron-dense **secretory vesicles** (also called **zymogen granules** in the pancreas). These are temporarily stored in the apical cytoplasm before release. Contents of mature secretory vesicles are discharged from apical parts of cells by *exocytosis:* a secretory vesicle membrane fuses with a cell's plasma membrane, which ruptures, so vesicle contents are discharged into the acinus lumen.

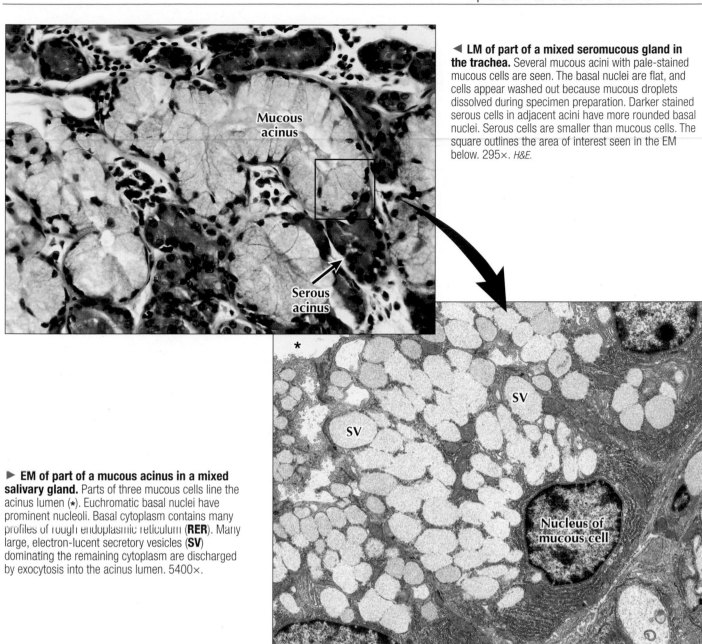

◀ **LM of part of a mixed seromucous gland in the trachea.** Several mucous acini with pale-stained mucous cells are seen. The basal nuclei are flat, and cells appear washed out because mucous droplets dissolved during specimen preparation. Darker stained serous cells in adjacent acini have more rounded basal nuclei. Serous cells are smaller than mucous cells. The square outlines the area of interest seen in the EM below. 295×. *H&E.*

▶ **EM of part of a mucous acinus in a mixed salivary gland.** Parts of three mucous cells line the acinus lumen (*). Euchromatic basal nuclei have prominent nucleoli. Basal cytoplasm contains many profiles of rough endoplasmic reticulum (**RER**). Many large, electron-lucent secretory vesicles (**SV**) dominating the remaining cytoplasm are discharged by exocytosis into the acinus lumen. 5400×.

2.16 STRUCTURE AND FUNCTION OF MUCOUS CELLS

Mucus, a secretion consisting in part of **mucin,** which contains highly viscous glycoproteins, protects and lubricates surfaces. Widely distributed mucus-producing cells are found either singly, as **goblet cells** in epithelia of the digestive, respiratory, and reproductive tracts, or grouped, as **tubules** or **acini.** Most notably, they occur in major and minor **salivary glands** of the oral cavity that are pure mucous or mixed seromucous. Mucous cells also line the stomach lumen and form small glands in the esophagus and duodenum. Several types of mucin exist, of different chemical compositions, but mucin-producing cells share similar histologic and ultrastructural features. Most histologic methods dissolve **mucous droplets** that dominate the cytoplasm, so in routine H&E sections the cytoplasm usually looks pale and vacuolated. The one **nucleus** in the basal part of a cell is usually flattened as the cell fills with mucous droplets. Lateral borders between cells in acini are usually more visible than they are in serous acini. Synthesis, temporary storage, and release of mucin involve mechanisms similar to those of serous cells. Mucous cells use ribosomes and **RER** for protein synthesis, and a supranuclear Golgi complex for addition of carbohydrates and then packaging of secretory product into large membrane-bound **secretory vesicles** or mucous droplets. The droplets are so densely packed that they often hide other cell organelles. Vesicles often coalesce before fusing with apical plasma membranes of the cells. Release of secretory product is by *merocrine secretion* (or *exocytosis*) to the free surface.

▼ **Position and structure of mammary gland.**

Anterolateral dissection

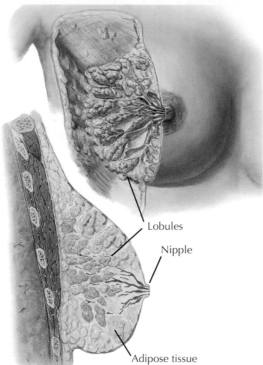

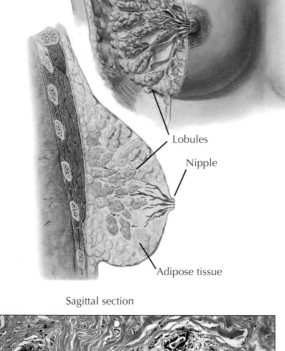

Lobules

Nipple

Adipose tissue

Sagittal section

▼ **Sagittal view of a mammary gland. Three lobes open separately by ducts into the nipple.** Each lobe contains many smaller lobules, which are secretory units of this compound tubuloalveolar gland.

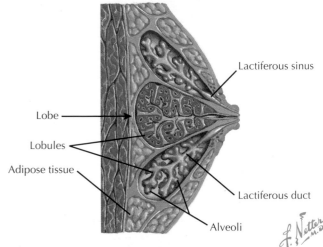

Lactiferous sinus

Lobe

Lobules

Adipose tissue

Lactiferous duct

Alveoli

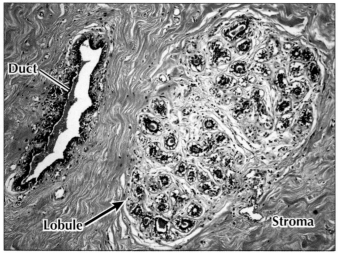

Duct

Lobule

Stroma

▲ **LM of a resting mammary gland.** Dense, prominent stroma surrounds a large duct next to an oval lobule. Small tubules of the terminal branching duct system in the lobule lie in loose connective tissue. 75×. *H&E.*

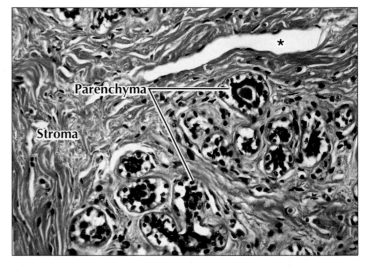

Parenchyma

Stroma

▲ **LM of a resting mammary gland at higher magnification.** Small tubules that make up the parenchyma are the terminal branching duct system. They are supported by connective tissue stroma, in which lies a small lymphatic channel (*). 300×. *H&E.*

2.17   STRUCTURE AND HISTOLOGY OF RESTING MAMMARY GLANDS

Each mammary gland comprises 12-20 irregular **lobes,** which radiate from the **nipple** and drain into it by separate **lactiferous ducts.** Each lobe is a separate **compound** (highly branched) **tubuloalveolar gland** whose size, shape, and histologic structure change with age and functional status of the reproductive system. In reproductive-age women who are not pregnant or lactating, the parenchyma (or epithelial component) of each lobe consists mostly of a branching network of ducts, which look like small tubules lined by epithelial cells. Only a few rudimentary **alveoli** may be present. The **lactiferous sinus,** a terminal expansion of each duct near the nipple, acts as a reservoir for milk. Smallest ducts are lined by *simple cuboidal epithelium,* which becomes *stratified cuboidal* as ducts get larger and closer to the sinus. *Stratified squamous epithelium* lines the duct as it approaches the nipple. **Adipose** and **dense fibrous connective tissues** of superficial fascia surround the lobes.

▼ **Functional changes and lactation.**

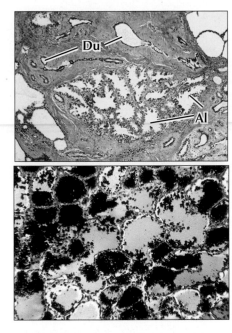

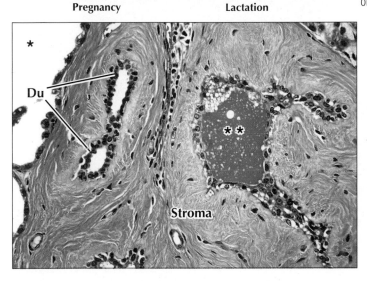

Pregnancy   Lactation

▲ **LMs of a lactating mammary gland. Top.** Ducts (**Du**) and irregular, closely packed secretory alveoli (**Al**) are prominent. 60×. *H&E.* **Bottom.** In a section of gland treated to detect lipid in milk, alveolar contents are black. 80×. *Osmium.*

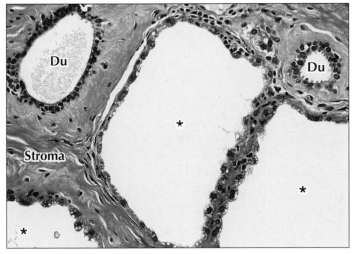

▲ **LMs of a lactating mammary gland.** Simple cuboidal epithelium lines well-developed alveoli and the ducts (**Du**). Myoepithelial cells, although present, are not easily seen in routine sections. An alveolus is filled with milk secretion (**Left**) (**✶✶**); others appear empty (✶) (**Right**). A high content of collagen makes the connective tissue stroma eosinophilic. 240×. *H&E.*

2.18 HISTOLOGY AND FUNCTION OF LACTATING (ACTIVE) MAMMARY GLANDS

During **pregnancy,** mammary glands complete development and differentiation to prepare for **lactation. Alveoli** get larger, and **alveolar epithelial cells** undergo *hypertrophy* and *hyperplasia.* In addition, the number and size of **ducts** increase, and the amount of connective and adipose tissue decreases. The secretory unit of each *lobe*—the *lobule*—consists of several clusters of alveoli around a small duct. Several lobules constitute a lobe. **Simple cuboidal epithelial cells** surrounded by a delicate basement membrane line alveoli. Basally located **myoepithelial cells** share a basement membrane with the epithelium and embrace alveoli in a basket-like pattern. At the end of pregnancy, alveoli are large, irregular in shape, and lined by cuboidal to low columnar epithelium. Lobules vary greatly in functional activity. Alveolar cells in an actively secreting lobule contain large fat droplets, and lumina of many alveoli may contain heterogeneous secretions, plus desquamated cells and cell debris. *Prolactin,* which is released from the anterior pituitary, stimulates cells to secrete **milk** components into alveoli lumina. During lactation, *oxytocin* from the posterior pituitary stimulates myoepithelial cells to contract to help expel secretions into ducts. Late in pregnancy, plasma cells in stroma around alveoli increase in number and add secretory IgA to mammary gland secretions to confer passive immunity to an infant.

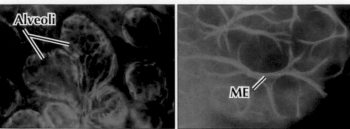

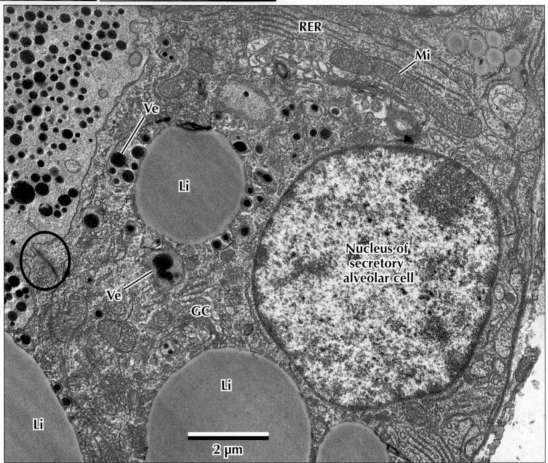

◄ **LMs of myoepithelial cells in lactating alveoli of a mouse mammary gland.** Outlines of stellate myoepithelial cells (**ME**) are visualized via fluorescently labeled actin. Cells form a basket-like network around each alveolus. **Left:** 110×; **Right:** 480×. NBD-phallacidin fluorescence. *(Courtesy of Drs. A. W. Vogl and J. T. Emerman)*

▲ **EM of part of a secretory alveolus in a lactating mouse mammary gland.** Parts of two secretory cells line the alveolar lumen (**above, left**), which contains many micelles and flocculent material. Lateral cell borders have intercellular junctions (**circle**); basal nuclei are euchromatic. The cytoplasm holds rough endoplasmic reticulum (**RER**), Golgi complex (**GC**), mitochondria (**Mi**), dark globular micelles in large vesicles (**Ve**), and lipid droplets (**Li**). 10,000×.

2.19 ULTRASTRUCTURE AND FUNCTION OF MAMMARY GLAND ALVEOLI

Milk consists of water (87%), lipids (4%), lactose (7%), and proteins (2%), which are mainly *casein, lactalbumin,* and *secretory IgA.* **Secretory alveolar cells** synthesize and secrete most components. Cell ultrastructure is consistent with active secretion of lipid, carbohydrate, and protein. Polarized cells have a spherical **nucleus** with a prominent **nucleolus.** Cytoplasm has many **free ribosomes** and **RER** at the base, a large supranuclear **Golgi complex,** and scattered **mitochondria.** In lactating glands, membrane-bound **secretory vesicles** packed with dense globular **micelles,** which contain protein, are moved from the Golgi complex to apical cell surfaces. Contents are released by *exocytosis* (or *merocrine secretion*) into alveolar lumina by fusion of vesicles with apical cell membranes, which contain short, irregular micro-villi. The disaccharide lactose is synthesized in the Golgi and released in the same vesicles that contain milk proteins. Droplets of lipid, mostly triglycerides, are taken to the apical part of cells, bulge into alveolar lumina, and are released from cells by *apocrine secretion.* They pinch off from cell surfaces along with a thin, investing rim of cytoplasm. Lateral cell borders interdigitate with those of adjacent cells and contain apical **junctional complexes.** The hormone *prolactin* from the anterior pituitary stimulates milk production. Elongated or stellate **myoepithelial cells** derive, like alveolar cells, from surface ectoderm. They are seen between the base of epithelial cells and the basement membrane and are dominated by bundles of actin-containing **cytoplasmic filaments,** which are usually parallel to the cells' long axis. *Oxytocin* from the posterior pituitary stimulates these cells to contract.

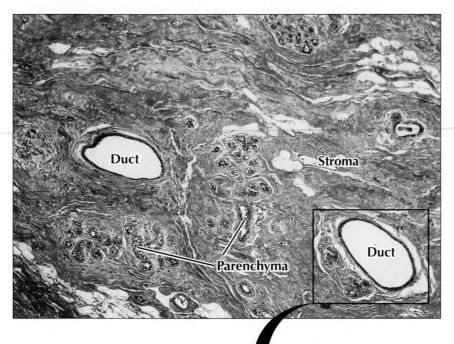

◄ **LM of an atrophic mammary gland from a postmenopausal woman at low magnification.** Regressive changes include involution of parenchyma with a few remaining secretory alveoli. Scattered ducts are in dense connective tissue stroma. The rectangle outlines the duct seen in lower left LM. 85×. *H&E.*

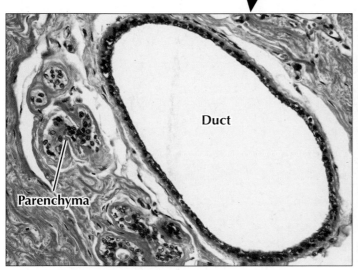

▲ **LM of an atrophic mammary gland at higher magnification.** The duct system is often abnormally enlarged. A few tubuloalveolar elements of parenchyma remain scattered in the stroma. 270×. *H&E.*

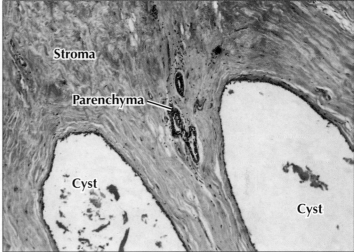

▲ **LM of an atrophic mammary gland from an elderly postmenopausal woman.** A few isolated tubular elements of parenchyma and parts of two large cysts are in thickened stroma. 85×. *H&E.*

2.20 HISTOLOGY OF ATROPHIC MAMMARY GLANDS

After *pregnancy* and *breast-feeding,* mammary glands atrophy and lobules degenerate. **Alveoli** shrink until they are no longer distinguishable, but some persist. Only larger **ducts,** embedded in a thicker **dense irregular connective tissue** accompanied by **adipose tissue,** remain. After *menopause,* mammary glands slowly undergo involution. Any remaining alveoli atrophy and are resorbed. Epithelial cells undergo *apoptosis* and are phagocytosed by macrophages in the stroma. Ducts also regress, but a few may remain; some ducts may proliferate and transform into **cysts.** Similarly, connective tissue atrophies, with the amount of adipose tissue reduced. Irregular secretory changes may also occur.

CLINICAL POINT

Parenchyma of mammary glands, uterine endometrium, and cervical epithelium respond to female sex hormones during adolescence, menstruation, pregnancy, and menopause. Knowledge of their histology is thus essential for interpretation of pathologic changes. **Breast cancer—mammary carcinoma**—is the most common malignancy in women and usually occurs after menopause. Most *invasive primary breast cancers* are **adenocarcinomas** that arise from epithelium of lactiferous ducts and may penetrate the basement membrane and invade the stroma. Immunocytochemistry can reveal the presence of nuclear hormone receptors for estrogen and progesterone, which suggests a good prognosis, and predict success of treatment with targeted hormonal agents such as *tamoxifen.*

3

CONNECTIVE TISSUE

▼ **Loose connective tissue.**

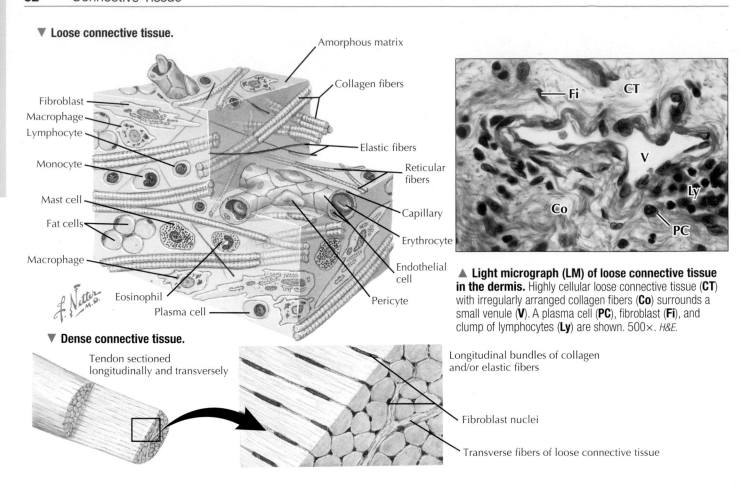

▲ **Light micrograph (LM) of loose connective tissue in the dermis.** Highly cellular loose connective tissue (**CT**) with irregularly arranged collagen fibers (**Co**) surrounds a small venule (**V**). A plasma cell (**PC**), fibroblast (**Fi**), and clump of lymphocytes (**Ly**) are shown. 500×. *H&E.*

▼ **Dense connective tissue.**

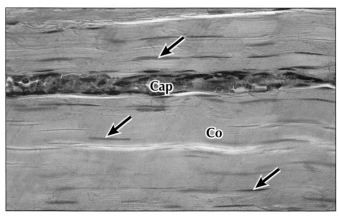

◄ **LM of a tendon in longitudinal section.** Fascicles of regularly arranged collagen (**Co**) are mixed with inactive fibroblasts (**arrows**). Collagen eosinophilia is due to a high protein content. A capillary (**Cap**) crossing the field of view supplies oxygen and nutrients to fibroblasts and surrounding tissue. 100×. *H&E..*

3.1   OVERVIEW

Adult connective tissue comprises a diverse family of tissues whose major function is to *provide form* and *support* to the body and organs and to connect and anchor parts. It is also a medium for *exchange* of nutrients, oxygen, and waste products between other tissues; it aids in *defense* and *protection;* and in certain sites, as in adipose tissue, it stores fat for cushioning and *thermoregulation.* Connective tissue, one of the four basic body tissues, is the most versatile, the types including **connective tissue proper** and the specialized *blood, cartilage,* and *bone.* Almost all connective tissue, regardless of form, arises embryonically from mesoderm; some connective tissue of the head originates from neural crest ecto-

derm. Like all body tissues, connective or supportive tissues consist of cells, both fixed and wandering, and an **extracellular matrix (ECM)** composed of fibers embedded in an **amorphous ground substance.** Cells of connective tissue include **fibroblasts, mast cells, macrophages, plasma cells, adipocytes (fat cells),** and **pericytes.** The many functions of connective tissue depend largely on the properties of the ECM, which predominates. Connective tissue proper includes a range of recognizable histologic types and can be classified as **loose (areolar)** or **dense,** mostly on the basis of the proportion and density of fibrous components of the ECM. Connective tissue may have a regular arrangement, as in a **tendon,** or an irregular arrangement, as in the **dermis.**

Classification of Connective Tissue Proper	
Type	*Principal locations*
Adult connective tissue	
Loose (areolar)	Most tissues and organs; mucous membranes; directly under epithelia
Dense	
• Irregular	Dermis of skin; capsules of organs; submucosa of hollow viscera
• Regular	Tendons; ligaments; aponeuroses; cornea of eye
Specialized forms of connective tissue	
Adipose (fat)	Subcutaneous tissue; omentum; mesenteries; breast; bone marrow
Elastic	Tunica media of large arteries; elastic ligaments (nuchae and flava); lungs
Reticular	Stroma of lymphoid organs, bone marrow, liver
Embryonic connective tissue	
Mesenchyme	Chiefly in embryo and fetus; perivascular sites in adult
Mucous	Umbilical cord (Wharton's jelly)

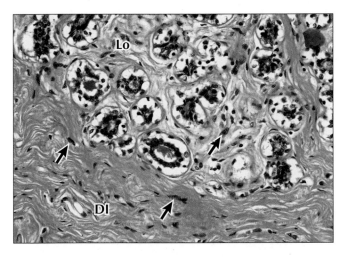

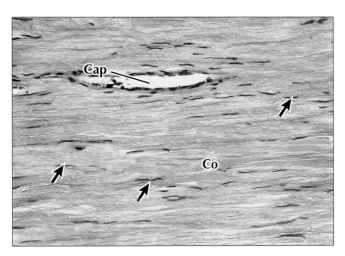

▲ **LM of part of the inactive mammary gland contrasting key features of dense irregular and loose connective tissue.** Dense irregular (**DI**) connective tissue shows an interwoven network of tightly packed collagen. Loose (**Lo**) connective tissue has a loose, delicate arrangement of collagen fibers. Fibroblasts (**arrows**) are the primary cell type of connective tissue. 220×. *H&E.*

▲ **LM of part of a ligament in longitudinal section.** The salient features of dense regular connective tissue are seen. Close, tightly packed bundles of collagen fibers (**Co**) are oriented in the same direction. Nuclei of flattened fibroblasts (**arrows**) are aligned in rows between the fibers. A capillary (**Cap**) courses between the collagen bundles. 300×. *H&E.*

3.2   CLASSIFICATION OF CONNECTIVE TISSUE PROPER

The composition of connective tissues varies greatly in different parts of the body. On the basis of appearance and related to function, connective tissue proper can be placed into different categories in the **adult** and **embryo**. The main criteria are the amount and type of extracellular matrix, arrangement and kinds of **fibers,** and abundance and types of **cells.** Many classification schemes exist, but they represent a continuum of tissue types and, being arbitrary, should not be interpreted too rigidly. The two main types of adult connective tissue proper are **loose (areolar)** and **dense.** Loose connective tissue, the most widespread, has the greatest variety of cells and fibers. It is highly cellular with few fibers and has great flexibility. The term areolar refers to small

fluid-filled spaces in this tissue. Much of the body's tissue fluid is found within loose connective tissue, and excessive accumulation of this fluid causes swelling, or edema. Dense connective tissue has a greater proportion of fibers, fewer cells, and less ground substance. Its division into two subtypes depends on the orientation of its fibers. **Dense irregular connective tissue** has randomly oriented, interwoven fibers that can respond to stress in many directions. In **dense regular connective tissue,** fibers are in parallel and can withstand prolonged stress from one direction. Three specialized types of connective tissue in the adult are **adipose, reticular,** and **elastic.** The **embryo** and **fetus** have two types of connective tissue: **mesenchymal connective tissue** occupies spaces between developing organs, and **mucous connective tissue** is in the **umbilical cord.**

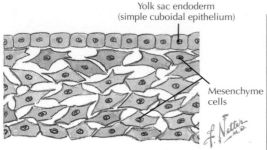

▲ **Schematic of the wall of the embryonic yolk sac.** Connective tissues derive from loose, undifferentiated embryonic connective tissue known as mesenchyme.

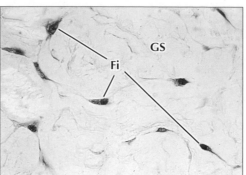

◀ **LM of the umbilical cord.** Highly viscous, gelatinous ground substance (**GS**) called Wharton's jelly surrounds a network of stellate fibroblasts (**Fi**) that resemble mesenchymal cells. Cells have branching cytoplasmic processes that emanate from nucleated cell bodies. 325×. *H&E.*

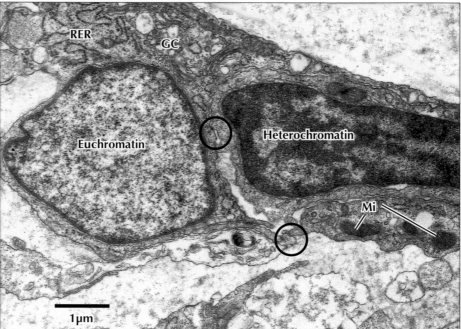

▲ **Electron micrograph (EM) of two apposed mesenchymal cells in the tendon of a fetus.** The nucleus of one cell is mainly euchromatic; that of the adjacent cell has relatively more heterochromatin, which reflects a different functional state. Profiles of rough endoplasmic reticulum (**RER**) and a prominent Golgi complex (**GC**) occupy the cytoplasm of one cell; mitochondria (**Mi**), in the other. Points of membrane contact between cells (**circles**), more common in developing tissue, are uncommon in adult connective tissue. 14,300×.

3.3 STRUCTURE AND FUNCTION OF MESENCHYMAL CELLS

Mesenchymal cells are primitive stem cells derived mostly from mesoderm or, in some sites, neural crest ectoderm. During embryonic development, they differentiate into various cell types for specific functions throughout the body; cells of connective tissue, bone, cartilage, blood, endothelium, and muscle derive from these undifferentiated cells. Also, some mesenchymal cells that retain plasticity persist in the adult and differentiate into diverse cell types when needed. Mesenchymal cells are often used as a source of *pluripotential stem cells* for *tissue repair* and *transplantation* because they can develop into other cell types. Tissue remodeling in response to injury depends on mesenchymal cells that differentiate into fibroblasts and myofibroblasts, but it is unknown whether mesenchymal cells that participate in remodeling originate locally or from circulating precursor cells. Mesenchymal cells are normally inconspicuous in connective tissue. They resemble active **fibroblasts** but are usually smaller. They produce cytokines and growth factors that may significantly influence the differentiation and aging of other cells in the body such as those of epithelium and muscle. Unlike epithelial cells, mesenchymal cells can invade and migrate through the extracellular matrix to create important cell transpositions. They are common in walls of capillaries outside the endothelium where they are known as *pericytes*.

CLINICAL POINT

Tumors of connective tissue or its mesenchymal precursors are known as **sarcomas.** The most common adult soft tissue sarcoma is **malignant fibrous histiocytoma.** The cellular origin is uncertain, but immunocytochemical marker evidence indicates that it derives from perivascular mesenchymal cells. A gene associated with this tumor, *MASL1,* has been identified. Electron microscopy reveals a mixture of cells resembling fibroblasts, myofibroblasts, macrophages, and primitive mesenchymal cells. Tumors typically arise in deep fascia, soft tissues of the neck or extremities, and skeletal muscle. Distant metastasis may spread to lung, bone, or liver. Treatment is usually by *radical resection.*

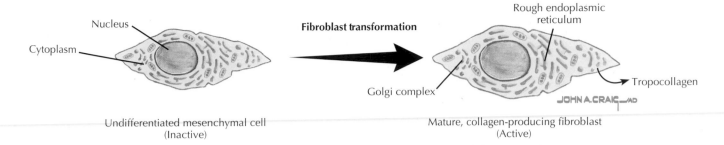

Nucleus

Cytoplasm

Fibroblast transformation

Rough endoplasmic reticulum

Golgi complex

Tropocollagen

JOHN A.CRAIG—AD

Undifferentiated mesenchymal cell
(Inactive)

Mature, collagen-producing fibroblast
(Active)

▲ **Undifferentiated mesenchymal cells.** can transform into active fibroblasts by developing organelles essential for collagen synthesis and secretion. This occurs during early development and is a hallmark of wound healing, when cell transformation and production of collagen accompany migration and proliferation of cells to wound sites.

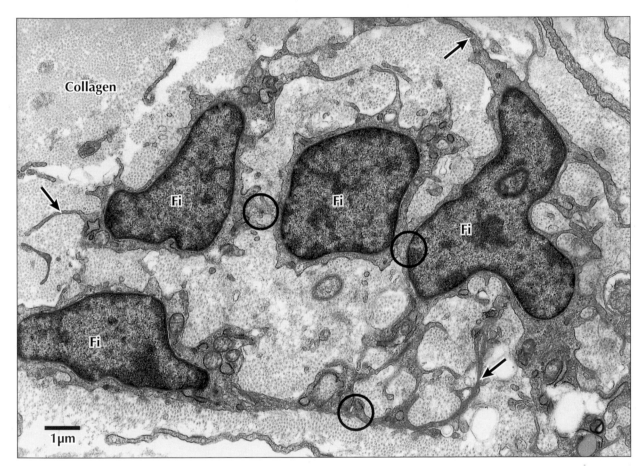

Collagen

▲ **EM of a growing tendon during the adolescent growth spurt.** Nucleated regions of several active fibroblasts (**Fi**) are evident. Euchromatin predominates in the nuclei. The cytoplasm contains many closely packed organelles. Many branching processes (**arrows**) emanate from the cell bodies. Collagen fibrils occupy the intervening ECM and are sectioned transversely. Cell-to-cell contacts between fibroblasts are circled. 9000×.

3.4 STRUCTURE AND FUNCTION OF FIBROBLASTS

Fibroblasts, the main cell type of connective tissue, are the most common cell of **loose (areolar) connective tissue** and virtually the only cell of **dense regular connective tissue** such as **tendon.** They function in synthesis and secretion of ground substance and, as their name implies, of connective tissue fibers, including **collagen** and elastic or reticular fibers, in the **ECM.** In mature connective tissue, these cells are relatively inactive and immobile and are often called *fibrocytes.* After injury and during *wound repair,* they rapidly proliferate and become active fibroblasts to synthesize new

ECM fibers and ground substance. Fibroblasts are ovoid or stellate cells with long, tapering **processes** that branch. They have one elliptical **nucleus,** usually euchromatic, with one or more distinct nucleoli. Light microscopy shows that staining attributes of their **cytoplasm** differ according to functional state. Active or immature cells have a weakly *basophilic,* relatively conspicuous cytoplasm. Mature cells have a weakly *acidophilic,* barely visible cytoplasm with a relatively homogeneous appearance, so that nuclei are seen mainly in histologic sections. Routine preparations typically cannot resolve their cell borders, which are better shown by electron microscopy.

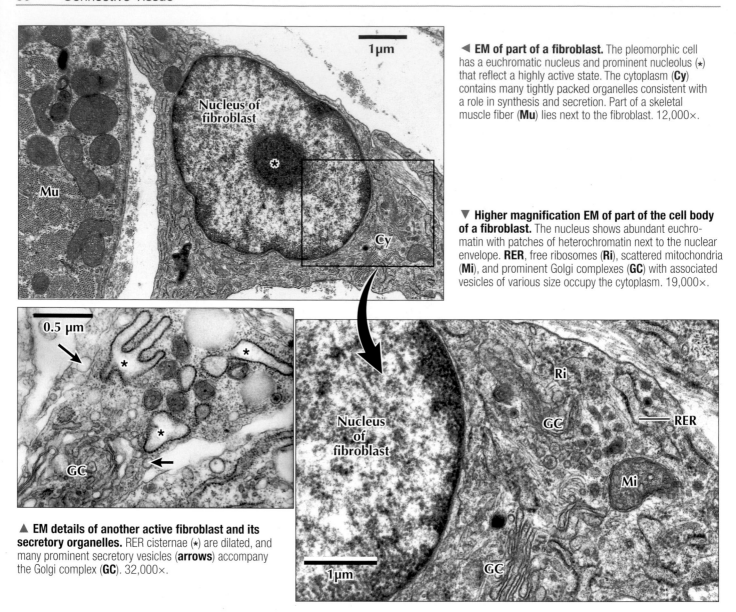

◀ **EM of part of a fibroblast.** The pleomorphic cell has a euchromatic nucleus and prominent nucleolus (⁎) that reflect a highly active state. The cytoplasm (**Cy**) contains many tightly packed organelles consistent with a role in synthesis and secretion. Part of a skeletal muscle fiber (**Mu**) lies next to the fibroblast. 12,000×.

▼ **Higher magnification EM of part of the cell body of a fibroblast.** The nucleus shows abundant euchromatin with patches of heterochromatin next to the nuclear envelope. **RER**, free ribosomes (**Ri**), scattered mitochondria (**Mi**), and prominent Golgi complexes (**GC**) with associated vesicles of various size occupy the cytoplasm. 19,000×.

▲ **EM details of another active fibroblast and its secretory organelles.** RER cisternae (⁎) are dilated, and many prominent secretory vesicles (**arrows**) accompany the Golgi complex (**GC**). 32,000×.

3.5 ULTRASTRUCTURE AND FUNCTION OF FIBROBLASTS

Electron microscopic features of fibroblasts, which synthesize connective tissue fibers including collagen, are typical of most protein-synthesizing cells. Cell shape varies in different areas, but cells are usually elongated with many tapering cytoplasmic processes. The one elongated **nucleus** contains **euchromatin,** with clumps of **heterochromatin** next to the **nuclear envelope.** Active cells have one or two **nucleoli** and a **cytoplasm** rich in **secretory organelles.** A prominent **Golgi complex** and a pair of centrioles sit near the nucleus. Many small **vacuoles** and **vesicles** associated with the Golgi complex may contain flocculent material that consists of precursors of collagen and other extracellular substances produced by the cell. Oval to rod-shaped **mitochondria** are scattered in the cytoplasm. Cytoplasmic filaments, microtubules, and small vesicles associated with the cell surface are abundant. An extensive **rough endoplasmic reticulum** (RER) and **free ribosomes** dominate in actively secreting cells. The RER consists of rounded to flat **cisternae** studded with ribosomes. An important

feature of connective tissue is an ability to provide repair after injury. *Scars* originate mainly from fibroblasts and their extracellular products. These cells have a capacity for *regeneration* throughout life.

CLINICAL POINT

Complex collagen synthesis can be impaired by **dietary deficiency** of **vitamin C** (ascorbic acid), producing scurvy, and by errors in critical genes or enzymes, leading to the rare **Ehlers-Danlos syndrome** (EDS). Lack of the vitamin causes nonhydroxylated, unstable collagen fibrils to fail to form a triple helix and have low tensile strength. Dentine (teeth), osteoid (bone), connective tissues, and tunica adventitia (blood vessel walls) are affected, but the typical *hemorrhage* and *poor wound healing* can occur anywhere. All of more than 10 forms of EDS involve a genetic defect in synthesis or assembly of collagen fibrils, the results being hyperelastic skin and hypermovable joints. Vascular EDS, the most severe, is caused by a *COL3A1* gene mutation that leads to abnormal type III collagen. Serious effects include *aortic rupture, colon perforation,* and *retinal detachment.*

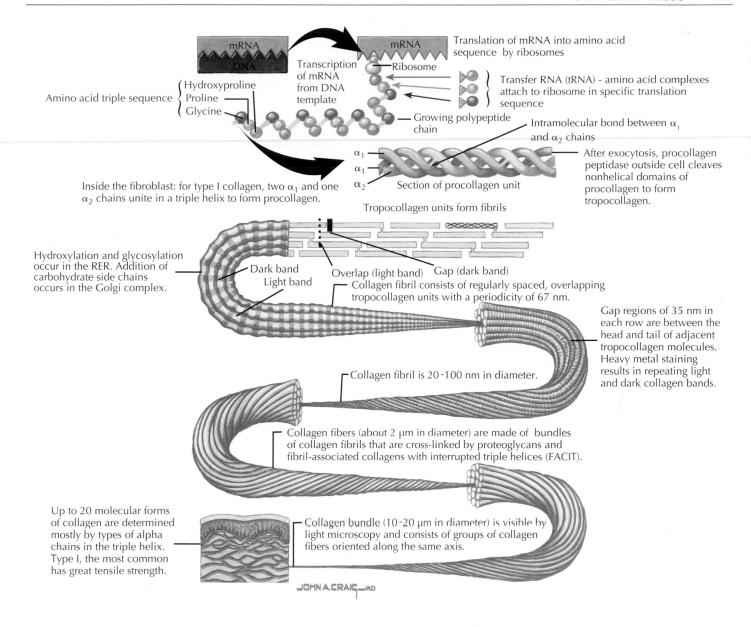

Translation of mRNA into amino acid sequence by ribosomes

Transcription of mRNA from DNA template

Transfer RNA (tRNA) - amino acid complexes attach to ribosome in specific translation sequence

Amino acid triple sequence { Hydroxyproline / Proline / Glycine

Growing polypeptide chain

Intramolecular bond between α_1 and α_2 chains

After exocytosis, procollagen peptidase outside cell cleaves nonhelical domains of procollagen to form tropocollagen.

Inside the fibroblast: for type I collagen, two α_1 and one α_2 chains unite in a triple helix to form procollagen.

α_1
α_1
α_2

Section of procollagen unit

Tropocollagen units form fibrils

Hydroxylation and glycosylation occur in the RER. Addition of carbohydrate side chains occurs in the Golgi complex.

Dark band
Light band

Overlap (light band)   Gap (dark band)
Collagen fibril consists of regularly spaced, overlapping tropocollagen units with a periodicity of 67 nm.

Gap regions of 35 nm in each row are between the head and tail of adjacent tropocollagen molecules. Heavy metal staining results in repeating light and dark collagen bands.

Collagen fibril is 20-100 nm in diameter.

Collagen fibers (about 2 μm in diameter) are made of bundles of collagen fibrils that are cross-linked by proteoglycans and fibril-associated collagens with interrupted triple helices (FACIT).

Up to 20 molecular forms of collagen are determined mostly by types of alpha chains in the triple helix. Type I, the most common has great tensile strength.

Collagen bundle (10-20 μm in diameter) is visible by light microscopy and consists of groups of collagen fibers oriented along the same axis.

JOHN A. CRAIG—AD

3.6 SYNTHESIS OF COLLAGEN

Collagen formation involves both intracellular and extracellular events known in protein synthesis. **Messenger RNA** (mRNA) is synthesized from a template of **DNA** in the **fibroblast** nucleus. mRNA molecules enter the cytoplasm and attach to **ribosomes** of the RER. Ribosomes translate the nucleotide sequence of the mRNA into an **amino acid sequence.** A polypeptide chain of a specific sequence of several amino acids is assembled is detached from the ribosome and enters the RER cisternae. **Hydroxylation** of **proline** and **lysine** residues in the RER requires ascorbic acid (vitamin C) as a cofactor. Three **alpha chains** form a **triple helix** to form **procollagen,** a precursor to collagen. Packaging of procollagen occurs in the **Golgi complex,** and secretory vesicles release procollagen by **exocytosis** at the cell surface. Outside the cell, **enzymatic cleavage** by procollagen peptidase produces **tropocollagen** molecules that aggregate to form cross-striated **collagen fibrils.** The fibrils then assemble into bundles to form **collagen fibers.**

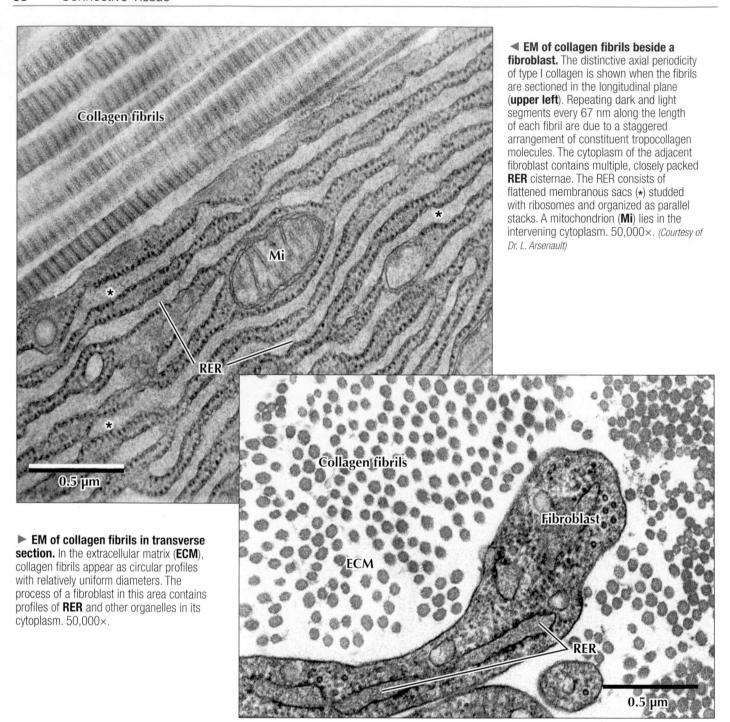

◀ **EM of collagen fibrils beside a fibroblast.** The distinctive axial periodicity of type I collagen is shown when the fibrils are sectioned in the longitudinal plane (**upper left**). Repeating dark and light segments every 67 nm along the length of each fibril are due to a staggered arrangement of constituent tropocollagen molecules. The cytoplasm of the adjacent fibroblast contains multiple, closely packed **RER** cisternae. The RER consists of flattened membranous sacs (⋆) studded with ribosomes and organized as parallel stacks. A mitochondrion (**Mi**) lies in the intervening cytoplasm. 50,000×. *(Courtesy of Dr. L. Arsenault)*

▶ **EM of collagen fibrils in transverse section.** In the extracellular matrix (**ECM**), collagen fibrils appear as circular profiles with relatively uniform diameters. The process of a fibroblast in this area contains profiles of **RER** and other organelles in its cytoplasm. 50,000×.

3.7   TYPES OF COLLAGEN AND ITS ULTRASTRUCTURE

At 30%-35% of the body's dry weight, collagen is the most abundant, ubiquitous structural protein. Its distribution is widespread: it occurs in all of the ordinary and specialized connective tissues. At least 20 genetically distinct types of collagen exist in this family of extracellular proteins that differ mainly in amino acid composition. **Type I collagen,** the most common, is found in the dermis, tendons, ligaments, fascia, bone, fibrocartilage, dentin, capsules of organs, and sclera. **Type II collagen** has a slightly different molecular composition and occurs in hyaline cartilage and the vitreous body of the eye. **Type III collagen** (or reticular fibers) is found in

several tissues. **Type IV collagen** is associated with basal laminae. Some collagens (types I, II, III, V, and IX) form **fibrils,** which may be several micrometers long; types IV, VIII, and X form sheets or meshworks. Other collagens (types VI, VII, IX, XII, XIV, and XVIII) have linking or anchoring roles, and two (types XIII and XVII) are transmembrane proteins. Diameters of individual collagen fibrils vary among tissues and with increasing age and range from 20 to 100 nm. Collagen fibrils in the stroma of the cornea are uniform in diameter and extremely thin, whereas those in tendon may be much thicker and more variable in diameter. Collagen has great *tensile strength,* and tissues that are subject to high tensile stress usually have very thick collagen fibrils.

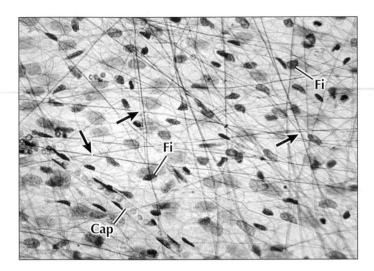

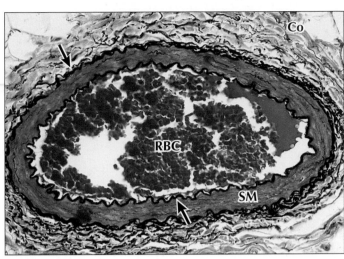

▲ **LM of the mesentery.** Elastic fibers (**arrows**) stain selectively as dark, thin branching fibers in loose connective tissue. Fibroblast nuclei (**Fi**) and a capillary (**Cap**) with erythrocytes are also seen. 475×. *Resorcin-fuchsin, spread preparation.*

▲ **LM of an arteriole in transverse section.** Elastic fibers (**arrows**) selectively stain dark purple. Collagen fibers (**Co**) are yellow to orange; smooth muscle (**SM**) and erythrocytes (**RBC**) in the lumen are red. 225×. *Modified van Gieson.*

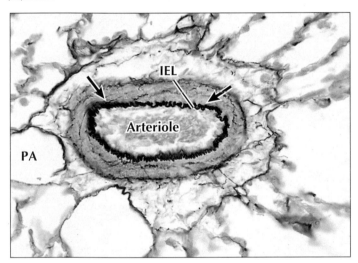

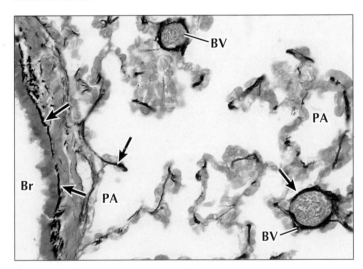

▲ **LMs showing the distribution of elastic fibers in the lung.** Elastic fibers (**arrows**) selectively stain dark purple to black. They are seen in the arteriole wall as an internal elastic lamina (**IEL**), in areas underlying the lumen of a bronchiole (**Br**), and in thin-walled pulmonary alveoli (**PA**) and small blood vessels (**BV**) as delicate strands. Cell details are not obvious, and the yellow counterstain is nonspecific. 360×. *Modified Gomori aldehyde fuchsin.*

3.8 HISTOLOGY OF ELASTIC CONNECTIVE TISSUE

Elastic connective tissue has a predominance of **elastic fibers** capable of stretching and returning to their original length. These stretchable fibers allow structures in which they are found to expand considerably, with return to an original shape by passive recoil. They cannot be distinguished with conventional methods; detection requires special stains such as orcein, **van Gieson,** or **Gomori aldehyde fuchsin.** They have widespread distribution and are abundant in **lungs,** skin, and urinary bladder. In walls of **arteries,** they form concentric **laminae,** or sheets. In these sites, smooth muscle cells produce the fibers; in other areas, **fibroblasts** do so. By electron microscopy, elastic fibers contain bundles of *microfibrils* that act as a scaffold during development and consist of the glycoprotein *fibrillin. Elastin,* an amorphous component, is added later and forms the major part of the fiber.

CLINICAL POINT

Marfan syndrome is an inherited *connective tissue disorder* caused by molecular defects in the *FBN1* gene that encodes the glycoprotein *fibrillin-1.* This extracellular protein is a component of microfibrils, which serve as scaffolds for elastic fiber deposition. Abnormal elastic tissues in the body mark the disease. Cardiovascular lesions, the most life-threatening, include mitral valve prolapse and weakening of the tunica media of the aorta, which may rupture spontaneously. Loss of connective tissue support in heart valves creates the so-called floppy valve that may contribute to heart failure.

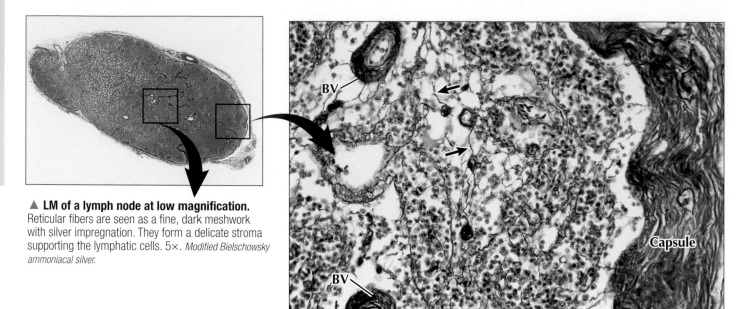

▲ LM of a lymph node at low magnification.
Reticular fibers are seen as a fine, dark meshwork
with silver impregnation. They form a delicate stroma
supporting the lymphatic cells. 5×. *Modified Bielschowsky
ammoniacal silver.*

**▲ LM of the cortex of a lymph node at
medium magnification.** Reticular fibers are
delicate black threads (**arrows**). These thin,
long branching fibers form the node's
structural framework. Collagen fiber bundles
in the capsule and blood vessels (**BV**) do not
have an affinity for silver and are reddish
brown. 280×. *Modified Bielschowsky ammoniacal
silver.*

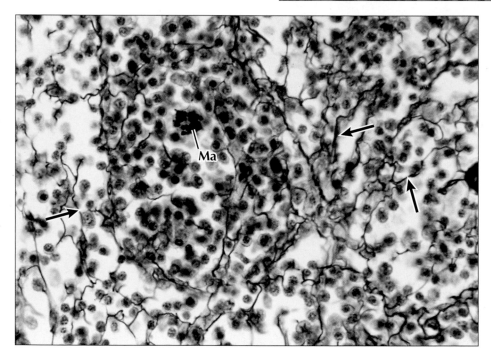

**◀ LM of the medulla of a lymph node at
high magnification.** Reticular fibers (**arrows**)
are the branching linear elements that are darkly
stained with silver. They form a loose network
associated with lymphoid cells, whose pale
nuclei can be seen. A large macrophage (**Ma**) is
recognizable by the presence of ingested
particles in its cytoplasm. 550×. *Modified
Bielschowsky ammoniacal silver.*

3.9 HISTOLOGY OF RETICULAR CONNECTIVE TISSUE

Reticular connective tissue, a specialized **loose connective tissue,**
has wide body distribution in **lymphatic** and **hematopoietic
organs**—bone marrow, **lymph node,** and spleen. This meshwork
forms the supportive **stroma** of many tissues and organs. A looser,
delicate network of **reticular fibers** is also closely associated with
adipocytes, hepatocytes, smooth muscle cells, endothelial cells of
blood vessels, and nerve fibers. Reticular fibers are long, thin
extracellular fibers, 100-150 nm in diameter. They do not form
bundles like collagen fibers but rather a felt-like aggregation of
branching fibers. Once thought to have a different composition
from collagen, they are now known to be thin **type III collagen

fibers.** Electron microscopy reveals a banding pattern similar to
that seen in other fibrillar forms of collagen. However, they stain
poorly with hematoxylin and eosin (H&E) and thus require special
light microscopic stains. They have an affinity for **silver salts,** a
property known as *argyrophilia,* and they are strongly PAS-
positive, indicating a high carbohydrate content. Their selective
staining with metallic silver is most likely due to precipitation of
reducible silver salts on an external coating of bound proteoglycans. Epithelial basement membranes also contain a reticular
lamina made of a fine meshwork of reticular fibers. During *wound
healing* in connective tissue, reticular fibers are the first to be synthesized by fibroblasts and are later replaced by type I collagen
fibers.

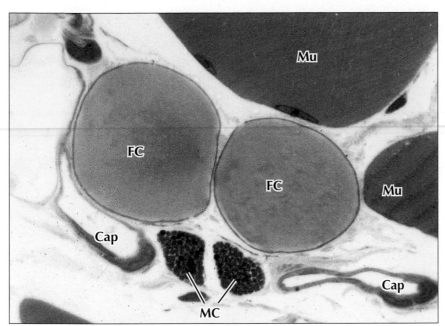

◄ **LM of two mast cells in connective tissue of skeletal muscle.** Mast cells (**MC**) have prominent metachromatic granules and sit close to capillaries (**Cap**). Metachromasia is the property whereby the granules stain with a color (magenta to purple) different from that of the dye itself (blue). Two adipocytes (**FC**), or fat cells, and parts of two skeletal muscle fibers (**Mu**) are nearby. 1000×. *Toluidine blue, plastic section.*

▼ **Mast cell and vascular response to injury.**

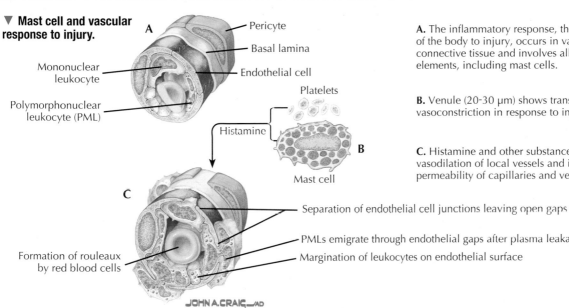

A. The inflammatory response, the basic reaction of the body to injury, occurs in vascularized connective tissue and involves all of its structural elements, including mast cells.

B. Venule (20-30 μm) shows transient vasoconstriction in response to injury.

C. Histamine and other substances cause active vasodilation of local vessels and increased permeability of capillaries and venules.

3.10 HISTOLOGY AND FUNCTION OF MAST CELLS

Mast cells are normal elements of the **connective tissues** and **lamina propria** of mucous membranes, where they trigger or maintain *inflammatory* and *immune* responses. Measuring 20-30 μm in diameter, they derive from bone marrow precursors. Their location near small **blood vessels** allows them to perform many sentinel functions for *host defense*. They are found at sites of *inflammation* and *neoplastic foci* and play a central role in *immediate allergic reactions*. They usually contain large, abundant **granules** of several biologically active substances. The highly heterogeneous tissue mast cells vary greatly in size, granule contents, and function. They release potent inflammatory mediators such as *histamine,* the anticoagulant *heparin, chemotactic factors, cytokines,* and metabolites of *arachidonic acid* that act on vasculature, smooth muscle, connective tissue, mucous glands, and inflammatory cells. Histamine, a potent vasodilator and proteolytic enzyme, can destroy tissue or cleave complement components. Histamine release from mast cells increases **permeability** of **capillaries** and **venules** and results in local **edema** and emigration of **leukocytes** and monocytes from circulation. They stimulate local cell proliferation, which leads to production of connective tissue elements involved in repair of damaged tissues. Chemotactic factors are important regulators of eosinophil and neutrophil function. Granules are **metachromatic** when stained with cationic dyes such as **toluidine blue** because they contain sulfated glycosaminoglycans.

CLINICAL POINT

Anaphylaxis is a life-threatening *allergic reaction.* It starts when antibodies to IgE bind with allergens. Mast cell membranes contain IgE receptors, and when the receptors bind to antigen, mast cells release contents of their granules—histamine and other stored molecules. Histamine dilates small blood vessels and increases their permeability so that plasma leaks out; the skin appears red and *edematous.* The *wheals* of **urticaria**, called **hives**, are caused by release of histamine from mast cells. These cells also activate a pathway leading to release of prostaglandin, leukotriene, and platelet-activating factor.

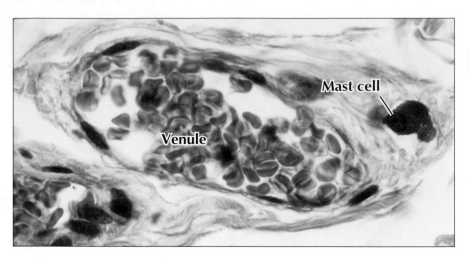

◀ **LM of a mast cell in connective tissue.** It has many granules in its cytoplasm and is close to a venule, which is filled with erythrocytes. 800×. *H&E.*

▼ **EM of a mast cell in connective tissue.** This section is at the level of the cell nucleus, which is euchromatic with peripheral patches of heterochromatin and a prominent nucleolus (⋆) at its center. An irregular cell border with filopodia (**arrows**) is a distinctive feature of the cell surface. Many prominent, moderately electron dense granules (**Gr**) fill the cytoplasm. Collagen fiber bundles (**Co**) are in the extracellular matrix. 10,500×.

▼ **EM of a mast cell in loose connective tissue.** The cytoplasm shows the granules (**Gr**) that vary in size, shape, and electron density. Short, stubby filopodia (**arrows**) project from the cell surface. Collagen fibrils (**Co**) occupy extracellular matrix. 10,000×.

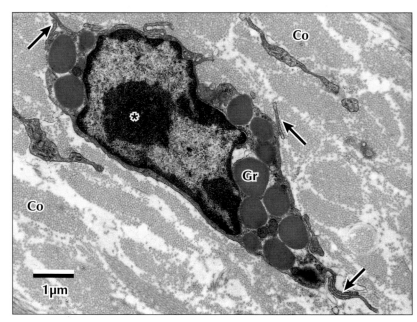

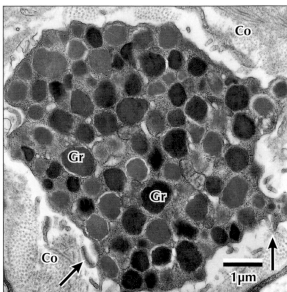

3.11 ULTRASTRUCTURE AND FUNCTION OF MAST CELLS

The usually ovoid mast cells, the largest **connective tissue** cells, are found in areas where antigens and foreign proteins are most likely to enter underlying tissues. Many **granules** in the **cytoplasm** often obscure the small, round to elongated **nucleus.** The cell has an irregular outline with many small surface projections, or **filopodia,** that extend into surrounding connective tissue and most likely increase surface area. The cell's plasma membrane has surface receptors for IgE. The membrane-bound granules, measuring 0.2-1 μm in diameter, vary in size, shape, and density of their internal contents, which may be finely granular, lamellar, or amorphous. The granules store various *inflammatory mediators* before discharge. The cytoplasm contains a small Golgi complex, scattered profiles of smooth and rough endoplasmic reticulum, and scattered mitochondria. The Golgi complex plays a role in synthesis and sulfation of glycosaminoglycans such as heparin that are packaged and stored in the granules. *Degranulation* of the granules is consistent with release of their contents into the extracellular space.

HISTORICAL POINT

Mast cells were first described by the German medical scientist, **Paul Ehrlich** (1854-1915). He named them *Mastzellen,* meaning well-fed cells, because the granules led him to the mistaken belief that the cells nourish surrounding tissues. Mast cells are now thought to be part of the *immune system.* Ehrlich obtained his doctorate of medicine with a dissertation on the theory and practice of staining tissues for histology; he showed how different dyes acted on cells. A pioneer for future work in hematology, immunology, and bacteriology, he won the Nobel Prize in Physiology or Medicine in 1908.

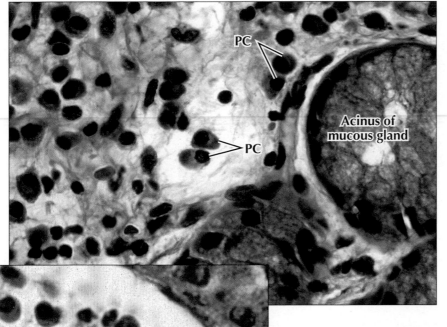

◄ **LM showing plasma cells in connective tissue underlying a palatine tonsil.** The typical features of plasma cells (**PC**) include an ovoid shape, basophilic cytoplasm, eccentrically placed nucleus, and coarse chromatin pattern. Collections of these cells are seen in connective tissue between mucous gland acini. 400×. *H&E.*

▼ **Bone marrow smear showing a plasma cell.** The plasma cell (**PC**) has an eccentrically placed heterochromatic nucleus. Its basophilic cytoplasm shows a juxtanuclear halo corresponding to the Golgi complex. Developing red (**RBC**) and white (**WBC**) blood cells and platelets (**P**) are nearby. 1000×. *Wright's.*

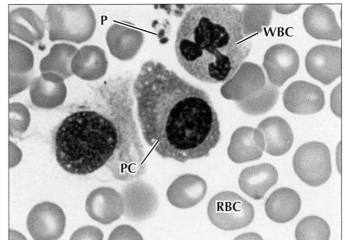

▲ **LM of plasma cells in a lymph node.** The clock–face nucleus and pale–staining Golgi are seen in the plasma cell (PC) in the center of the field. 600×. *H&E.*

3.12 HISTOLOGY AND FUNCTION OF PLASMA CELLS

Plasma cells are mature B lymphocytes that are specialized for antibody (immunoglobulin) production. Lymphocytes that enter **connective tissue** from the circulation differentiate into plasma cells when activated. Plasma cells are free cells of the connective tissues, able to move slowly through them. Most are distributed widely throughout the body, especially in the lamina propria of the gastrointestinal tract and in lymphatic organs. They rarely occur in peripheral blood and normally constitute 0.2%-2.8% of the bone marrow leukocyte count. The typically oval mature plasma cells measure 10-20 μm in diameter. Their **cytoplasm** is deeply **basophilic,** the color depending on the stain and ribosomal content of the cell. A clear area near the eccentric, round **nucleus** is a **juxtanuclear halo (negative Golgi image),** which corresponds to the **Golgi complex.** The **nuclear chromatin** is mostly condensed and **heterochromatic,** alternating with light areas, to give a spoke-wheel or clock–face appearance. A prominent nucleolus is often seen. Plasma cells actively synthesize protein. They produce antibodies that are released locally and circulate in blood. They play an important role in defense against infection. Increased numbers of plasma cells are seen in many hematologic disorders such as plasma cell leukemia.

CLINICAL POINT

Of several types of plasma cell malignancies or neoplasms, the most common is **multiple myeloma.** In this disorder, abnormal plasma cells—*myeloma cells*—accumulate in bone marrow and form multiple *tumors,* mostly in bones. As the number of such cells increases, other hematopoietic stem cells in the bone marrow are compromised. Many serious conditions, including an erythrocyte shortage, or *anemia,* result. Improved prognosis is due to novel treatment modalities such as pulse corticosteroids, thalidomide, and allogeneic stem cell transplantation, as well as chemotherapy.

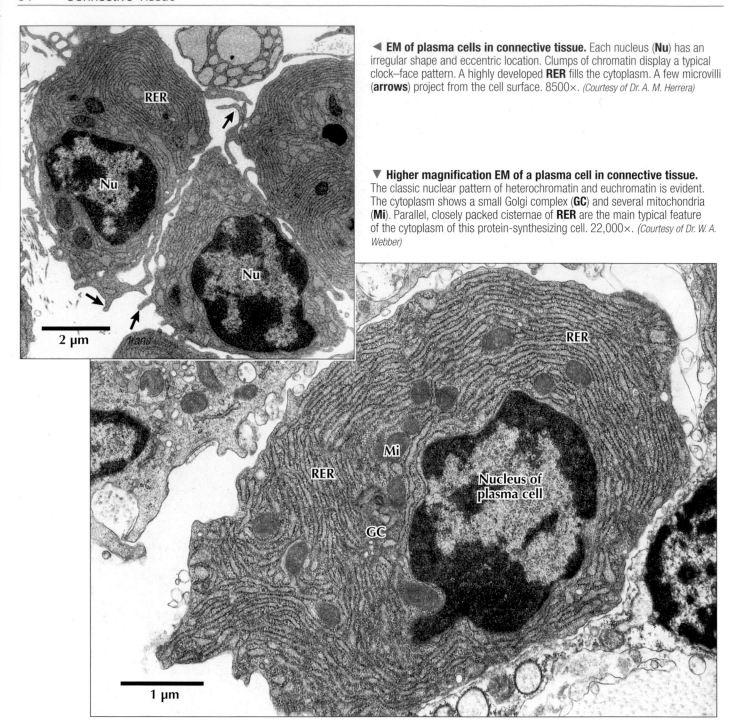

◄ **EM of plasma cells in connective tissue.** Each nucleus (**Nu**) has an irregular shape and eccentric location. Clumps of chromatin display a typical clock–face pattern. A highly developed **RER** fills the cytoplasm. A few microvilli (**arrows**) project from the cell surface. 8500×. *(Courtesy of Dr. A. M. Herrera)*

▼ **Higher magnification EM of a plasma cell in connective tissue.** The classic nuclear pattern of heterochromatin and euchromatin is evident. The cytoplasm shows a small Golgi complex (**GC**) and several mitochondria (**Mi**). Parallel, closely packed cisternae of **RER** are the main typical feature of the cytoplasm of this protein-synthesizing cell. 22,000×. *(Courtesy of Dr. W. A. Webber)*

3.13 ULTRASTRUCTURE OF PLASMA CELLS

By electron microscopy, the cytoplasm of the plasma cell has abundant free ribosomes and an extensive RER. The small juxtanuclear Golgi complex consists of flattened sacs and a few associated vesicles. Two centrioles are often close to the Golgi complex. The prominent RER is studded externally by ribosomes and is usually organized as closely spaced, flattened cisternae in parallel stacks. The cisternae are often dilated and contain flocculent, moderately electron-dense material that is probably newly synthesized immunoglobulin. A single cell normally releases one class of immunoglobulin molecules, specific for one epitope of an anti-body, known as a monoclonal antibody. From the RER, this molecule is delivered to the Golgi complex, where it is packaged into small vesicles that are shuttled to the cell periphery and released by exocytosis at the surface. Unlike most other protein-secreting cells in the body, plasma cells lack large secretory granules, which reflects continuous delivery and discharge of secretory product at the cell surface. The nucleus shows peripheral clumps of heterochromatin intermixed with prevailing euchromatin in a clock–face pattern. The nuclear membrane-associated heterochromatin has wide spaces for rapid movement of mRNA through nuclear pores, which results in the typical low electron-dense cartwheel form.

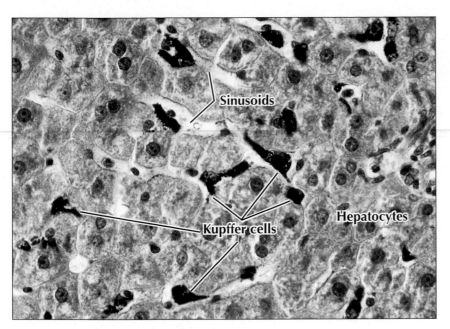

◀ **LM of rat liver showing macrophages that have ingested India ink.** One hour after a rat was injected with India ink, the liver was removed and processed for conventional histology. Macrophages in the liver, called Kupffer cells, ingested carbon particles in the ink, so that the pleomorphic cells appear black. They line the small sinusoids that are close to hepatocytes. 400×. *H&E.*

▼ **Phagocytosis and antigen processing by macrophage.**

A. After emigration from circulation across blood vessel wall, a monocyte becomes a macrophage, which is attracted to a wound area or inflammatory site by chemotaxis.

B. Antibody receptors on a macrophage cell membrane bind antibody-coated foreign material. The phagocytic cell forms pseudopods around antigen or debris particles.

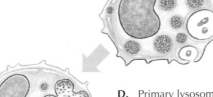

C. Membranes of pseudopods fuse, enclosing debris in a vacuole.

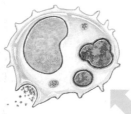

E. At the end of phagocytosis, the cell shows few primary lysosomes and contains many dense residual bodies, or tertiary lysosomes. The phagocytic vacuole fuses with cell membrane; antigen is presented to a T lymphocyte (CD4⁺ helper T cell) next to the macrophage.

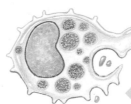

D. Primary lysosomes of a phagocytic cell fuse with the vacuole and extrude enzymes into the resulting digestive vacuole. Antigen is degraded into small peptide fragments that bind to a receptor molecule known as class II major histocompatability complex.

JOHN A. CRAIG—AD

3.14 STRUCTURE AND FUNCTION OF MACROPHAGES

After fibroblasts, macrophages—or histiocytes (an older term for tissue macrophage)—are the most numerous cell type in **loose connective tissue.** They belong to a family of **monocyte-derived cells** with wide distribution in the body: **Kupffer cells** in liver, alveolar dust cells of lung, microglia in brain, Langerhans cells in epidermis, dendritic cells in lymphatic tissue, and osteoclasts of bone. These avidly **phagocytic cells** have a more variable appearance and shorter cytoplasmic processes than fibroblasts. They may be fixed cells attached to connective tissue fibers of the matrix or wandering cells that are motile and migratory. Some macrophages derive from differentiating mesenchymal cells within connective tissue, but most originate from hematopoietic stem cells in bone marrow that circulate as monocytes and migrate across blood vessel walls to enter connective tissues. The small **nucleus** has an irregular outline and finely dispersed **chromatin.** In addition to engulfing and digesting particulate matter, infectious microorganisms such as bacteria, and damaged cells, macrophages synthesize and secrete various biologically active molecules. Cytokines, growth factors, and complement proteins produced by these cells exert profound effects on other cells. Macrophages are attracted to sites of *inflammation* and are involved in the *immune response* by *antigen processing* and *presentation.*

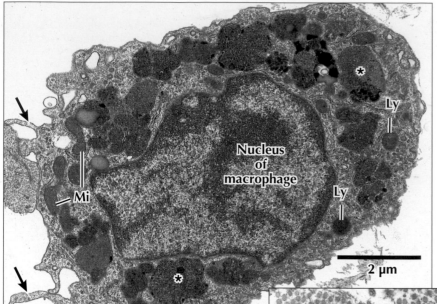

◀ **EM of a macrophage.** The cell is sectioned at the level of its nucleus, which has an irregular outline, slightly eccentric location, and finely dispersed chromatin. The cytoplasm contains many vesicles, mitochondria (**Mi**), and other closely packed organelles. Numerous lysosomes at various developmental stages are scattered throughout the cytoplasm and range from small primary (**Ly**) to large tertiary (⋆) lysosomes. The cell surface bears many cytoplasmic processes, or pseudopods (**arrows**). 11,000×.

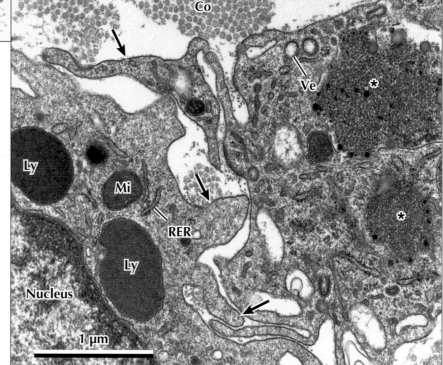

▶ **EM of parts of two macrophages.** Primary lysosomes (**Ly**), close to the nucleus, have a dense, homogeneous electron-dense core. The larger tertiary lysosomes (⋆), more irregular in shape, contain a heterogeneous collection of particulate matter. Cell surfaces have many pseudopodia (**arrows**) that vary in size and shape. Cytoplasm shows abundant vesicles (**Ve**), a few mitochondria (**Mi**), and elements of rough endoplasmic reticulum (**RER**). A prominent cytoskeleton composed mostly of irregularly arranged filaments makes remaining cytoplasm stain densely. Collagen fibrils (**Co**) are in surrounding extracellular matrix. 32,000×.

3.15 ULTRASTRUCTURE AND FUNCTION OF MACROPHAGES

Ultrastructure of macrophages reflects their ability to phagocytose, synthesize various secretory products, and engage in ameboid movement and migratory activity. The cell's functional state determines whether electron microscopy shows many primary lysosomes, phagosomes that have ingested exogenous material, secondary lysosomes, or tertiary lysosomes (residual bodies) with indigestible remnants. Primary lysosomes derive from the Golgi complex, which is usually near the nucleus. Also associated with the Golgi complex are many smooth and coated vesicles. Macrophages are motile in many areas of the body, so a striking feature of their cytoplasm is an extensive cytoskeleton, with abundant microtubules, actin filaments, and intermediate filaments. The filaments, often arranged in bundles, are especially prominent just under the plasma membrane. This membrane has an irregular surface consisting of many finger-like extensions called pseudopodia. Pseudopodia are numerous in actively phagocytic cells, change their shape, and often contact surrounding cells during cell movement. Cells phagocytose by adhering to particulate matter before its uptake by invagination of plasma membrane. Mitochondria, free ribosomes, and variable amounts of rough endoplasmic reticulum are also scattered in the cytoplasm. The one nucleus is often indented or kidney shaped, and, depending on its functional state, usually has abundant euchromatin. In chronic inflammation, fusion of macrophages may form multinucleated foreign body giant cells that are protective (sequester material).

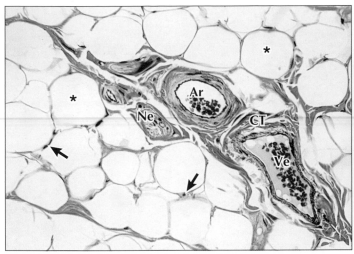

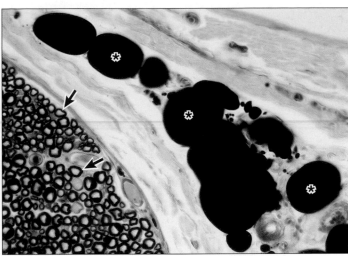

▲ **LM of white adipose tissue.** A fibrous septum of connective tissue (**CT**) is between closely packed adipocytes (∗). Adipocytes are large globular cells distended by lipid content. Tissue processing removes lipid, with clear empty spaces left in the cells. Between the cells is a rich network of capillaries (**arrows**). An arteriole (**Ar**), venule (**Ve**), and nerve fascicle (**Ne**) are in view. 340×. *Masson trichrome.*

▲ **LM of adipocytes in the epineurium of a peripheral nerve.** The fat in the adipocytes (∗) has been preserved, so they appear black. These spherical cells vary in size. The myelin sheaths of adjacent peripheral nerve fibers (**arrows**) have high lipid content and are thus also preserved in this preparation. 360×. *Osmium.*

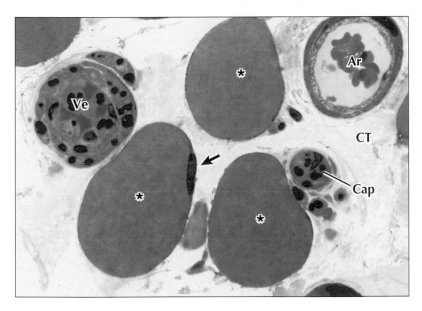

◀ **LM of adipocytes in white adipose tissue.** The lipid of the cells is preserved by glutaraldehyde and osmium fixation and fills the cytoplasm (∗). The signet ring appearance typical of these cells is in the lower left cell: the cytoplasm forms a thin rim around the fat, and the nucleus, when in the plane of section, is flattened at the cell periphery (**arrow**). Adipose tissue is richly vascularized, and an arteriole (**Ar**), venule (**Ve**), and capillary (**Cap**) filled with blood cells in intervening connective tissue (**CT**) are seen here. Adipocytes have an average diameter of 70 μm in lean adults; in obese persons, the diameter may reach 170-200 μm. 670×. *Toluidine blue, plastic section.*

3.16   HISTOLOGY OF ADIPOSE TISSUE

Adipose tissue is a specialized **loose connective tissue** that contains large numbers of **adipocytes.** It functions in *insulation* and *padding* and provides a ready source of *fuel* for metabolic processes. Except in emaciated or obese states, adipose tissue normally constitutes 10%-15% of body weight. It is a highly labile tissue, specialized for synthesis and storage of **lipids.** Fat may be formed directly from carbohydrates in adipocytes or taken up by micropinocytosis from the blood; it has a rapid and continuous turnover rate. Closely associated with small **blood vessels,** adipocytes occur singly or in clusters that are usually arranged in lobules surrounded by **fibrous septa** and thus resemble a bunch of grapes. A delicate network of reticular fibers supports each cell. In routine preparations treated with alcohol and xylol, fats are extracted, so

cells appear to have holes. Each cell has a thin rim of **cytoplasm**— a signet ring appearance with a flattened, peripheral **nucleus.** Fat can be shown in frozen sections treated with special stains or in tissue fixed and stained with osmium. The two types of adipose tissue, **white** or **unilocular** and **brown** or **multilocular,** differ in distribution, metabolic activity, histologic appearance, vascularity, and color. White adipose tissue, the most widely distributed, has large cells with average diameters of 70 μm. Cells have one unilocular **fat droplet,** which is formed during development by coalescence of multiple small droplets. Brown adipose tissue is restricted to the embryo and fetus and, after birth, to limited body locations. Its cells measure up to 60 μm and are multilocular, with several small fat droplets in the cytoplasm.

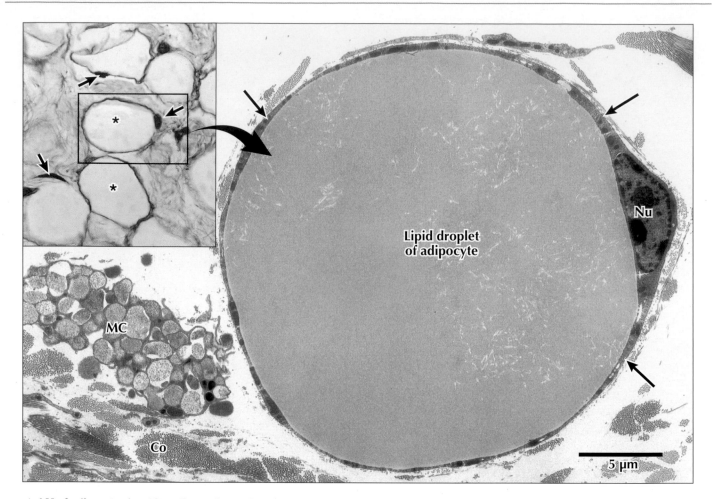

▲ **LM of adipocytes in white adipose tissue.** Each cell holds one fat droplet (∗) that appears to be empty space because of the organic solvents used in tissue preparation. The nuclei (**arrows**) are pushed to the periphery of each cell. 400×. *H&E.*

▲ **EM of a white (unilocular) adipocyte.** One large lipid droplet displaces the nucleus (**Nu**) to one side of the cell and flattens it against the cell membrane. The cytoplasm is reduced to an extremely attenuated rim (**arrows**). Surrounding connective tissue contains collagen fibrils (**Co**) and a degranulated mast cell (**MC**). 4400×.

3.17 ULTRASTRUCTURE AND FUNCTION OF UNILOCULAR ADIPOCYTES IN WHITE FAT

Adipocytes are specialized for synthesis, storage, and mobilization of neutral fats called *triglycerides. Hormones,* such as *insulin,* and the *sympathetic nervous system,* which innervates adipose tissue, control these activities. These fats are stored in non-membrane-bound **lipid droplets.** When fats are needed to provide fuel for cells in other tissues, adipocytes release them as fatty acids into circulation. Dietary lipids from the intestine also circulate in blood as water-soluble lipoproteins called *chylomicrons.* Together with *very-low-density lipoproteins* (VLDLs) from the liver, they reach the adipocyte surface via capillaries. *Lipoprotein lipase,* an enzyme produced by adipocytes, releases fatty acids and monoglycerides from chylomicrons and VLDLs that are then moved to the adipocyte cytoplasm. Re-esterification into triglycerides occurs in the smooth endoplasmic reticulum, followed by storage in lipid droplets. Some fatty acids are also produced from glycogen in adipocytes. Scattered mitochondria, a small Golgi complex, and cytoskeletal filaments are other organelles in the cytoplasm. Adipocytes also secrete steroid hormones, cytokines, and *leptin,* a peptide hormone, which functions in *appetite regulation* by acting on the hypothalamus.

CLINICAL POINT

A global epidemic of obesity—an increase in adipose tissue above normal body needs—exists. A major public health problem, it leads to serious disorders such as hypertension, diabetes, and myocardial infarction, as well as poor surgical outcomes. The etiology is multifactorial, but ultimately it is a disorder of *energy imbalance:* long-term caloric intake exceeds energy expenditure. Excess calories are stored as triglycerides in adipocytes, whose size can distend or shrink in response to various stimuli. *Leptin,* a cytokine produced by adipocytes, functions in energy homeostasis. After entering the bloodstream and crossing the blood-brain barrier, it binds to receptors in neurosecretory cells of the hypothalamus that affect appetite and energy expenditure.

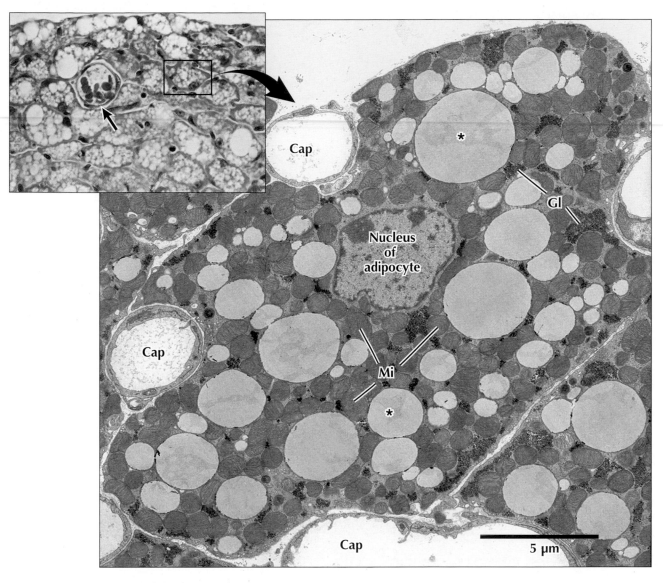

▲ **LM of several adipocytes in brown adipose tissue.** The many lipid droplets of various size give the cells a frothy appearance. A rich vasculature (**arrow**) characterizes this tissue. 300×. *H&E.*

▲ **EM of a multilocular adipocyte in brown fat.** Cytoplasm replete with mitochondria (**Mi**), lipid droplets (∗), and glycogen (**Gl**) deposits surrounds the nucleus. Capillaries (**Cap**) are in close contact with adipocyte surfaces. 6000×.

3.18 ULTRASTRUCTURE AND FUNCTION OF MULTILOCULAR ADIPOCYTES IN BROWN FAT

Brown adipose tissue is recognized by a characteristic color, which is due to rich vascularity and to lipochromes in numerous **mitochondria** within adipocytes. Brown fat constitutes about 2% of body weight in newborns but becomes more limited in extent with age; animals that hibernate have large quantities of brown fat. In humans, its main function is heat generation, or nonshivering thermogenesis. Its cells are smaller and more polygonal than cells in white adipose tissue, and the **nucleus** is more centrally located. The **cytoplasm** contains multiple **lipid droplets** of various sizes that give the cell a multilocular appearance, as well as many large, rounded mitochondria that possess well-developed cristae extending across the entire width of these organelles. Mitochondria sit between the lipid droplets and play a role in mediating heat production by oxidation of fatty acids. Aggregates of **glycogen particles** are also found in the cytoplasm. Adipocyte **plasma membranes** are in intimate contact with abundant **capillaries.** Multilocular adipocytes are directly innervated by the sympathetic nervous system, and noradrenergic unmyelinated axons are often seen in close contact with cell surfaces. Similar to unilocular adipocytes in white fat, multilocular adipocytes in brown fat originate from primitive mesenchymal cells. Unlike unilocular adipocytes that respond mainly to fasting, a cold environment primarily activates these multilocular adipocytes.

4

MUSCLE TISSUE

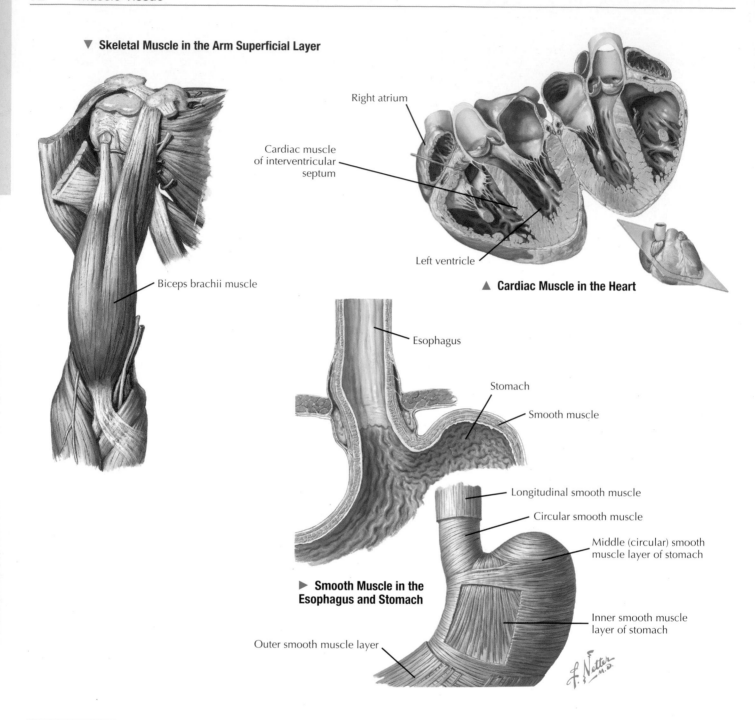

▼ **Skeletal Muscle in the Arm Superficial Layer**

Biceps brachii muscle

Right atrium

Cardiac muscle of interventricular septum

Left ventricle

▲ **Cardiac Muscle in the Heart**

Esophagus

Stomach

Smooth muscle

Longitudinal smooth muscle

Circular smooth muscle

Middle (circular) smooth muscle layer of stomach

Inner smooth muscle layer of stomach

▶ **Smooth Muscle in the Esophagus and Stomach**

Outer smooth muscle layer

4.1 OVERVIEW

Muscle tissue in the body is classified into one of three major categories according to structure, function, and location. **Skeletal muscle** is the most common and characteristic type; the other two kinds are **cardiac muscle** and **smooth muscle.** Skeletal muscle produces purposeful movements of the skeleton. Cardiac muscle forms the **myocardium** and is responsible for beating of the heart to pump blood. Smooth muscle provides the motile force for many vital activities including *peristalsis* in the gut, emptying of the urinary bladder, *pupillary constriction,* and childbirth *(parturition)* by contraction of the uterus. The *voluntary nervous system* controls skeletal muscle function, whereas cardiac and smooth muscles are known as involuntary muscles and are innervated by the *autonomic nervous system.* Although most cells can undergo

shape change and generate motile forces, *contractility* (cell shortening) is a property that is most highly developed in muscle cells. Under the microscope, the specialized contractile cells of skeletal muscle show an alternating series of transverse bands or striations, which result from the arrangement of contractile filaments; smooth muscle cells, which have a less orderly array of filaments and are found, for example, in internal organs and blood vessels, lack these striations. Cardiac muscle is striated and has characteristics that are intermediate between skeletal and smooth muscle. The principal cellular and functional unit of muscle tissue is the **muscle fiber,** an elongated and highly differentiated cell. Each fiber has a parallel array of cytoplasmic **filaments** containing the proteins **myosin** and **actin.** Filaments interact and slide past each other to cause contraction or shortening of muscle fibers.

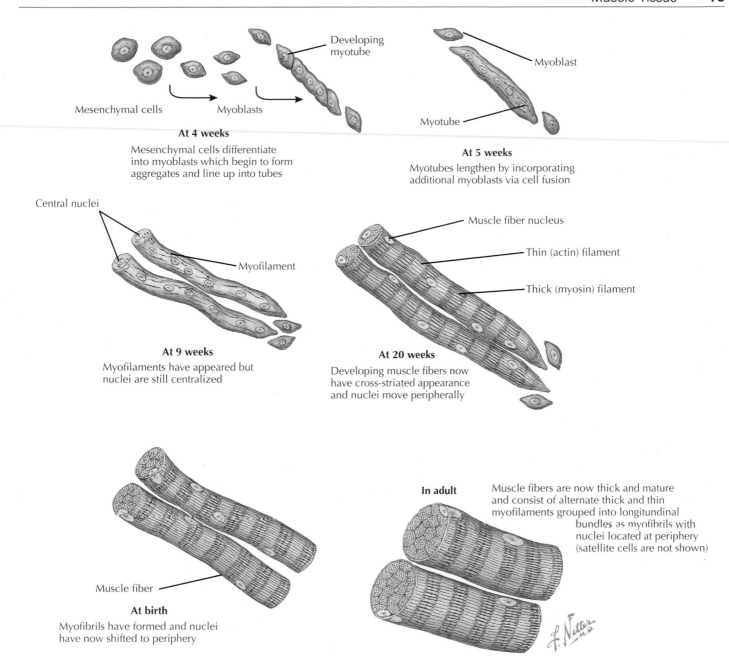

At 4 weeks

Mesenchymal cells differentiate into myoblasts which begin to form aggregates and line up into tubes

At 5 weeks

Myotubes lengthen by incorporating additional myoblasts via cell fusion

At 9 weeks

Myofilaments have appeared but nuclei are still centralized

At 20 weeks

Developing muscle fibers now have cross-striated appearance and nuclei move peripherally

At birth

Myofibrils have formed and nuclei have now shifted to periphery

In adult

Muscle fibers are now thick and mature and consist of alternate thick and thin myofilaments grouped into longitundinal bundles as myofibrils with nuclei located at periphery (satellite cells are not shown)

4.2 EMBRYONIC DEVELOPMENT OF SKELETAL MUSCLE FIBERS

Muscle tissue originates from mesoderm (middle primary germ layer). In the human embryo, most skeletal muscles develop from segmented paraxial mesoderm, organized as myotomes of somites (each becoming innervated by a spinal nerve). Other muscles may develop from mesoderm of branchial arches on each side of the embryonic head (become innervated by cranial nerves), or in situ from local areas of condensed mesenchyme. In the 4-week embryo, **mesenchymal cells** at genetically predetermined sites proliferate, elongate, and differentiate into **myoblasts.** Aggregation and end-to-end fusion of myoblasts produce syncytial, multinucleated **myotubes.** At 5 weeks, myotubes lengthen by incorporating more myoblasts. Some myoblasts fail to fuse, retain an ability to undergo

mitosis, and become future **satellite** (or **myosatellite**) **cells.** At 9 weeks, myotubes synthesize two sets of longitudinally oriented **myofilaments,** which align in parallel arrays. By 20 weeks, myofilaments continue to proliferate, and nuclei become peripherally located as cells increase in both **circumference** and length. Myofilaments are arranged in alternating, overlapping bands, so muscle fibers have a cross-striated appearance. At birth, **thick** (**myosin**) and **thin** (**actin**) myofilaments have collected into cylindrical bundles called **myofibrils,** and muscle fibers can *contract* as they become innervated by motor neurons. A single motor neuron and all the skeletal muscle fibers it innervates are known as a motor unit. Myosatellite cells, capable of division, remain closely associated with the plasma membrane, or sarcolemma, of each **muscle fiber** throughout life.

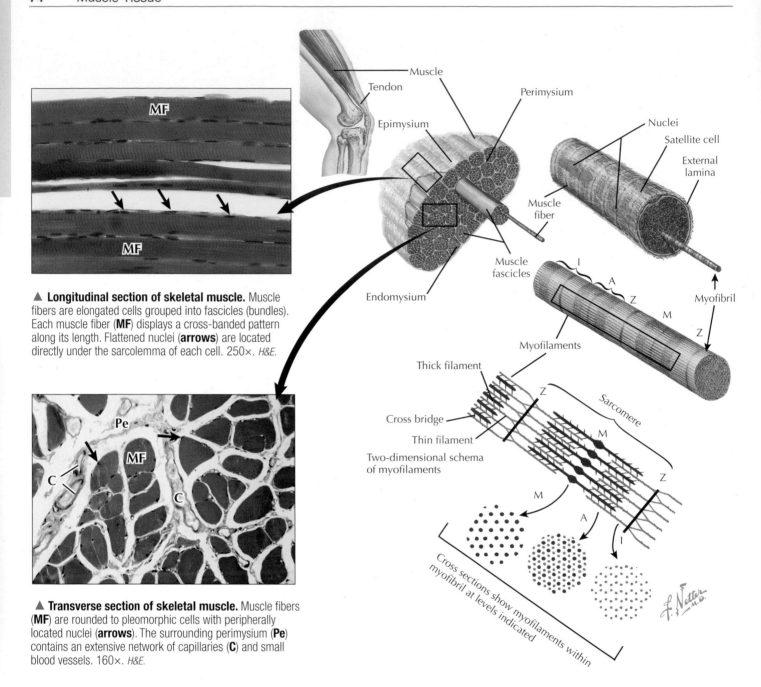

▲ **Longitudinal section of skeletal muscle.** Muscle fibers are elongated cells grouped into fascicles (bundles). Each muscle fiber (**MF**) displays a cross-banded pattern along its length. Flattened nuclei (**arrows**) are located directly under the sarcolemma of each cell. 250×. *H&E.*

▲ **Transverse section of skeletal muscle.** Muscle fibers (**MF**) are rounded to pleomorphic cells with peripherally located nuclei (**arrows**). The surrounding perimysium (**Pe**) contains an extensive network of capillaries (**C**) and small blood vessels. 160×. *H&E.*

4.3   ORGANIZATION OF SKELETAL MUSCLE

Although individual skeletal muscles have remarkably diverse functions, their fundamental role is to produce movement and generate force. To do so, skeletal muscle contains elongated, thread-like multinucleated cells called **muscle fibers.** The ends of the fibers insert into tendons, which attach to bones across joints. A dense connective tissue sheath—the **epimysium**—surrounds the whole muscle externally. Connective tissue septa that make up the **perimysium** subdivide the muscle internally into bundles, or **fascicles,** each containing several muscle fibers. A more delicate, looser connective tissue—the **endomysium**—surrounds individual muscle fibers. The vascular supply follows the connective tissue into the muscle, where **capillaries** run parallel with the longitudinal axis of the muscle fibers. Each muscle fiber is invested by a thin **external lamina** (basement membrane), which also encloses **satellite cells** that closely adhere to the plasma membrane, or **sarcolemma,** of the muscle fibers. The most striking features of skeletal muscle fibers are an orderly arrangement of contractile **myofilaments** into **myofibrils** and a characteristic striation pattern. Each myofibril has alternating **light** (**I,** for isotropic) and **dark** (**A,** for anisotropic) **bands** along its length. Two sets of myofilaments, thick and thin, that make up each myofibril are organized into repeating units of contraction known as **sarcomeres.** Dark, transverse **Z** *(Zwischenscheibe)* **bands** mark the ends of each sarcomere and anchor the thin filaments. The center of the sarcomere contains the **thick** (myosin-containing) **filaments,** which form the A band; **thin** (actin-containing) **filaments,** which form the I bands, are at the ends of each sarcomere.

▼ **Segment of a skeletal muscle fiber enlarged to show its major components.**

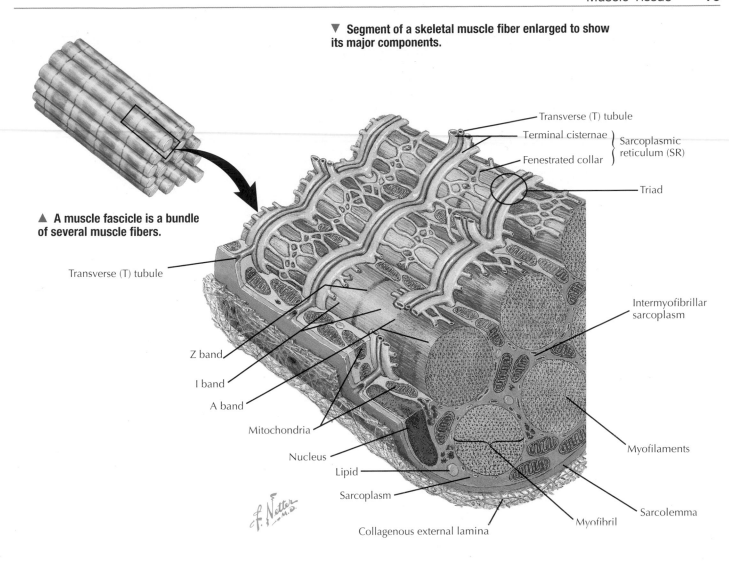

▲ **A muscle fascicle is a bundle of several muscle fibers.**

Transverse (T) tubule

Terminal cisternae } Sarcoplasmic reticulum (SR)

Fenestrated collar

Triad

Transverse (T) tubule

Intermyofibrillar sarcoplasm

Z band

I band

A band

Mitochondria

Nucleus

Lipid

Sarcoplasm

Myofilaments

Sarcolemma

Myofibril

Collagenous external lamina

4.4 MAJOR COMPONENTS OF SKELETAL MUSCLE FIBERS

The **sarcolemma** is the plasma membrane of the **muscle fiber** enveloped by an outer layer of *glycoproteins* and a fine network of *reticular fibers*, all constituting an **external lamina.** The sarcolemma and its tubular invaginations, called **transverse (T) tubules,** play a role in initiation of contraction. The **myofibrils,** each of which is 1-2 μm in diameter, constitute about 80% of the cell volume. Each myofibril contains a closely packed, orderly, overlapping longitudinally arranged array of **myofilaments** with a highly regular banding pattern. Each **sarcomere** of a myofibril consists of an **A band** and half of two contiguous **I bands.** A relaxed sarcomere is about 2.5 μm long, with the A band being about 1.6 μm long, and the I band on each side of the **Z band** about 1 μm long. Organelles, including **mitochondria** and tubular elements of the smooth-surfaced sarcotubular system, are interposed between myofibrils. Mitochondria are pleomorphic, and their density and distribution vary markedly in different muscle fiber types. The **sarcotubular system** is composed of two separate and distinct membrane systems of the muscle fiber, known as the **sarcoplasmic reticulum** (SR) and the transverse tubular system.

The SR, similar to the smooth endoplasmic reticulum of other cells, is an elaborate, anastomosing network of tubules and cisternae that surround the myofibrils. At regular intervals relative to the sarcomeres, two flattened sacs of the SR, known as **terminal cisternae (lateral sacs),** closely associate with a central transverse tubule and form a **muscle triad,** which is the main site for excitation-contraction coupling. The remaining **sarcoplasm** contains ribosomes, glycogen, and **lipid** droplets.

CLINICAL POINT
Duchenne muscular dystrophy is a genetic disorder caused by a deficiency of *dystrophin*, a large membrane-associated cytoskeletal protein. It is the most common of a group of muscular dystrophies characterized by rapid progression of skeletal muscle degeneration occurring early in life. Dystrophin is encoded by a gene on the short arm of the X chromosome (Xp21) and is linked to the cytoplasmic side of the sarcolemma of the muscle fiber. Dystrophin maintains mechanical integrity of the cell during contraction by anchoring cytoskeletal elements. Mainly young boys are affected, and symptoms, including muscle weakness and wasting and heart involvement, worsen with age.

▶ **Light micrograph (LM) of part of a skeletal muscle fiber in longitudinal section.** The regular cross-striation pattern is clear. Alternating dark and light segments cross the fiber from one side to the other. The dark stripes correspond to A bands (**A**) of myofibrils, whereas the light stripes are the I bands (**I**) bisected by very thin Z bands. Several elongated nuclei (**N**) are located in the peripheral areas of the cell. The surrounding loose connective tissue (**CT**) constitutes the endomysium, which contains nuclei of scattered fibroblasts. 1200×. *H&E.*

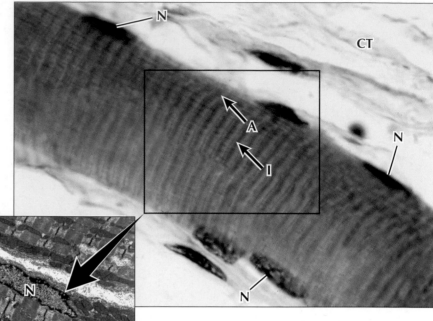

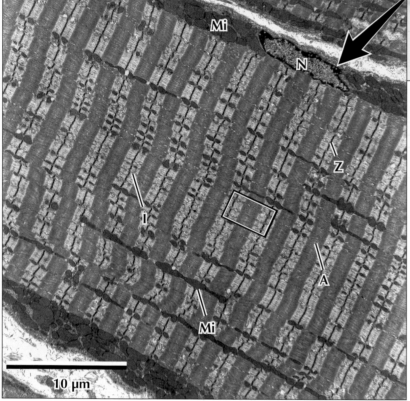

◀ **Low-magnification electron micrograph (EM) of part of a skeletal muscle fiber in longitudinal section.** Details of the organization and banding pattern are visible. Alternating dark (**A**) and light (**I**) bands of myofibrils are arranged in series along the length of the muscle fiber and show lateral registration with bands in adjacent myofibrils. An elongated nucleus (**N**) is close to the sarcolemma, with its long axis parallel to that of the cell. Mitochondria (**Mi**) are found in the peripheral sarcoplasm or in rows between the myofibrils. The rectangle marks a sarcomere. 3000×.

4.5   HISTOLOGY AND ULTRASTRUCTURE OF SKELETAL MUSCLE FIBERS IN LONGITUDINAL SECTION

Skeletal muscle constitutes 40%-50% of the body weight. As its name implies, it is mostly attached to the skeleton. It is also called **striated,** or **voluntary,** muscle, because its cells appear striated or cross-banded under the microscope. Skeletal **muscle fibers** are elongated, cylindrical cells, 50-200 μm in diameter, with tapered ends. They are **multinucleated,** the nuclei occupying peripheral positions in the cell. Their cytoplasm, known as sarcoplasm, is packed with **myofibrils,** which are cylindrical bundles of **myofila-ments** along the length of the fiber. Each myofibril has a uniform diameter and consists of identical repeating units, called **sarco-**

meres. Sarcomeres are composed of longitudinally oriented thick and thin filaments and perpendicular **Z** bands. In longitudinal section, skeletal muscle fibers show transverse striations because adjacent myofibrils are in lateral register with each other across the width of the fiber. The greater density of the **A bands** is due mainly to the presence of **thick (myosin-containing) filaments,** whereas the lighter density of the **I bands** is due to the prevalence of **thin (actin-containing) filaments.** In the center of each A band is a lighter **H zone** (the central part of thick filaments not over-lapped by thin filaments), which is bisected by a thin, dark **M band.** The width of the I band and H zone in each sarcomere varies and depends on the extent to which the muscle fiber is contracted or stretched.

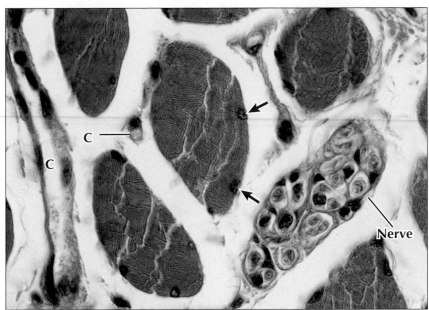

► **LM of skeletal muscle showing parts of several muscle fibers in transverse section.** Eosinophilic staining characteristics and punctate appearance are due to the contractile proteins, which constitute much of the sarcoplasm of each cell. Multiple rounded to oval nuclei (**arrows**) sit under the sarcolemma of each cell. Nuclei of satellite cells are not visible in conventional H&E sections, but they lie between the sarcolemma and the thin external lamina. Nerve fascicles (**Nerve**) of various sizes and capillaries (**C**) abound in surrounding endomysium. 700×. *H&E.*

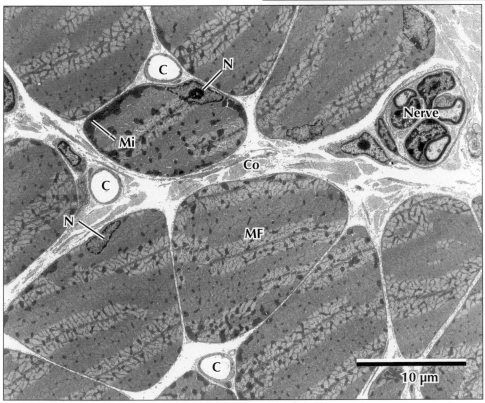

◄ **EM of skeletal muscle in transverse section.** The close relationship of a muscle fiber (**MF**) in the center of the field to surrounding capillaries (**C**) and neighboring muscle fibers is seen. Muscle fibers are pleomorphic, and myofibrils pack the sarcoplasm of each cell. Mitochondria (**Mi**) occur singly between myofibrils or in clusters under the sarcolemma. The peripheral nuclei (**N**) of muscle fibers are typically euchromatic and often contain nucleoli. A small nerve fascicle and collagen (**Co**) are in the perimysium between muscle fibers. 3000×.

4.6 HISTOLOGY AND ULTRASTRUCTURE OF SKELETAL MUSCLE FIBERS IN TRANSVERSE SECTION

Adult skeletal muscle fibers are polygonal, although in infancy they tend to be rounded, as are those of the extrinsic eye muscles and some muscles of facial expression. In transverse sections stained with hematoxylin and eosin (H&E), the **sarcoplasm** of each fiber is intensely **eosinophilic** and looks punctate because of tightly packed **myofibrils.** Myofibrils constitute the bulk of each fiber and mostly contain the major contractile proteins **myosin** and **actin,** which make up the **myofilaments.** In cross section, myofibrils are often seen grouped together and form irregularly shaped Cohnheim's fields, which are probably artifacts of preparation caused by shrinkage. The surrounding endomysium supports a rich vascular and nerve supply, which consists of **capillaries** and **nerve fascicles** close to the muscle fibers. Electron microscopy clarifies further details of ultrastructure. Myofibrils are rounded to irregular in shape, and the intervening, intermyofibrillar sarcoplasm contains a variety of other organelles, **mitochondria** being the most conspicuous at low magnification.

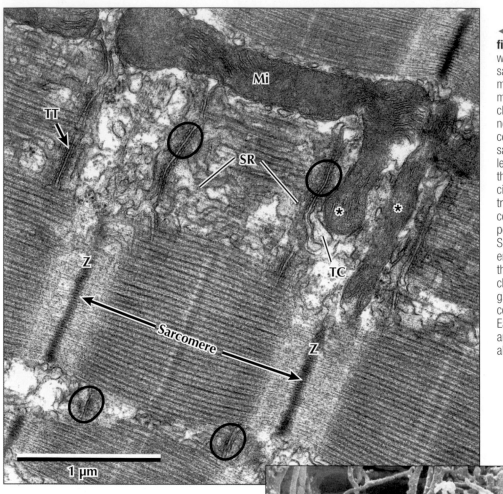

◀ **EM of part of a skeletal muscle fiber in longitudinal section.** Associated with each sarcomere are elements of the sarcotubular system. Because this elaborate membranous system closely encircles each myofibril, it is adequately revealed only by chance. This section shows the interlacing network of tubules and cisternae that constitutes the SR in relation to the sarcomere's banding pattern. At the A band level, a fenestrated collar courses toward the A-I junctions where tubules form terminal cisternae (**TC**) adjacent to T tubules (**TT**). Two triads (**circles**) occur per sarcomere, each composed of a central T tubule linked by periodic densities to terminal cisternae of the SR. The densities correspond to junctional end-feet and give a scalloped appearance to the triad junction. Intermyofibrillar mitochondria (**Mi**) are often oriented in the longitudinal plane with side branches (⋆) that course transverse to the level of the I band. Each sarcomere is bounded by Z bands (**Z**) and is formed by the precise and orderly alignment of myofilaments. 38,000×.

▶ **High-resolution scanning electron micrograph (HRSEM) showing the spatial arrangement of the sarcotubular system and mitochondria in a skeletal muscle fiber.** The SR forms a fenestrated collar opposite the central regions of two sarcomeres. Triads (**circles**) consisting of a central T tubule and a lateral pair of terminal SR cisternae are opposite the A-I junctions of the sarcomeres. Mitochondria (**Mi**) are pleomorphic and branched. Myofilaments were selectively extracted to highlight the SR. 30,000×.

4.7 ULTRASTRUCTURE OF THE SARCOTUBULAR SYSTEM IN SKELETAL MUSCLE

Two membranous components of skeletal muscle fibers, the **sarcotubular system** and **mitochondria,** are closely associated with **myofibrils.** The sarcotubular system, comprising the **T tubules** and the SR, plays a critical role in *excitation-contraction coupling.* These elements are not continuous with each other but are closely associated and have a specific orientation to the **sarcomere. T tubules,** a membrane system external to the muscle fiber at the junction of A and I bands, penetrate the fiber interior at regular intervals, mostly in a transverse plane. They rapidly convey electrical impulses from the **sarcolemma** to the cell interior. The SR, an internal membrane system that stores intracellular *calcium ions,* consists of a repeating array of longitudinally oriented tubules and flattened sacs, the **terminal cisternae,** surrounding the myofibrils. At A-I junctions, two terminal SR cisternae lie very close to a central T tubule, with an intervening gap of 15 nm, to form a tripartite complex called a **muscle triad.** Action potentials are propagated along T tubules. At the interface of the T tubule with the SR in the triad, calcium ions are released from the SR into the **sarcoplasm,** which initiates *contraction.* Junctional **end-feet** link the T tubule with the SR and are composed of a voltage-sensing *dihydropyridine receptor* on the T tubule connected to a *ryanodine receptor calcium release channel.* The elongated to pleomorphic mitochondria, an aerobic energy source, produce *ATP,* which is needed for contraction. They are aligned at strategic sites within muscle fibers; they usually occur at I band levels or in aggregates at the periphery of the fibers. Their density, location, and distribution in muscle fibers depend on muscle fiber type.

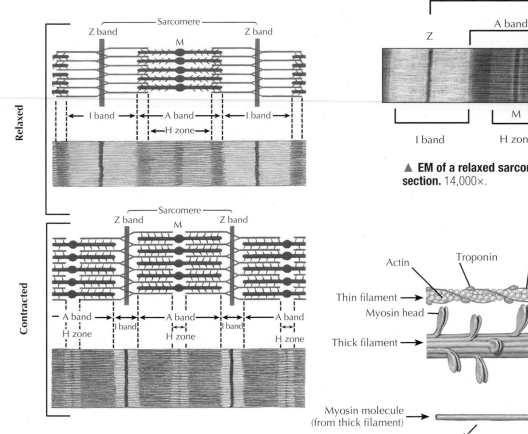

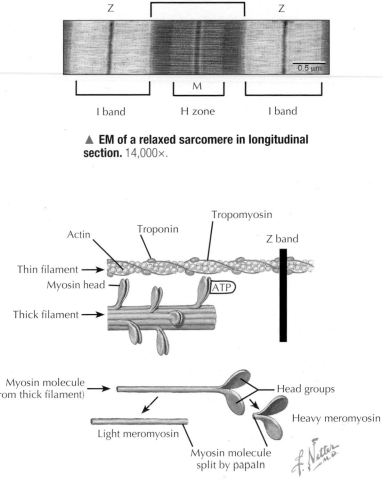

▲ **EM of a relaxed sarcomere in longitudinal section.** 14,000×.

▲ **Muscle contraction and relaxation.** Interdigitation of thick and thin filaments allows sarcomere contraction, which is best explained by the sliding filament model in which actin filaments slide along myosin filaments. During contraction, both sets of filaments retain their normal length, A bands remain unchanged in length, I bands shorten, and H zones are narrowed.

▲ **Schematic showing interaction of myosin and actin filaments at rest and during contraction.** The Z band is drawn closer to the edge of the A band by the sliding of filaments, and the I band region narrows.

4.8 THE SARCOMERE AND MYOFILAMENTS IN CONTRACTION

Parallel arrays of **thin filaments** span the **I band** and overlap **thick filaments** of the **A band.** A third filament system is made of single molecules of *titin,* one of the largest known proteins, that connects the **Z band** to the **M band.** Titin contains elastic elements that act as molecular springs and contribute to the passive elasticity of muscle. *Nebulin,* another giant protein, spans the length of thin filaments and forms a fourth filament system in skeletal muscle. At Z bands, thin filaments, nebulin, and titin are anchored to the protein α-*actinin.* Myosin molecules are polarized and have a globular head and a tail region. The globular head, or *S1 region,* contains an *ATPase* that facilitates binding to actin to move the head and produce a power stroke. Antiparallel association of **myosin** molecules forms thick filaments. In half of the thick fila-ment, myosin heads are oriented in one direction; those in the other half are in the opposite direction. The tails of the myosin molecules overlap, which yields a bare central shaft. Each thick filament is 1.6 μm long and 15 nm in diameter. Each thin fila-ment, about 1 μm long and 5 nm in diameter, consists of a double helix of filamentous **actin.** Two proteins associated with actin, **tropomyosin** and the **troponin** complex, respond to varying *calcium ion* concentrations by acting as a switch to enable or disable the interaction and formation of *cross bridges* between actin and the myosin heads. Myosin heads bind to actin and draw the thin filament a short distance past the thick filament. Then, linkages break and re-form farther along the thin filament to repeat the process. Filaments are thus pulled past each other in a ratchet-like action.

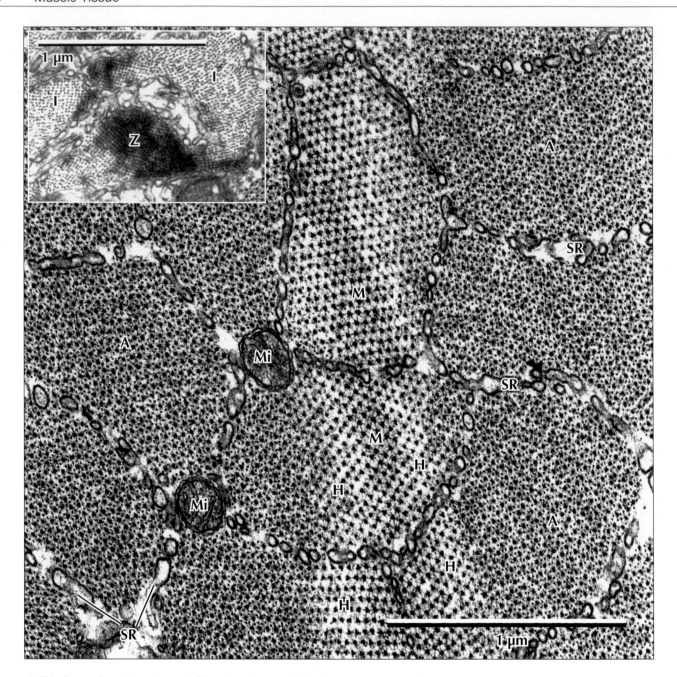

▲ **EM of part of a skeletal muscle fiber showing myofibrils in transverse section.** Tubular components of the sarcoplasmic reticulum (**SR**) with intervening mitochondria (**Mi**) encircle myofibrils. The section passes through different parts of A bands of sarcomeres and shows an orderly arrrangement of myofilaments in each region (**A**, the thick and thin filament overlap zone; **H**; **M**). 63,000×. The inset shows the square lattice pattern of the Z band (**Z**) and associated thin filaments in nearby I band (**I**). 45,000×.

4.9 ULTRASTRUCTURE OF SKELETAL MYOFILAMENTS IN TRANSVERSE SECTION

By high-magnification electron microscopy, transverse sections reveal the precise arrangement of two sets of myofilaments at different levels of the sarcomere. Myofilaments in cross section are electron-dense, punctate profiles; the diameter of **thick filaments** is more than twice that of **thin filaments.** Cross sections of I bands show only thin filaments, whereas **A bands** show both thick and thin filaments, which appear as hexagonal networks with myosin fixed at the **M band.** Where the two sets of filaments overlap, the networks mesh so that each thick filament is in the center of a hexagon made of six neighboring thin filaments. The interval between thick and thin filaments in the double hexagonal array is 10-20 nm. Regularly spaced globular heads of the myosin cross bridges radiate from each thick filament toward the thin filaments; however, cross bridges are not well resolved by routine electron microscopy, so thick filaments show a roughened surface. In pale **H zones,** the central segment of each thick filament lacks cross bridges. M bands, which are in the center of the H zones, show thick filaments with fine interconnections. **Z bands** in cross section show a typical square lattice pattern, and thin filaments in the immediate vicinity are organized in a regular array.

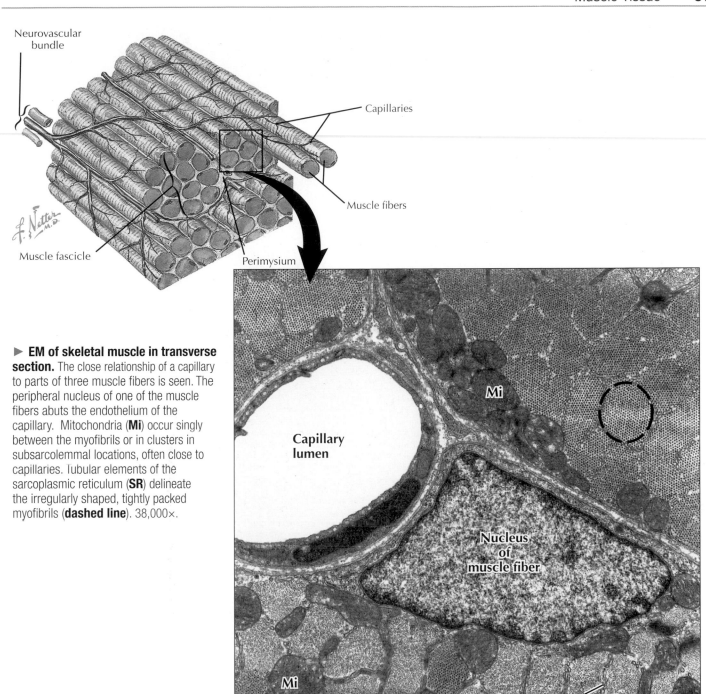

Neurovascular bundle

Capillaries

Muscle fibers

Muscle fascicle

Perimysium

► **EM of skeletal muscle in transverse section.** The close relationship of a capillary to parts of three muscle fibers is seen. The peripheral nucleus of one of the muscle fibers abuts the endothelium of the capillary. Mitochondria (**Mi**) occur singly between the myofibrils or in clusters in subsarcolemmal locations, often close to capillaries. Tubular elements of the sarcoplasmic reticulum (**SR**) delineate the irregularly shaped, tightly packed myofibrils (**dashed line**). 38,000×.

Mi

Capillary lumen

Nucleus of muscle fiber

Mi

SR

1 µm

4.10 INTRINSIC BLOOD SUPPLY OF SKELETAL MUSCLE

Because of their high O_2 consumption and energy requirements, skeletal muscles are richly vascularized. **Arteries** supplying and **veins** draining blood usually enter a muscle with the nerves and together are called a **neurovascular bundle**. Main **distributing** (or **muscular**) **arteries** typically pierce the epimysium and course longitudinally within the connective tissue of the **perimysium** to form a radiating pattern of collateral branches. They become progressively smaller, bifurcate, and give rise to **arterioles** that run in the **endomysium** within **muscle fascicles**. **Capillaries** emanating from the terminal arterioles are in close contact with surfaces of muscle fibers in a plane parallel to the longitudinal axis of the fibers and form a richly anastomosing network of vascular loops. Electron microscopy shows most capillaries to be the tight nonfenestrated type, although occasional fenestrated capillaries are seen. Different muscles, as well as muscles of trained versus untrained athletes, show marked variations in capillary density. *Type I* muscle fibers also have a higher capillary density than *type II* fibers. **Lymphatic vessels** are seen only in the perimysium and epimysium.

Histochemical and Functional Classification

Fiber Type	ATPase Stain (pH 9.4)	SDH Stain
IIB. Fast-twitch, Fatiguable, Glycolytic, White Stains deeply for myofibrillar ATPase at alkaline pH, poorly for succinate dehydrogenase (SDH)	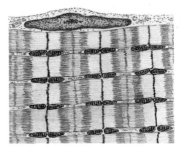	
IIA. Fast-twitch, Fatigue-resistant, Intermediate Stains deeply for both myofibrillar ATPase at alkaline pH and SDH		
I. Slow-twitch, Fatigue-resistant, Red Stains poorly for myofibrillar ATPase at alkaline pH but deeply for SDH		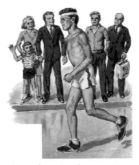

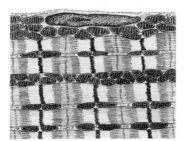

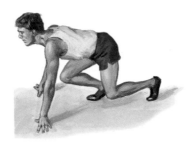

Type I: Dark or red fiber. Large profuse mitochondria beneath sarcolemma and in rows as well as paired in interfibrillar regions. Z bands wider than in type II.

Type II: Light or white skeletal muscle fiber in longitudinal section on electron microscopy. Small, relatively sparse mitochondria, chiefly paired in interfibrillar spaces at Z bands.

Sprinter
Type IIB fibers predominate

Marathon (endurance) runner
Types I and IIA fibers predominate

4.11 SKELETAL MUSCLE FIBER TYPES

Skeletal muscles contain various fiber types specialized for particular tasks. Most muscles contain a mixture of fiber types, with one type usually predominating. Muscle fibers have a typical mosaic pattern when examined histochemically, and fiber typing via histochemical and immunocytochemical staining has clinical significance for health and disease and is done routinely for both diagnosis and treatment. Sections are obtained by *muscle biopsy,* a rather simple procedure. Fiber typing is also used to determine functional properties of a particular muscle on the basis of the distribution and percentage of fiber types. Postural muscles, for example, have a higher percentage of **type I fibers** for endurance, whereas high-power output muscles have a higher percentage of **type II fibers.** Genetic differences in the same muscle group pre-dispose people to a preference for certain types of activity. Marathon runners have more **type IIA fibers** than power lifters, who have a higher percentage of **type IIB fibers.** The plasticity of muscle in response to exercise pattern is clearly shown by a shift in metabolic properties. Training can change the percentage of fiber types, mostly in one direction; training for marathons, for example, produces more type IIA fibers. Physiotherapists determine how to train a muscle on the basis of knowing the function of a muscle and the percentage of its fiber types. For example, the transversus abdominis, a postural or stabilizer muscle, would be trained with a low-force, high-endurance activity. Power muscles such as the biceps would be trained with high force or load and a low number of repetitions.

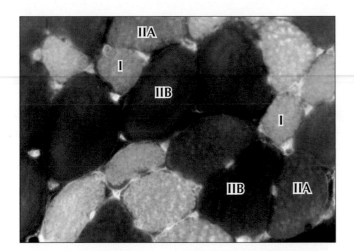

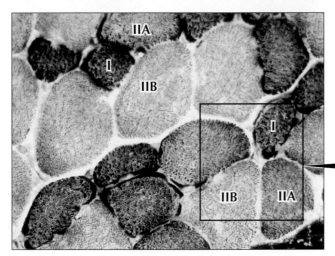

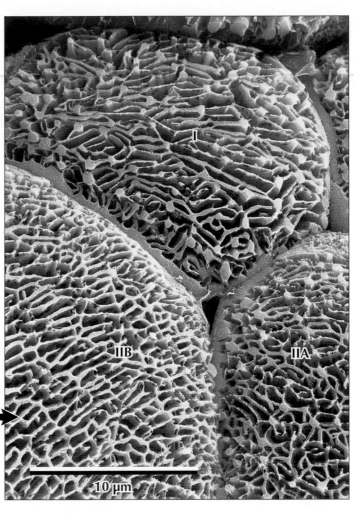

▲ **Serial transverse frozen sections of skeletal muscle.** These sections were treated histochemically to detect activities of myofibrillar ATPase at pH 9.4 (**top**) and SDH (**bottom**). These staining methods clearly demonstrate fiber types. Type I fibers are small and correspond to slow oxidative fibers. Type IIA are intermediate and are fast, oxidative-glycolytic fibers. Type IIB are white, fast, glycolytic fibers. 370×.

▲ **HRSEM of the three fiber types of skeletal muscle in transverse section.** After cytosol extraction, whereby myofilaments are selectively removed, the delicate honeycomb pattern of the sarcotubular system and mitochondria surrounding myofibrillar spaces is revealed. Differences in the content and distribution of these membranous organelles are seen in the three types. 4500×.

4.12 HISTOCHEMISTRY AND ULTRASTRUCTURE OF SKELETAL MUSCLE FIBER TYPES

In humans, at least three types of muscle fibers can be distinguished within each muscle on the basis of functional, metabolic, and ultrastructural features. Small-diameter **type I, or red, fibers** are *aerobic*, slowly contracting, very resistant to fatigue, and capable of long and continued activity. They have a high content of **mitochondria** and *myoglobin*, low *glycogen* content, and low *myofibrillar ATPase* activity. Large numbers of these fibers are found in muscles used for aerobic activities requiring low force production, such as walking and maintaining posture. **Type IIB, or white, fibers** are anaerobic, contract rapidly, and are very sensitive to *fatigue*. They have low mitochondrial density and *oxidative*

enzyme activity but high myofibrillar ATPase and *phosphorylase* activity. They are used for short *anaerobic* and high force production activities such as jumping and sprinting. **Type IIA, or intermediate, fibers** show fast contraction, moderate resistance to fatigue, medium mitochondrial density, and high *glycolytic* and oxidative enzyme activity. They are used for prolonged anaerobic activities with a relatively high force output, such as racing 400 m. Histochemical fiber type diversity is mostly based on the differential expression pattern of specific *isoforms* of myofibrillar and other related proteins. Ultrastructural features that also distinguish fiber types include density and spatial distribution of mitochondria, sarcomere banding patterns, and organization of the **sarcotubular system.**

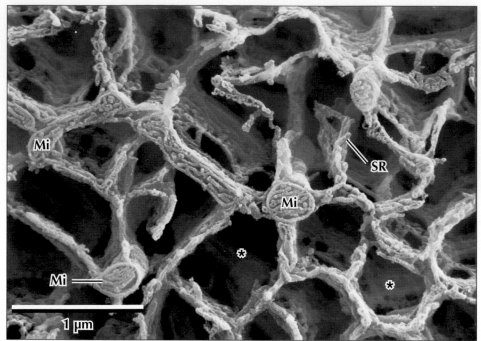

◀ **HRSEM of part of a type IIA (intermediate) fiber fractured in the transverse plane.** An extensive tubular network made of the **SR** embraces the polygonal myofibrillar spaces (★), which appear empty because of myofilament extraction. Mitochondria (**Mi**), seen in both longitudinal and transverse planes, are fractured open to reveal internal cristae. 35,000×.

▶ **HRSEM of part of a type IIA (intermediate) fiber fractured in the longitudinal plane.** A highly anastomosing, uniformly sized, tubular network of A band (**A**) and I band (**I**) sarcoplasmic reticulum is revealed at the level of a sarcomere. A triad, shown at the A-I junction (**circle**), consists of a central T tubule and two terminal cisternae of the SR. The mitochondrion (**Mi**) in this fiber is elongated, pleomorphic, and branched. It is closely surrounded by elements of the sarco-tubular system. Note a small bridge of SR (**arrow**) connecting the two terminal cisternae in the region of A-I junction. Myofilaments in the muscle fiber were selectively extracted by the preparation procedure. 34,000×.

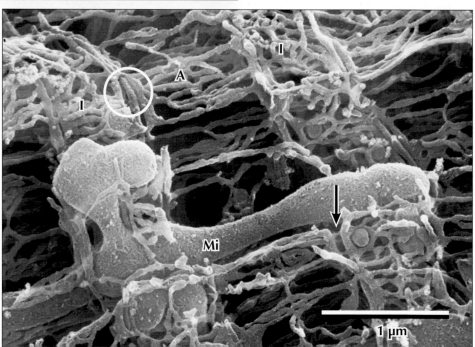

4.13 HIGH-RESOLUTION SCANNING ELECTRON MICROSCOPY OF SKELETAL MUSCLE

Because tightly packed myofibrils predominate in the **muscle fiber** sarcoplasm, appreciation of the spatial relationship of the other, noncontractile components of the cell is difficult with conventional two-dimensional electron microscopy. *High-resolution scanning electron microscopy*, in combination with selective cytosol extraction and *freeze fracture* of muscle fibers, provides novel views of a cell interior with a greater depth of field. This methodology selectively removes myofibrils, which often obscure other organelles in the sarcoplasm, but leaves membranous components of the muscle fiber intact. Examination of high-resolution scanning electron microscopy specimens clarifies the three-dimensional arrangement and distribution of **mitochondria** and elements of the **sarcotubular system** inside a fiber. Subtle differences in internal architecture of the three types of skeletal muscle fibers, which reflect functional diversity, are also revealed. Mitochondria in **type I fibers** are usually larger, more numerous, and more highly branched than those in **type II fibers,** in which mitochondria are thinner, simpler in structure, and more cylindrical. These variations most likely reflect differences in energy demand and utilization of fiber types. The density, arrangement, and distribution of the sarcotubular system also vary in fiber types. A more highly developed and extensive SR in type II (fast-twitch) fibers than in type I (slow-twitch) fibers correlates with speeds of contraction and relaxation.

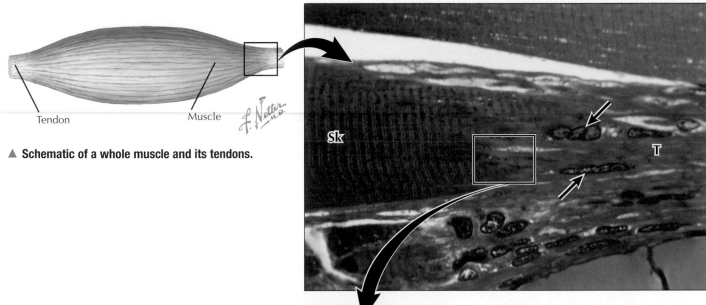

▲ Schematic of a whole muscle and its tendons.

▲ **LM of the muscle-tendon junction in longitudinal section.** At the tapering end of a skeletal muscle fiber, terminal finger-like extensions of the muscle fiber (**Sk**) insert into the dense regular connective tissue of the tendon (**T**). Fibroblasts (**arrows**) are interspersed with regularly arranged collagen fibers in the tendon. 840×. *Toluidine blue, plastic section.*

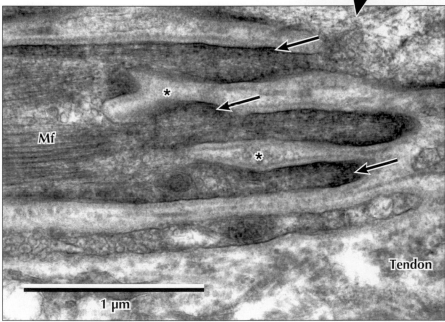

▲ **EM of the muscle-tendon junction in longitudinal section.** The end of a muscle fiber splits into several villus-like terminal projections, which contain a network of myofilaments (**Mf**) that run toward subsarcolemmal densities (**arrows**). The sarcolemma is highly indented and invested by a prominent external lamina. Extracellular clefts (∗) invaginate the sarcolemma of the fiber. Collagen fibrils of the adjacent tendon penetrate intervillous clefts and are in close contact with the sarcolemma. 48,000×.

4.14 HISTOLOGY AND ULTRASTRUCTURE OF THE MUSCLE-TENDON JUNCTION

The muscle-tendon junction marks the end of the skeletal muscle fiber and its insertion into collagenous **connective tissue** of a tendon. It is an interface between two diverse yet interconnected tissues with a complicated communication system and a high shear component. Biomechanically, this area involves a concentration of *tensile forces* and marks a site of abrupt change in the *modulus of elasticity,* which represents the point of maximum stress in this unit. Developmentally, it is the rapidly growing area of the muscle fiber during postnatal life. Light and electron microscopy can show that the interface between muscle and tendon is highly interdigitated and consists of branching finger-like extensions of **myofibrils** that interlock with projections of adjacent tendon—like the fingers of a hand inserted into a tight-fitting glove. The extensive infolding of the **sarcolemmal membrane** increases surface area, which enhances mechanical stability at the site of force transmission and in response to junctional stress. Specific membrane-associated proteins including *α-actinin, vinculin, talin,* and *integrins* are found at these sites. Muscle injuries often occur at or near the muscle-tendon junction. Immobilization reduces the tensile strength of the junction and predisposes it to *strain injuries.*

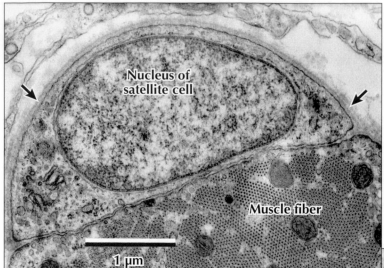

◄ **EM of a satellite cell in fetal skeletal muscle.** The euchromatic nucleus is typical of active, protein-synthesizing cells. The cytoplasm contains scattered free ribosomes, and a few profiles of rough and smooth endoplasmic reticulum. A narrow gap separates the cell from the underlying muscle fiber, where plasma membranes of the two cells are parallel to each other. The underlying muscle fiber contains tightly packed but poorly defined myofibrils and a few mitochondria. The satellite cell and muscle fiber share an external lamina (**arrows**). 24,000×.

▶ **EM of a satellite cell in adult skeletal muscle.** The cell sits on the surface of a mature muscle fiber. They share a thin, common external lamina (**arrows**). The narrow space between their apposed membranes is difficult to distinguish at this magnification. The cytoplasm contains a sparse collection of mitochondria, rough endoplasmic reticulum, and free ribosomes. Well-defined myofibrils with intervening elements of sarcoplasmic reticulum and mitochondria characterize the underlying muscle fiber. 24,000×.

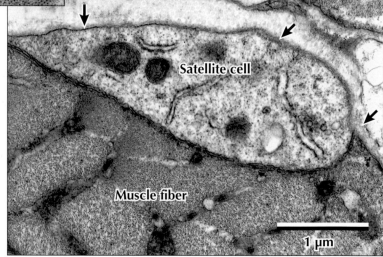

4.15   STRUCTURE AND FUNCTION OF SATELLITE CELLS

Satellite cells are small, flattened mononucleated cells located between the sarcolemma of a skeletal muscle fiber and the **external lamina.** The close location of these cells to the surface of a fiber, with an intervening space of about 15 nm, makes them identifiable by electron microscopy or by immunocytochemical staining and molecular markers. Satellite cells serve as a population of reserve stem cells, or resting myoblasts, either for normal postnatal growth or for *repair* and *regeneration* of damaged segments of the skeletal muscle fiber after injury. They are most abundant during early development and growth. Also, more satellite cells occur in slow-twitch muscles than in fast-twitch muscles. Although the cells are normally quiescent in adults and their numbers and *mitotic capacity* decline with age, they have proliferative potential throughout life, and they increase in number in response to *denervation,* in mildly traumatized muscle, and in regenerating diseased muscle. They typically have a high nucleus-to-cytoplasm ratio. A single **nucleus** contains clumped peripheral *heterochromatin;* the cytoplasm normally contains a paucity of organelles. Free **ribosomes,** scattered small **mitochondria,** occa-

sional **rough endoplasmic reticulum,** and Golgi complex are the only distinguishing features. Activation of satellite cells after *muscle injury* leads to cell *proliferation,* followed by *differentiation* and *fusion* to either form new muscle fibers or repair damaged ones. Advances in our knowledge of satellite cell dynamics hold promise for progress in treatment of diseases, such as *muscular dystrophy,* that affect skeletal muscle.

CLINICAL POINT
Myotonic dystrophy is a rare hereditary disorder characterized by progressive weakness and wasting of skeletal muscle, accompanied by delayed relaxation after contraction *(myotonia).* The most common adult muscular dystrophy, it often occurs in early adulthood and has an extremely variable degree of severity. Other features are mental retardation, cardiac disease, hair loss, and cataracts. The gene associated with myotonic dystrophy is on the long arm of chromosome 19 and encodes for a protein kinase normally found in skeletal muscle, where it most likely has a regulatory role. Although the etiology of this disorder remains enigmatic, a cell membrane defect is suspected as the major cause.

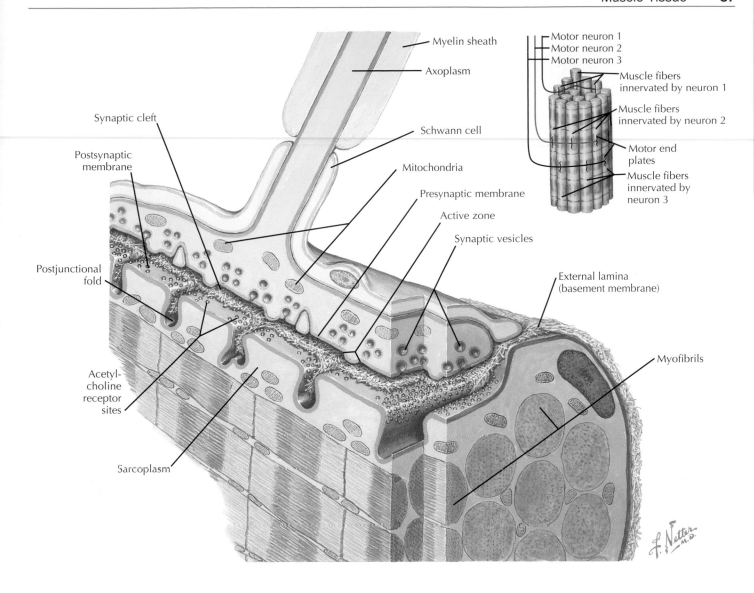

4.16 ORGANIZATION OF NEUROMUSCULAR JUNCTIONS

Skeletal muscle is under direct control of the **voluntary,** or somatic, **nervous system.** A motor nerve terminates on the surface of a muscle fiber at a specialized site—the **neuromuscular junction (motor endplate).** This site is the synaptic contact between the motor axon and the muscle fiber. Histologic visualization of motor endplates requires special techniques, the best being electron microscopy. As the motor axon approaches the sarcolemma of the muscle fiber, it loses a **myelin sheath** but retains an investment of the terminal **Schwann cell.** Several branches of the axon terminal emanate from the parent axon to end on the muscle fiber. Each bulbous **axon terminal** sits in a trough or depression on the muscle fiber surface called the **synaptic trough,** in which lie acetylcholine receptor sites. A narrow, intervening intercellular space—the **primary synaptic cleft**—separates the plasma membrane of the axon terminal from the sarcolemma of the muscle fiber. At the site of the junction, the highly folded sarcolemma of the muscle fiber forms **postjunctional folds** (also called secondary synaptic clefts or subneural apparatus) that markedly increase the surface area of the muscle fiber. The **external lamina** of the muscle fiber fuses with that of the terminal Schwann cell and extends into synaptic clefts. The subsarcolemmal sarcoplasm is replete with **mitochondria,** free ribosomes, and rough endoplasmic reticulum. Nuclei and a prominent Golgi complex also occur in this part of the muscle cell.

CLINICAL POINT

Myasthenia gravis is the most common hereditary disorder of neuromuscular transmission, but this *autoimmune* disease most often results from an acquired immunologic abnormality. Symptom onset commonly occurs after the age of 30 years in women and somewhat later in men. Muscle weakness often fluctuates but is usually progressive. In the acquired disorder, a distortion of the postsynaptic sarcolemmal membrane of the neuromuscular junction is accompanied by a reduction in the concentration of acetylcholine receptors. Antibodies are attached to the postsynaptic membrane, which makes it less sensitive to acetylcholine and leads to a reduced muscle action potential in response to a nerve impulse.

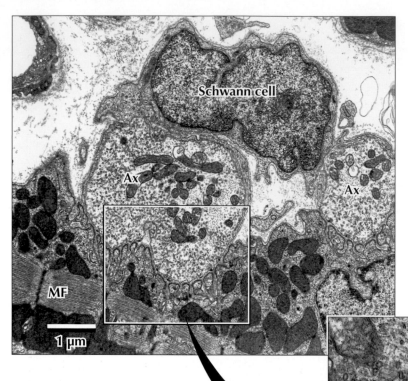

◀ **EM of a neuromuscular junction in skeletal muscle.** Processes of a Schwann cell cover external aspects of two axon terminals (**Ax**), which end close to the corrugated surface of a muscle fiber (**MF**). Mitochondria and smaller synaptic vesicles are clustered in the axon terminals. The postjunctional sarcoplasm contains abundant mitochondria and a nearby nucleus of the muscle fiber. 12,000×.

▶ **EM of part of a neuromuscular junction in skeletal muscle at higher magnification.** The axon terminal contains abundant membrane-bound synaptic vesicles, many in the region of the presynaptic membrane. Mitochondria (**Mi**) are also plentiful in the terminal axoplasm, as well as in the underlying sarcoplasm of the muscle fiber. The underlying postsynaptic region of the junction contains numerous infoldings of the muscle fiber sarcolemma. Both primary (**Pr**) and secondary (**Se**) synaptic clefts contain a thin external lamina (**arrow**) between the presynaptic and postsynaptic areas of the junction. 35,000×.

4.17 ULTRASTRUCTURE OF NEUROMUSCULAR JUNCTIONS

The neuromuscular junction has five principal components. First, a **Schwann cell** process forms a cap above the nerve terminal; here, it does not face the synaptic region. Second, the **axon terminal,** which is devoid of myelin, contains many clear, rounded **synaptic vesicles** filled with the *neurotransmitter acetylcholine.* These membrane-bound vesicles are 50-60 nm in diameter and are concentrated near the **presynaptic membrane** in regions known as *active zones.* Acetylcholine is stored in the vesicles and released by *exocytosis.* Recycling of vesicles by *endocytosis* occurs after neurotransmitter release. Neurofilaments, microtubules, smooth endoplasmic reticulum, lysosomes, scattered glycogen particles, and **mitochondria** occupy other regions of the axon terminal. The third component is the **synaptic cleft,** which is a narrow space between nerve terminal and muscle fiber surface, about 70 nm wide. It consists of a primary cleft and several smaller secondary clefts at right angles to it. The synaptic cleft is lined by a basement membrane, which plays a role in development and regeneration of the neuromuscular junction. The fourth component is the **postsynaptic membrane** of the muscle fiber, which contains intramembrane particles that can be revealed by freeze-fracture techniques. These particles contain *nicotinic receptors* for acetylcholine. The fifth component is the **postjunctional sarcoplasm** of the muscle fiber, which is critical for structural and metabolic support of the junction.

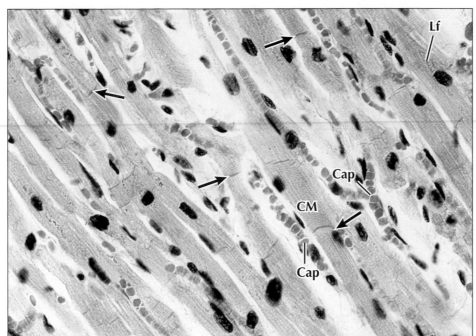

◄ **Longitudinal section of cardiac muscle.**
Cardiac muscle fibers (**CM**) are branched and
contain a single, centrally placed nucleus. In
some cells, lipofuscin (**Lf**) pigment is concentrated at the nuclear poles. The cells
are eosinophilic and possess cross-striations.
Cells are linked by intercalated discs (**arrows**),
which appear as dark, jagged transverse lines
between the cells or their branches. Numerous
capillaries (**Cap**) in surrounding connective tissue
form an extensive, branching network. Lying
close to the muscle fibers, many capillaries
can be identified by erythrocyte content.
475×. *H&E.*

▶ **Transverse section of cardiac muscle.**
The irregularly shaped cardiac muscle cells
(**CM**) are grouped in bundles and surrounded
by richly vascularized connective tissue. When
in the plane of section, nuclei occupy a central
position in the cells. An arteriole (**A**) filled with
erythrocytes occupies the interstitial connective
tissue. Smooth muscle (**SM**) is seen in the wall
of the arteriole 440×. *H&E.*

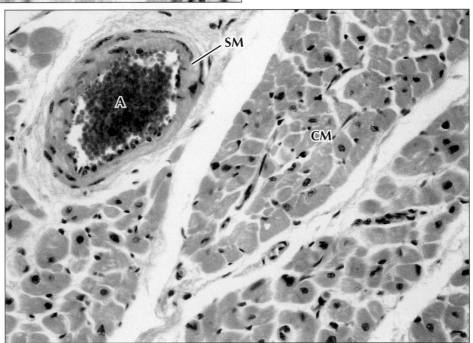

4.18 HISTOLOGY OF CARDIAC MUSCLE

Cardiac muscle is striated, involuntary muscle in the **myocardium** whose cells are similar to those of skeletal muscle. Cardiac muscle cells, also known as **myocytes (myocardial cells),** have the same basic organization as skeletal muscle—myofibrils, myofilaments, and cross striations—and a primarily contractile function. Measuring 10-20 μm in diameter and 80-100 μm long, the cells are branched and joined end to end and side to side at specialized sites, unique to cardiac muscle, known as **intercalated discs.** Each cell has an **eosinophilic sarcoplasm** surrounding a single, centrally placed, ovoid **nucleus,** but occasional binucleated cells are seen. The nuclei are usually larger and more euchromatic than nuclei of skeletal muscle fibers. Cardiac muscle fibers are orga-nized in a complex, three-dimensional, spiral arrangement of layers and form an intercommunicating, anastomosing network of contiguous cells. When they contract in synchrony, blood is expelled from the heart chambers and forced into systemic, pulmonary, and coronary vascular circuits. In transverse section, cardiac muscle fibers are closely apposed; they have irregular cellular outlines with cross-sectional profiles of various sizes. Because the cells are long-lived, with advancing age they accumulate **lipofuscin,** a "wear-and-tear" pigment. Of the three kinds of muscle tissue, cardiac muscle is the most richly vascularized. Regeneration of cardiac muscle cells after injury does not readily occur, as no satellite cells are associated with the cells.

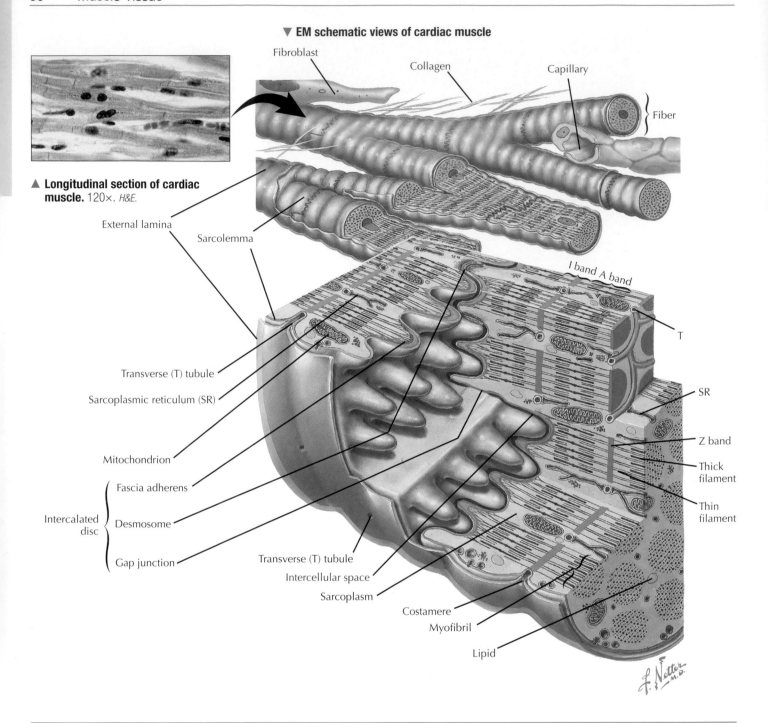

▼ EM schematic views of cardiac muscle

Fibroblast

Collagen

Capillary

Fiber

▲ Longitudinal section of cardiac muscle. 120×. *H&E.*

External lamina

Sarcolemma

I band A band

T

Transverse (T) tubule

Sarcoplasmic reticulum (SR)

SR

Z band

Thick filament

Mitochondrion

Thin filament

Fascia adherens

Intercalated disc

Desmosome

Gap junction

Transverse (T) tubule

Intercellular space

Sarcoplasm

Costamere

Myofibril

Lipid

4.19   ULTRASTRUCTURAL COMPONENTS OF CARDIAC MUSCLE

Cardiac muscle cells are cylindrical, with irregular ends, and are elongated in the direction of force generation. Numerous **capillaries,** bundles of **collagen,** and occasional **fibroblasts** separate them. Each cell is enveloped by a **plasma membrane,** or **sarcolemma,** covered by a thin **external lamina** (basement membrane). The size of cardiac muscle cells is intermediate between that of skeletal muscle cells and smooth muscle cells. Cardiac muscle cells have loose **myofilament** bundles, or **myofibrils,** and closely packed **mitochondria.** Myofibrils, like those in skeletal muscle, are the *contractile* parts of the cell. They are long and parallel and have a regular banding pattern. **Costameres** are sites at which **Z bands** of the outermost myofibrils contact the sarcolemma and

probably play a mechanical role. **Intercalated discs** join cardiac muscle cells where cell borders interdigitate in rectangular steps of irregular width and length. Discs are aggregates of three **junctional specializations: desmosomes** provide mechanical stability; **fascia adherentes** are sites of attachment and insertion of thin filaments of myofibrils. Both of these junctions are perpendicular to the longitudinal axis of a cell. **Gap junctions** are oriented parallel to the long axis. Many large mitochondria occupy a significant volume in the cell and are closely associated with **lipid** droplets and glycogen particles. The **sarcotubular system** consists of **transverse (T) tubules** and **SR.** T tubules, which are invaginations of the sarcolemma, surround myofibrils at Z band levels of the sarcomeres, whereas the SR forms an anastomosing network of tubules and thereby a sleeve around the myofibrils.

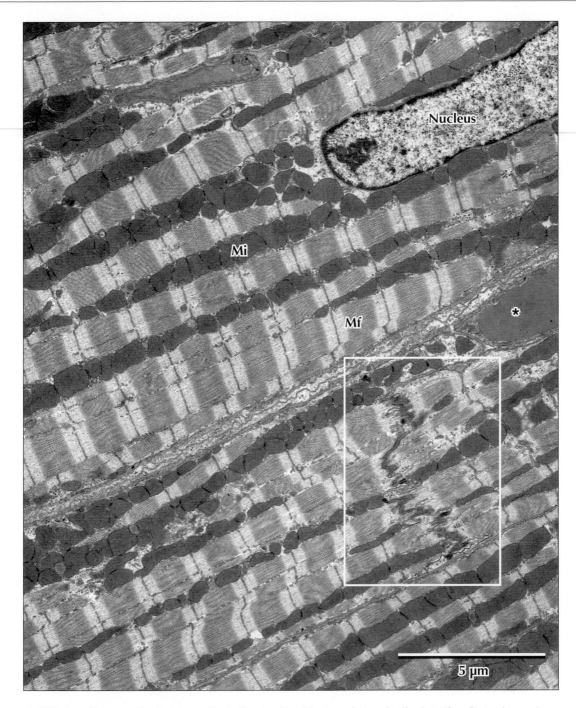

▲ **EM of cardiac muscle showing salient ultrastructural features in longitudinal section.** Parts of several cardiac muscle cells are seen here. A large, euchromatic nucleus with a prominent nucleolus has a central location. Numerous mitochondria (**Mi**) occupy intermyofibrillar spaces. Myofibrils (**Mf**) are not as linearly arranged as those in skeletal muscle fibers. Adjacent cardiac muscle cells are joined by intercalated discs (**boxed area**). A capillary (∗) contains an erythrocyte. 8000×.

4.20   ULTRASTRUCTURE OF CARDIAC MUSCLE IN LONGITUDINAL SECTION

Electron microscopy reveals the regularly repeating array of **myofibrils** and **mitochondria** of cardiac muscle fibers. The banding pattern of each fiber is similar to that of skeletal muscle, as is the *sliding filament mechanism* that causes cell *contraction*. Also as in skeletal muscle cells, in cardiac muscle cells the sarcomeres are the main functional unit of contraction, although they form branching columns instead of single columns of skeletal muscle myofibrils. A supporting network of intermediate filaments and microtubules helps maintain cell shape. Mitochondria are large, numerous, and arranged in continuous longitudinal rows between the irregularly shaped myofibrils. Mitochondria make up 20%-25% of the volume of the cells. Glycogen and lipid droplets, an important alternative energy source, are abundant in sarcoplasm and are also found, with Golgi complexes, at poles of centrally placed nuclei. Unlike skeletal muscle fibers, which are solitary and independent units, cardiac muscle cells are joined by **intercalated discs,** which mechanically and electrically link the cells and allow them to function in a coordinated way.

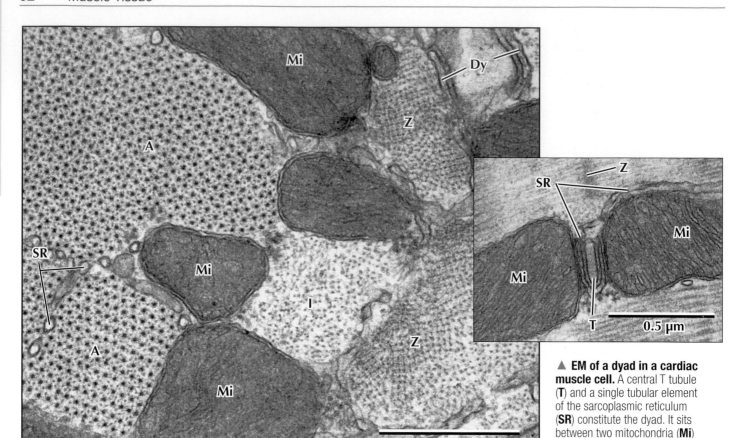

▲ **EM of a dyad in a cardiac muscle cell.** A central T tubule (**T**) and a single tubular element of the sarcoplasmic reticulum (**SR**) constitute the dyad. It sits between two mitochondria (**Mi**) and at the Z band (**Z**) of the sarcomere. 56,000×.

▲ **EM of part of a cardiac muscle cell in transverse section.** Several myofibrils are sectioned at different levels of the sarcomere. The overlap region of A bands (**A**) shows the typical double hexagonal array of thick and thin filaments, whereas the I band (**I**) contains only thin filaments. Z bands (**Z**) in cross section show a typical square lattice pattern. Large mitochondria (**Mi**) and sarcoplasmic reticulum (**SR**) tubules lie between myofibrils. Dyads (**Dy**), which are unique to cardiac muscle, sit at Z band levels. 74,000×.

4.21 ULTRASTRUCTURE OF CARDIAC MUSCLE IN TRANSVERSE SECTION

Actively contracting cardiac muscle is the most energy-demanding tissue in the body. Cardiac muscle cells have large **mitochondria** with tightly packed cristae. Mitochondria are seen along and between myofibrils, and their abundance reflects dependence on aerobic metabolism and a continuous need for ATP. Cardiac muscle, like skeletal muscle, shows an orderly arrangement of **thick (myosin)** and **thin (actin) filaments,** plus unique isoforms of the regulatory proteins *troponin* and *tropomyosin*. Thin filaments are anchored to **Z bands,** which demarcate each **sarcomere.** Sarcomere contraction involves interaction of myosin and actin initiated by calcium binding to troponin C. Stimulation of *ATPase* activity in the myosin head produces force along actin filaments. As in skeletal muscle, *excitation-contraction coupling* involves a **sarcotubular system** that is closely associated with **myofibrils. Transverse (T) tubule** diameters are larger than those in skeletal muscle. These tubules, like those in skeletal muscle fibers, penetrate muscle fiber interiors at regular intervals and rapidly transmit action potentials to inner cell cores. Rather than forming triads with the SR, a T tubule in cardiac muscle contacts a single tubular component of the SR to form a two-component junctional coupling—a **dyad.** Dyads sit at Z band levels of sarcomeres, with a 15-nm gap between the apposing membranes of the SR and T tubule. **Junctional end-feet** are not as abundant as those in skeletal muscle.

CLINICAL POINT

Hypertrophic cardiomyopathy is a primary disorder of the myocardium and often produces sudden cardiac death. It is most often a familial disorder (55%), with autosomal dominant transmission. It is caused by mutations in genes encoding sarcomeric proteins, including β-myosin heavy chain, myosin binding protein C, and cardiac troponins, the result being defective contraction. Abnormal growth and hypertrophy of cardiac muscle cells lead to ventricular wall thickening, with myocytes in disarray instead of showing a normal arrangement. Focal myocardial ischemia frequently produces anginal pain. The interstitium shows variable fibrosis that can result in impaired cardiac conduction.

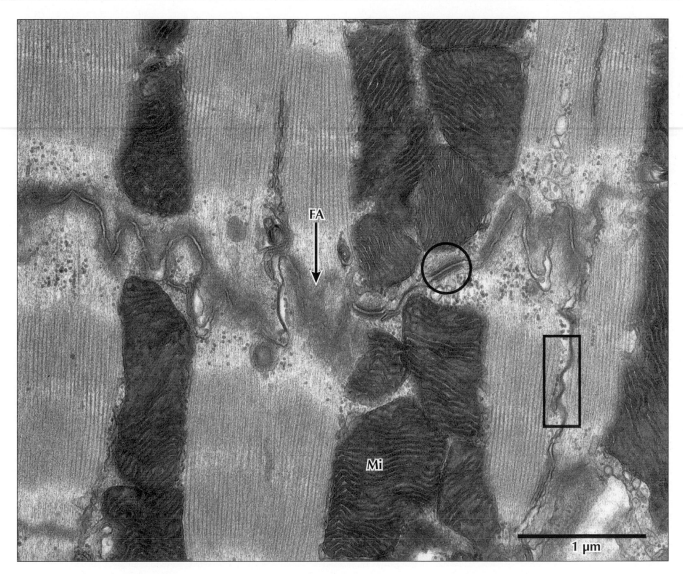

▲ **EM of an intercalated disc, showing its stepwise configuration, with transverse and longitudinal portions.** Fascia adherentes (**FA**) and desmosomes (**circle**) are seen in transverse parts of the disc, whereas gap junctions (**rectangle**) are in the longitudinal part. Adjoining myocytes contain mitochondria (**Mi**) with tightly packed cristae. 34,000×.

4.22 ULTRASTRUCTURE OF INTERCALATED DISCS

Intercalated discs of cardiac muscle cells are anchors that contain three main types of special junctions where cells and their branches meet end-to-end; the discs have the appearance of steps in a stair-case. **Gap junctions,** in longitudinal areas of the disc, where apposing sarcolemmal membranes are parallel to the long axis of the cells, chemically and electrically couple neighboring **myocytes** to facilitate spread of excitation in the myocardium. They allow chains of individual cells to act as a syncytium so that the contraction signal passes quickly from cell to cell. **Fascia adherentes,** in transverse parts of the disc that are subject to mechanical stress, connect the actin **cytoskeleton** and terminal I band filaments to the sarcolemma. They are unique to cardiac muscle cells. *N-cadherin,* a transmembrane protein, links the sarcolemmal membrane to the contractile apparatus at these sites and stabilizes attachments of myofibrils to muscle terminals. **Desmosomes,** in transverse areas of the disc, attach intermediate filaments to muscle terminals and prevent the constantly contracting cells from being pulled apart. The disc serves three main functions: cellular adhesion, electrical and ionic cell coupling, and transmission of tension and contraction from cell to cell.

CLINICAL POINT

In familial **dilated cardiomyopathy** (DCM), a heritable form of heart failure, mutations exist in cytoskeletal proteins that disrupt intercalated disc morphology by dissociating junctions between myocytes and disrupting myofibrillar organization and contractile function. DCM is the most common type of cardiomyopathy, in which there is stretching of disease-affected myocytes, which leads to enlargement of one or more chambers of the heart and thinning of ventricular walls. These changes progressively weaken the heart's pumping ability. Usually, DCM is idiopathic, is most common in middle age, and occurs more in men than in women.

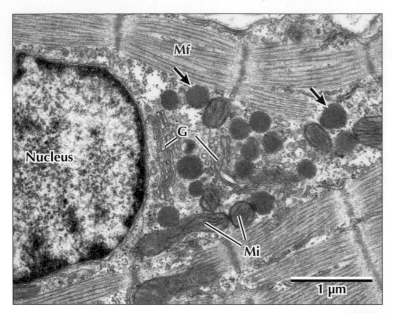

◀ **EM of an atrial cardiac muscle cell.** The sarcoplasm next to the nucleus contains well-developed Golgi complexes (**G**), free ribosomes, and scattered mitochondria (**Mi**). A collection of moderately electron-dense, membrane-bound specific granules (**arrows**) lies in the area of the Golgi complex. Myofibrils (**Mf**) occupy other areas of the cell, some close to the sarcolemma (**top**). 21,000×.

▶ **Higher magnification EM of an atrial cardiac muscle cell next to a capillary.** Several atrial-specific granules (**straight arrows**) lie between a Golgi complex (**G**) and the sarcolemma (**S**) of the cell. Most are moderately electron dense; one (**curved arrow**) appears to have just released its contents into the extracellular space. The endothelium (**E**) of the capillary (**Cap**) is linked by tight junctions (**circles**) and contains many pinocytotic vesicles and a Weibel-Palade body (**WP**), a bundle of microtubules. 27,000×.

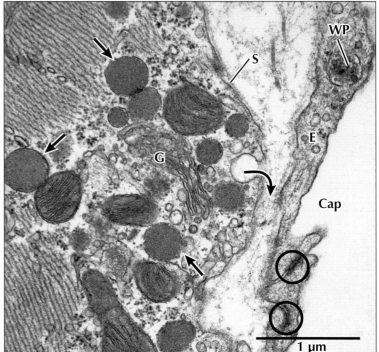

4.23 ULTRASTRUCTURE OF ATRIAL MYOCYTES

In addition to a role in *contraction* to enable the heart to operate as a mechanical pump, cardiac muscle cells in the **atrial** wall are specialized to synthesize and secrete a *hormone* with diverse biologic functions. Known as *atrial natriuretic hormone,* this potent *polypeptide* has a critical role in cardiovascular *homeostasis*, blood pressure regulation, and fluid-electrolyte balance. It promotes *natriuresis* (sodium excretion) and *diuresis* (excretion of urine). A conspicuous electron microscopic feature of the juxtanuclear region of these cells is the presence of distinctive membrane-bound, electron-dense vesicles known as *atrial-specific granules.* Most numerous in myocytes of the right atrium, these sites store the precursor of the hormone, also known as *atrial natriuretic*

peptide (ANP). These rounded organelles are 300-500 nm in diameter, are derived from the formative (trans) face of the **Golgi complex,** and are closely associated with profiles of rough endoplasmic reticulum. The granules are released by *exocytosis* when cells are stretched. Vesicles are transported to the cell surface, where their membranes fuse with the **sarcolemma** to discharge the contents into extracellular spaces. The prohormone is then converted to its active form before it reaches the circulation in nearby **capillaries.** Circulating ANP increases *glomerular filtration* and promotes sodium excretion by acting on collecting ducts in the kidney. The hormone has beneficial effects: it is important in compensation for *congestive heart failure,* with its vasodilating, natriuretic, and antiproliferative properties.

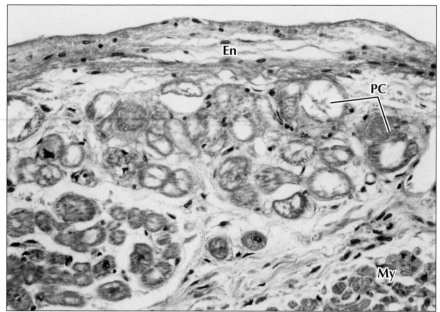

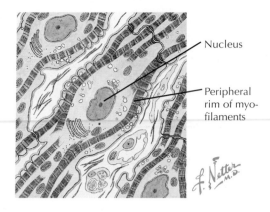

▲ Schematic of an EM of a Purkinje fiber.

▲ **LM of Purkinje fibers in the heart in transverse section.** The cells (**PC**) lie between the endocardium (**En**) and myocardium (**My**) of the interventricular septum. Purkinje fibers are larger and paler than ordinary myocytes. 300×. *H&E.*

▶ **EM of Purkinje fibers in transverse section.** A group of four apposed Purkinje cell profiles sits close to the endothelium (**E**) lining the heart chamber (⋆). In cross section, profiles of the cells have an irregular shape; neighboring cells appear to interlock like overlapping pieces of a jigsaw puzzle. Scattered myofibrils (**Mf**) and numerous mitochondria (**Mi**), many of which occur in clumps, occupy the cytoplasm. The surrounding connective tissue (**CT**) contains scattered cells and collagen fibers. 6500×.

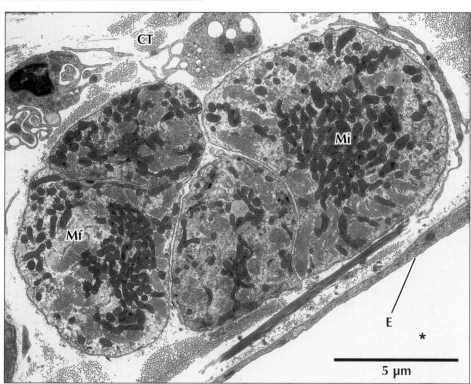

4.24 HISTOLOGY AND ULTRASTRUCTURE OF PURKINJE FIBERS

Purkinje fibers, which are formed of modified cardiac muscle cells, are scattered along the innermost part of the myocardium adjacent to the endocardium. They are found especially in the interventricular septum, organized into discrete bundles and embedded in connective tissue. Part of the cardiac conduction system, these fibers are specialized for conduction of electrical impulses. Purkinje fibers are larger and thicker than ordinary cardiac muscle cells and have scattered myofibrils around the cell periphery. A notable feature is the presence of various amounts of glycogen in the sarcoplasm around the centrally placed nucleus. Purkinje fibers thus appear pale and washed-out in routine H&E

sections. Their electron microscopic characteristics are consistent with their role in rapid impulse conduction. Sparse, disorganized myofilament bundles are located under the sarcolemma. Mitochondria, an important energy source in addition to glycogen, are a dominant and typical feature. Purkinje fibers have an unusually well-developed cytoskeleton, which consists mainly of desmin-containing intermediate filaments. The sarcoplasm contains various numbers of lipid droplets but lacks a transverse tubular (T) system. Intercalated discs are not common, but at least two kinds of intercellular junctions link neighboring Purkinje fibers: desmosomes promote cell adhesion, and extensive gap junctions permit intercellular communication.

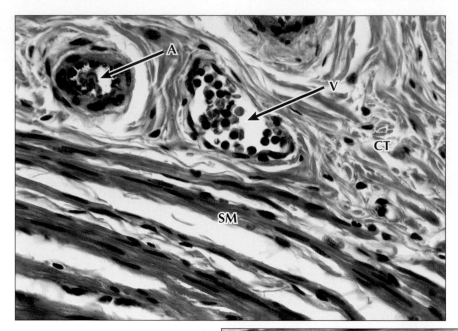

◀ **LM of the wall of the ureter showing organization of vascular and visceral smooth muscle.** A small arteriole (**A**), seen in transverse section, contains a layer of vascular smooth muscle cells in its wall. An accompanying venule (**V**) is in the surrounding connective tissue (**CT**). For comparison, a bundle of visceral smooth muscle cells (**SM**) in the wall of the ureter is shown in longitudinal section. Cell borders are difficult to distinguish because cells are packed tightly and bound together by connective tissue. Their nuclei conform to the elongated, spindle-like shape of the cells. 435×. *H&E.*

▶ **LM of smooth muscle in the wall of the appendix.** Two aggregate layers of smooth muscle occupy the field of view. Longitudinal (**LS**) and cross-sectional (**XS**) profiles of smooth muscle cells show their characteristic appearance. Because of the staggered arrangement of the cells, cross-sectional profiles vary in size, and only the largest profiles contain sections of nuclei. A small myenteric plexus (**MP**) of autonomic nerve fibers is situated between the two layers of smooth muscle. 480×. *H&E.*

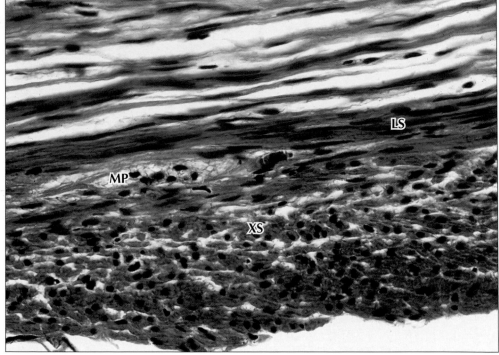

4.25   HISTOLOGY OF SMOOTH MUSCLE

Smooth muscle lacks striations and, as its activity is not under conscious control, is an *involuntary muscle.* It is found in walls of hollow tubes, sacs, and internal viscera. Although it represents only about 2% of adult body weight, smooth muscle is one of the most ubiquitous tissues. As **visceral smooth muscle,** it regulates the luminal caliber of many hollow organs. Also, because of its presence in blood vessel walls, where it is known as **vascular smooth muscle,** it ultimately controls functions of all organs and organ systems. Smooth muscle cells, through *contraction* and *relaxation,* regulate physiologic functions such as digestion, respiration, reproduction, and blood flow. Smooth muscle consists of **mononucleated cells** that have a relatively simple cytoplasmic structure. The cells are elongated and tapering, with a relatively homogeneous, **eosinophilic** cytoplasm. The single **nucleus** is found in the widest part of the cell. In contracted cells, the nucleus looks wrinkled or pleated; in relaxed cells the nucleus is more elongated. Smooth muscle cells have a smaller diameter, usually 3-10 µm, than skeletal muscle fibers. Cell length varies: cells are shortest in walls of blood vessels, at 20 µm long, and much longer in the pregnant uterus, where they may be up to 500 µm long. They rarely occur as isolated fibers but are organized either as sheets, with cells arranged in parallel, or as aggregated bundles oriented in different directions. To achieve closest packing, adjacent cells overlap in a staggered fashion and are bound together by **loose connective tissue.**

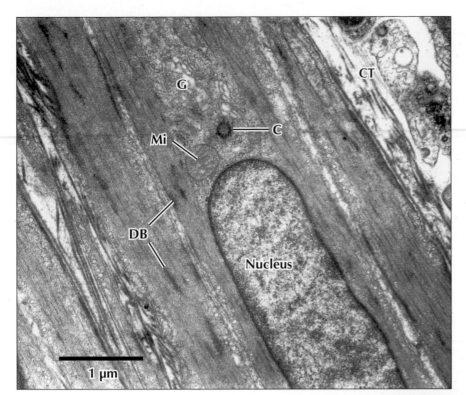

◀ **EM of smooth muscle in longitudinal section.**
The single nucleus is in the widest part of the cell and
conforms to its shape. The juxtanuclear sarcoplasm
contains a mixture of organelles, including Golgi
complex (**G**), ribosomes, mitochondria (**Mi**), and
centriole (**C**). Filaments make up the bulk of the
sarcoplasm and are densely packed and oriented
parallel to the long axis of a cell. Dense bodies (**DB**)
are regularly distributed along the perimeter of the
cell and are dispersed throughout the sarcoplasm.
The surrounding connective tissue (**CT**), some of which
is produced by the smooth muscle cell, contains
collagen and elastic fibrils. 23,000×.

▶ **Three-dimensional schematic of smooth
muscle cells in relaxed and contracted states.**

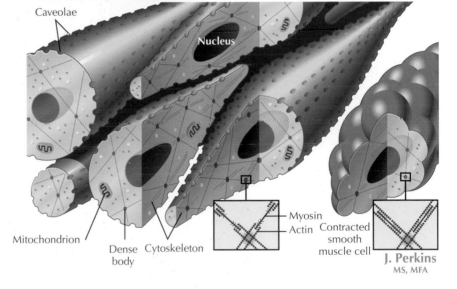

4.26 ULTRASTRUCTURE OF SMOOTH MUSCLE

The ultrastructure and architecture of smooth muscle cells are
markedly different from those of skeletal muscle. Although smooth
muscle can produce *contractile force* comparable to that of skeletal
muscle, it has a much slower and more variable speed of contraction, which can be sustained for long periods. Its cells are also very
efficient in terms of energy expended and show less fatigue. As its
name implies, smooth muscle lacks visible striations or sarcomeres, in contrast to striated skeletal and cardiac muscle. By electron microscopy, the **sarcoplasm** of smooth muscle cells has three
sets of **filaments** that are oriented obliquely and longitudinally in
each cell. **Thick filaments,** containing **myosin,** are 14 nm in diameter; **thin filaments,** composed of **actin,** are 6-8 nm in diameter.
Myosin filaments run parallel to actin filaments, with a myosin-
to-actin ratio of 1 : 12. The 10-nm **intermediate filaments** contain
desmin or *vimentin* and form an intersecting **cytoskeletal** network.
Dense bodies, unique to smooth muscle cells, are found in all
parts of a cell, either scattered in **cytoplasm** or attached to the
undersurface of the **sarcolemma,** where they link thin and intermediate filaments to the cell membrane. The attachment of thin
filaments to dense bodies and their content of the protein α-
actinin are similar to those found at Z bands of skeletal muscle.
Intermediate filaments function as a strong cable-like system that
probably harnesses the force generated during contraction.

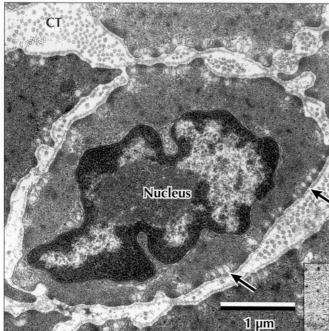

◄ **EM of a smooth muscle cell in the region of its nucleus in transverse section.** Caveolae (**arrows**) are found along the sarcolemma, and filaments are tightly packed. Dense bodies are scattered in the sarcoplasm or attached to the undersurface of the sarcolemma. An external lamina covers each cell, and connective tissue (**CT**) is seen in intercellular spaces. 19,000×.

► **EM of parts of several smooth muscle cells in transverse section.** The sarcoplasm is tightly packed with filaments, dense bodies (**DB**), and scattered mitochondria (**Mi**). Caveolae (**arrows**) are a dominant feature of the cell surfaces; intercellular junctions (**circles**) link neighboring cells. A prominent external lamina envelops the sarcolemma of each cell, and surrounding connective tissue (**CT**) contains collagen fibers, which are probably produced by smooth muscle cells. 40,000×.

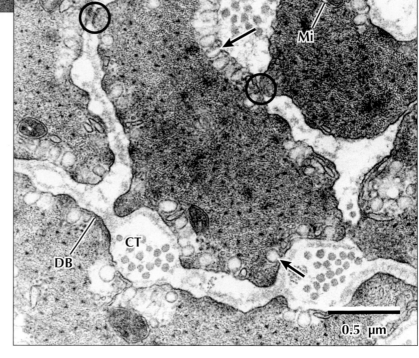

4.27 ULTRASTRUCTURE OF SMOOTH MUSCLE IN TRANSVERSE SECTION

Caveolae, which are flask-shaped invaginations of the **sarcolemma,** are a dominant feature of smooth muscle cells. They are 70-120 nm in diameter and regular in shape and increase the cell surface area up to 70%. Because they open to the surface and are just under the sarcolemma, caveolae have been likened to T tubules in skeletal muscle. They probably serve a critical role in *calcium transport* to initiate smooth muscle cell *contraction,* which requires *phosphory-lation* of *myosin light chains.* After *calcium ions* enter the cell, they bind to *calmodulin,* which enables myosin to interact with actin. Actin filaments in smooth muscle, unlike those in skeletal muscle, do not contain troponin. Formation of *cross bridges* between myosin and actin is followed by hydrolysis of *ATP,* which leads to

contraction. Smooth muscle cells show two types of **intercellular junctions. Intermediate junctions (zonulae adherentes)** provide adhesion and anchor cells during contraction. Numerous **gap (communicating) junctions** provide electrical coupling. Smooth muscle cells synthesize and secrete many components of surrounding extracellular matrix, including **collagen** and elastin. Its organelles, most located at poles of the nucleus, include a small Golgi complex, smooth and rough endoplasmic reticulum, and scattered **mitochondria,** which make up 3%-10% of cell volume. Cisternae and tubules of SR occur under the sarcolemma or scattered throughout the cytoplasm and serve a function similar to the SR in skeletal muscle. Smooth muscle activity includes maintenance of tone, sustained partial contraction, and *peristalsis* (a series of alternate and synchronous contractions).

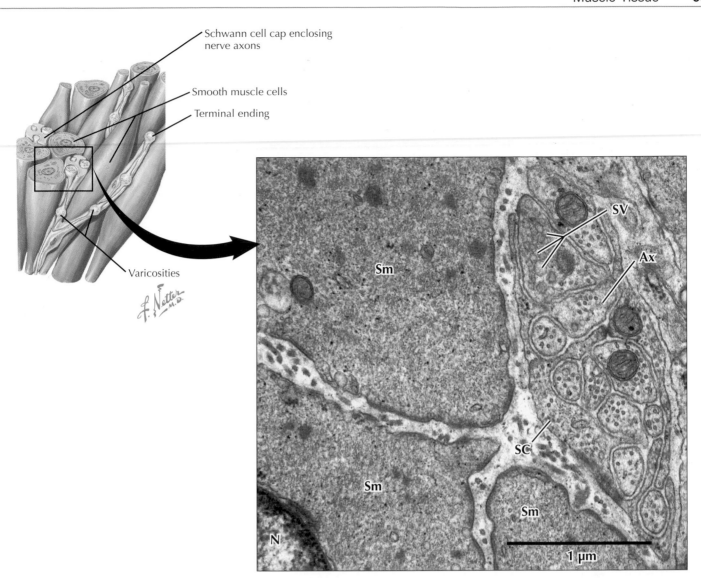

Schwann cell cap enclosing nerve axons

Smooth muscle cells

Terminal ending

Varicosities

f. Netter
M.D.

SV

Ax

Sm

SC

Sm

Sm

N

1 μm

▲ **EM of smooth muscle cells close to nerve axons in transverse section.** Several smooth muscle cells (**Sm**) are in the field of view; one is sectioned at the level of its nucleus (**N**). A group of unmyelinated axons (**Ax**) supported by the process of a Schwann cell (**SC**) is seen in surrounding interstitial connective tissue. An axonal varicosity contains a cluster of synaptic vesicles (**SV**). 37,000×.

4.28 INNERVATION OF SMOOTH MUSCLE

Unlike skeletal muscle fibers, each having a discrete neuromuscular junction, smooth muscle cells possess a different, less complex *innervation*. Regulation of smooth muscle activity often occurs via the *autonomic nervous system,* whereby **axonal varicosities** containing **synaptic vesicles** come into close contact with the sarcolemma of a smooth muscle cell. At such sites, innervation of the cell has a relatively simple structure, and synapses are *en passant* (along its course). The intervening synaptic cleft of 20-100 nm or more between the axon plasma membrane and the sarcolemma of the muscle cell has no postjunctional specialization. Although the axon varicosity is **unmyelinated,** a **Schwann cell** cap supports it. The varicosity typically contains focal accumulations of synaptic vesicles of various sizes and electron densities, microtubules, and mitochondria. The vesicles may store *acetylcholine, norepinephrine,* or other *neurotransmitters* before release. In some sites, smooth muscle cells are individually innervated by efferent nerve endings. In most areas, however, not all smooth muscle cells are innervated, and the branch of an autonomic nerve fiber supplies groups of several cells. Gap junctions between cells allow *excitation* to spread among adjacent cells, which results in *synchronous contractions.* Many other extrinsic factors control smooth muscle activity. Circulating hormones such as *oxytocin* stimulate contraction in the uterus during birth, and local substances such as *histamine* and *serotonin* or physical factors such as *stretching* can affect muscle activity.

CLINICAL POINT

Because mature smooth muscle cells can undergo *hyperplasia* and *hypertrophy,* contractile and proliferative abnormalities of smooth muscle cells are major causes of disease. **Asthma** and **hypertension** are often due to sustained contraction of bronchial and vascular smooth muscle, respectively. Excess histamine in **allergy,** for example, frequently induces increased excitation of smooth muscle activity, thereby narrowing the airways. In **atherosclerosis,** arterial smooth muscle cells accumulate cholesterol, which often leads to formation of plaques that compromise normal blood flow. Many therapeutic drugs, such as bronchodilators and vasodilators, influence contractile regulatory mechanisms affecting smooth muscle.

5

NERVOUS TISSUE

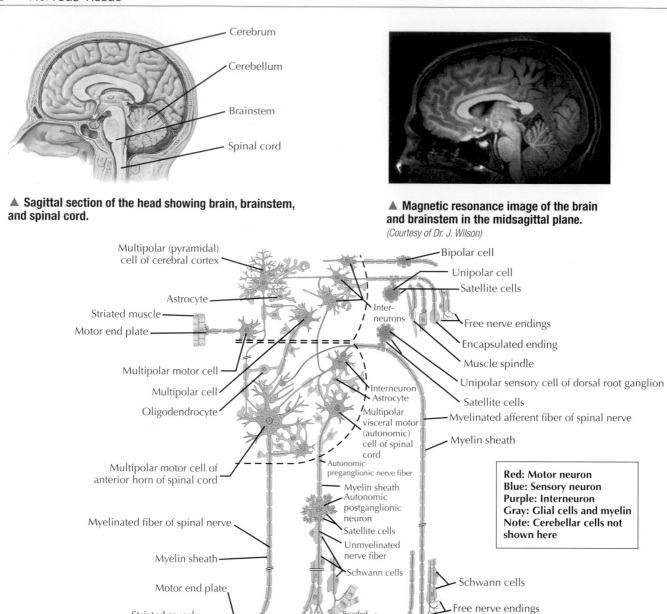

▲ Sagittal section of the head showing brain, brainstem, and spinal cord.

Cerebrum
Cerebellum
Brainstem
Spinal cord

▲ Magnetic resonance image of the brain and brainstem in the midsagittal plane.
(Courtesy of Dr. J. Wilson)

Multipolar (pyramidal) cell of cerebral cortex
Astrocyte
Striated muscle
Motor end plate
Multipolar motor cell
Multipolar cell
Oligodendrocyte
Multipolar motor cell of anterior horn of spinal cord
Myelinated fiber of spinal nerve
Myelin sheath
Motor end plate
Striated muscle

Bipolar cell
Unipolar cell
Satellite cells
Inter-neurons
Free nerve endings
Encapsulated ending
Muscle spindle
Unipolar sensory cell of dorsal root ganglion
Satellite cells
Myelinated afferent fiber of spinal nerve
Myelin sheath

Interneuron
Astrocyte
Multipolar visceral motor (autonomic) cell of spinal cord
Autonomic preganglionic nerve fiber
Myelin sheath
Autonomic postganglionic neuron
Satellite cells
Unmyelinated nerve fiber
Schwann cells
Beaded varicosities and endings on smooth muscle and gland cells

Schwann cells
Free nerve endings
Encapsulated ending
Muscle spindle

Red: Motor neuron
Blue: Sensory neuron
Purple: Interneuron
Gray: Glial cells and myelin
Note: Cerebellar cells not shown here

▲ Schematic showing organization of main cell types in the CNS and PNS.

5.1 OVERVIEW

The nervous system is divided anatomically into the **central** (CNS) and **peripheral** (PNS) nervous systems. The CNS comprises the **brain, brainstem,** and **spinal cord;** the PNS, all **nerve fibers** (**axons** and **dendrites**), **nerve endings,** and collections of their cell bodies that lie outside the CNS. The **autonomic nervous system,** a subdivision of the PNS, is connected to the CNS through **spinal** and **cranial nerves.** Its **sympathetic** and **parasympathetic** portions innervate organs and tissues that are under autonomic, or involuntary, control such as glands, smooth muscle, and cardiac muscle. The CNS and PNS contain **nervous tissue,** one of the four basic body tissues, which possesses two major cell types: **nerve cells,** or **neurons,** and supporting cells, or **glia.** Neurons can gen-

erate *nervous impulses* in response to stimuli and transmit them along cellular processes. More than 50 billion neurons are estimated to be in the nervous system. The types of neurons are classified on the basis of appearance, shape, and number of processes as multipolar, bipolar, or pseudounipolar. Despite their variability, all neurons conform to a common histologic plan: highly specialized cells with several parts to carry out functions of receiving signals and then transmitting information as nerve impulses to other neurons or effector organs. *Conductivity* and *irritability* are best developed in neurons; glial cells are non-impulse-conducting cells that represent interstitial tissue and mostly support and protect neurons.

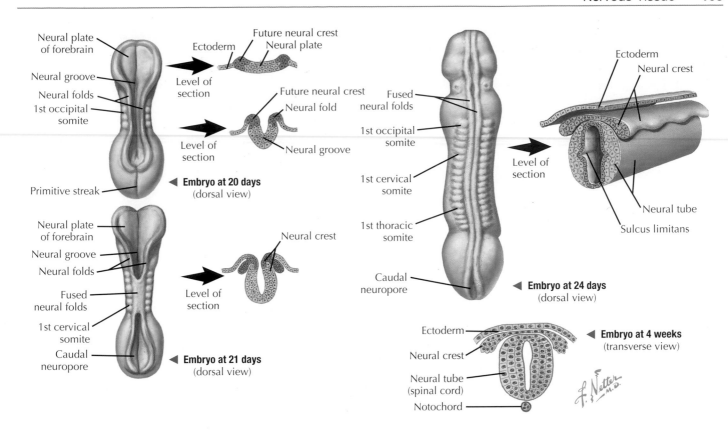

5.2 EMBRYONIC DEVELOPMENT

The nervous system develops from a thickening of dorsal **ecto-derm** of the early embryo. At 14-16 days, a **neural plate** of surface ectoderm appears in the dorsal midline. It becomes indented and forms a longitudinal **neural groove** with **neural folds** on each side. By 24 days, the neural folds fuse dorsally to form a **neural tube,** which becomes the CNS, including the brain rostrally and **spinal cord** more caudally. The neural tube is first open at both ends, but at 24-26 days it closes. Isolated cells not incorporated into the neural tube form a strip of neuroectodermal cells—the **neural crest.** These cells migrate ventrolaterally along each side of the neural tube to form a series of **somites.** The neural crest ecto-derm ultimately gives rise to PNS components, including **dorsal root ganglia** of **spinal nerves,** comparable **sensory ganglia** of **cranial nerves, autonomic ganglia,** and **chromaffin cells** of the adrenal medulla. Neuron bodies inside the CNS are derived from the neural tube; those outside, in the PNS, the neural crest. Axons and dendrites sprout from neuron bodies and grow long dis-tances. Supporting satellite cells envelope neuron bodies in the PNS, whereas cells around neuron peripheral processes or nerve fibers are Schwann cells. The neural tube lumen gives rise to fluid-filled ventricles of the brain and central canal of the spinal cord. Coverings of the brain and spinal cord, known as meninges, develop later. They are composed of three distinct layers: an out-ermost dura mater, arachnoid, and innermost pia mater.

CLINICAL POINT

Malformations of the developing nervous system may arise during closure and later growth of the neural tube and result in various neural tube defects. **Anencephaly** is a congenital malformation caused by failure of fusion of neural folds in rostral regions. Degeneration of unfused folds leads to failure of development of neural tissue and absence of most of the brain, the result being stillbirth or premature death. A defect at more caudal levels of the primitive spinal cord is called **spina bifida.** This condition typically produces paralysis depending on the level of the lesion and is usually not life-threatening.

▼ **Meninges and reflection of dura mater.**

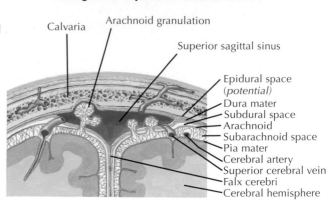

Branches of middle meningeal artery
Superior sagittal sinus
Dura mater
Superior cerebral veins (penetrating arachnoid and passing through subdural space to enter superior sagittal sinus)
Inferior anastomotic vein (of Labbé)
Superficial middle cerebral vein
Middle meningeal artery and veins

▼ **Meninges and superficial cerebral veins.**

Calvaria
Arachnoid granulation
Superior sagittal sinus
Epidural space (potential)
Dura mater
Subdural space
Arachnoid
Subarachnoid space
Pia mater
Cerebral artery
Superior cerebral vein
Falx cerebri
Cerebral hemisphere

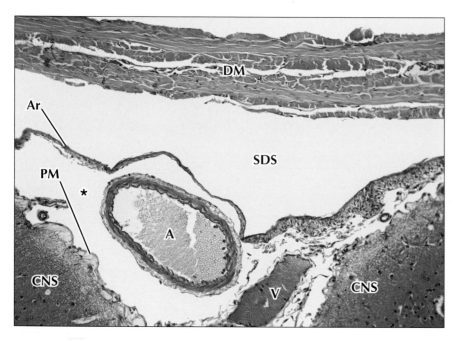

◄ **Light micrograph (LM) of the meninges covering the monkey brain.** The dura mater (**DM**), the most superficial meningeal layer, is dense, fibrous connective tissue. Underlying the arachnoid (**Ar**), a more delicate connective tissue, is the subarachnoid space (∗), which, in life, contains cerebrospinal fluid. Arterial (**A**) and venous (**V**) branches of cerebral vessels traverse this space. The pia mater (**PM**) is the innermost, thinnest meningeal layer. Although not well seen at this magnification, tissue of the **CNS** is separated from the pia by a thin layer, called the outer glia limitans, which is formed by astrocyte end-feet. The subdural space (**SDS**) (between dura and arachnoid) is a preparation artifact. 270×. *H&E.*

5.3   STRUCTURE AND FUNCTION OF THE MENINGES

The term meninges derives from the Greek *meninx*, meaning membrane. The three layers of the meninges stabilize and protect the brain and spinal cord. The **dura mater** invests the brain, spinal cord, and optic nerves. The thickest and toughest layer, the dura, is dense, fibrous **connective tissue** consisting of interlacing bundles of collagen and elastic fibers associated with flattened fibroblasts. The outer aspect of the dura attaches to the periosteum of the skull; the inner dural surface is lined by a layer of flattened fibroblasts. The dura contains large **blood vessels,** nerves, and lymphatics. Two potential spaces associated with it are the *epidural space* (exterior) and **subdural space** (between dura and arachnoid). These normally potential spaces can in some pathologic conditions accumulate fluid such as blood. The **arachnoid** and **pia mater** are thinner and more delicate than the dura and are known together as the *leptomeninges*. The arachnoid comprises several layers of flattened, closely packed fibroblasts linked by tight junctions with some intervening collagen. The arachnoid, so named because it resembles a spider's web, sends inward pro-

jections, the arachnoid trabeculae, into the **subarachnoid space** to form a "cobweb" that merges with the pia. This space is filled with cerebrospinal fluid (CSF) and contains branches of cerebral arteries and veins. Peripherally, the arachnoid is continuous with the *perineurium* around peripheral nerve fascicles. The pia mater intimately invests all external surfaces of the CNS and extends into its folds, fissures, and convolutions. At certain sites, the pia protrudes into the ventricles close to modified ependymal cells to form the *choroid plexus.*

CLINICAL POINT

Meningitis, or inflammation of the meninges, is most often caused by bacteria or viruses. Other pathogens such as fungi or parasites are also causes. *Bacterial meningitis* is less common than the viral form, can be life-threatening, and is characterized by exudates of polymorphonuclear leukocytes in the CNS. *Viral hepatitis* is marked mostly by lymphocyte infiltration in the brain and raised numbers of T cells in CSF. A leading cause of meningitis in children is *Haemophilus influenzae type b,* and a vaccine for it has dramatically reduced its incidence. Meningitis may occur at any age, but it is most common in children, the elderly, and immunocompromised people.

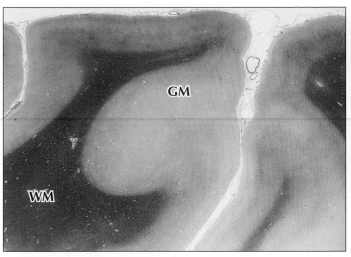

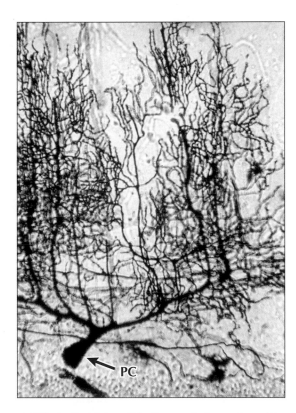

▲ **LM of the cerebrum showing external gray matter (GM) and internal white matter (WM).** The shading difference is due mainly to the amount of myelin, which stains darker in the white matter. 4×. *Luxol fast blue and cresyl violet.*

▲ **LM of the cerebellum showing its corrugated surface.** The outer cortex of gray matter (**GM**) covers an inner medullary region of white matter (**WM**). 12×. *H&E.*

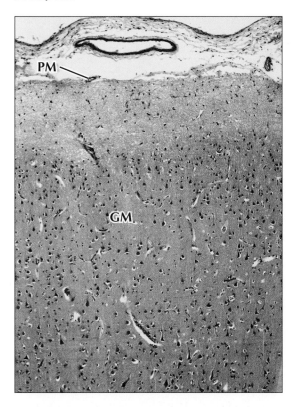

▲ **LM of cerebral cortex showing pia mater (PM) and cortical gray matter (GM).** Neuronal somas in the cortex are surrounded by the neuropil consisting of a feltwork of intermingled axons, dendrites, and glia. 60×. *H&E.*

▲ **LM of a Purkinje cell in the cerebellar cortex.** This heavy metal impregnation highlights the cell body (**PC**) with a black deposit and reveals the elaborate dendritic arborization that characterizes this cell. 270×. *Golgi silver.*

5.4 NEUROCYTOLOGY: CYTOARCHITECTURE

The unique cytoarchitecture of the CNS varies regionally. By inspection with the naked eye, the CNS is made up of **gray matter** and **white matter.** Unmyelinated neuronal processes and **glial cells,** tracts of myelinated nerve fibers, and associated glia dominate the white matter, whereas gray matter consists mostly of neuron bodies. The CNS also has a rich vascular supply that includes a profuse network of capillaries, which are more abun-

dant in gray matter. In the spinal cord, gray matter is located internally and is enveloped by an external layer of white matter. In other regions of the CNS, such as **cerebrum** and **cerebellum,** an outer **cortex** of gray matter covers an internal **medullary** region of white matter. Because of the complexity and intricate nature of nervous tissue, ordinary staining methods have limited value when used alone to examine its cytologic features.

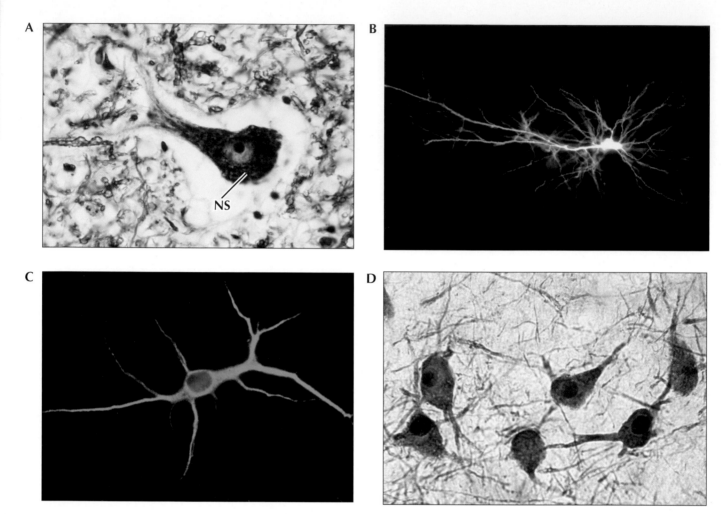

▲ **LMs of central nervous system neurons treated with different staining methods to demonstrate salient features. A.** Anterior motor neuron in the human spinal cord stained with Luxol fast blue and cresyl violet to show Nissl substance (**NS**). 500×. **B.** Pyramidal cell in the rat hippocampus injected iontophoretically with a fluorescent marker to highlight the soma and multiple dendrites. 200×. *Lucifer yellow. (Courtesy of Dr. J. Church)* **C.** A mouse neocortical neuron immunofluorescently labeled with microtubule-associated protein and fluorescein. 300×. *(Courtesy of Drs. M. A. Ozog and C. C. Naus)* **D.** Multipolar neurons in the base of the human forebrain stained immunocytochemically with an antibody to calbindin, a calcium-binding protein. The light brown demonstrates the spatial distribution of calbindin in somas, axons, and dendrites. These cholinergic neurons project to the cerebral cortex and are commonly affected in Alzheimer disease. 400×. *Immunoperoxidase-diaminobenzidine. (Courtesy of Dr. K. G. Baimbridge)*

5.5 NEUROCYTOLOGY: STAINING METHODS

Special techniques with varied and selective stains, which provide a composite view of nervous tissue, are often used in *neurohistology* and *neuropathology*. Basic cationic dyes such as *cresyl violet* and *toluidine blue* elucidate cell nuclei and neuronal **Nissl substance** (rough endoplasmic reticulum and ribosomes). *Luxol fast blue* and other reagents such as *osmium* can demonstrate myelin sheaths. *Metal impregnation* with reduced gold and silver demonstrates the intricate nature of **axons** and **dendrites**. *Histochemistry* and *immunocytochemistry* permit localization of specific substances and molecules within different types of **neurons** and glia. Electron microscopy has proved to be quite useful for revealing fine structural details beyond the resolution power of light microscopy.

CLINICAL POINT

Senile dementia of the Alzheimer type, or **Alzheimer disease,** which is characterized by progressive *memory loss,* is increasingly common in developed countries as populations include more elderly persons. Definitive diagnosis is made by microscopic examination of the brain at autopsy, with the histopathologic hallmark being an increased number of *neuritic,* or *senile, plaques,* which occur mostly in the cerebral cortex. They consist of tortuous neuritic processes formed mainly by degenerative presynaptic endings, which surround a central amyloid core. Reactive astrocytes and microglia may appear at a plaque periphery. Another important histologic feature is proliferation of intracytoplasmic *neurofibrillary tangles.*

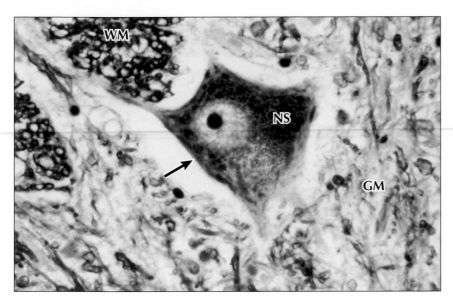

◄ **LM of part of the spinal cord.** The large multipolar neuron (**arrow**) in the gray matter (**GM**) has an irregularly shaped soma with dispersed Nissl substance (**NS**), which makes the cytoplasm basophilic. A lightly stained, spherical nucleus is eccentrically placed and contains a prominent, dark nucleolus. The neuron is close to the white matter (**WM**), consisting of bundles of myelinated nerve fibers. Small round nuclei in the gray matter are those of glial cells. 750×. *Luxol fast blue and cresyl violet.*

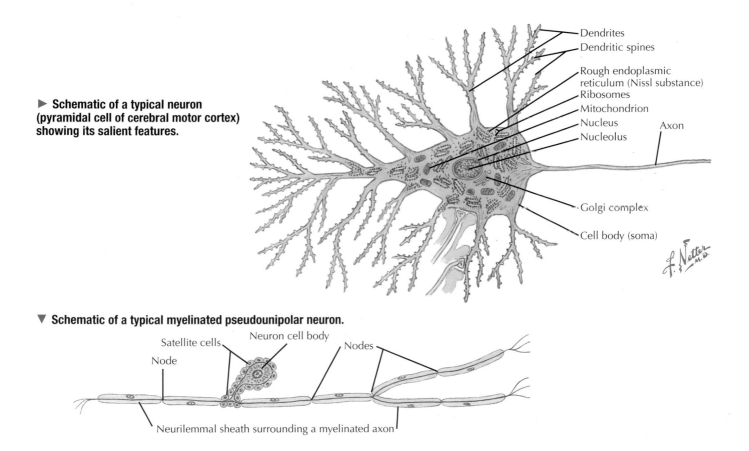

► **Schematic of a typical neuron (pyramidal cell of cerebral motor cortex) showing its salient features.**

Dendrites
Dendritic spines
Rough endoplasmic reticulum (Nissl substance)
Ribosomes
Mitochondrion
Nucleus
Axon
Nucleolus
Golgi complex
Cell body (soma)

▼ **Schematic of a typical myelinated pseudounipolar neuron.**

Satellite cells
Neuron cell body
Node
Nodes
Neurilemmal sheath surrounding a myelinated axon

5.6   STRUCTURE OF A NEURON

The **neuron** is a highly polarized cell that consists of a **soma,** or **cell body,** from which cytoplasmic processes arise. The processes, known as **nerve fibers,** vary greatly in size, some being up to 1.5 m long. Processes conducting impulses toward cell bodies are **dendrites,** whereas a single process conveying impulses away from cell bodies is an **axon.** The soma consists of a **nucleus** and the surrounding **cytoplasm,** known as the **perikaryon.** Soma sizes, which depend on cell type and function, vary from 5 to 150 μm. **Anterior motor neurons** of the **spinal cord** are among the largest in

the CNS, whereas granule cells in the cerebellar cortex are among the smallest. Irregularly shaped masses of basophilic material known as **Nissl substance** are scattered in the cytoplasm of the body and the dendrites. Neurons are classified into three types on the basis of the number of processes. **Multipolar** neurons are the most common and characteristic and have one axon and several dendrites. **Bipolar** neurons have two processes, an axon and a dendrite, and are found in the visual, auditory, and olfactory systems. **Pseudounipolar** neurons have one short process, which bifurcates into an axon and a dendrite.

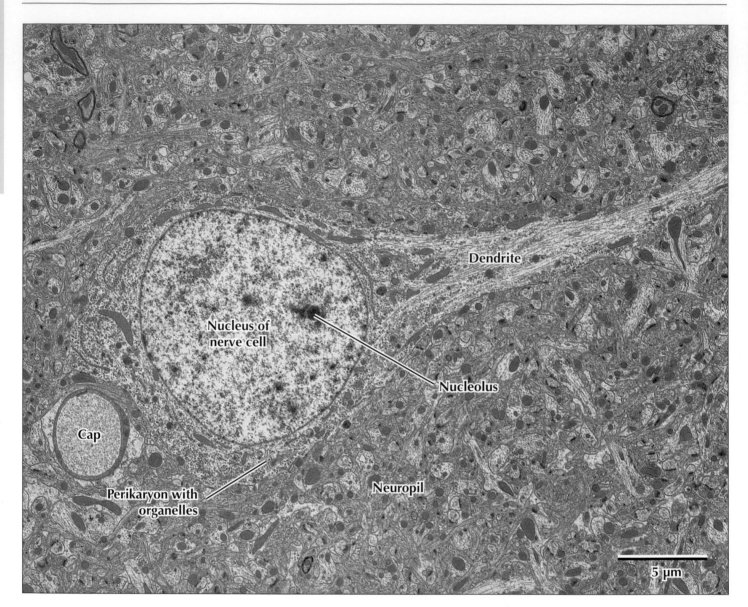

▲ **Electron micrograph (EM) of part of the cerebral cortex showing typical features of a neuron in gray matter.** The soma contains a large, spherical, euchromatic nucleus surrounded by a rim of cytoplasm—the perikaryon. Projecting from the soma is a large dendrite, which is an extension of the cell body. The cytoplasm of both the soma and the dendrite is replete with various organelles. The pyramid-shaped neuron is surrounded by tightly packed neuron processes and parts of glial cells. They collectively constitute the neuropil of gray matter. A capillary (**Cap**) is seen in transverse section. Very little intervening extracellular space is in the surrounding area. 4500×.

5.7 ULTRASTRUCTURE OF A NEURON IN GRAY MATTER IN RELATION TO SURROUNDING STRUCTURES

The **soma** is the trophic center of the **neuron** and varies greatly in size and shape. Reflecting its role in *genetic regulation* and *transcription,* the *euchromatic* **nucleus** of a typical neuron has small patches of heterochromatin, peripherally displaced, just under the nuclear envelope. The nucleus is usually spherical to ovoid, and it is large relative to the surrounding **perikaryon.** A characteristic feature is one or more prominent nucleoli, seen in fortuitous sections; they have a role in synthesizing ribosomal RNA. The surrounding cytoplasm is the site of synthesis of most of the structural and secretory proteins, enzymes, and organelles needed for diverse functions of the cell. Dominating the cytoplasm are multiple flattened cisternae of rough endoplasmic reticulum between which are numerous free ribosomes (the basophilic Nissl substance seen in light micrographs). Their major function is protein synthesis for internal use and export. A highly developed Golgi complex with multiple stacks of flattened sacs and associated vesicles and vacuoles is usually seen near the nucleus. This organelle is responsible for packaging and concentration of secretory products, post-translational modification of macromolecules, and supply of lysosomes, which accumulate wear-and-tear lipofuscin pigment in these long-lived cells with advancing age.

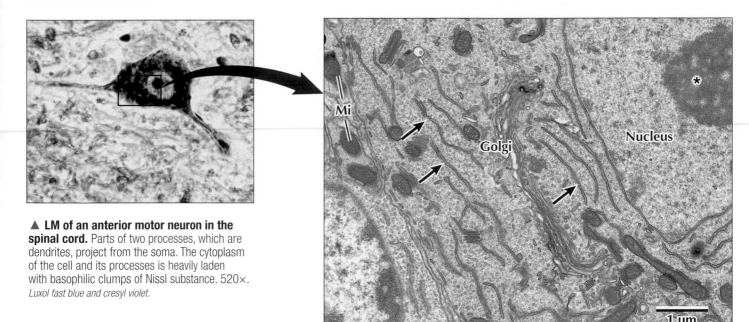

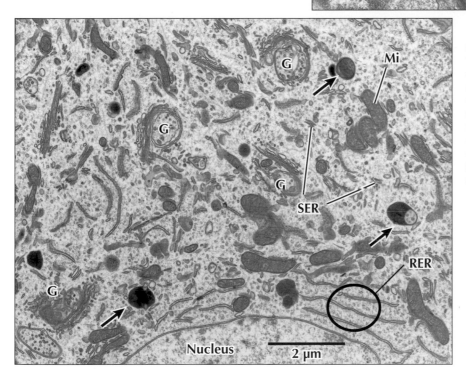

▲ **LM of an anterior motor neuron in the spinal cord.** Parts of two processes, which are dendrites, project from the soma. The cytoplasm of the cell and its processes is heavily laden with basophilic clumps of Nissl substance. 520×. *Luxol fast blue and cresyl violet.*

◄ ▲ **EMs showing ultrastructural features of the neuron soma. Above.** The euchromatic nucleus contains a prominent nucleolus (*). A striking feature of the cytoplasm is the presence of multiple cisternae of rough endoplasmic reticulum (**RER**) (**arrows**) and an elaborate juxtanuclear Golgi complex. The cytoplasm also contains many slender mitochondria (**Mi**) and free ribosomes. 13,000× **Left.** Throughout the cytoplasm are numerous elements of smooth endoplasmic reticulum (**SER**) and **RER** interspersed with mitochondria (**Mi**). Several lysosomes (**arrows**) and Golgi complexes (**G**) are also seen. 10,000×.

5.8   ULTRASTRUCTURE OF A SPINAL CORD NEURON SOMA

Mitochondria, the source of *ATP* to meet energy requirements for the metabolically active neuron, are abundant throughout the **soma** and in peripheral processes of the cell. They are especially numerous in axon terminals close to synapses. Neuronal **cytoplasm** has a well-developed cytoskeleton consisting of microtubules, actin filaments, and neurofilaments (an intermediate type). These organelles, found throughout the soma and extending into the axon and **dendrites,** help maintain cell shape and structural stability. Microtubules provide intracellular axoplasmic transport of organelles, most notably of mitochondria and membrane-bound vesicles containing precursors of *neurotransmitters.* Intra-cellular neuronal transport is bidirectional: *anterograde transport* is directed away from the soma and into cytoplasmic processes, whereas *retrograde transport* transports organelles and other material toward the soma. Microtubules and neurofilaments also play roles in *axonal growth* and guidance during development and in *regeneration* after injury. Neurofilaments are best seen by electron microscopy and can be detected by immunocytochemistry, but an affinity for heavy metals is the basis for metal impregnation staining techniques developed more than a century ago. Neuronal cytoplasm also contains lipid droplets, **smooth endoplasmic reticulum, lysosomes,** peroxisomes, **Golgi complexes, ribosomes,** and sometimes melanin pigment granules.

► **Types of synapses in the central nervous system.**

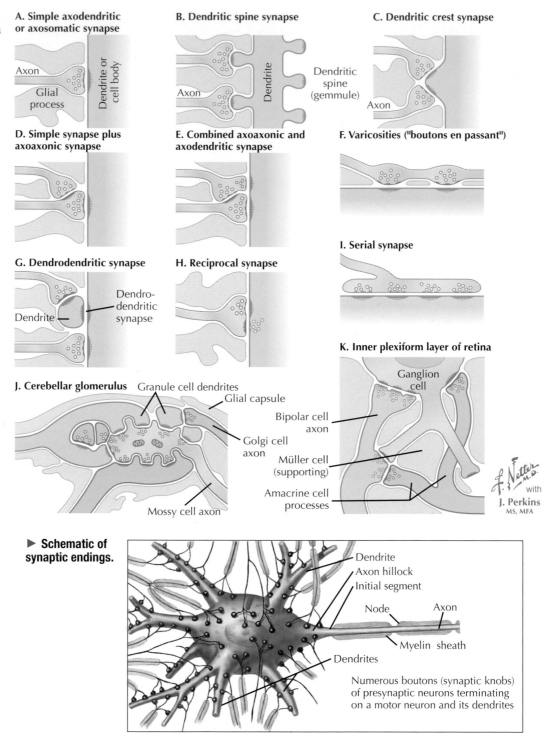

A. Simple axodendritic or axosomatic synapse

Axon · Glial process · Dendrite or cell body

B. Dendritic spine synapse

Axon · Dendrite

C. Dendritic crest synapse

Dendritic spine (gemmule) · Axon

D. Simple synapse plus axoaxonic synapse

E. Combined axoaxonic and axodendritic synapse

F. Varicosities ("boutons en passant")

G. Dendrodendritic synapse

Dendrite · Dendro-dendritic synapse

H. Reciprocal synapse

I. Serial synapse

K. Inner plexiform layer of retina

Ganglion cell · Bipolar cell axon · Golgi cell axon · Müller cell (supporting) · Amacrine cell processes

J. Cerebellar glomerulus

Granule cell dendrites · Glial capsule · Mossy cell axon

► **Schematic of synaptic endings.**

Dendrite · Axon hillock · Initial segment · Node · Axon · Myelin sheath · Dendrites · Numerous boutons (synaptic knobs) of presynaptic neurons terminating on a motor neuron and its dendrites

5.9 TYPES OF SYNAPSES

Synapses are specialized sites for chemical or electrical *transmission* for communication between **neurons** or between neurons and other **effector cells** such as skeletal muscle fibers. Most synapses in humans involve chemical neurotransmitters, which are released from presynaptic terminals of one **axon** or **dendrite** to affect receptors on the postsynaptic membrane of the target cell. Various *neurotransmitters* exist and include amino acids such as *glutamate,* catecholamines such as *epinephrine* and *norepinephrine, serotonin, neuropeptides,* and *acetylcholine.* In functional terms, two main types of synapses occur: *excitatory* and *inhibitory.*

In excitatory synapses, neurotransmitter release from the presynaptic neuron depolarizes the postsynaptic membrane; in inhibitory synapses, the postsynaptic membrane is hyperpolarized. Most CNS synapses are between an axon of one neuron and the dendrite of another—**axodendritic.** Other types include **axosomatic** and, less commonly, **axoaxonic** synapses. In some sites, such as hypothalamus and posterior pituitary, large vesicles in presynaptic terminals may contain polypeptide hormones, for example, oxytocin or vasopressin, that are neurosecretory products, not neurotransmitters.

► **Schematic showing the main features of a CNS synapse.**

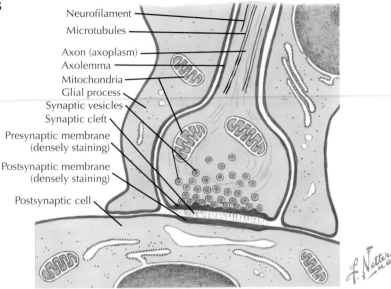

Neurofilament

Microtubules

Axon (axoplasm)

Axolemma

Mitochondria

Glial process

Synaptic vesicles

Synaptic cleft

Presynaptic membrane (densely staining)

Postsynaptic membrane (densely staining)

Postsynaptic cell

► **High-magnification EM of a typical synapse in the brain.** Clear, round synaptic vesicles are abundant in the presynaptic terminal; some are clustered near the presynaptic membrane in areas called active zones. The postsynaptic membrane exhibits electron densities at two such zones (**arrows**). A narrow synaptic cleft separates the two cell processes. Mitochondria (**Mi**) with well-developed cristae are found in both presynaptic and postsynaptic areas of the synapse and provide ATP to meet high-energy demands. 100,000×.

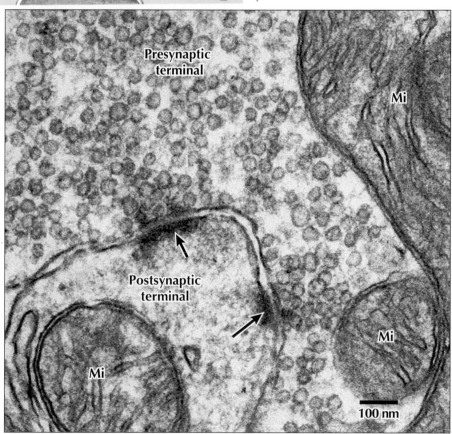

Presynaptic terminal

Mi

Postsynaptic terminal

Mi

Mi

100 nm

5.10 ULTRASTRUCTURE OF SYNAPSES

A typical synapse in the CNS consists of three major components: **presynaptic terminal, synaptic cleft,** and **postsynaptic membrane.** The presynaptic terminal aligns closely with the postsynaptic membrane of the target cell. In the area of membrane apposition, presynaptic and postsynaptic membranes are separated by a narrow **synaptic cleft** 12-30 nm wide. Clusters of large numbers of **synaptic vesicles** in the presynaptic terminal contain *neurotransmitter* that is released by *exocytosis* to mediate *synaptic transmission*. By electron microscopy, synaptic vesicles are 40-60 nm in diameter and are membrane-bound. Whether they have a clear center or an electron-dense core depends on the chemical nature of the neurotransmitter. Pre- and postsynaptic membrane specializations contain electron-dense material that extends into underlying cytoplasm and is usually thicker in the postsynaptic area. An *action potential* causes presynaptic vesicles to fuse with the presynaptic membrane and discharge neurotransmitter into the synaptic cleft. Neurotransmitter then diffuses across the cleft to interact with receptor molecules on the postsynaptic membrane, which changes postsynaptic *membrane conductance*. **Mitochondria,** sacs of **smooth endoplasmic reticulum, microtubules,** and **neurofilaments** are also seen in axon terminals.

▼ **Schematic of the cellular topography of the brain showing the four types of glial cells and their relationships to a neuron, a capillary, and the pia mater.**

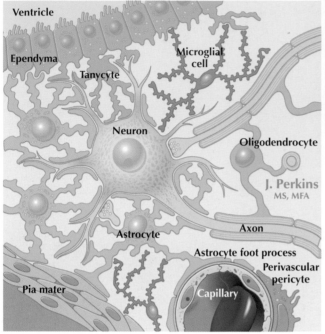

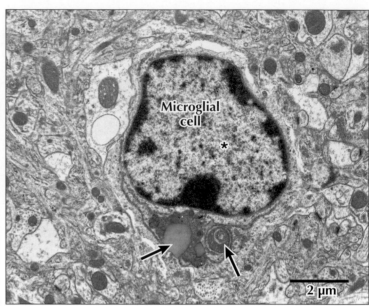

▲ **EM of a microglial cell in the brain.** The irregularly contoured, euchromatic nucleus (✶) has a peripheral rim of heterochromatin. Lysosomes of various sizes and large inclusions with lipofuscin (**arrows**) dominate the cytoplasm. These morphologic features are associated with phagocytic cells. 6900×.

5.11 STRUCTURE AND FUNCTION OF GLIAL CELLS

Glial cells outnumber neurons by at least 10 : 1 and make up more than 50% of the total volume of the **brain** and **spinal cord.** Their existence has been known for more than 100 years. They are ubiquitous but are not easily detected by conventional stains; special, improved techniques are required to reveal them. The four types of cells bear descriptive names: **astrocytes, oligodendrocytes, ependymal cells,** and **microglial cells.** Except for microglia, which originate from blood monocytes, glial cells are derived from neural ectoderm. Smaller than neurons, with cell bodies 3-10 μm in diameter, these nonconducting cells of the CNS have diverse structural, protective, and nutritive roles, as they ensure an interstitial milieu compatible for neuronal function. Astrocytes, the most abundant glial cell, are stellate cells with various critical functions in the CNS, such as maintaining homeostasis. Their delicate processes terminate either on surfaces of the brain and spinal cord or on walls of blood vessels. Main functions of oligodendrocytes are to provide support to nerve fibers and produce myelin sheaths that insulate them. Ependymal cells are remnants of embryonic neuroepithelium and form a closely packed cuboidal or columnar epithelium lining the **ventricles** of the brain and central canal of the spinal cord. Microglia, as their name implies, are the smallest glial cell. They act as *phagocytes* and remove CNS debris, protect the brain from invading microorganisms, and constitute the brain's immune system. Unlike neurons, glia retain a postnatal ability to divide and are the source of most intracranial tumors, known as *gliomas.*

HISTORICAL POINT
The renowned Spanish neurohistologist Santiago Ramón y **Cajal** (1852-1934) was the first to meticulously describe the cytoarchitecture of the nervous system and the histology of the neuron and its interconnections. The Italian Camillo **Golgi** (1843-1926) made his greatest contribution with his famous *reazione nera*, or black reaction, which permitted neurons and glial cells to be stained with osmium and silver. Cajal's student, Pio del **Rio-Hortega** (1882-1945), developed his own silver carbonate stain that selectively labeled glia. He discovered oligodendrocytes and microglia and viewed the latter as distinct from other neuroglia. For their pioneering work on the nervous system, Cajal and Golgi shared the Nobel Prize in Physiology or Medicine in 1906.

◄ **Immunofluoresence staining of human astrocytes in culture.** Cells were immunolabeled with an antibody to GFAP, which is unique to astrocytes in the CNS. Because this intermediate filament protein fills the cell bodies and extends into the thin cytoplasmic processes, the stellate cell shapes are clearly visualized with a Texas red secondary antibody. The cells in vitro are known to be linked by gap junctions, which is similar to the in vivo condition. 200×. *Texas red.*

► **EM of parts of two neighboring astrocytes.** The cytoplasm is replete with filaments (**Fi**). Most are glial filaments, although actin filaments, as well as microtubules, may also occupy the cell interior. A few profiles of rough endoplasmic reticulum (**RER**) and glycogen particles (**Gl**) are scattered in the cytoplasm. The plasma membranes (**PM**) of adjacent glial cells are in close apposition and show areas of increased density, which are intercellular junctions (see area in rectangle). Although not well resolved at this magnification, gap junctions are an important junction type that electrically links the cells. 13,000×.

5.12 STRUCTURE AND FUNCTION OF ASTROCYTES

Astrocytes are the largest and most numerous glial cell in the CNS. This heterogeneous population includes fibrous and protoplasmic astrocytes in the brain and spinal cord, Müller cells in the retina, and pituicytes in the posterior pituitary. In the embryo, they induce formation of capillary endothelial cell tight junctions in the CNS. Many elaborate, branched **cell processes** extend from the stellate **cell bodies** into the surrounding parenchyma of the brain and spinal cord. Terminal expansions of the processes, known as **perivascular end-feet,** form an intimate relationship with surfaces of small blood vessels, with a complete covering forming around capillaries. At these sites, they are part of the blood-brain barrier. They are also found around initial segments of neurons and bare axonal segments, the nodes of Ranvier. The cytoplasm contains abundant, tightly packed **intermediate filaments** with a unique amino acid sequence—**glial fibrillary acidic protein** (GFAP). In the CNS, this endogenous protein is exclusive to astrocytes and is thus used routinely as an immunocytochemical marker for these cells in normal brain and in diagnosis of tumors derived from the cells. Astrocytes perform many diverse and critical functions. Because of the presence of gap junctions, they form a structural syncytium in the CNS and provide metabolic and physical support for neurons. They control the ionic milieu by taking up excess potassium ions, and they regulate GABA (γ-aminobutyric acid) and inactivate neurotransmitters such as glutamate. In response to CNS injury, astrocytes undergo mitosis and are the main source of gliotic scar tissue (*gliosis*), which may impede neural regeneration.

CLINICAL POINT

Astrocytomas are CNS neoplasms derived from astrocytes. It is the most common type of **glioma** (tumor of glial cells) and can occur in most parts of the brain or spinal cord. It usually develops in the frontal and parietal lobes of the cerebrum and is most common in adults, especially middle-aged men. At least three different types exist, the most malignant of which is **glioblastoma multiforme**. This type usually grows quickly and spreads to other parts of the brain, so it is difficult to treat. As for most brain tumors, the etiology is unknown, and research attempting to discover possible causes is under way.

▼ Schematic showing salient features of the blood-brain barrier.

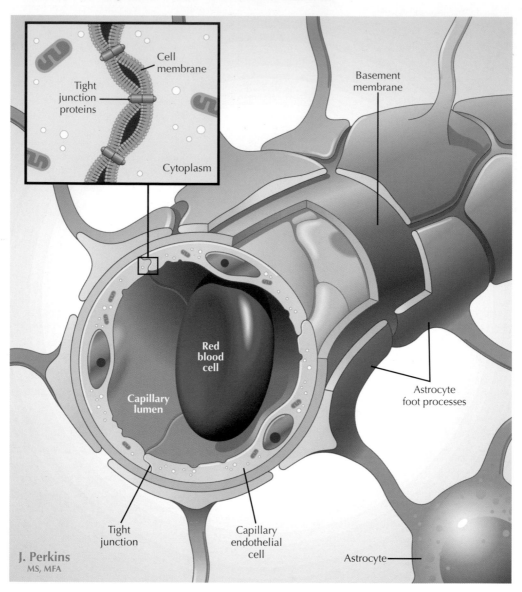

J. Perkins
MS, MFA

5.13 STRUCTURE AND FUNCTION OF THE BLOOD-BRAIN BARRIER

The **brain** receives about 15% of the cardiac output, about 750 mL of blood per minute, mostly for maintenance of cell function. Structural and functional characteristics of **capillaries** in the CNS are markedly different from those of capillaries elsewhere. The **blood-brain barrier** (BBB) is a physiologic barrier that restricts indiscriminate access of certain substances in the bloodstream to the brain, which normally requires homeostasis of its environment for optimal function. The BBB consists of **capillary endothelial cells** sealed by extensive **tight junctions** and an overlying **basement membrane,** with a narrow perivascular space. These endothelial cells have sparse pinocytotic vesicles, which participate in active, unidirectional transport of protein and fluids from blood to brain. Capillaries are also covered by **astrocyte end-feet (foot processes),** which induce BBB characteristics in the endo-

thelium. The end-feet cover more than 85% of the surface of the basement membrane; between the end-feet are gap junctions, which allow transport of potassium and other ions between the blood and the neuronal microenvironment.

CLINICAL POINT

Encephalitis is an inflammation of the brain parenchyma. *Acute* encephalitis is most commonly a *viral infection,* whereas a form that leads to abscess formation usually implies a highly destructive *bacterial infection.* Swift identification and immediate treatment can save lives. In herpes simplex encephalitis, a sporadic, relatively rare and lethal disease in neonates, the virus replicates outside the CNS and gains entry to the brain either via the bloodstream or traveling along neural or olfactory pathways. Once across the BBB, the virus enters neurons and disrupts cell functioning. A diffuse inflammatory response commonly affects gray matter disproportionately compared with white matter.

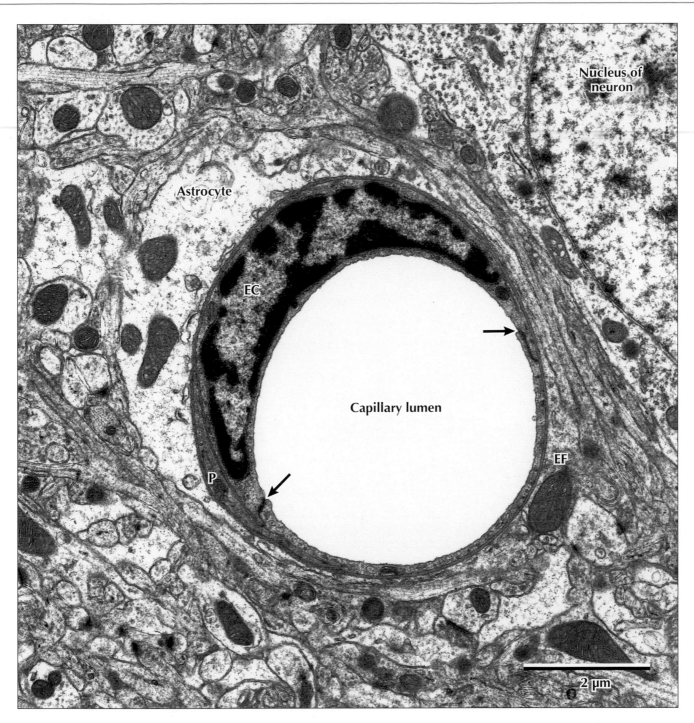

▲ **EM of a capillary in the brain in transverse section.** The endothelium of this capillary is attenuated, except where an endothelial cell (**EC**) is sectioned at the level of its nucleus. Tight junctions (**arrows**) link adjacent endothelial cells. Part of a pericyte (**P**) sits on the external aspect of the endothelium. Overlying basement membrane is barely visible at this magnification, and the perivascular space is very narrow. An astrocyte's pale perivascular end-feet (**EF**) abut the external aspect of the capillary. Scattered organelles, including several mitochondria of various sizes, occupy cytoplasm of the astrocyte. Surrounding nervous tissue, known as the neuropil, consists of many tightly packed processes of neurons and glia. The nucleus of a neuron is at the upper right. 15,500×.

5.14   ULTRASTRUCTURE OF THE BLOOD-BRAIN BARRIER

The BBB restricts passage of large molecules from the **capillary lumen** to the surrounding tissue, but it allows free passage of gases and selected molecules such as *glucose*. The barrier protects **neurons** in the CNS from toxins, drugs, and other potentially harmful substances that may be in the bloodstream. Most *antibiotics* such as penicillin do not cross the barrier in sufficient quantities because of their large *molecular size* and low degree of *lipid solubility*. A few brain regions—pineal gland, posterior pituitary, and parts of the hypothalamus—lack this barrier and contain capillaries that are highly permeable and fenestrated.

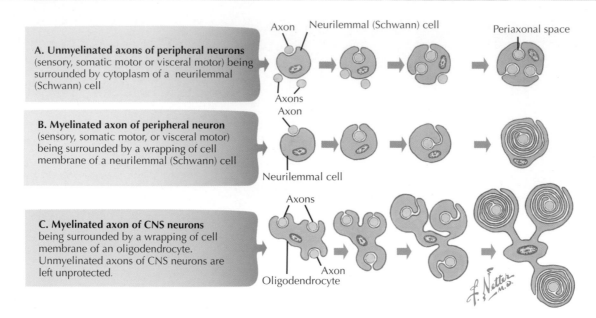

A. Unmyelinated axons of peripheral neurons (sensory, somatic motor or visceral motor) being surrounded by cytoplasm of a neurilemmal (Schwann) cell

B. Myelinated axon of peripheral neuron (sensory, somatic motor, or visceral motor) being surrounded by a wrapping of cell membrane of a neurilemmal (Schwann) cell

C. Myelinated axon of CNS neurons being surrounded by a wrapping of cell membrane of an oligodendrocyte. Unmyelinated axons of CNS neurons are left unprotected.

Axon   Neurilemmal (Schwann) cell   Periaxonal space

Axons
Axon

Neurilemmal cell

Axons

Oligodendrocyte   Axon

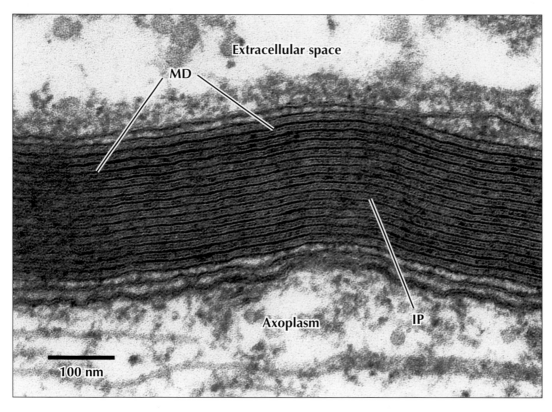

Extracellular space

MD

Axoplasm   IP

100 nm

◄ **High-magnification EM of part of a myelinated axon in the PNS.** Concentric rings of Schwann cell membrane that form the multilayer myelin sheath surround the axon. Alternate fusion of inner and outer leaflets of the cell's plasma membrane creates major dense lines (**MD**) and intraperiod lines (**IP**), respectively, of myelin lamellae; this fusion also squeezes out the cytoplasm. Major dense lines contain myelin basic protein, constituting about 10% of PNS myelin and 30% of CNS myelin. Myelin-associated glycoprotein is an important transmembrane protein of the CNS and PNS. Axoplasm (cytoplasm of the axon) of the nerve fiber and the surrounding extracellular space are seen. 165,000×.

5.15 MYELINATION OF AXONS IN THE CENTRAL AND PERIPHERAL NERVOUS SYSTEMS

Oligodendrocytes and **Schwann cells** are responsible for synthesis and maintenance of **myelin** in the CNS and PNS, respectively. Myelin is an electrical insulator that increases *conduction velocity* of **nerve fibers** and is the physical basis for rapid *saltatory conduction* (in which impulses jump from one node of Ranvier to another). Myelination, a series of complex events, begins in the third fetal trimester and ends during early childhood. The two main PNS populations of Schwann cells, which are morphologically and molecularly distinct, are derived from the neural crest.

They are called *myelinating* and *nonmyelinating* Schwann cells, although differentiation into two groups is probably mediated by **axons:** nonmyelinating cells collectively ensheath groups of several small axons; myelinating cells are most often associated with one large axon. Like oligodendrocytes in the CNS, they produce a myelin sheath by wrapping around axons. Unlike oligodendrocytes that wrap around numerous axons, one Schwann cell myelinates one segment of an axon. Schwann cells also aid debris removal and serve as guides for sprouts of regenerating axons after injury. Damage to myelin is common in neurologic diseases and leads to blocked axonal conduction, secondary damage to axons, and possibly permanent neurologic deficits.

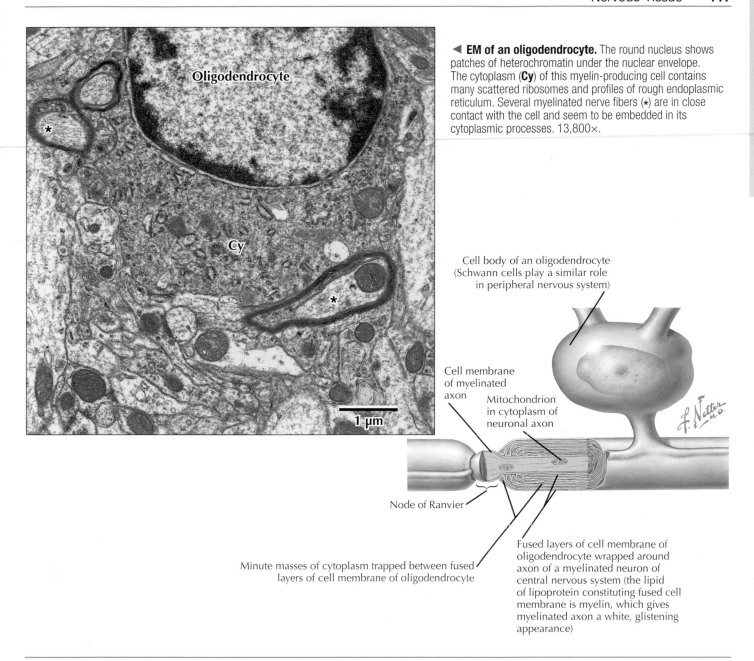

◄ **EM of an oligodendrocyte.** The round nucleus shows patches of heterochromatin under the nuclear envelope. The cytoplasm (**Cy**) of this myelin-producing cell contains many scattered ribosomes and profiles of rough endoplasmic reticulum. Several myelinated nerve fibers (∗) are in close contact with the cell and seem to be embedded in its cytoplasmic processes. 13,800×.

Cell body of an oligodendrocyte (Schwann cells play a similar role in peripheral nervous system)

Cell membrane of myelinated axon

Mitochondrion in cytoplasm of neuronal axon

Node of Ranvier

Minute masses of cytoplasm trapped between fused layers of cell membrane of oligodendrocyte

Fused layers of cell membrane of oligodendrocyte wrapped around axon of a myelinated neuron of central nervous system (the lipid of lipoprotein constituting fused cell membrane is myelin, which gives myelinated axon a white, glistening appearance)

5.16 OLIGODENDROCYTES AND MYELINATION IN THE CENTRAL NERVOUS SYSTEM

Oligodendrocytes are smaller than astrocytes and have fewer and shorter processes. A small spherical **cell body** houses a darkly stained, rounded nucleus. Several thin **cytoplasmic processes** emanate from the cell body, so, as its name implies, the oligodendrocyte resembles a tree with a few branches. Unlike astrocytes, oligodendrocytes are more numerous in white matter than in gray matter of the **CNS**. Oligodendrocytes occur in interfascicular rows among **myelinated axons**; as **satellite** oligodendrocytes, they are closely associated with neuronal somas. Their **cytoplasm** contains abundant **free ribosomes** and **rough endoplasmic reticulum**, scattered **mitochondria**, and a Golgi complex; the cytoplasm is also replete with microtubules but lacks intermediate filaments and glycogen. These cells produce and maintain **myelin sheaths** in the CNS. During *myelination*, the **plasma membrane** of the oligodendrocyte becomes tightly wrapped around axons, the number of layers determining the thickness of the myelin sheath. The **nodes of Ranvier** occur in intervals between adjacent oligo-

dendrocytes. In contrast to their Schwann cell counterparts in the PNS, one oligodendrocyte can myelinate up to 60 axons, they do not envelop unmyelinated axons in the CNS, and they are not enveloped by a basal lamina, which may contribute to relatively poor *regeneration* after CNS injury. By using the enzyme *carbonic anhydrase,* oligodendrocytes also help control extracellular pH in the CNS, a role critical for *acid-base equilibrium.*

CLINICAL POINT

Multiple sclerosis (MS) is a chronic inflammatory disease of the CNS characterized by a loss of myelin; damaged patches called plaques appear in seemingly random areas of the white matter. The disease course is unpredictable, and the type and severity of symptoms can vary greatly. During periods of MS activity, leukocytes (T cells) are drawn to regions of the white matter, which initiates an *inflammatory response* accompanied by loss of oligodendrocytes and axon demyelination. Although its etiology remains enigmatic, a leading theory proposes an *autoimmune* or *viral* cause. No cure exists, but certain medications are used to treat symptoms.

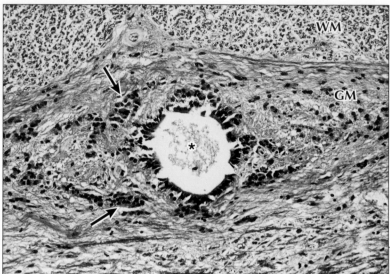

◀ **LM of the central canal of the spinal cord in transverse section.** In life, CSF normally fills the lumen (∗) of this canal. A single continuous layer of ependymal cells lines the lumen. A few isolated ependymal cell nests (**arrows**) are also seen nearby, and their presence is normal in the adult. The central canal of the spinal cord is usually patent in the child and young adult but with advancing age often becomes obliterated. Areas of white (**WM**) and gray (**GM**) matter of the spinal cord are indicated. 160×. *H&E.*

▶ **LM of part of the lateral ventricle of the brain.** The ventricular lumen (∗) has a ciliated ependymal lining composed of closely apposed cuboidal cells, some of which bear apical cilia (**arrows**). Because this specimen is fixed with osmium, myelin sheaths of nerve fibers in the underlying white matter (**WM**) are seen to good advantage and appear as hollow tubes. Nucleated cells in the white matter are other glial cells (**GC**). 920×. *Toluidine blue, semithin plastic section.*

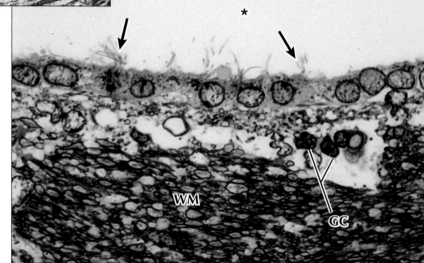

5.17   STRUCTURE AND FUNCTION OF THE EPENDYMA

The ependyma is a continuous simple cuboidal to columnar **epithelium** that lines the brain **ventricles** and the **central canal** of the spinal cord. Luminal surfaces of ependymal cells are in direct contact with CSF, a modified plasma ultrafiltrate with low protein content, which fills the ventricles and cushions the brain. These cells bear apical **microvilli** to increase surface area, and most also have motile **cilia** that project into the ventricular lumen. The cilia beat in a coordinated manner to sweep foreign particles in the same direction as bulk CSF flow. Ciliary movement also aids in metabolite exchange between CSF and extracellular spaces of the brain and spinal cord. The ependyma mainly serves as a protective and selective barrier between the brain and CSF and prevents passage of potentially neurotoxic substances to the brain. Characteristic of the ependyma is the presence of apical intercellular junctions between lateral borders of contiguous cells; other types of junctions are adherens, tight, and gap junctions. The ependyma becomes highly modified in brain regions known as the choroid plexus, where the cells serve a secretory role and produce and secrete components of the CSF. About 500 mL of CSF is produced daily. Ependymal cells also possess structural and enzymatic characteristics needed for scavenging and detoxifying many substances in CSF, thus forming a metabolic barrier at the brain-CSF interface. Specialized elongated ependymal cells known as tanycytes are juxtaposed to blood vessels, neurons, and pia mater and form a *blood-CSF barrier.*

CLINICAL POINT
Ependymomas are *glial tumors* derived from ependymal cells within the CNS. The four subtypes represent 6%-9% of primary CNS neoplasms. Intracranial lesions, arising from the roof of the fourth ventricle, usually occur in children, whereas spinal cord tumors typically occur in adults. Treatment depends on neurosurgical intervention to facilitate definitive diagnosis. Postoperative adjuvant therapy includes radiation of the brain or spinal cord, chemotherapy, or radiosurgery. Ependymomas have no known environmental cause, but they are associated with a number of genetic mutations. A causal relationship between these mutations and tumor progression has not yet been proved, however.

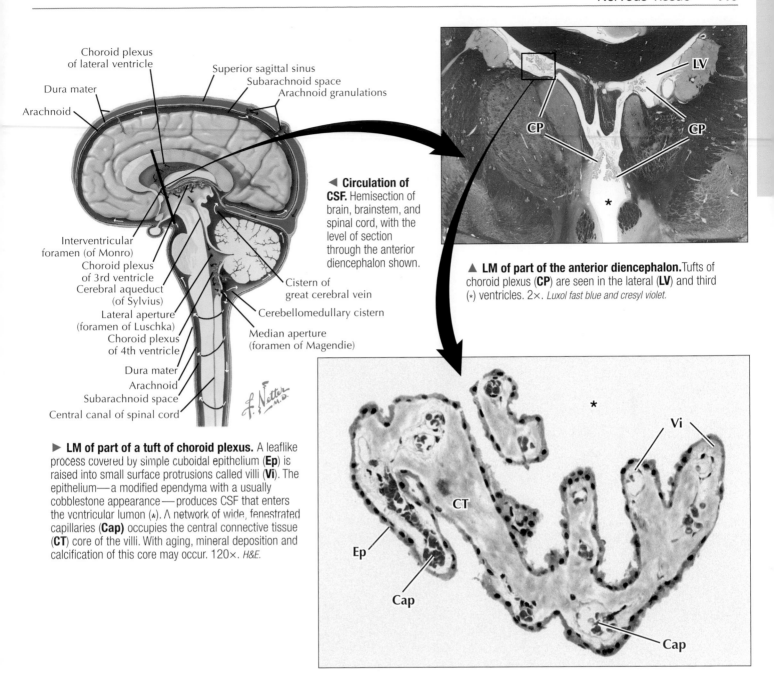

Choroid plexus
of lateral ventricle

Dura mater

Arachnoid

Superior sagittal sinus
Subarachnoid space
Arachnoid granulations

Interventricular
foramen (of Monro)
Choroid plexus
of 3rd ventricle
Cerebral aqueduct
(of Sylvius)
Lateral aperture
(foramen of Luschka)
Choroid plexus
of 4th ventricle

Dura mater
Arachnoid
Subarachnoid space
Central canal of spinal cord

Cistern of
great cerebral vein

Cerebellomedullary cistern

Median aperture
(foramen of Magendie)

◀ **Circulation of CSF.** Hemisection of brain, brainstem, and spinal cord, with the level of section through the anterior diencephalon shown.

▲ **LM of part of the anterior diencephalon.** Tufts of choroid plexus (**CP**) are seen in the lateral (**LV**) and third (*) ventricles. 2×. *Luxol fast blue and cresyl violet.*

▶ **LM of part of a tuft of choroid plexus.** A leaflike process covered by simple cuboidal epithelium (**Ep**) is raised into small surface protrusions called villi (**Vi**). The epithelium—a modified ependyma with a usually cobblestone appearance—produces CSF that enters the ventricular lumen (*). A network of wide, fenestrated capillaries (**Cap**) occupies the central connective tissue (**CT**) core of the villi. With aging, mineral deposition and calcification of this core may occur. 120×. *H&E.*

5.18 STRUCTURE AND FUNCTION OF THE CHOROID PLEXUS

The choroid plexus is a highly specialized tissue in the roof of the **third** and **fourth ventricles** of the brain and walls of **lateral ventricles.** It produces **CSF,** a slightly viscous clear fluid, which circulates in the ventricles, central canal of the spinal cord, and subarachnoid space. The choroid plexus consists of highly branched leaf-like folds of vascularized pia mater covered by a modified **ependyma,** which is a secretory and ion-transporting **epithelium.** This simple cuboidal or low simple columnar epithelium rests on a thin basement membrane. A core of loose **connective tissue** of the pia mater contains a tortuous network of large **fenestrated capillaries** that are highly permeable. The polarized epithelial cells bear apical **microvilli** that increase surface area for elaboration of CSF. This process involves active transport of

sodium ions and passive diffusion of water. Tight junctions link lateral borders of epithelial cells, and basal membranes of the cells have many infoldings similar to those seen in other ion-transporting epithelial cells. The total amount of CSF in adults is 80-150 mL. CSF is produced continuously and is resorbed in small projections in the subarachnoid space called arachnoid granulations, which return CSF to the venous circulation. When production of CSF exceeds resorption, *hydrocephalus* results. CSF serves mainly as a shock absorber to cushion and protect the CNS from trauma. It also removes metabolic waste products from the CNS. CSF protein level is normally low (0.18-0.58 g/L), so elevated levels indicate neurologic disease, infections, or CNS abnormalities. With age, lightly eosinophilic and calcified concretions, known as *corpora arenacea,* may accumulate in the choroid plexus.

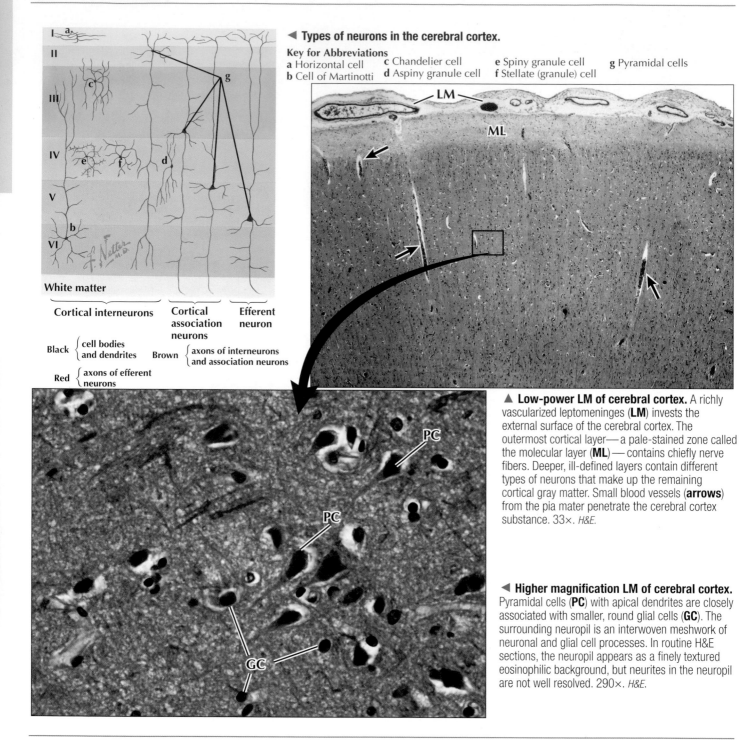

◀ Types of neurons in the cerebral cortex.

Key for Abbreviations
a Horizontal cell   **c** Chandelier cell   **e** Spiny granule cell   **g** Pyramidal cells
b Cell of Martinotti   **d** Aspiny granule cell   **f** Stellate (granule) cell

White matter

Cortical interneurons   Cortical association neurons   Efferent neuron

Black { cell bodies and dendrites

Brown { axons of interneurons and association neurons

Red { axons of efferent neurons

▲ Low-power LM of cerebral cortex. A richly vascularized leptomeninges (**LM**) invests the external surface of the cerebral cortex. The outermost cortical layer—a pale-stained zone called the molecular layer (**ML**)—contains chiefly nerve fibers. Deeper, ill-defined layers contain different types of neurons that make up the remaining cortical gray matter. Small blood vessels (**arrows**) from the pia mater penetrate the cerebral cortex substance. 33×. *H&E.*

◀ Higher magnification LM of cerebral cortex. Pyramidal cells (**PC**) with apical dendrites are closely associated with smaller, round glial cells (**GC**). The surrounding neuropil is an interwoven meshwork of neuronal and glial cell processes. In routine H&E sections, the neuropil appears as a finely textured eosinophilic background, but neurites in the neuropil are not well resolved. 290×. *H&E.*

5.19 CYTOARCHITECTURE OF THE CEREBRAL CORTEX

The **cerebrum** consists of two **hemispheres** with an outer cortex of **gray matter** and a central region of **white matter**. The **cerebral cortex**, 1.5-4.5 mm thick and with more than 15 billion neurons, constitutes 40% of the weight of the human brain. The outer surface is highly folded to increase the surface area, estimated at about 2000 cm². The convolutions are known as **sulci** and the intervening grooves, **gyri**. Different types of neurons and fibers are arranged in horizontal layers, so the cortex appears laminated. Despite regional variations, the cortex typically consists of six ill-defined layers, which differ in neuronal population density. As many as five types of cortical neurons exist, but **pyramidal cells** and **stellate cells** are most numerous. Nerve fibers are oriented tangentially and radially, establish complex intracortical circuits, and transmit *impulses* at multiple synaptic sites. Many neurons make connections with other cortical neurons or project to other areas of the brain and spinal cord. Pyramidal cell bodies, shaped like isosceles triangles, range from 10 to 50 μm in diameter. A large **dendrite** projects apically, is oriented at right angles to the surface, and branches repeatedly as it climbs to the surface. Emerging from the base of each cell is a single axon that penetrates to deeper cortical layers and enters the medullary white matter. In certain cortical regions, giant pyramidal neurons, called Betz cells, have diameters up to 100 μm.

▼ **Types of neurons in the cerebellar cortex.**

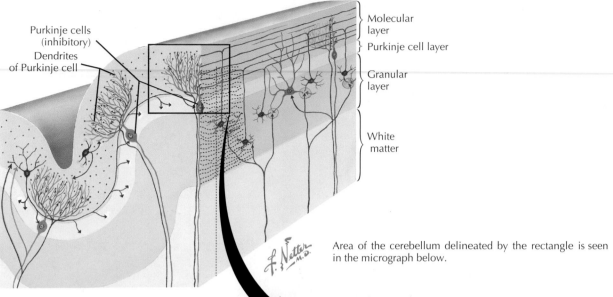

Purkinje cells (inhibitory)
Dendrites of Purkinje cell

Molecular layer
Purkinje cell layer
Granular layer
White matter

Area of the cerebellum delineated by the rectangle is seen in the micrograph below.

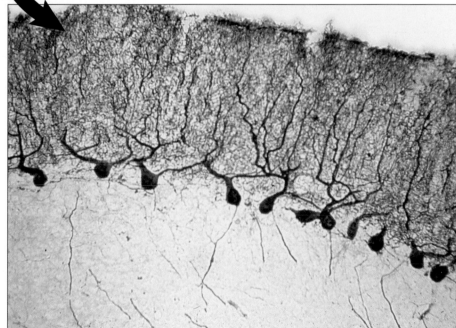

▶ **Immunocytochemical staining of Purkinje cells in the cerebellar cortex.** An antibody to parvalbumin selectively labels Purkinje cells, so that their cell bodies, basal axons, and elaborate apical fan-like dendritic tree are clear. 135×. *Immunoperoxidase-diaminobenzidine. (Courtesy of Dr. K. G. Baimbridge)*

5.20 CYTOARCHITECTURE OF THE CEREBELLUM

The cerebellum is a bilaterally symmetric part of the brain with an extensively folded surface that has thin transverse folds known as folia, which resemble leaves of a tree. It consists of a surface layer of cortex of **gray matter** and a medullary center of **white matter.** Its name is misleading as it implies that it is a small part of the brain, but the **cerebellar cortex** is three-fourths the size of the cerebral cortex. Also, the cerebellar cortex most likely contains more neurons than the cerebral cortex. The cerebellar cortex has a remarkably uniform trilaminar organization: an outer **molecular layer,** an inner layer of **granule cells,** and a middle monolayer of large pear-shaped neurons known as **Purkinje cells.** The molecular layer is a pale-stained zone with relatively few neuron bodies. It contains a network of profusely branching **dendrites** of

Purkinje cells and represents mainly a *synaptic* field. These dendritic branches are not readily seen in conventional preparations; more specialized techniques, such as *metal impregnation* or *immunocytochemistry*, are required for elucidation.

CLINICAL POINT

Nervous tissue in the CNS is mostly cellular and has an intricate, tightly packed topography of neurons, axons, dendrites, and associated glia. Its extracellular matrix (ECM) constitutes only about 10% of brain volume. Unlike other organs, the brain has very little connective tissue, and the limited amount of ECM is fluid-filled. **Cerebral edema**— swelling caused by accumulation of fluid in the ECM of the brain—is a common clinical condition after head injury. If edema is not treated quickly, neurons in the brain are irreparably damaged; once injured, neurons cannot repair themselves and undergo mitosis.

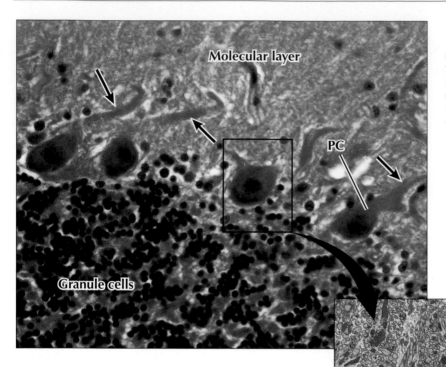

▶ **EM of part of the cerebellar cortex.** Ultrastructural features —soma and apical dendrite— of a Purkinje cell are clearly seen. The spherical nucleus is euchromatic and contains a nucleolus. The perikaryon contains abundant rough endoplasmic reticulum, free ribosomes, scattered mitochondria, and lysosomes. A primary dendrite projects apically. Small round granule cells are also visible. The surrounding neuropil contains neuronal processes of various size interspersed with glial cell processes. 3100×.

5.21 HISTOLOGY AND ULTRASTRUCTURE OF THE CEREBELLUM

Cerebellar **Purkinje cells** have a unique flask-like shape and, with soma diameters of 50-80 μm, are one of the largest neurons in the CNS. At 15-30 million, they are also among the most numerous in the brain. They form a single row of uniformly arranged, large neuron bodies on the outer surface of the **granule cell layer.** Light microscopy shows a single, vesicular **nucleus** with prominent Nissl substance in surrounding cytoplasm. By electron microscopy, **primary** and **secondary dendrites** are smooth surfaced; small tertiary branches have short, stubby spines. Each Purkinje cell has more than 100,000 dendritic spines that markedly increase its surface area for synaptic contact. A single myelinated axon projects from the base of each Purkinje cell and descends to the underlying medullary white region. **Granule cells** are densely packed, round to oval, small neurons, about 5 μm in diameter. Only the nucleus is readily seen, as there is very little surrounding cytoplasm. Several short dendrites project from the base of each granule cell, and one apical axon extends into the **molecular layer,** loses its myelin sheath, and bifurcates up to 3 mm in each direction. Because of their orientation parallel to the surface, unmyelinated axons are known as parallel fibers. They establish multiple synaptic contacts with dendritic spines of Purkinje cells.

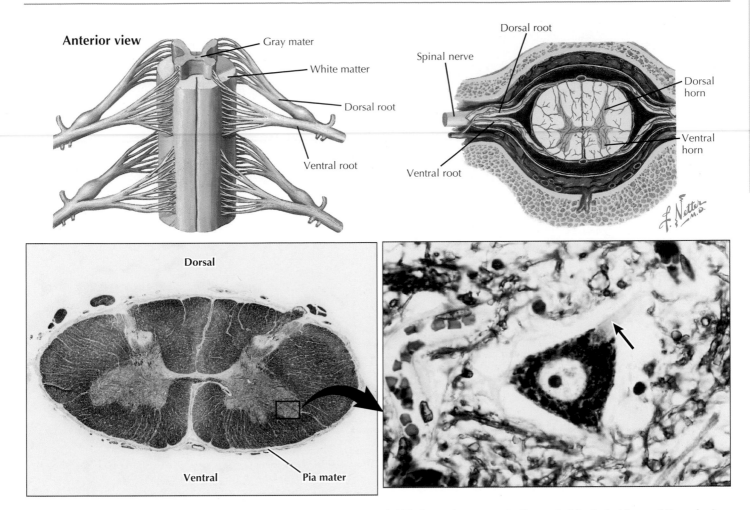

Anterior view — Gray mater
— White matter
— Dorsal root
Ventral root

Dorsal root
Spinal nerve
Dorsal horn
Ventral horn
Ventral root

Dorsal

Ventral   **Pia mater**

▲ **The spinal cord in transverse section.** The gray matter is the butterfly-shaped area, whereas the peripherally located white matter is composed of tracts of myelinated nerve fibers. 8×. *Luxol fast blue and cresyl violet.*

▲ **LM of a motor neuron in the ventral (anterior) horn of the spinal cord.** An axon (**arrow**) lacking Nissl substance projects from the soma of this multipolar neuron. 840×. *Luxol fast blue and cresyl violet.*

5.22 ANATOMY AND HISTOLOGY OF THE SPINAL CORD

Specific spinal cord anatomy varies according to the cord level, but in cross section the cord is roughly oval to cylindrical with a ventral fissure. The **white matter** of the spinal cord, unlike that in other CNS areas, is peripherally located; the **gray matter** occupies an H-shaped central region. White matter is so named because of large amounts of myelin, the fatty insulating substance that forms sheaths around individual nerve fibers. White matter consists of ascending and descending tracts of **myelinated nerve fibers.** Gray matter consists chiefly of cell bodies and unmyelinated nerve fibers, so to the naked eye, they appear pinkish gray compared with myelinated fibers of the white matter. Gray matter has two **ventral horns** and two **dorsal horns** connected at the center by an isthmus of gray commissures surrounding a small central canal, which is lined by ependymal epithelium. Sensory nerve fibers enter the spinal cord via the dorsal horns, and motor nerve fibers exit from the ventral horns in discrete bundles known as spinal nerves. The PNS comprises 31 pairs of **spinal nerves,** which are divided into cervical, thoracic, lumbar, sacral, and coccygeal groups. Two enlargements of the ventral horns—in the cervical and the lumbar regions—provide motor innervation to upper and lower limbs, respectively. A unique feature of the thoracic and upper lumbar levels of the spinal cord is small lateral horns of gray matter, which are the source of efferent sympathetic neurons of the *autonomic nervous system.* The spinal cord is covered by **connective tissue meninges**—an outer **dura,** middle **arachnoid,** and inner **pia mater.**

CLINICAL POINT

Amyotrophic lateral sclerosis (ALS), also known as **Lou Gehrig's disease,** is a progressive *neuromuscular disorder* caused by destruction of specific neurons in the brain and spinal cord. ALS belongs to a class of disorders known as *motor neuron diseases* and results in loss of nervous control of skeletal muscles, which leads to degeneration and atrophy of muscle fibers. Respiratory muscles are ultimately affected; death is thus due to an inability to breathe. ALS mostly affects men, although women also get the disorder, with the progression rate varying among individuals. Its cause is uncertain, but several proposed hypotheses include *glutamate toxicity, mitochondrial dysfunction,* and *autoimmune mechanisms.*

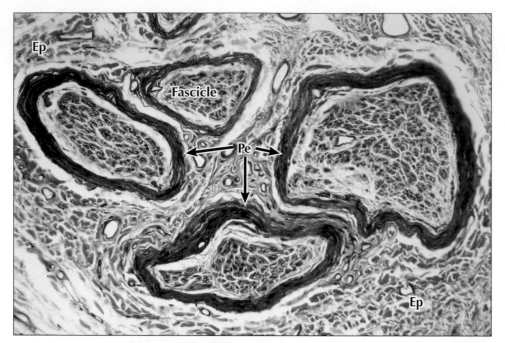

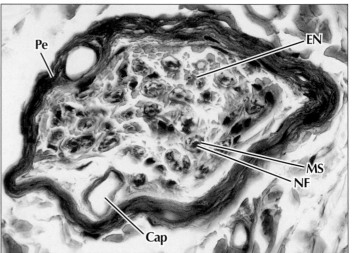

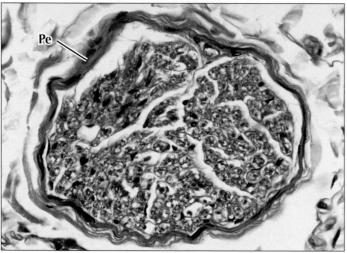

◄ **LM of a peripheral nerve in transverse section.** Several fascicles that make up this nerve are enveloped by connective tissue of the epineurium (**Ep**), which merges imperceptibly with surrounding loose connective tissue. A more deeply stained perineurium (**Pe**) encloses the fascicles. Each fascicle consists of large numbers of nerve fibers, which are embedded in a more delicate endoneurium (not well resolved at this magnification). 200×. *Masson trichrome.*

▲ **LM of one peripheral nerve fascicle in transverse section at medium magnification.** The perineurium (**Pe**) forms an investment around the fascicle. This small nerve has a single fascicle in the connective tissue, so it lacks an epineurium. The interior has numerous nerve fibers sectioned transversely or obliquely and embedded in loose connective tissue of the endoneurium. Many nerve fibers are surrounded by myelin sheaths, which appear washed out because of lipid content. Within the fascicle are nuclei of occasional fibroblasts, Schwann cells, and capillary endothelial cells between nerve fibers. 280×. *H&E.*

▲ **LM of a nerve fascicle at higher magnification.** Here, the perineurium (**Pe**) is dark blue and the endoneurium (**En**), light blue. Nerve fibers (**NF**) are densely stained structures surrounded by a myelin sheath (**MS**), which is red. A capillary (**Cap**) is shown. 465×. *Masson trichrome.*

5.23 HISTOLOGY OF PERIPHERAL NERVES IN TRANSVERSE SECTION

A peripheral nerve consists of one or more bundles of nerve fibers. Each bundle, or fascicle, contains a mixture of fibers, either efferent (motor) or afferent (sensory). In peripheral nerves consisting of more than one fascicle, an outer layer of dense irregular connective tissue, the epineurium, binds the fascicles together and forms a strong cylindrical sheath around the whole nerve. Surrounding each fascicle is a very condensed layer of specialized connective tissue called the perineurium, which is made of multiple concentric layers of flattened cells with intervening, longitu-

dinal collagen fibrils. The perineurium acts as a selective, metabolically active diffusion barrier. It restricts passage of many macromolecular substances, thereby regulating the internal microenvironment of the nerve. Perineurial cells are modified fibroblasts, most likely of neural crest origin, which are linked together by tight junctions and help contribute to a blood-nerve barrier between highly permeable blood vessels in the exterior of each fascicle and the interior tight capillaries. Individual nerve fibers and their support cells within each fascicle are firmly embedded in a delicate packing of loose connective tissue called endoneurium.

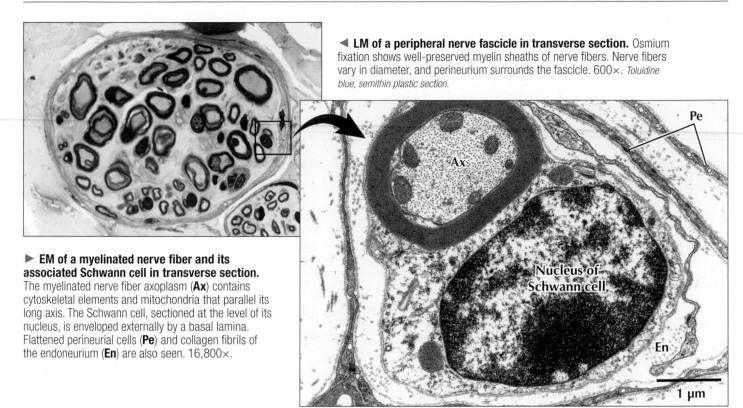

◀ **LM of a peripheral nerve fascicle in transverse section.** Osmium fixation shows well-preserved myelin sheaths of nerve fibers. Nerve fibers vary in diameter, and perineurium surrounds the fascicle. 600×. *Toluidine blue, semithin plastic section.*

▶ **EM of a myelinated nerve fiber and its associated Schwann cell in transverse section.** The myelinated nerve fiber axoplasm (**Ax**) contains cytoskeletal elements and mitochondria that parallel its long axis. The Schwann cell, sectioned at the level of its nucleus, is enveloped externally by a basal lamina. Flattened perineurial cells (**Pe**) and collagen fibrils of the endoneurium (**En**) are also seen. 16,800×.

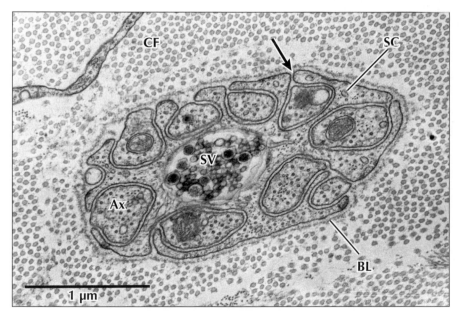

◀ **EM of a Schwann cell associated with several unmyelinated nerve fibers in transverse section.** Nerve fibers (**Ax**) occupy channel-like invaginations of Schwann cell cytoplasm (**SC**). Most nerve fibers contain neurofibrils and microtubules. One nerve fiber in the center contains clear, dense core synaptic vesicles (**SV**). A basal lamina (**BL**) covers the outer aspect of the Schwann cell, and a mesaxon is indicated (**arrow**). Surrounding endoneurial connective tissue contains collagen fibrils (**CF**). 33,000×. *(Courtesy of Dr. A. M. Herrera)*

5.24 ULTRASTRUCTURE OF MYELINATED AND UNMYELINATED NERVE FIBERS IN THE PERIPHERAL NERVOUS SYSTEM

Schwann cells, the principal supporting cells of the peripheral nervous system, surround all nerve fibers, **myelinated** and **unmyelinated.** Myelin acts as an electrical insulator and permits nerve impulses to be transmitted rapidly by *saltatory conductance* along nodes of Ranvier. A direct relationship exists among speed of nerve conduction, axon size, and thickness of the **myelin sheath** (number of concentric myelin lamellae). In myelinated fibers, the speed of conduction may vary from 5 to 100 m/s, which is much higher than that in smaller unmyelinated fibers, with conduction speeds of 0.2-2 m/s. The association of Schwann cells to nerve fibers differs for myelinated and unmyelinated fibers. Small-diameter nerve fibers composed of both axons and dendrites are grouped together by a Schwann cell that either completely or partly envelops them in groove-like invaginations that open to the surface. Schwann cells associated with unmyelinated nerve fibers may invest up to 20 fibers, and the outer surface of the Schwann cell is covered by a **basal lamina.** The narrow cleft from the external surface of the Schwann cell to the nerve fiber is the **mesaxon.**

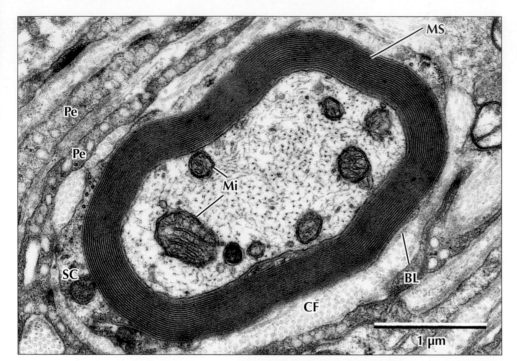

◀ **EM of a PNS nerve fiber in transverse section.** The axon is surrounded by a myelin sheath (**MS**) composed of multiple lamellae formed by the plasma membrane of a Schwann cell. A thin rim of Schwann cell cytoplasm (**SC**) envelops the myelin and is invested externally by a thin basal lamina (**BL**). Collagen fibrils (**CF**) of the endoneurium and flattened perineurial cells (**Pe**) are in the surrounding area. The nerve fiber axoplasm contains mitochondria (**Mi**), neurofilaments, and a few microtubules. 30,000×.

▶ **High-resolution scanning electron micrograph of a myelinated nerve fiber fractured in the transverse plane.** The axon, fractured open, reveals mitochondria (**Mi**) and cytoskeletal elements in the axoplasm (**Ax**). A peripheral rim of Schwann cell cytoplasm (**SC**) is outside the myelin sheath (**MS**). Collagen fibrils (**CF**) of the surrounding endoneurium are shown well. A flattened perineurial cell (**Pe**) is also fractured open. 15,000×.

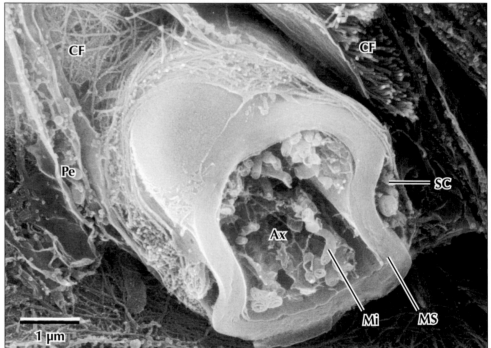

5.25 ULTRASTRUCTURE OF MYELINATED NERVE FIBERS IN THE PERIPHERAL NERVOUS SYSTEM

Further ultrastructural details of **peripheral nerve fibers** and **internodal myelin** are provided by transmission and high-resolution scanning electron microscopy. The close relationship of the **Schwann cell** to the segment of nerve fiber that it myelinates is clear. Along the length of a nerve fiber, consecutive segments of myelin between nodes of Ranvier are called internodal myelin. When viewed at high resolution, the myelin is composed of regularly repeating, concentric layers (**lamellae**) of Schwann cell **plasma membrane** that wrap around the nerve fiber during devel-

opment. The layers repeat radially at a period of about 12-15 nm. Myelin is a *lipoprotein* with a high proportion of lipid (70%) to protein (30%), a proportion different from that elsewhere in the body (35% lipid, 65% protein). Myelin lipid consists of phospholipids, glycolipids, and cholesterol. The composition of PNS myelin and specific kinds of *myelin basic proteins* also appear different from those of CNS myelin. The German pathologist Rudolph Virchow first coined the term from the Greek *myelos*, meaning marrow. It reflects his observation more than a century ago that myelin is abundant in the marrow, or core, of the brain, spinal cord, and peripheral nerves.

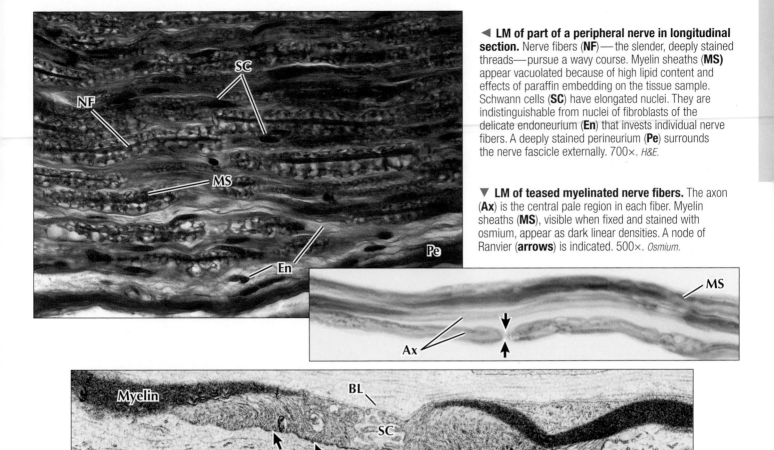

◄ **LM of part of a peripheral nerve in longitudinal section.** Nerve fibers (**NF**)—the slender, deeply stained threads—pursue a wavy course. Myelin sheaths (**MS**) appear vacuolated because of high lipid content and effects of paraffin embedding on the tissue sample. Schwann cells (**SC**) have elongated nuclei. They are indistinguishable from nuclei of fibroblasts of the delicate endoneurium (**En**) that invests individual nerve fibers. A deeply stained perineurium (**Pe**) surrounds the nerve fascicle externally. 700×. *H&E.*

▼ **LM of teased myelinated nerve fibers.** The axon (**Ax**) is the central pale region in each fiber. Myelin sheaths (**MS**), visible when fixed and stained with osmium, appear as dark linear densities. A node of Ranvier (**arrows**) is indicated. 500×. *Osmium.*

▲ **EM of a node of Ranvier in longitudinal section.** Adjacent segments of myelin terminate at the node with terminal loops of Schwann cell cytoplasm (**arrows**) attached to the axolemma in paranodal regions. The axoplasm contains cytoskeletal elements and scattered mitochondria (**Mi**). A thin basal lamina (**BL**) invests interdigitating processes of Schwann cells (**SC**). 16,000x. *(Courtesy of Dr. J. Dupree)*

5.26 NERVE FIBERS IN LONGITUDINAL SECTION AND NODES OF RANVIER IN THE PERIPHERAL NERVOUS SYSTEM

Nodes of Ranvier are short, periodic interruptions of **myelin sheath** that occur at regular intervals along myelinated **nerve fibers** (or **axons**) of the CNS and PNS. The French physician Louis-Antoine Ranvier (1835-1922) described them in 1876 as *etranglements annulaires du tube.* He suggested that they were miniscule gaps that allow diffusion of extracellular nutrients to the cytoplasm of nerve fibers. These nodes are specialized sites, about 1 μm long, where glial cells (**Schwann cells** in the PNS or processes of oligodendrocytes in the CNS) meet. Except for a few ultrastructural differences, PNS and CNS nodes are similar. In the PNS, slender processes of adjacent Schwann cells interdigitate and cover nerve fibers at the node. The myelin sheath in the paranodal

region (on both sides of the node) ends as deep furrows produced by bulbous, loop-like expansions of Schwann cell cytoplasm. These cytoplasmic loops, close to the axon surface, contain many mitochondria, which likely reflect high energy needs at the node. Freeze-fracture electron microscopy and electrophysiology show that the plasma membrane of the nerve fiber at the node contains a high density of *voltage-gated sodium channels.* During nerve impulse transmission, these ionic channels play a critical role in *saltatory conduction.* At these nodes, nerve fiber diameters are slightly narrowed and branching of the fibers is typical; axoplasm contains microtubules, neurofilaments, mitochondria, vesicles, and lysosomes. Although each node in the PNS is invested by the **basal lamina** of Schwann cells, nodes in the CNS are covered by astrocyte end-feet lacking an overlying basal lamina.

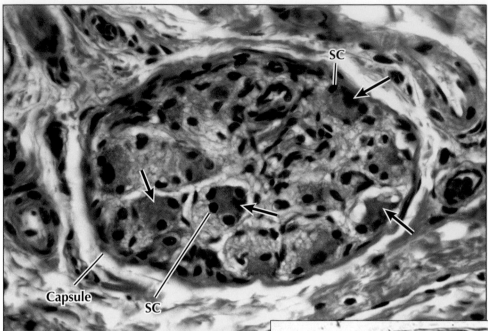

◀ **LM of an autonomic ganglion in the wall of the urinary bladder.** A well-defined capsule covers the ganglion. Darkly stained somas (**arrows**) are surrounded by small satellite cells (**SC**). The frothy appearance of intervening areas is due to abundant myelinated and unmyelinated nerve fibers that course in different directions within the ganglion. Nuclei of Schwann cells are closely associated with the nerve fibers. Nuclei other than Schwann cell nuclei are most often of fibroblasts. 450×. *H&E.*

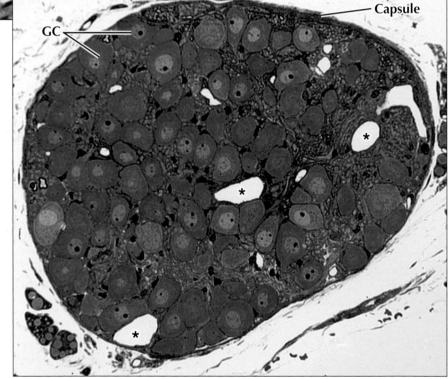

▶ **LM of a prevertebral ganglion associated with the aorta.** Tightly packed ganglion cells (**GC**) are in the interior of the ganglion, whose outer aspect is invested by a thin capsule. Neuronal somas are circular to pleomorphic and show eccentric euchromatic nuclei with prominent nucleoli. Several thin-walled blood vessels and capillaries with clear lumina (∗) are in intervening areas. 270×. *Toluidine blue, semithin plastic section.*

5.27 HISTOLOGY OF PERIPHERAL AUTONOMIC GANGLIA

Ganglia are discrete aggregations of **neuron bodies** located outside the CNS. All derived from neural crest, they include **sensory ganglia** of cranial nerves, **dorsal root ganglia** of spinal nerves, and **autonomic ganglia** at various peripheral sites. Regardless of ganglion site and size, an outer, dense connective tissue **capsule** continuous with epineurium and perineurium associated with entering or emerging nerve fibers invests all ganglia. Neuron bodies within cranial or spinal sensory ganglia are usually pseudounipolar, whereas those in autonomic ganglia are multipolar,

an important differentiating feature. Autonomic ganglia usually contain *cholinergic* synapses between pre- and postganglionic neurons; synapses do not occur in spinal ganglia. Most **ganglion cells** in autonomic ganglia are *adrenergic* and contain dense core vesicles in the bodies and dendrites. In H&E sections, most ganglia appear pale and foamy, which is due to the presence of **myelinated nerve fibers**—because myelin is not preserved and appears washed out—and abundant **unmyelinated nerve fibers,** which course in different directions within the ganglion. Internally, a richly vascularized loose connective tissue stroma surrounds neuronal ganglion elements and provides protection and support.

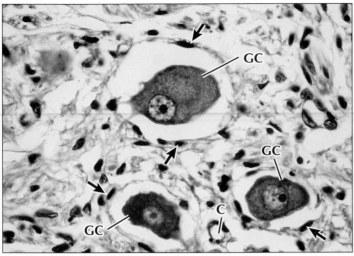

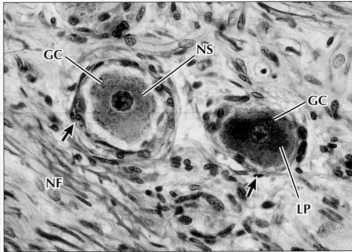

▲ **LM of part of a sympathetic ganglion.** Three large ganglion cells (**GC**) in the field of view possess pale, vesicular, eccentrically placed nuclei with prominent nucleoli. Their cytoplasm contains various amounts of basophilic Nissl substance and golden brown lipofuscin pigment. Flattened satellite cells (**arrows**) with small, dark nuclei surround the ganglion cells. Interstitial connective tissue shows nerve fibers, Schwann cell nuclei, and capillaries (**C**). 730×. *H&E.*

▲ **LM of part of a dorsal root ganglion.** In contrast to cells in sympathetic ganglia, ganglion cells (**GC**) in dorsal root ganglia have centrally placed nuclei. Their cytoplasm contains Nissl substance (**NS**) and lipofuscin pigment (**LP**). Satellite cells (**arrows**) surround ganglion cells. Interstitial connective tissue contains nerve fibers (**NF**) and nuclei of Schwann cells. 630×. *H&E.*

▶ **EM part of a sympathetic ganglion.** Satellite cells (**SC**) closely surround a large ganglion cell (**GC**) the center of the field. An eccentric, euchromatic nucleus contains a prominent nucleolus. An axon emanating from the soma is covered by a Schwann cell (**arrow**). Surrounding areas contain many unmyelinated nerve fibers and their associated Schwann cells (∗). 3400×.

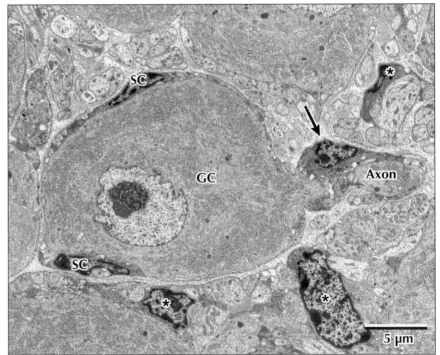

5.28   HISTOLOGY AND ULTRASTRUCTURE OF PERIPHERAL GANGLIA

Ganglion cells are large with spherical, pale-stained **nuclei,** often eccentric in location, which contain a prominent **nucleolus.** As in most neurons, ganglion cell **cytoplasm** has abundant **Nissl substance,** so the soma appears dark. Within the ganglion, a single layer of neural crest-derived **satellite cells** usually surrounds, to form a continuous investment around, each neuron body—arranged like satellites around a central planet. The investment is usually less complete in autonomic ganglia than in dorsal root ganglia, which allows passage of terminal parts of preganglionic axons that form synapses on ganglion cells. Satellite cells are flattened, modified **Schwann cells** with heterochromatic nuclei that are small compared with those of neurons. A basement membrane encloses the outer aspect of the satellite cells, which are linked by gap junctions. These cells are next to surfaces of ganglion somas, although an artifact in conventional paraffin sections often leaves an artificial space between the neuronal soma and satellite cell.

6

CARTILAGE AND BONE

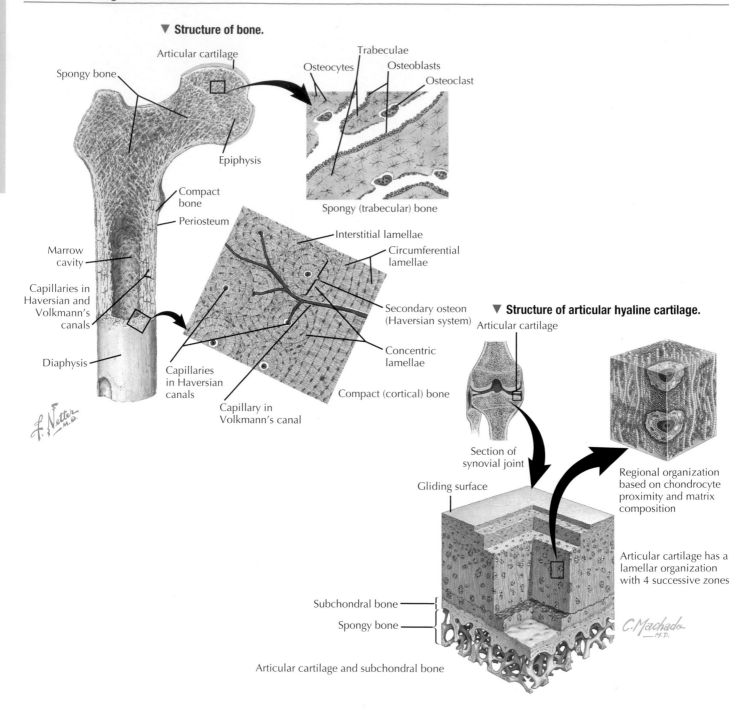

▼ **Structure of bone.**

Articular cartilage

Spongy bone

Osteocytes — Trabeculae — Osteoblasts — Osteoclast

Epiphysis

Compact bone

Periosteum

Spongy (trabecular) bone

Marrow cavity

Capillaries in Haversian and Volkmann's canals

Diaphysis

Interstitial lamellae

Circumferential lamellae

Secondary osteon (Haversian system)

Concentric lamellae

Compact (cortical) bone

Capillaries in Haversian canals

Capillary in Volkmann's canal

▼ **Structure of articular hyaline cartilage.**

Articular cartilage

Section of synovial joint

Gliding surface

Regional organization based on chondrocyte proximity and matrix composition

Articular cartilage has a lamellar organization with 4 successive zones

Subchondral bone

Spongy bone

Articular cartilage and subchondral bone

6.1 OVERVIEW

Cartilage and **bone** are specialized forms of connective tissue that have critical roles in providing the skeletal framework of the body. Although they share similarities, many important differences set them apart. As with other connective tissues, they derive from embryonic mesenchyme; both consist of cells embedded in an **extracellular matrix.** Cartilage matrix is a firm yet resilient gel, with physical attributes of a plastic; it is not as rigid as matrix of bone and gives cartilage a solid, firm consistency. Cartilage matrix is highly hydrated, being 70%-75% water. The rest of the matrix is composed of **collagen** (15%-20%), for *tensile strength*, and **proteoglycans** (2%-10%), for *resilience.* Cartilage provides structural support for soft tissues and a sliding area for joints and allows for growth in long bone length. Cartilage performs diverse and varied functions, but it lacks attributes of most other tissues: it is avascular and has no nerve or lymphatic supply. Bone is the *calcified* component of the skeleton, which in the human comprises 206 individual bones. The matrix of bone, as a rigid connective tissue, consists of collagen embedded in a ground substance on which is deposited a complex inorganic mineral, *hydroxyapatite.* As a tissue, compared with cartilage, bone has a higher metabolic rate, is richly vascularized, and receives up to 10% of cardiac output. Bone has good regenerative potential for self-repair throughout life, whereas cartilage has a very limited capacity for regeneration in response to traumatic injury or disease.

▼ Structure of three types of cartilage.

Articular hyaline cartilage

Histology (H&E) Orientation of collagen fibers

Zone I Tangential

Zone II Oblique

Zone III Vertical

Zone IV Vertical (calcified)

Matrix

Chondrocytes in lacunae

Calcified cartilage

Subchondral bone

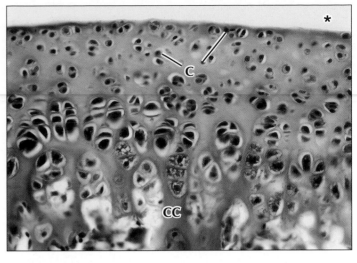

▲ **LM of articular hyaline cartilage from a developing rat knee joint.** Articular cartilage has a complex internal structure, as well as sharing features with other types of hyaline cartilage. Of its four poorly demarcated zones, the most superficial, uppermost zone forms the gliding surface and is in contact with the synovial cavity (∗) of the joint. Small round chondrocytes (**C**) are oriented parallel to the surface; chondrocytes in deeper zones are larger, more rounded, and arranged in vertical columns. The deepest zone contains calcified cartilage (**CC**), which separates hyaline cartilage from subchondral bone. The term chondron encompasses the chondrocyte and its pericellular and territorial matrix. Lacking a perichondrium, articular cartilage is a variant of hyaline cartilage found elsewhere (e.g., in the trachea, nasal septum, and larynx). 100×. *Hematoxylin and phloxine orange G.*

Fibrocartilage

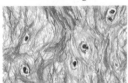

Interlacing strands of fibrous tissue throughout matrix (H&E)

Elastic cartilage

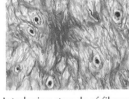

Dark-staining elastic fibers between and around lacunae (H&E)

6.2 STRUCTURE OF CARTILAGE

The three types of cartilage—hyaline cartilage, elastic cartilage, and fibrocartilage—differ mostly in histologic appearance and properties of **extracellular matrix. Hyaline cartilage,** the most common and characteristic type, has a matrix with a translucent, glassy appearance because the *refractive index* of its **collagen** is similar to that of the ground substance in which it is embedded. In the fetus, hyaline cartilage forms a provisional skeleton, which is replaced by bone during endochondral bone formation. Soon after birth and up to adolescence, hyaline cartilage is an integral component of epiphyseal growth plates, which control the growth and shape of long bones. In addition, hyaline cartilage lines articular surfaces of **synovial joints,** where it acts as a self-lubricating shock absorber with low friction properties. Hyaline cartilage also provides semirigid support to walls of some respiratory airways. Damaged hyaline cartilage is unable to be repaired because in the adult its cells—**chondrocytes**—cannot undergo mitosis. **Elastic cartilage** contains chondrocytes embedded in a matrix dominated by **elastic fibers.** Firm but flexible, it contributes structural integ-

rity to the auricle of the ear, epiglottis, and eustachian (auditory) tube and allows bending. **Fibrocartilage** has great tensile strength because of the number of collagen fibers in its matrix. It attaches bone to tendon and, because it has load-distributing properties, it is found in menisci of synovial joints and in intervertebral discs. **Dense fibrous connective tissue** replaces damaged fibrocartilage.

CLINICAL POINT

Osteoarthritis, the most common form of arthritis, is a major cause of long-term disability in adults in North America. It is primarily a disease of *articular cartilage,* its hallmarks being extracellular matrix degradation and altered chondrocyte metabolism. The disorder is associated with decreased glycosaminoglycan content of the matrix accompanied by increased water content. Enhanced matrix metalloproteinase enzyme activity appears to play a major role in matrix degradation and to participate in breakdown of both proteoglycans and collagen. Loss of cartilage leads to bone-on-bone contact in synovial joints with rapid deterioration of movement and function.

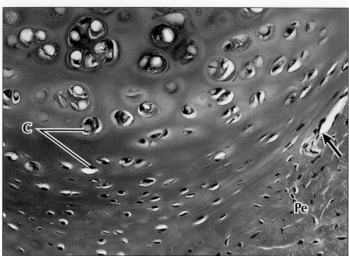
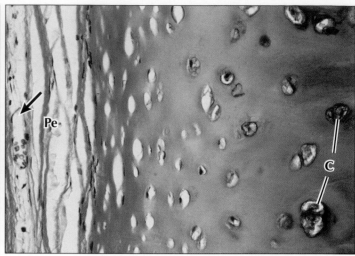

▲ **LM of hyaline cartilage.** In both rib (costal) (**Left**) and tracheal (**Right**) cartilage, a perichondrium (**Pe**) surrounds the cartilage matrix. Blood vessels (**arrows**) in the perichondrium provide oxygen and nutrients, which diffuse into the avascular cartilage. Chondrocytes (**C**) in lacunae are surrounded by a glassy matrix. Peripheral flattened cells are cells added recently by appositional growth. In deeper regions, the cells are more spherical and occur in isogenous nests, indicative of interstitial growth. A fixation artifact causes shrinkage of chondrocytes, with clear spaces around them. 225×. *H&E.*

▶ **Higher magnification LM of hyaline cartilage from the trachea.** Groups of chondrocytes (**C**), the isogenous nests, sit in lacunae. Preparation artifact causes some lacunae to appear empty (∗). In other lacunae, chondrocytes shrank away from walls to leave a clear pericellular halo. Each cell has a slightly irregular shape and contains a single nucleus, often eccentric in location. A thin rim of basophilic territorial matrix (**TM**) is in the immediate vicinity of lacunae, which indicates a high concentration of newly synthesized sulfated GAGs. Between the chondrocytes, the interterritorial matrix (**IM**) appears more eosinophilic and has a typical glassy appearance. 480×. *H&E.*

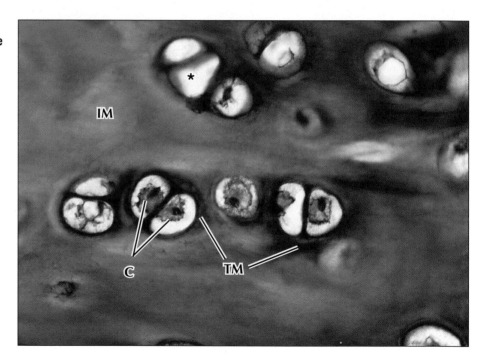

6.3 HISTOLOGY OF HYALINE CARTILAGE

Except where hyaline cartilage serves as articular cartilage and is exposed to synovial fluid, it is enclosed by a layer of **dense connective tissue**—the **perichondrium**—which is essential for cartilage growth. This connective tissue investment is rich in fibroblasts, undifferentiated mesenchymal cells, **blood vessels,** and nerves. During growth, the perichondrium consists of an inner chondrogenic layer surrounded by a fibrous layer. In the embryo, hyaline cartilage arises from loose connective tissue when the oxygen supply is low, whereas bone arises from the same tissue when oxygen is plentiful. **Chondrocytes** are flattened near the perichondrium and more round in deeper regions. Chondrocytes in hyaline cartilage are often arranged in pairs or groups of four to six. Cells of a group are known as an **isogenous nest** because they are progeny of a single chondrocyte during development. Type II collagen fibers, water, and ground substance constitute the **matrix.** *Collagen fibers* impart *eosinophilia* to the matrix but are not visible by light microscopy because their refractive index is similar to that of ground substance. *Basophilia* of this cartilage is due to the presence of *glycosaminoglycans* (GAGs), such as chondroitin sulfate, in ground substance. The basophilic, metachromatic matrix immediately surrounding chondrocytes is the **territorial matrix,** which is rich in **sulfated GAGs** but contains few collagen fibers. A paler, less basophilic **interterritorial matrix** between chondrocytes is older synthetically and contains a fine basket-like network of type II collagen fibers.

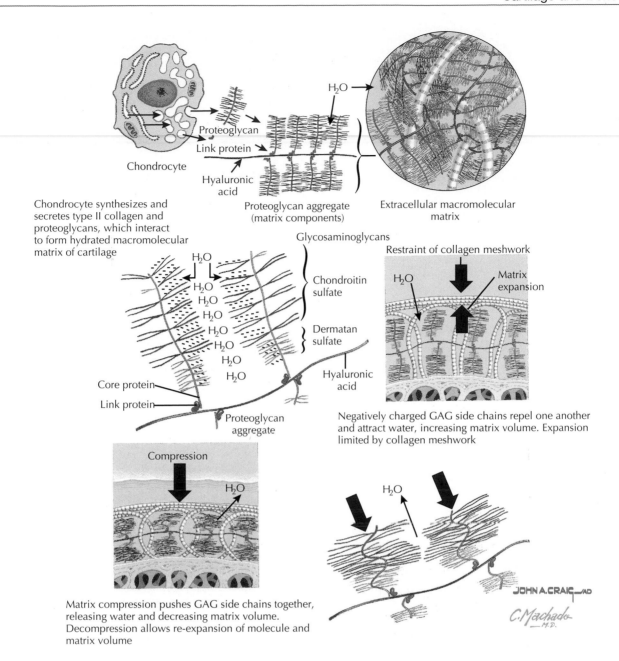

Chondrocyte synthesizes and secretes type II collagen and proteoglycans, which interact to form hydrated macromolecular matrix of cartilage

Proteoglycan aggregate (matrix components)

Extracellular macromolecular matrix

Negatively charged GAG side chains repel one another and attract water, increasing matrix volume. Expansion limited by collagen meshwork

Matrix compression pushes GAG side chains together, releasing water and decreasing matrix volume. Decompression allows re-expansion of molecule and matrix volume

6.4 COMPOSITION OF HYALINE CARTILAGE MATRIX

Chondrocytes of hyaline cartilage are highly specialized cells that synthesize and maintain all components of the **extracellular matrix.** The matrix has a unique, highly ordered molecular organization. Depending on age and location of the cartilage, 60%-70% of its wet weight is water. Water and inorganic salts give cartilage its *resilience* and *lubricating* capabilities. Remaining constituents are structural **macromolecules: collagens, proteoglycans** (PGs), and noncollagenous **proteins.** Of the dry weight of cartilage matrix, 40%-70% is collagen. **Type II** collagen accounts for 90%-95% of the collagen in hyaline cartilage and forms a fibrillar meshwork that mainly provides *tensile strength* and shape. At least two other types—**IX** and **XI**—help stabilize the network of type II fibrils. PGs in the matrix are negatively charged and hold large amounts of positively charged water ions. PGs are composed of a core protein with complex carbohydrates, known as GAGs, that radiate from the core and resemble bristles of a brush. GAGs consist of repeating, negatively charged disaccharide units of various lengths and may be *sulfated* or not. Sulfated PGs, mainly **chondroitin sulfate, dermatan sulfate,** and **keratan sulfate,** in turn attach noncovalently to **hyaluronic acid,** a nonsulfated GAG, to form large PG aggregates known as *aggrecans.* Interactions of aggrecans, water, and collagen fibril network give cartilage its resistance to compression (stiffness) and resilience. Chondrocytes scattered throughout the matrix attach via transmembrane proteins to the macromolecular framework they synthesize.

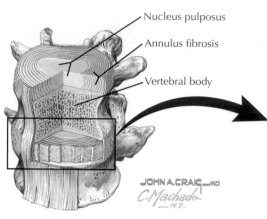

▲ **An intervertebral disc connects bodies of adjacent vertebrae.** The disc has two parts: a central nucleus pulposus consisting of collagen and hydrated PGs and an outer annulus fibrosis of fibrocartilage composed of concentric lamellae of collagen fibers.

▲ **Low-magnification LM of an intervertebral disc in longitudinal section.** The disc is between bodies of two vertebrae (**V**), which are made of spongy bone. A central nucleus pulposus (**NP**) is surrounded by an annulus fibrosis (**AF**). 5×. *H&E.*

▶ **LM of fibrocartilage of the annulus fibrosis of an intervertebral disc.** Between the chondrocytes (**C**) in the matrix (**M**) are coarse bundles of dense, intensely eosinophilic collagen fibers (**arrows**), which are all oriented in the same direction. The elongated chondrocytes, found in short rows, are surrounded by a narrow zone of basophilic ground substance. Fibrocartilage lacks a perichondrium. Part of the nucleus pulposus (**NP**), seen in the upper right, has an amorphous appearance. 380×. *H&E.*

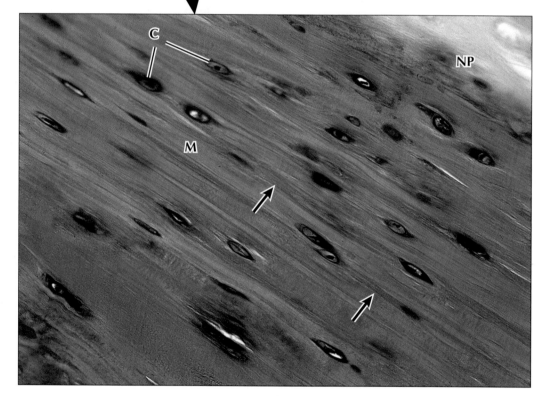

6.5 HISTOLOGY OF FIBROCARTILAGE

Fibrocartilage is found in the symphysis pubis, the **annulus fibrosis** of **intervertebral discs,** and at points of attachment of tendons to bone. It is a mixture between dense regular connective tissue (similar in many respects to tendon or ligament) and hyaline cartilage. It combines the tensile strength, firmness, and durability of tendon with resistance to compression of cartilage. In contrast to other types of cartilage, fibrocartilage lacks a distinct **perichondrium,** which blends imperceptibly with surrounding connective tissue or hyaline cartilage. Its **matrix** is intensely *eosinophilic* because numerous **collagen fibers** are present. Arranged in parallel bundles, often in line with the direction of pull or stress applied, they give a characteristic fibrous appearance to the matrix, which

is readily seen in routine histologic preparations. The matrix contains a minimal amount of amorphous **ground substance,** which is usually seen at boundaries of lacunae, where it is slightly **basophilic** or stains positively for periodic acid-Schiff (PAS). **Chondrocytes** are thinly dispersed in the matrix and are arranged in short, parallel rows between collagen fiber bundles. In contrast to hyaline cartilage, with type II collagen in its matrix, fibrocartilage is composed of *type I collagen*. Fibrocartilage initially forms from dense connective tissue that is rich in fibroblasts, some of which differentiate into chondrocytes. Thus, a mixture of chondrocytes and fibroblasts is characteristic of mature fibrocartilage. At any location, damaged hyaline or elastic cartilage is repaired via formation of fibrocartilage.

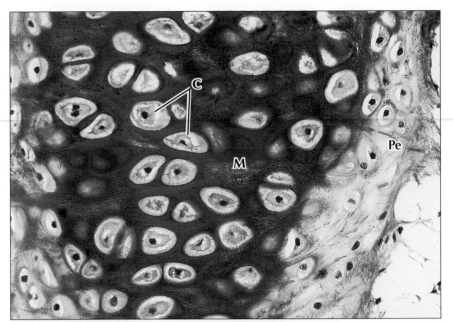

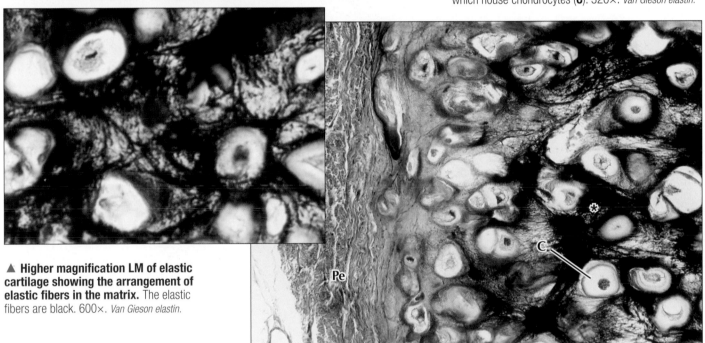

◄ **LM of elastic cartilage in the epiglottis of a child.** A pale-staining perichondrium (**Pe**) encloses the cartilage externally. Pleomorphic chondrocytes (**C**) with small, dark nuclei occupy lacunae and are regularly arranged throughout the matrix (**M**). Because of cell shrinkage, lacunae appear as clear spaces around each chondrocyte. The matrix has a fibrillar appearance and consists of a network of elastic fibers that are dark violet because of selective staining by resorcin-fuchsin. 300×. *Resorcin-fuchsin, nuclear fast red.*

▼ **LM of elastic cartilage in the adult epiglottis.** The section passes through the perichondrium (**Pe**) made mostly of regularly arranged collagen fibers that stain green. The black elastic fiber bundles (∗) in the matrix of this cartilage form whorls around the lacunae, which house chondrocytes (**C**). 320×. *Van Gieson elastin.*

▲ **Higher magnification LM of elastic cartilage showing the arrangement of elastic fibers in the matrix.** The elastic fibers are black. 600×. *Van Gieson elastin.*

6.6 HISTOLOGY OF ELASTIC CARTILAGE

Fresh elastic cartilage appears more opaque and yellow than hyaline cartilage because of abundant **elastic fibers** in its **matrix.** Elastic cartilage is resilient, easily returning to its original shape after bending or distortion, and has more flexibility and elasticity than other cartilage types. Its matrix contains a dense, interwoven network of elastic fibers embedded in a small amount of amorphous extracellular ground substance. This network is denser in the interior than at the periphery. The spherical **chondrocytes,** which sit in **lacunae,** appear similar to chondrocytes of hyaline cartilage, except that they are more closely packed and often found singly in the lacunae (only a few isogenous nests are present). The high refractive index of elastic fibers imparts a lightly eosinophilic staining pattern in conventional preparations. With methods that stain selectively for *elastin,* the branching and anastomosing of the elastic fibers are seen more clearly. The matrix also contains a small number of **type II collagen fibers** that are masked by ground substance and intermingle with the more abundant elastic fibers. Like hyaline cartilage (other than that on articular surfaces of joints), elastic cartilage is enveloped by a **perichondrium.** Blood vessels and lymphatics in the perichondrium do not penetrate the cartilage interior. Elastic cartilage undergoes either appositional growth, from the perichondrium, or interstitial growth, by chondrocyte mitosis. In contrast to other types of cartilage, elastic cartilage does not calcify with age.

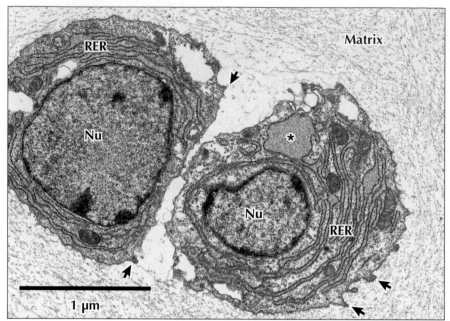

◀ **Electron micrograph (EM) of an isogenous nest in hyaline cartilage.** Cartilage matrix surrounds a pair of chondrocytes. Each cell has a single nucleus (**Nu**) and an irregular cell border with short, stubby foot-like extensions (**arrows**) of plasma membrane. The cytoplasm has abundant **RER** with both flattened and dilated (*) cisternae. Surrounding extracellular matrix has a finely fibrillar appearance. 35,000×. *(Courtesy of Dr. B. J. Crawford)*

▶ **EM of a chondrocyte in hyaline cartilage of the trachea.** The eccentrically placed nucleus (**Nu**) has euchromatin and patches of heterochromatin and is surrounded by a well-defined nuclear envelope. The cytoplasm is replete with organelles involved in synthesis and secretion. **RER** and a well-developed Golgi complex (**GC**) are prominent. The RER consists of parallel arrays of narrow cisternae studded with ribosomes. Mitochondria (**Mi**) lie scattered among elements of the RER. The surrounding matrix contains a meshwork of type II collagen fibrils. 35,000×. *(Courtesy of Dr. B. J. Crawford)*

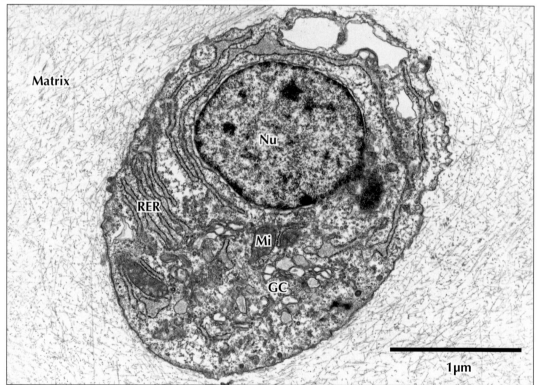

6.7 ULTRASTRUCTURE OF CHONDROCYTES

Ultrastructural features of chondrocytes reflect function: synthesis and secretion of all components of the **extracellular matrix.** These features are similar to those of other cells such as fibroblasts and osteoblasts that synthesize and secrete proteins such as collagen as well as carbohydrates that make up ground substance. In optimal electron microscopic preparations, a chondrocyte completely fills its lacuna. Its **plasma membrane** has small, irregular extensions, or **footlets,** that project at various points around the periphery. In active cells, a single, irregularly ovoid **nucleus** is mostly euchromatic with peripheral clumps of **heterochromatin** close to the **nuclear envelope.** The cytoplasm contains abundant free ribo-somes and well-developed **rough endoplasmic reticulum** (RER) with dilated **cisternae.** The prominent juxtanuclear **Golgi complex** contains expanded saccules and vacuoles of various sizes. **Mito-chondria** are sporadic, which most likely reflects their energy utilization from *glycolytic,* or anaerobic, rather than aerobic mech-anisms. Fat droplets and extensive clusters of glycogen are present, especially in mature, less active cells. Delicate **type II collagen fibrils** dispersed in the matrix have a faintly cross-banded appear-ance at high magnification but lack the 64-nm periodicity char-acteristic of type I collagen in other sites. Type II fibrils form a loose three-dimensional network throughout the matrix and do not assemble into coarse bundles.

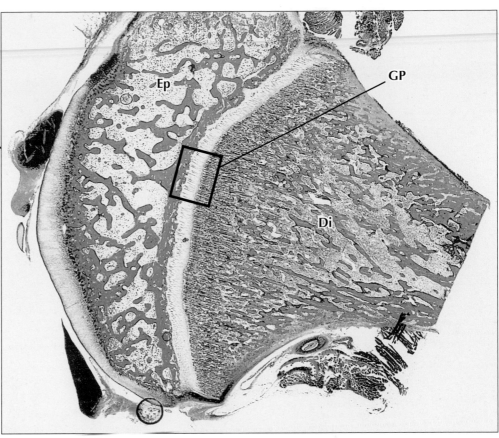

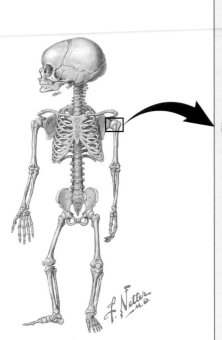

▲ **Skeleton of full-term newborn.** At birth, skeletal ossification centers are mostly primary centers; secondary centers are found in the distal femur, proximal tibia, and head of the humerus. Many secondary centers do not form until a number of years after birth.

▲ **LM of the head of the developing humerus at low magnification.** The section passes through the epiphysis (**Ep**) and part of the diaphysis (**Di**) of this long bone. Growth in length of the bone depends on the epiphyseal growth plate (**GP**), which is the basis for endochondral bone formation. 10×. *Masson trichrome.*

6.8 OVERVIEW OF BONE FORMATION (OSTEOGENESIS)

Bone formation, or osteogenesis, is an astounding, complex series of interrelated, simultaneously occurring processes: *cell migration, mitosis, differentiation, modulation, synthesis, secretion, extracellular mineralization,* and *resorption.* Development of the skeleton begins in the early embryo and fetus, with growth continuing after birth and up to adolescence. Bones are formed by either **intramembranous** or **endochondral ossification.** These two types of osteogenesis refer only to the initial environment in which a bone forms—whether bone forms on the basis of a cartilage model (endochondral) or not (intramembranous)—not the microscopic structure of completely developed bone. Intramembranous ossification occurs in areas of ordinary mesenchyme where osteoblasts, or bone-forming cells, differentiate directly within richly vascularized mesenchymal connective tissue. Flat bones of the cranium, part of the mandible, and the clavicles develop in this way. Most **long bones** (of the extremities), vertebral column, ribs, and pelvis develop by endochondral ossification in preexisting hyaline cartilage models. Here, mesenchymal cells differentiate into chondrocytes. A cartilage template is modified to facilitate mineralization, vascular invasion, and replacement by bone. Both kinds of osteogenesis have the same mechanism of bone matrix deposition and mineralization by first producing spongy (cancellous, or trabecular) bone. Much of this bone later develops into dense (compact, or cortical) bone. After bone forms, it remains dynamic throughout life to allow growth and serve as a source of mineral ions for homeostasis.

▼ Initial bone formation in mesenchyme.

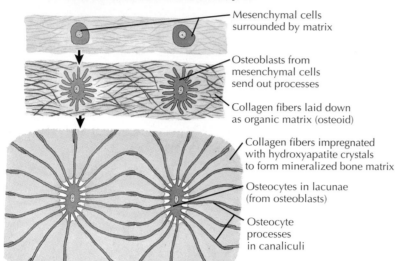

Mesenchymal cells surrounded by matrix

Osteoblasts from mesenchymal cells send out processes

Collagen fibers laid down as organic matrix (osteoid)

Collagen fibers impregnated with hydroxyapatite crystals to form mineralized bone matrix

Osteocytes in lacunae (from osteoblasts)

Osteocyte processes in canaliculi

▼ Successive stages in formation of secondary osteon (Haversian system) during transformation of trabecular to compact bone.

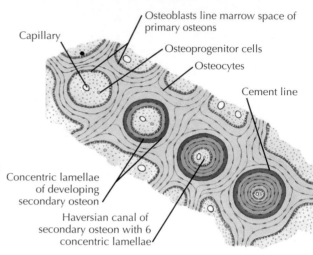

Osteoblasts line marrow space of primary osteons

Capillary

Osteoprogenitor cells

Osteocytes

Cement line

Concentric lamellae of developing secondary osteon

Haversian canal of secondary osteon with 6 concentric lamellae

Early Stages of Flat Bone Formation

Trabeculae lined by osteoblasts

Capillaries in marrow spaces

Dense layer of subperiosteal bone surrounds primary trabecular bone

Periosteum of condensed mesenchyme

Marrow spaces (primary osteons)

Bony trabeculae lined with osteoblasts

▼ Secondary osteon with 6 concentric lamellae (greatly enlarged).

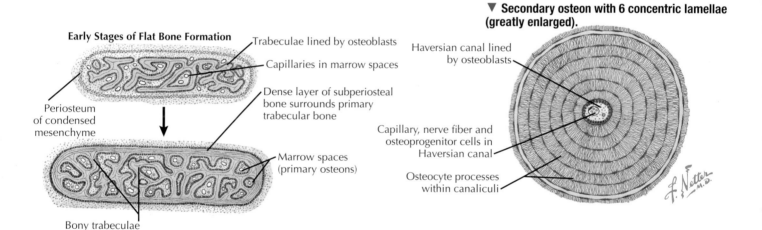

Haversian canal lined by osteoblasts

Capillary, nerve fiber and osteoprogenitor cells in Haversian canal

Osteocyte processes within canaliculi

6.9 INTRAMEMBRANOUS BONE FORMATION

Intramembranous bone formation begins during gestation when **mesenchymal cells** aggregate at sites of richly vascularized connective tissue and differentiate into **osteoblasts.** They secrete **osteoid,** which is an organic matrix of proteoglycans and **type I collagen fibers.** Osteoblasts also secrete alkaline phosphatase, which induces *mineralization* of osteoid via precipitation of inorganic calcium phosphate salts. **Hydroxyapatite** is the dominant mineral of the bony **matrix.** During ossification, osteoblasts are entrapped in the matrix and become **osteocytes**—mature cells of bone. These spider-shaped cells reside in small spaces called **lacunae** and are connected with neighboring osteocytes by slender processes that lie in small channels called **canaliculi.** Small islands, or **trabeculae,** of newly formed bone are initially laid down.

Osteoblasts arrange themselves on trabeculae surfaces and continue to produce bony matrix. Trabeculae thicken and merge to produce a three-dimensional latticework of **trabecular (spongy) bone.** Intervening spaces contain loose, highly vascularized, hematopoietic connective tissue that becomes primary bone **marrow.** Large multinucleated cells called **osteoclasts** migrate to trabeculae surfaces to begin resorbing bony matrix, which provides a mechanism for constant bone remodeling. Conversion of spongy bone to **compact bone** occurs in selected regions. Bony matrix fills in spaces between trabeculae. Deposition of concentric layers, or **lamellae,** of matrix around trapped **blood vessels** forms **osteons.** A layer of specialized connective tissue invests developing bone to become the **periosteum.**

▼ **Growth and ossification of long bones (humerus, midfrontal section).**

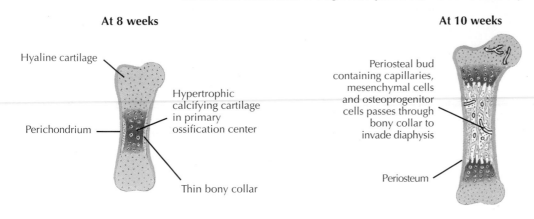

At 8 weeks

Hyaline cartilage

Perichondrium

Hypertrophic calcifying cartilage in primary ossification center

Thin bony collar

At 10 weeks

Periosteal bud containing capillaries, mesenchymal cells and osteoprogenitor cells passes through bony collar to invade diaphysis

Periosteum

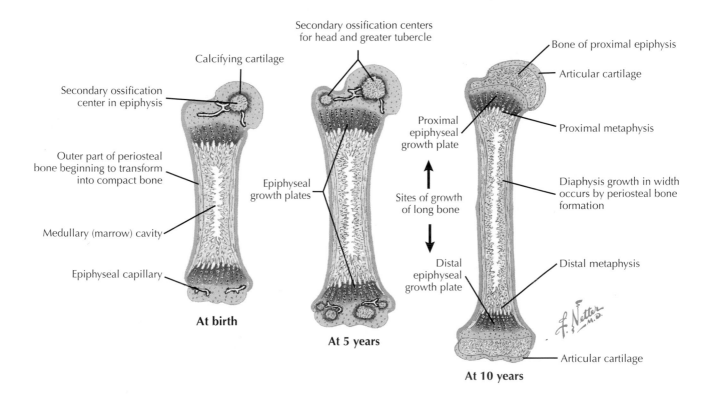

Secondary ossification centers for head and greater tubercle

Calcifying cartilage

Secondary ossification center in epiphysis

Outer part of periosteal bone beginning to transform into compact bone

Medullary (marrow) cavity

Epiphyseal capillary

At birth

Epiphyseal growth plates

Sites of growth of long bone

At 5 years

Proximal epiphyseal growth plate

Distal epiphyseal growth plate

Bone of proximal epiphysis

Articular cartilage

Proximal metaphysis

Diaphysis growth in width occurs by periosteal bone formation

Distal metaphysis

Articular cartilage

At 10 years

6.10 ENDOCHONDRAL BONE FORMATION

Endochondral bone formation begins with hyaline cartilage replicas of future adult bone. Having developed from mesenchyme, cartilage templates take the shape of the later bone. The first of two or more ossification centers appears in the shaft, or diaphysis, of the cartilage template. A thin bony collar appears around the diaphysis by intramembranous ossification as bone is laid down directly by connective tissue perichondrium of the cartilage. After the delicate collar of bone forms around the center of the diaphysis, the perichondrium becomes a periosteum. Deep to the new collar, cartilage matrix begins to calcify, and chondrocytes hypertrophy and die. From the periosteum, blood vessels, collectively termed the periosteal bud, invade the diaphysis interior and bring in associated mesenchymal and osteoprogenitor cells. Erosion of cartilage in the center and formation of a primitive marrow cavity also occur. Incoming blood vessels carry in primitive bone marrow cells. Because the interior diameter of the diaphysis remains constant, interstitial proliferation of remaining chondrocytes causes the two ends, or epiphyses, to grow longitudinally. Chondrocytes are thus arranged in columns and appear as two fronts on both sides of the central region. They eventually form the epiphyseal growth plates at the junction between epiphysis and diaphysis. Growth plates of hyaline cartilage determine the longitudinal diaphysis growth. Toward the end of fetal life and continuing into puberty, ossification centers appear in the two epiphyses of long bones. After adolescence, growth plates close and growth ceases.

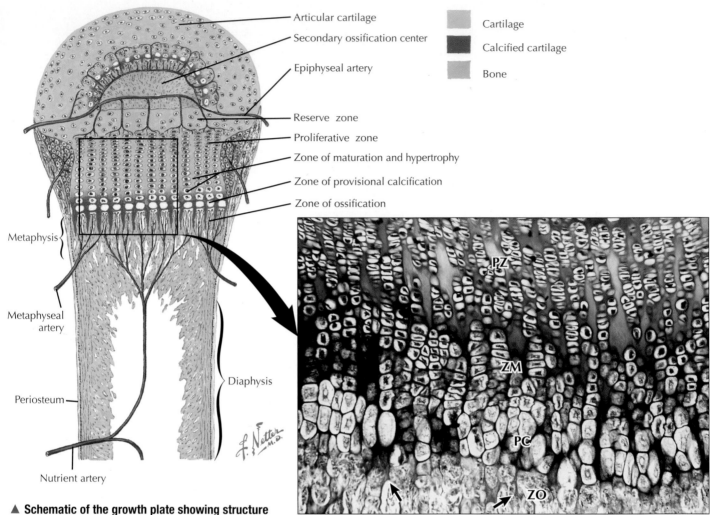

Articular cartilage
Secondary ossification center
Epiphyseal artery
Reserve zone
Proliferative zone
Zone of maturation and hypertrophy
Zone of provisional calcification
Zone of ossification

Cartilage
Calcified cartilage
Bone

Metaphysis
Metaphyseal artery
Periosteum
Diaphysis
Nutrient artery

▲ **Schematic of the growth plate showing structure and blood supply.** The two growth plates in a typical long bone are peripheral extensions of the primary ossification center. The primary center grows and expands centrifugally in all directions until it becomes confined to the bone ends. A growth plate consists mostly of a cartilagenous portion with various histologic zones and a bony component known as the metaphysis.

▲ **Low-magnification LM of the growth plate in longitudinal section.** The proliferative zone (**PZ**) shows closely packed stacks of flattened chondrocytes. Zones of maturation and hypertrophy (**ZM**) contain enlarged cells, which create small open cavities in the provisional calcification (**PC**) zone. The cartilage matrix becomes more basophilic as it calcifies and gives rise to slender spicules (**arrows**) of the zone of ossification (**ZO**) that project into the marrow cavity. 150×. *Wright's.*

6.11 STRUCTURE AND FUNCTION OF GROWTH PLATES

Cartilagenous growth plates in a typical long bone are confined to its two ends and provide temporary scaffolding on which new bone is laid down. The plate promotes appositional growth of **hyaline cartilage** at the end facing the **epiphysis.** Cartilage destruction in lower regions and replacement with primary spongy bone in the deepest region, the **metaphysis,** follow. Five histologically distinct, transverse zones of the growth plate reflect the sequence of events in endochondral ossification. 1) The **reserve zone (resting cartilage)** consists of small clusters of flattened or rounded, randomly arranged, quiescent **chondrocytes.** 2) In the **proliferative zone,** chondrocytes undergo rapid mitosis under influence of growth hormone. No lateral cellular displacement occurs; daughter cells are stacked into columns, resembling stacks of coins, and are parallel to the long axis of the future bone. 3) In the **zone of maturation and hypertrophy,** mitosis ceases, and cells and their lacunae enlarge, followed by cellular accumulation of lipid, glycogen, and alkaline phosphatase. 4) In the relatively narrow **zone of provisional calcification,** thin partitions, or **spicules,** of deeply basophilic **calcified cartilage matrix** are left behind. Dead chondrocytes are resorbed; lacunae erode. Richly vascularized primary marrow extends into the newly opened spaces, and osteoblasts differentiate from mesenchymal cells in the marrow. 5) In the **ossification zone** at the metaphysis, osteoblasts gather on exposed plates, or spicules, of calcified cartilage. Osteoblasts secrete osteoid, which becomes mineralized.

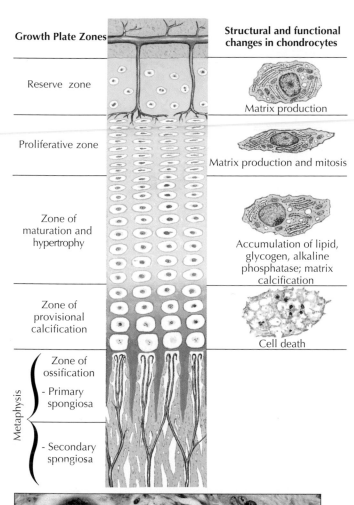

Growth Plate Zones

Reserve zone

Proliferative zone

Zone of maturation and hypertrophy

Zone of provisional calcification

Zone of ossification
- Primary spongiosa

Metaphysis

- Secondary spongiosa

Structural and functional changes in chondrocytes

Matrix production

Matrix production and mitosis

Accumulation of lipid, glycogen, alkaline phosphatase; matrix calcification

Cell death

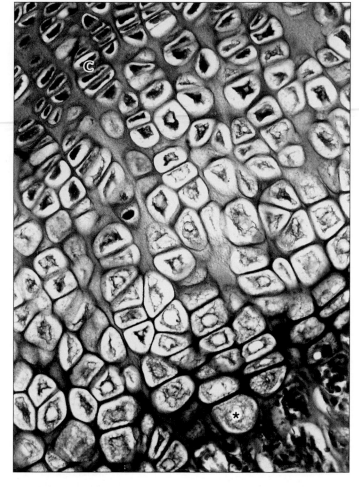

▲ **LM showing details of the growth plate in longitudinal section.** Chondrocytes (**C**), arranged in columns, progressively enlarge (from top to bottom) and leave empty spaces (✶) in calcified matrix. The metaphysis and zone of ossification are in the lower right. 350×. *H&E.*

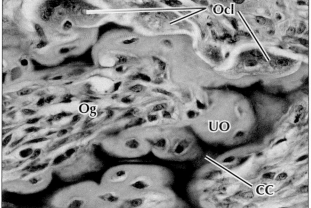

◄ **High-magnification LM of part of the metaphysis in endochondral bone formation.** Newly formed, unmineralized osteoid (**UO**) forms a thin layer on surfaces of calcified cartilage spicules (**CC**). The osteoid contains small osteoblasts. The intensely stained spicules will eventually be resorbed by osteoclasts (**Ocl**). The large multinucleated osteoclasts sit in resorption cavities—Howship lacunae—on the osteoid. Small elongated cells in surrounding areas are osteogenic cells (**Og**). 500×. *Wright's.*

6.12 HISTOLOGY OF THE GROWTH PLATE AND THE METAPHYSIS

The metaphysis, at the distal end of the growth plate between the epiphysis and diaphysis, is formed by slender **calcified cartilage spicules.** These spicules project from the epiphyseal growth plate into the marrow cavity of the diaphysis and thus may be likened to hanging stalactites. The metaphysis is invaded by numerous **capillary loops** that transport cells that become **osteoblasts,** which deposit a veneer of **bony matrix** on calcified cartilage remnants. The metaphysis is divided into two functionally distinct regions. In the upper one—the **primary spongiosa**—primary spongy bone

forms. It contains capillary sprouts between mixed spicules, which consist of a core of calcified cartilage covered by a thin layer of newly formed bone. The lower end of the metaphysis is the **secondary spongiosa,** in which calcified cartilage in the mixed spicules is ultimately resorbed by **osteoclasts,** followed by secondary remodeling of spongy bone. These events result in the lengths of the spicules remaining nearly constant as the marrow cavity volume gradually increases. Growth in length continues until puberty under the influence of *growth hormone, thyroid hormone, parathyroid hormone,* and *androgens.* At skeletal maturity, epiphyseal growth ceases, and bony union of epiphysis and diaphysis occurs.

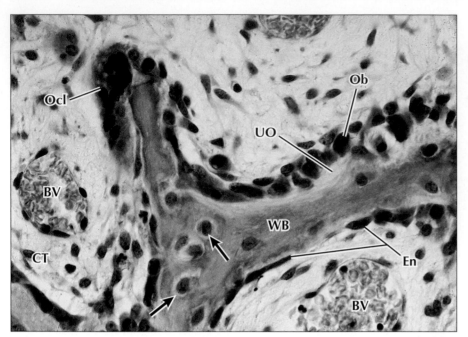

◄ **LM of fetal bone showing a developing bony trabecula undergoing bone deposition and resorption.** Osteoblasts (**Ob**) engage in active bone formation and form a monolayer of plump, cuboidal cells on the trabecular surface. Unmineralized osteoid (**UO**) is the thin, pale layer between these cells and the more deeply stained matrix of woven bone (**WB**). Osteocytes in the woven bone are large, round cells within clear lacunae (**arrows**). A large, multinucleated osteoclast (**Ocl**) lies in another part of the trabecula. Surrounding loose connective tissue (**CT**) is highly vascular and contains many thin-walled blood vessels (**BV**) and mesenchymal stem cells, some of which will become osteoprogenitor cells. Cells of the endosteum (**En**), which include osteogenic cells and inactive osteoblasts, are on the lower surface of the trabecula. 500×. *H&E.*

► **LM of mature spongy bone showing part of a bony trabecula.** The intensely eosinophilic trabecula is made of lamellar bone (**LB**). Embedded in the bony matrix are osteocytes (**arrows**) and their lacunae, which are small and spindle shaped. Flattened cells on the trabecular surface make up the delicate endosteum (**En**) and appear to be inactive. Surrounding bone marrow (**BM**) contains abundant small hematopoietic cells and occasional fat cells (**FC**). Because of the high mineral content and hardness of bone, conventional histologic preparations require decalcification, whereby chelation of calcium permits tissue sectioning and staining. 240×. *H&E.*

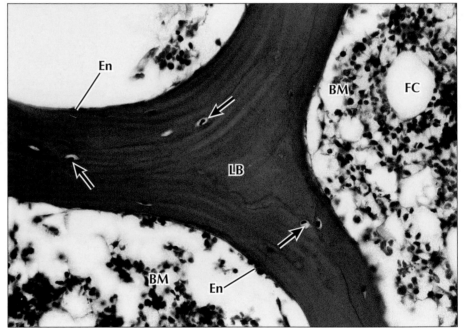

6.13 HISTOLOGY OF TRABECULAR BONE DESPOSITION AND RESORPTION

Orientation of collagen fibers in the bony matrix determines whether bone is either **primary (woven)** or **mature (lamellar) bone.** Woven bone is found in bones of fetuses and young children and has coarse collagen fibers that are oriented randomly. Lamellar bone begins to form soon after birth and actively replaces woven bone by 4 years. In lamellar bone, collagen fibers are in parallel layers, which are readily apparent when viewed by polarization microscopy. Bone **resorption** begins as soon as bone is first formed, and both deposition and resorption continue throughout life, determine the adaptable structure of mature lamellar bone, and affect homeostasis of calcium and phosphate ions between bone and blood. **Osteoblasts** are the main bone-producing cells, whereas **osteoclasts** are specialized multinucleated cells whose major role is to resorb bone. In spongy bone, osteoblasts produce new lamellae on one surface of a **trabecula.** Osteoclasts in resorption cavities, or **Howship lacunae,** on other surfaces actively resorb bone. Several parallel lamellae make up each trabecula and are not penetrated by **blood vessels.** Nourishment of **osteocytes** entrapped in lamellae depends on diffusion of nutrients from vascular **bone marrow.** Bony matrix can be likened to reinforced concrete and consists of both organic and inorganic components. The organic portion, comprising 30%-40% of the matrix, consists mostly of type I collagen and associated glycoproteins and provides *tensile strength* and *resilience.* The remaining 60%-70% of the matrix is inorganic and consists of minerals, mostly crystals of hydroxyapatite, for *hardness* and *rigidity.*

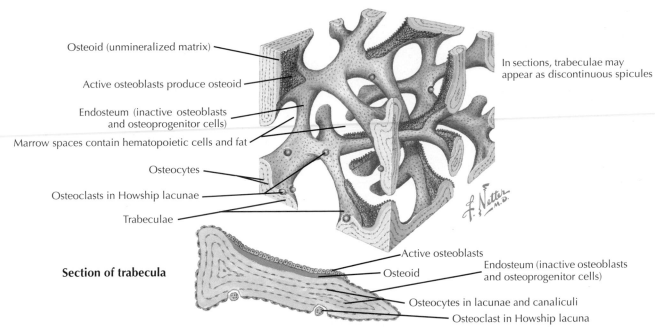

Osteoid (unmineralized matrix)

Active osteoblasts produce osteoid

Endosteum (inactive osteoblasts and osteoprogenitor cells)

Marrow spaces contain hematopoietic cells and fat

Osteocytes

Osteoclasts in Howship lacunae

Trabeculae

In sections, trabeculae may appear as discontinuous spicules

Section of trabecula

Active osteoblasts

Osteoid

Endosteum (inactive osteoblasts and osteoprogenitor cells)

Osteocytes in lacunae and canaliculi

Osteoclast in Howship lacuna

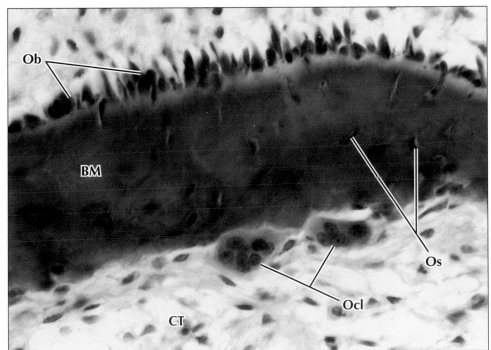

► **LM of part of a bony trabecula in fetal spongy bone.** In this developing trabecula, a row of basophilic osteoblasts (**Ob**) is on one surface, with osteoid (stained lighter) immediately below; two osteoclasts (**Ocl**) in Howship lacunae are on another surface. Osteocytes (**Os**) in lacunae are in the bony matrix (**BM**). Its intense eosinophilia is due to the presence of type I collagen. Surrounding connective tissue (**CT**) contains undifferentiated stem cells, including osteoprogenitor cells. 500×. *H&E.*

6.14 HISTOLOGY AND FUNCTION OF THE CELLS OF TRABECULAR BONE

The four cell types are **osteoprogenitor cells, osteoblasts, osteocytes,** and **osteoclasts.** The first are undifferentiated mesenchymal stem cells that, depending on the stimulus, can modulate into osteoblasts, fibroblasts, or chondroblasts. These flattened cells, which resemble fibroblasts, reside in the periosteum, perivascular **connective tissue, endosteum** lining all internal surfaces of bone, and **bone marrow.** They are not easily recognized in conventional preparations. Osteoblasts, the bone-forming cells derived from osteoprogenitor cells, produce **collagen** of the **osteoid** and induce matrix *mineralization* during bone development and remodeling. With diameters of 15-30 μm, these cuboidal to columnar cells with intensely basophilic cytoplasm are aligned in rows along bone surfaces and maintain contact with each other by gap junctions. Cells are polarized, with a nucleus at the end of the cell opposite the surface of newly formed bone. Once an osteoblast is surrounded by mineralized bony matrix, it becomes an osteocyte, or mature bone cell. Residing in **lacunae,** osteocytes are spider-shaped cells whose slender processes occupy canaliculi that radiate from the lacunae. Osteoclasts are large, multinucleated cells that originate by fusion of monocytes derived from bone marrow. They function in bone *resorption* by removing local mineralized matrix. They lie in **resorption cavities,** or **Howship lacunae,** which are created by digestion of underlying bony matrix by lysosomal enzymes of the cells.

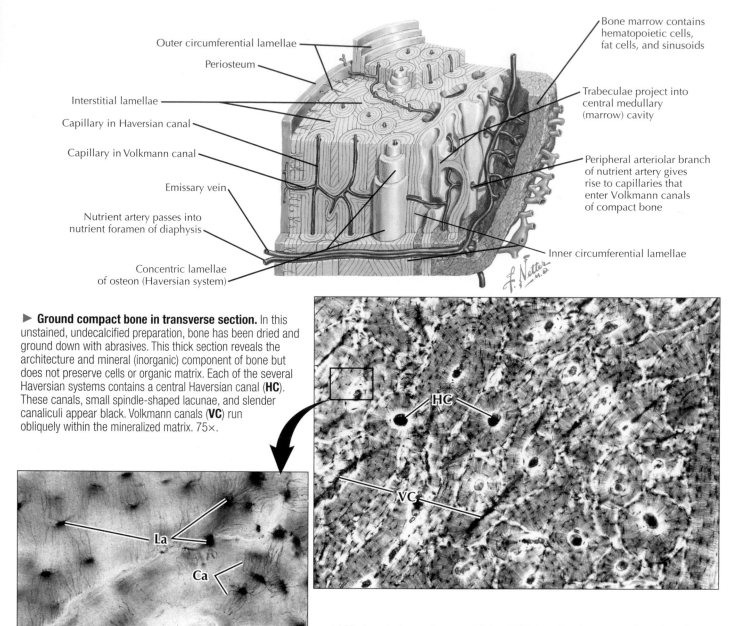

Outer circumferential lamellae

Periosteum

Interstitial lamellae

Capillary in Haversian canal

Capillary in Volkmann canal

Emissary vein

Nutrient artery passes into nutrient foramen of diaphysis

Concentric lamellae of osteon (Haversian system)

Bone marrow contains hematopoietic cells, fat cells, and sinusoids

Trabeculae project into central medullary (marrow) cavity

Peripheral arteriolar branch of nutrient artery gives rise to capillaries that enter Volkmann canals of compact bone

Inner circumferential lamellae

F. Netter M.D.

▶ **Ground compact bone in transverse section.** In this unstained, undecalcified preparation, bone has been dried and ground down with abrasives. This thick section reveals the architecture and mineral (inorganic) component of bone but does not preserve cells or organic matrix. Each of the several Haversian systems contains a central Haversian canal (**HC**). These canals, small spindle-shaped lacunae, and slender canaliculi appear black. Volkmann canals (**VC**) run obliquely within the mineralized matrix. 75×.

◀ **LM of part of an osteon and interstitial lamellae in a ground section of compact bone.** A Haversian canal (**HC**) occupies the center of an osteon. Canaliculi (**Ca**) form an extensive network of slender tunnels that connect spider-like lacunae (**La**). Lacunae and canaliculi appear black. 525×.

6.15 MICROARCHITECTURE OF COMPACT BONE

Two basic architectural types of bone are recognized macroscopically: **compact** (or **cortical**) and **spongy** (or **cancellous**). Compact bone is limited to the outer shell, or cortex, of bone. It is composed of many adjacent **Haversian systems,** or **osteons,** that appear round to oval in transverse section and are usually oriented in the long axis of the bone. Each osteon is a cylindrical unit, about 250 μm in diameter, that consists of a central **Haversian canal,** which contains small **blood vessels** and nerves and is surrounded by 4-20 concentric **lamellae.** Osteocytes in **lacunae** are arranged circumferentially around the central canal. Lacunae are oriented parallel to lamellae and are connected by fine **canaliculi** containing slender osteocyte processes. Haversian canals connect with other canals and with the **medullary,** or **marrow, cavity.** Transverse **Volkmann canals** connect neighboring Haversian canals and penetrate from the periosteal surface to carry blood vessels from one osteon to another. Irregular areas of lamellar bone, called **interstitial lamellae,** between the osteons are remnants of previously formed osteons that were disrupted during remodeling. Cement lines mark boundaries between osteons and interstitial lamellae. Found in internal areas of bone, spongy bone has a relatively simple structure of interconnecting **trabeculae,** composed of lamellar bone, that form a three-dimensional latticework aligned along areas of stress. They impart a large surface area for metabolic activities and provide mechanical strength without undue weight. An attenuated layer of flattened cells—the endosteum—covers trabeculae surfaces.

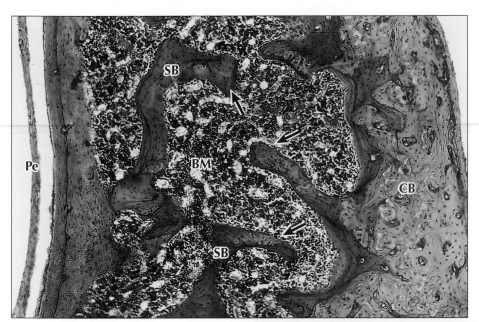

◀ **LM of decalcified diaphysis of a long bone in longitudinal section.** The outer cortex is made of dense compact bone (**CB**), whereas trabeculae of spongy bone (**SB**) protrude into the bone marrow (**BM**) cavity. Compact bone appears as a solid mass; spongy bone shows a network of plate-like trabeculae (**arrows**) bordering spaces occupied by richly cellular bone marrow. Part of the periosteum (**Pe**), at the left, is separated by an artifactual space from the outer bone surface. 100×. *H&E.*

▶ **LM of decalcified compact bone at higher magnification.** Each of three adjacent osteons, shown in transverse section, consists of several lamellae concentrically arranged around a circular Haversian canal (**HC**). Each canal is a conduit for a capillary (**Cap**). Although not apparent here, collagen fibers within each lamella are parallel to one another and pursue a helical course, whereas fibers in adjacent lamellae are oriented at right angles. Osteocytes (**Os**) in their lacunae are arranged circumferentially around each Haversian canal. Thin, lightly basophilic cement lines (**CL**) are seen at edges of the osteons. Canaliculi (**Ca**) connect adjacent lacunae. They appear as fine striations within the bony matrix (see the small encircled area). 240×. *H&E.*

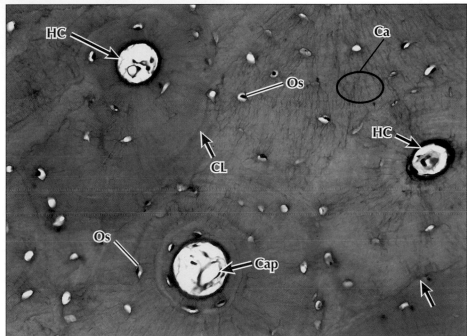

6.16 HISTOLOGY AND FUNCTION OF SPONGY AND COMPACT BONE

Most bones contain both spongy and compact bone, their relative amounts and distribution varying with age and according to function. Bone architecture is a result of physical forces acting on it and the vascularization pattern that develops as a result of these forces. Bone tissue performs many vital functions. It provides skeletal support for the body and limbs and protects vital organs. It secures skeletal muscles for movement and locomotion and houses hematopoietic tissue of **bone marrow**. It serves a vital metabolic role, as a storage reservoir of calcium, phosphate, and other important ions, which it releases in a closely regulated manner to maintain mineral homeostasis. Throughout life, bone undergoes constant turnover as it remodels itself, so fatigued areas are continuously repaired and bone strength is adjusted in response to stress. Spongy bone withstands stress and compression applied from many directions and remodels along internal lines of stress in the bone. Remodeling occurs by osteoblasts laying down bone on one part of a trabecula, while osteoclasts resorb another part. Its trabecular framework also protects the marrow cells. Compact bone can form or resorb beneath the **periosteum** or on the endosteum. With aging, bone girth increases but thickness and density of the cortex decrease. Compact bone also remodels by forming **osteons**, which are all aligned in the same direction to resist bending forces. The outer periosteum provides a route for vessels and nerves and actively participates in bone growth and repair after fracture.

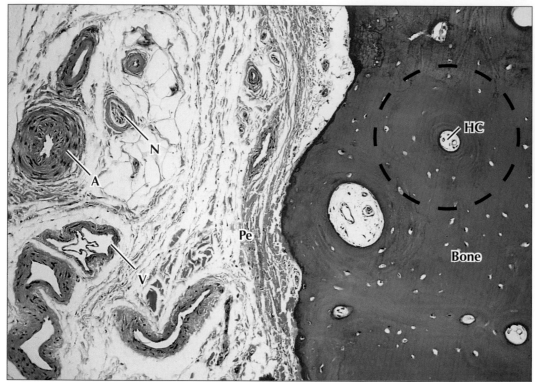

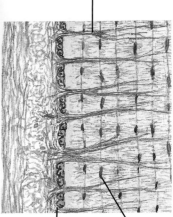

Schematic section of decalcified bone shows attachment of periosteum to bone by perforating (Sharpy) fibers

Inner (cambium) layer (osteoblasts)

Osteocyte in lacuna

▲ **LM showing the periosteum on the surface of a bone (decalcified) from an elderly person.** The outer cortex, to the right, contains many closely packed osteons and Haversian canals (**HC**). The bony matrix is intensely eosinophilic because of the high collagen content. The periosteum (**Pe**) consists of an outer fibrous layer with densely packed collagen fibers. Its inner surface contains cells that vary in morphology depending on age and functional state. Here, bone growth is complete, and these cells are fibroblasts that seem inactive. Surrounding connective tissue, to the left, shows several neurovascular structures—arterioles (**A**), venules (**V**), and a small nerve fascicle (**N**). 130×. *H&E.*

6.17 STRUCTURE AND FUNCTION OF THE PERIOSTEUM

Except where a bone articulates with other bones in joints, the outer surface is covered by a tough, fibrous, highly specialized connective tissue. Known as the periosteum, it consists of two poorly demarcated layers that differ histologically. An outer layer of dense, irregular, connective tissue consists mostly of **fibroblasts** interspersed with type I collagen fibers and a smaller proportion of elastic fibers. It contains many large **blood vessels, nerves,** and lymphatics. An inner (**cambium**) layer of loose, richly vascularized connective tissue contains osteogenic cells and **osteoblasts** in direct contact with the bone surface. Blood vessels have a small caliber and give rise to branches that supply Volkmann and **Haversian canals.** From the outer layer of periosteum, bundles of **collagen (Sharpey) fibers** penetrate underlying bone at regular intervals to anchor it firmly to bone. These fibers are especially prominent at sites of attachment of tendons and ligaments to bone. The marked variation in microscopic appearance of the periosteum depends on the functional state of the bone. During bone development and growth, the inner layer shows increased cellular activity. In addition, after bone injury or fracture, an increased number of osteoblasts is found in this layer with the potential to form new bone. The inner surfaces of bone, including marrow spaces of the diaphysis, surfaces of bony trabeculae of spongy bone, and Haversian canals, are lined by a thin, single layer of flattened cells with osteogenic potential, known as the endosteum.

CLINICAL POINT

Bone structure and function are maintained by bone remodeling—a balance between bone resorption by osteoclasts and bone formation by osteoblasts. **Osteoporosis** is a systemic skeletal disease caused by imbalance between these two processes. Low bone mass and micro-architectural deterioration of bone tissue lead to increased *bone fragility* and susceptibility to *fracture*. The disease is exacerbated by **estrogen deficiency** in postmenopausal women, which causes rapid bone loss and predisposes them to fractures. Postmenopausal *hormone replacement therapy* (HRT) is effective in slowing the rate of bone loss but may have deleterious side effects on the cardiovascular system. Administration of *calcitonin* also inhibits bone resorption and can prevent postmenopausal bone loss.

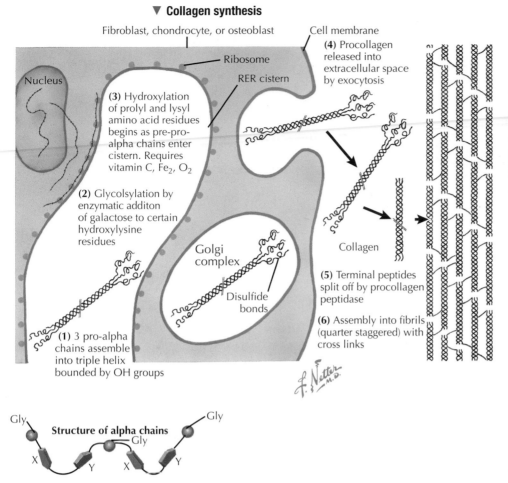

▼ **Collagen synthesis**

Fibroblast, chondrocyte, or osteoblast

Cell membrane

Ribosome

RER cistern

Nucleus

(3) Hydroxylation of prolyl and lysyl amino acid residues begins as pre-pro-alpha chains enter cistern. Requires vitamin C, Fe_2, O_2

(4) Procollagen released into extracellular space by exocytosis

(2) Glycolsylation by enzymatic additon of galactose to certain hydroxylysine residues

Golgi complex

Disulfide bonds

Collagen

(5) Terminal peptides split off by procollagen peptidase

(6) Assembly into fibrils (quarter staggered) with cross links

(1) 3 pro-alpha chains assemble into triple helix bounded by OH groups

f. Netter M.D.

Structure of alpha chains

Gly   Gly

Gly

X   Y   X   Y

Each alpha chain is made of about 1000 amino acids. Every third amino acid in chain is glycine, smallest of amino acids. Glycine has no side chains, which permits tight coil. X and Y indicate other amino acids (X often proline; Y often hydroxyproline). Proline and hydroxyproline, respectively, constitute about 20% and 25% of total amino acids in each chain.

Fibril

0.1 µm

▲ **EM of type I collagen fibrils at high magnification.** Cross-banding patterns, a result of staggered alignment of tropocollagen molecules in fibrils, are visible. Hole zones (**arrows**) between adjacent molecules provide sites for deposition of hydroxyapatite crystals as mineralization begins. 100,000×. *(Courtesy of Dr. L. Arsenault)*

6.18   FORMATION AND COMPOSITION OF COLLAGEN

Collagen, the most ubiquitous family of proteins in the body, is also the most abundant, with more than 20% of lean body mass. It is the major component of extracellular matrix and the structural foundation of all **connective tissues. Osteoblasts, chondrocytes,** and **fibroblasts** produce it. Its synthesis uses a common pathway for many extracellular molecules that consists of both intracellular and extracellular events. The genetically distinct types of collagen differ according to the types of polypeptide **alpha chains,** the basic building blocks, that are compiled to form a **triple helix. Type I** collagen, the most abundant, found in bone, tendon, ligament, and skin, is synthesized as a **prepropeptide** containing **lysine** and **proline** residues, some of which are enzymatically hydroxylated. Resulting polypeptide is moved into the lumen of RER, and **procollagen** is assembled from three alpha chains in the triple helix. It is then taken to the **Golgi complex** and packaged for secretion by exocytosis at the cell surface. Outside the cell, **peptidases** cleave terminal peptides to produce **tropocollagen,** which assembles in staggered arrays to form **collagen fibrils** with a distinct 64-nm banding pattern. Collagen contains high

concentrations of **hydroxyproline** and **hydroxylysine,** which stabilize triple helixes and cross-link tropocollagen monomers. Type I collagen of bone differs from that found elsewhere, in that transverse spacings, or internal **hole zones,** provide space for deposition of **hydroxyapatite crystals,** inducing nucleation and later matrix **mineralization.** Articular cartilage and cartilagenous parts of growth plates contain type II collagen.

CLINICAL POINT

Osteogenesis imperfecta is a hereditary disorder characterized by bone *fragility* and *deformability* and recurrent *fractures,* with four clinical subtypes. It results from abnormalities in type I collagen. The structure of normal collagen shows a left-handed helix of intertwining pro-alpha-1 and pro-alpha-2 chains. Mutations in loci encoding for these chains cause osteogenesis imperfecta I, the most common type. The number of osteoblasts per unit of bone is higher, but their activity is greatly reduced. About 50,000 people in North America have the disease, a progressive condition that needs lifelong management to prevent deformity and complications.

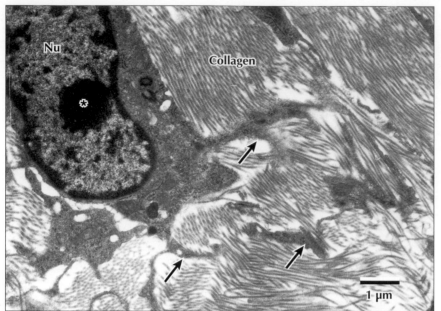

◀ ▼ **EMs of parts of active osteoblasts adjacent to osteoid.** At low magnification (**Left**), the cuboidal cell contains many tightly packed cytoplasmic organelles, which is consistent with a role in osteoid synthesis and secretion. Its euchromatic nucleus (**Nu**) shows a prominent nucleolus (*). Cytoplasmic processes (**arrows**) of the osteoblast extend into surrounding osteoid. An irregular array of type I collagen fibrils occupies the matrix, which is not yet mineralized. At higher magnification (**Below**), the cytoplasm includes many profiles of RER and mitochondria (**Mi**). The nucleus contains light euchromatin, darker clumps of heterochromatin, and a prominent nucleolus (*). The matrix shows collagen fibrils. **Left**: 9700×; **Below**: 27,000×.

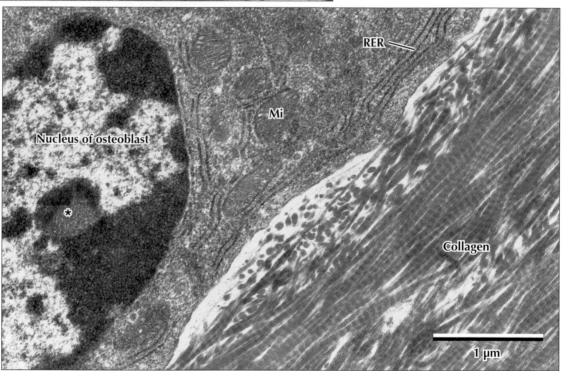

6.19 ULTRASTRUCTURE OF OSTEOBLASTS

Osteoblasts are polarized cells that synthesize and secrete unmineralized **osteoid,** which consists mainly of **type I collagen** and noncollagenous glycoproteins such as osteocalcin and osteopontin. These cells also synthesize alkaline phosphatase, a cell surface protein that promotes *mineralization.* The most distinctive feature of the cells is intense *cytoplasmic basophilia,* which corresponds to an extensive RER, seen by electron microscopy. Osteoblasts contain other **organelles** for glycosylation and secretion of protein, including a well-developed Golgi complex near the **nucleus** and assorted secretory vesicles for exocytosis of secretory product. Long, branched **cytoplasmic processes** extend from cell bodies at the side where bone matrix is formed and penetrate deeply into osteoid. Gap junctions between adjacent cells most likely play a role in propagation of signals related to mineral metabolism. Osteoblasts have membrane receptors for parathyroid hormone, estrogen, and progesterone.

CLINICAL POINT

Osteomalacia is a metabolic bone disorder caused by vitamin D deficiency, characterized by excessive amounts of unmineralized osteoid tissue: mineral is not deposited in normally formed bone matrix. Osteoid accounts for less than 5% of normal bone but 40%-50% of bone in this disorder. Reduced bone strength results in *fractures* and *bone pain.* In children, the disorder, known as **rickets,** especially affects epiphyseal growth plates and leads to *bowed legs* and *deformed skull* and *ribs.* Causes of this deficiency are many, but most cases result from toxins or poor dietary intake leading to decreased serum vitamin D levels.

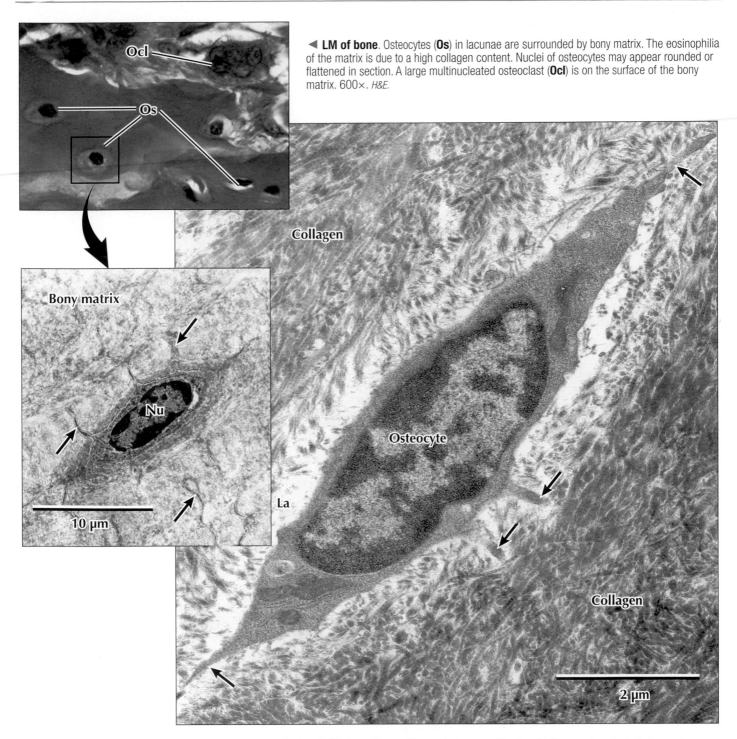

◀ **LM of bone**. Osteocytes (**Os**) in lacunae are surrounded by bony matrix. The eosinophilia of the matrix is due to a high collagen content. Nuclei of osteocytes may appear rounded or flattened in section. A large multinucleated osteoclast (**Ocl**) is on the surface of the bony matrix. 600×. *H&E.*

▲ **EMs of osteocytes in decalcified sections of bone.** At low magnification (**Left**), an osteocyte in its lacuna is surrounded by bony matrix; minerals and some collagen have been removed for sectioning. The ellipsoidal cell has a prominent nucleus (**Nu**), which is surrounded by a small amount of cytoplasm. Slender cytoplasmic processes (**arrows**) extend from the cell body. Higher magnification (**Right**) shows a more detailed osteocyte, including the thin cytoplasmic processes (**arrows**). The cell is bounded by a lacuna (**La**) that, in turn, is surrounded by type I collagen of the bony matrix. **Left**: 3000×; **Right**: 17,500×.

6.20 ULTRASTRUCTURE OF OSTEOCYTES

Osteocytes, the mature cells of bone, possess a high nucleus-to-cytoplasm ratio and relatively few cytoplasmic organelles. They reside, with extracellular fluid, in **lacunae.** Each cell displays many slender **cytoplasmic processes** that extend into thin channels, or canaliculi, in the mineralized matrix. Processes of one cell are linked to those of adjacent cells by gap junctions. Extracellular fluid in canaliculi permits transfer of molecules, oxygen, and nutrients by *diffusion.* Osteocytes actively maintain bone matrix. They participate in exchange of calcium ions and other minerals with extracellular fluid, a process known as *osteocytic osteolysis.*

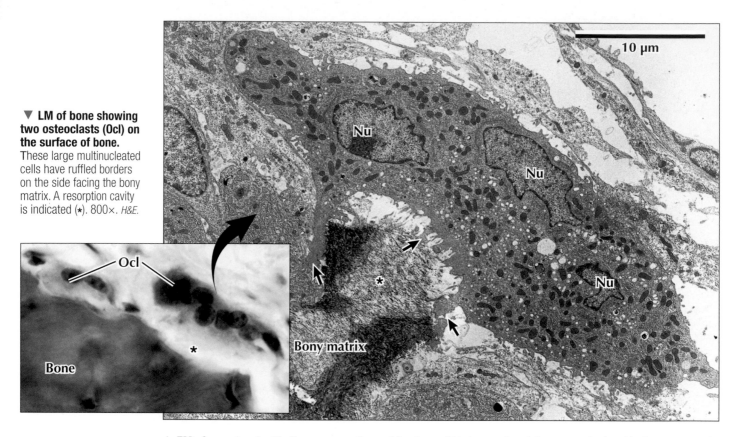

▼ **LM of bone showing two osteoclasts (Ocl) on the surface of bone.** These large multinucleated cells have ruffled borders on the side facing the bony matrix. A resorption cavity is indicated (∗). 800×. *H&E.*

▲ **EM of an osteoclast in the process of resorbing bone.** This large cell contains many mitochondria, lysosomes, and vesicles of various sizes, and several nuclei (**Nu**). Its cell membrane has an irregular outline, with a prominent ruffled border (**arrows**) in contact with bone that is being resorbed (∗) in Howship lacuna. Parts of the bony matrix under the border are undergoing demineralization and dissolution. 3300×. *(Courtesy of Dr. W. L. Hunter)*

6.21 ULTRASTRUCTURE AND FUNCTION OF OSTEOCLASTS

The giant **multinucleated** osteoclasts have a diameter of 40 to more than 100 μm and up to 50 nuclei. Cells are highly polarized, and nuclei congregate away from bone-resorbing areas. Their unique ultrastructure is consistent with a role in bone *resorption.* Actively resorbing osteoclasts are found in or near surface cavities known as **Howship lacunae.** By light microscopy, their cytoplasm either is eosinophilic or appears foamy, and the cell surface near the bone looks striated. By electron microscopy, numerous **mitochondria, lysosomes,** and membrane-bound **vesicles** and vacuoles are located throughout the cell, as are small amounts of rough endoplasmic reticulum and multiple Golgi complexes. The **ruffled border** at the ultrastructural level corresponds to the striated cell surface. Composed of extensive infoldings of **plasma membrane,** this border facilitates bone resorption by increasing surface area. An area of the cytoplasm rich in actin filaments but poor in other organelles underlies the ruffled border and facilitates its motility during bone resorption. The membrane of the border contains a proton pump that keeps pH low in the resorption cavity. Secretion of H^+ ions into the extracellular space dissolves inorganic minerals in the matrix. Also, lysosomes release hydrolytic enzymes, including collagenase, into extracellular space to degrade organic matrix components. Small vesicles at the ruffled border take up degraded collagen fibers and crystals of calcium salts, move them across the cell, and release them into extracellular fluid and then the circulation.

CLINICAL POINT

Osteopetrosis is a rare hereditary bone disease in which failure of osteoclastic bone resorption leads to *increased bone mass.* Patients, usually diagnosed in early infancy, have thickened and sclerotic bones with poor mechanical properties. Three distinct forms of the disease are based on age and clinical features. Greater bone fragility results from defective remodeling of woven bone to compact bone. Several treatments have been studied for the infantile malignant form of the disease, which is usually fatal if untreated. The only potentially curative therapy is *hematopoietic stem cell* or *bone marrow transplant* from an allogenic donor.

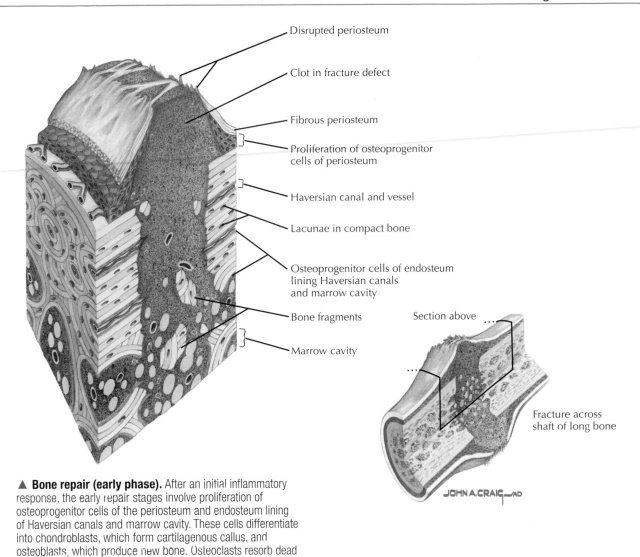

Disrupted periosteum

Clot in fracture defect

Fibrous periosteum

Proliferation of osteoprogenitor cells of periosteum

Haversian canal and vessel

Lacunae in compact bone

Osteoprogenitor cells of endosteum lining Haversian canals and marrow cavity

Bone fragments

Marrow cavity

Section above

Fracture across shaft of long bone

JOHN A.CRAIG—AD

▲ **Bone repair (early phase).** After an initial inflammatory response, the early repair stages involve proliferation of osteoprogenitor cells of the periosteum and endosteum lining of Haversian canals and marrow cavity. These cells differentiate into chondroblasts, which form cartilagenous callus, and osteoblasts, which produce new bone. Osteoclasts resorb dead bone and bone fragments. The periosteal reaction extends beyond the local fracture site.

6.22   BONE FRACTURE REPAIR: EARLY EVENTS

Bone can repair itself, and its dynamic nature is best appreciated in response to a **fracture.** Successful bone regeneration requires a viable **periosteum,** with effective *apposition* and *immobilization* of broken fragments. New bone formation recapitulates osteogenesis during embryonic development and growth. Repair of **long bones,** unlike flat bones of the skull and facial skeleton, occurs by both intramembranous and endochondral ossification. Healing involves successive and overlapping morphologic phases: an *inflammatory phase* is followed by a *reparative phase,* and then a *remodeling phase.* In bone, as in other tissues, immediate responses to injury are inflammation and edema. Torn blood vessels near the fracture cause bleeding from the **marrow cavity** and surrounding tissues. Within a few hours, a **blood clot,** or **hematoma,** forms at the site. Circulation to osteons in the area is disrupted; death of osteocytes and necrosis of bone fragments result. Infiltration of fibroblasts and new capillaries from periosteum is followed by migration of leukocytes, monocytes, and macrophages to form granulation tissue. **Osteoprogenitor cells** from both periosteum and **endosteum** also migrate and proliferate at the wound site. This tissue becomes more fibrous and then develops around and between fragment ends to form a bridge, or callus, to unite the fragments.

Bone Repair (Intermediate Phase)

Fibrous periosteum covering external callus

External cartilagenous callus formed by chondroblasts

Osteogenic layer of periosteum

New bone and osteoprogenitor cells of external callus replacing cartilage

Clot in fracture defect

New bone and osteoprogenitor cells of internal callus bridging fracture site

Section above

New bone

Cartilage

External callus

Internal callus

JOHN A. CRAIG—MD

▲ **External callus of bone or cartilage is formed by osteoprogenitor cells of the periosteum.** Cells form bone in areas of high vascularity and form cartilage in areas of low vascularity. As new capillaries grow, new bone replaces cartilagenous callus. **Internal callus** is formed by osteoprogenitor cells of endosteum and is primarily new bone because of high oxygen tension.

Bone Repair (Late Phase)

Fibrous periosteum

Osteogenic layer of periosteum

New woven bone in external callus

Residual islands of cartilage in woven bone

Mineralization of new bone with formation of osteons

Woven bone in internal callus

Section above

▲ **New bone of external callus extends centripetally to join new bone of internal callus and bridge the defect.** Bone is remodeled as osteoclasts resorb callus. Concentric layers of bone laid down around blood vessels form new Haversian canals.

6.23   BONE FRACTURE REPAIR: INTERMEDIATE AND LATE EVENTS

Internal callus—between ends of bone fragments and marrow cavities—and **external callus**—around opposing ends of bone fragments—temporarily stabilize and bind together bone fragments. Because **osteoprogenitor** cells in the callus are pleuripotential, their fate depends on vascularity and oxygen tension of their immediate microenvironment: cells close to blood vessels become osteoblasts, which directly form trabeculae of new woven bone. This process usually occurs internally in the medullary cavity as well as in the innermost layer of the **periosteum.** In contrast, pleuripotential cells far from capillaries, at a lower oxygen

tension, differentiate into chondroblasts, which become chondrocytes that form hyaline **cartilage.** This cartilage typically develops externally in the callus and is later replaced by **woven spongy bone** by a process similar to endochondral bone formation. Bony union occurs when new spongy bone from two fragments meets and becomes continuous across the fracture line. The later remodeling of woven to lamellar bone occurs over time. In the last stage of repair, primary spongy bone is resorbed, and new bony lamellae are laid down. Eventually, new **osteons** of compact bone destined for the cortex are constructed and the medullary cavity is reestablished. Forces of stress in healed bone influence progressive remodeling.

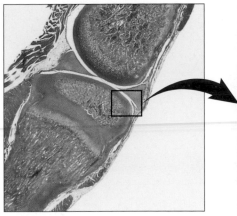

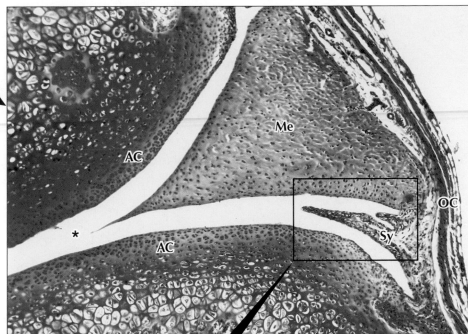

▲ **Low-magnification LM of a rat knee joint.** Articulating ends of two bones are separated by a synovial cavity. 5×. *H&E.*

▲ **Medium-magnification LM of part of a rat knee joint.** Articulating ends of two bones are covered by articular hyaline cartilage (**AC**). A triangular meniscus (**Me**) projects into the synovial cavity (∗). Highly folded synovium (**Sy**) lines the inner surface of the fibrous outer capsule (**OC**) of the joint. 75×. *H&E.*

◀ **High-magnification LM showing details of a synovial villus and the synovium.** Synoviocytes (**arrows**) form the intimal synovial lining. The subintimal layer is highly vascularized loose connective tissue (**CT**). The villus projects into the synovial cavity (∗). Parts of the meniscus (**Me**) and articular cartilage (**AC**) are shown. 500×. *H&E.*

6.24 HISTOLOGY OF SYNOVIAL JOINTS

Synovial joints are freely moveable, or *diarthrodial*, joints between articular surfaces of bones that allow gliding movement facilitated by efficiently lubricated cartilagenous surfaces with minimal friction and wear. A marvel of construction, they share a common structural design and consist of separate tissues with different functions. Each joint has a fluid-containing **synovial cavity** that confers mobility. It also contains a confining sheet of tissue—the **synovium**—that produces **synovial fluid,** and **articular cartilage** that slides and transmits weight. A tough, outer **capsule** of dense, regular connective tissue encases these structures plus vasomotor and sensory nerves. Except for sternoclavicular and temporomandibular joints that are lined with fibrocartilage, most synovial joints are lined with a specialized articular **hyaline cartilage.** In some joints, wedges of fibrocartilage, known as articular discs or **menisci,** lie between articular surfaces of the bones. They function in shock absorption and load distribution. The meniscus has an interlacing network of chondrocytes and type I collagen fibers but no perichondrium. The synovium, or synovial membrane, is a specialized connective tissue that lines inner surfaces of joint capsules and all other intraarticular surfaces except articular cartilage and meniscus. Synovium comprises a highly cellular **intimal layer** in contact with the joint cavity and a **subintimal layer** made of fibrous and adipose **connective tissue.** The membrane surface is smooth and moist and may have a few small fringe-like folds, or villi, that increase surface area.

▼ **Structure of the synovium.**

Areolar synovium   Fibrous synovium

f. Netter m.d.

Synovium

Meniscus

Synovium

Adipose synovium

Articular
cartilage

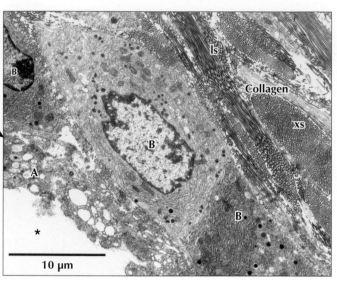

▲ **EM of fibrous synovium.** Part of a type A (**A**) and several type B (**B**) synoviocytes make up this area of the synovium. Underlying matrix consists of collagen fibrils sectioned transversely (**xs**) and longitudinally (**ls**). The synovial cavity (★) is shown. 2600×.

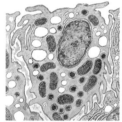 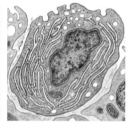

▲ **Schematic EMs of type A (left) and type B (right) cells of the synovium.** Type A cell has numerous lysosomes for phagocytosis; type B cell, abundant rough endoplasmic reticulum for secretion.

6.25   HISTOLOGY AND FUNCTION OF THE SYNOVIUM

Synovium is a delicate, highly vascularized lining of the **synovial joint.** It is normally about 100 μm thick. Contrary to expectations, the intimal lining cells, known as **synoviocytes,** are modified **connective tissue cells,** not epithelial cells. They form one or two cellular layers along the luminal surface, seemingly a continuous epithelial cellular membrane, but they are not joined by intercellular junctions and lack a basement membrane. Subintimal matrix consists of **loose connective tissue,** and the associated synovium may be **areolar, fibrous,** or **adipose.** The subintimal interstitial matrix has numerous fenestrated capillaries close to the free surface. Thus, extravasated blood can readily enter synovial fluid from a minor joint injury. Primary functions of the synovium are to produce synovial fluid and to remove cellular and connective tissue debris from joint cavities. Cells of the synovium are either type A or B. **Type A synoviocytes,** 20%-30% of the lining cells, are modified phagocytes derived from blood monocytes that engulf and clear particulate matter. **Type B synoviocytes** are modified fibroblasts that synthesize and secrete

glycosaminoglycans and glycoproteins. Synovial fluid is mainly an ultrafiltrate of blood, with less protein but similar electrolyte concentrations. Fenestrated capillaries under the surface generate this ultrafiltrate. Type B synoviocytes actively secrete two lubricating molecules—hyaluronic acid in large quantities and lubricin in smaller amounts—into synovial fluid. In the joint, synovial fluid supplies nutrients to the avascular articular cartilage.

CLINICAL POINT

Rheumatoid arthritis is a chronic, inflammatory, systemic disease with greatest effects in diarthrodial joints. Persistent and progressive *synovitis* develops in peripheral joints. Histologically, the primary inflammatory joint lesion involves the synovium; earliest changes are injury to synovial microvasculature with luminal occlusion and endothelial swelling. Both type A and type B synoviocytes undergo hyperplasia; edema and fibrin exudation also occur. Small nodular aggregates of CD4+ T lymphocytes and diffuse infiltrates of CD8+ cells characterize synovial matrix. Inflammation causes synovium to become hypertrophic and granulation tissue to invade and destroy periarticular bone and cartilage.

7

BLOOD AND BONE MARROW

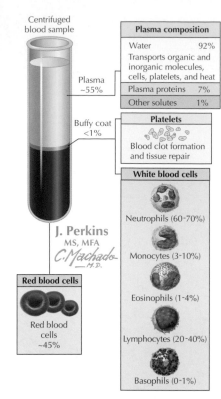

Centrifuged blood sample

Plasma ~55%

Buffy coat <1%

Plasma composition	
Water	92%
Transports organic and inorganic molecules, cells, platelets, and heat	
Plasma proteins	7%
Other solutes	1%

Platelets
Blood clot formation and tissue repair

White blood cells
Neutrophils (60-70%)
Monocytes (3-10%)
Eosinophils (1-4%)
Lymphocytes (20-40%)
Basophils (0-1%)

J. Perkins
MS, MFA
C. Machado
—M.D.

Red blood cells
Red blood cells ~45%

► **LM of a blood smear showing typical erythrocytes and leukocytes.** Two kinds of granular leukocytes seen are an eosinophil (**Eo**) and a basophil (**Ba**). They are distinguished by the staining pattern of their granules. A lymphocyte (**Ly**), an agranular leukocyte, has a densely stained nucleus and lacks cytoplasmic granules. Erythrocytes (**RBC**), the most numerous formed elements of blood, lack nuclei and have a uniform size: 7–10 μm in diameter and 2 μm wide. They are eosinophilic, with pale centers because of their biconcave disc-like shapes. 690×. *Wright's.*

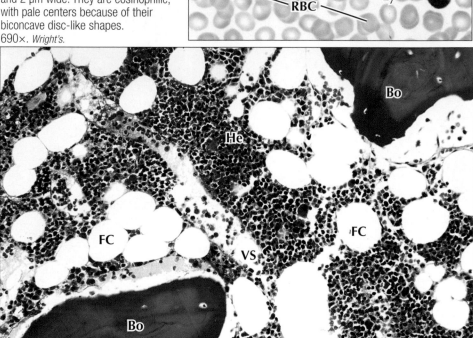

► **LM of bone marrow obtained via needle biopsy from the medullary cavity of the iliac crest.** In the adult, bone marrow is the major organ of hematopoiesis. It produces erythrocytes, granular and agranular leukocytes, and platelets. This highly cellular, richly vascularized connective tissue consists of small hematopoietic stem cells (**He**) and larger adipocytes (fat cells, **FC**). Bony trabeculae (**Bo**) are closely associated with the marrow. Abundant thin-walled venous sinusoids (**VS**) provide the main exit route for newly formed blood cells that move directly into circulation. 180×. *H&E.*

7.1   OVERVIEW

Blood is a specialized type of **connective tissue** that consists of cells suspended in a circulating fluid known as **plasma.** The total amount of circulating blood in men is 5-6 L; that in women, 4-5 L. Fresh blood is a red, viscous fluid, whereas plasma is translucent and yellow. Cellular elements of blood constitute about 45% of blood volume in adults, with plasma making up the other 55%. These elements include **erythrocytes** (or **red blood cells**), granular and agranular **leukocytes** (or **white blood cells**), and circulating cytoplasmic fragments known as **platelets** (or **thrombocytes**). Plasma consists of **plasma proteins,** such as fibrinogens, globulins, and albumin, and a ground substance called **serum. Bone marrow,** a highly vascularized tissue in **medullary cavities** of bones, consists of both vascular and *hematopoietic* (blood-forming) compartments. Like most other connective tissue types, blood and bone marrow derive embryonically from mesoderm. In the first few weeks of gestation, blood islands in the yolk sac are the first sites of *hematopoiesis,* or production of blood cells.

During the rest of fetal life until about 2 weeks after birth, blood cells form in the liver and spleen. In children and adults, bone marrow is the major site of hematopoiesis. **Lymphocytes** are also produced in lymphoid organs. Bone marrow is a large tissue and accounts for 4%-5% of body weight. Its total weight exceeds that of the liver and has been estimated at 1.6-3.7 kg in the adult.

CLINICAL POINT

A **complete blood count** (CBC) is a valuable screening test in medical practice that is used to diagnose and manage many conditions and diseases such as acute and chronic infections, allergies, and anemias. It measures the number of erythrocytes (RBCs) and leukocytes, total amount of blood *hemoglobin,* and fraction of blood composed of RBCs—the *hematocrit.* The CBC also includes other information about RBCs, such as *mean corpuscular hemoglobin* (MCH) and *mean corpuscular hemoglobin concentration* (MCHC), as well as the *platelet count.*

Features of Erythrocytes and Platelets in Wright-Stained Blood Smears						
Cells	**Diameter (μm)**	**Life span (days)**	**No. of cells/ L of blood**	**Shape and nucleus type**	**Cytoplasm**	**Functions**
Erythrocyte (red blood cell)	7–10	120	5×10^{12} in males; 4.5×10^{12} in females	Biconcave disc, anucleate	Pink because of acidophilia of hemoglobin; halo in center	Transports hemoglobin that binds O_2 and CO_2
Platelet (thrombocyte)	2–4	10	150 to 400×10^9	Oval biconvex disc, anucleate	Pale blue; central dark granulomere, peripheral less dense hyalomere	In hemostasis, promotes blood clotting; plugs endothelial damage

C. Machado —M.D.

Features of Leukocytes in Wright-Stained Blood Smears (Total Number: $5-10 \times 10^9$/L Blood)					
Cells	**Diameter (μm)**	**Differential count (%)**	**Nucleus**	**Cytoplasm**	**Functions**
Granulocytes					
Neutrophil	9–12	60–70	Segmented, 3–5 lobes, densely stained	Pale, finely granular, evenly dispersed specific granules	Phagocytoses bacteria; increases in number in acute bacterial infections
Eosinophil	12–15	1–4	Bilobed, clumped chromatin pattern, densly stained	Large homogeneous red granules that are coarse and highly refractile	Phagocytoses antigen-antibody complexes and parasites
Basophil	10–14	0–1	Bilobed or segmented	Large blue specific granules that stain with basic dyes and often obscure nucleus	Involved in anticoagulation, increases vascular permeability
Agranulocytes					
Monocytes	12–20	3–10	Indented, kidney shaped, lightly stained	Agranular, pale blue cytoplasm, with lysosomes	Is motile; gives rise to macrophages
Lymphocyte • Small • Medium to large	6–10 11–16	20–40	Small, round or slightly indented, darkly stained	Agranular, faintly basophilic, blue to gray	Acts in humoral (B cell) and cellular (T cell) immunity

7.2 FORMED ELEMENTS OF BLOOD

Blood cells can be studied via tissue sections, but a **blood film or smear** is preferred for routine microscopic evaluation. The procedure for a blood film involves placing a drop of blood on a glass slide, spreading it thinly and evenly over the surface with another slide on edge, and then air-drying and staining it. Rather than using a conventional hematoxylin and eosin (H&E) stain, special stains that utilize a combination of *acid* (eosin), *basic* (methylene blue), and *neutral dyes* better demonstrate the formed elements. Many blood stains are available, but **Giemsa** and **Wright** stains are superior for elucidating different blood cell types with an oil immersion objective lens. In blood films so stained, **erythrocytes** (RBCs) are typically orange-red to pink, and nuclei of **leukocytes**, with an affinity for basic dyes, stain blue. Various types of **granules** in granular leukocytes show different affinities for stains, and cells containing them are thus named **eosinophils, basophils,** or **neutrophils.** Determining RBC numbers, shapes, and sizes in blood smears provides useful data for diagnosis and treatment of many diseases such as microcytic and macrocytic *anemias.* Normal RBCs are usually uniform in size and shape, but **poikilocytes**— RBCs with distorted shapes—occur in certain conditions. Many pathologic conditions can alter the number of leukocytes. To determine relative proportions of leukocytes, a **differential white blood count** is obtained via a blood smear; normal values are listed in the table.

CLINICAL POINT

A valuable clinical test is the **hematocrit.** It is determined via centrifugation of a freshly drawn blood sample in a test tube with added anticoagulant (e.g., heparin). Three layers typically appear in the tube. The top layer of plasma constitutes about 55% of the column. A thin, white, middle layer—the buffy coat—consists of leukocytes and platelets and is only 1%. The hematocrit is represented by the lowest layer of packed red blood cells, normally about 45% of the volume. Significant changes in its value may be a sign of disease.

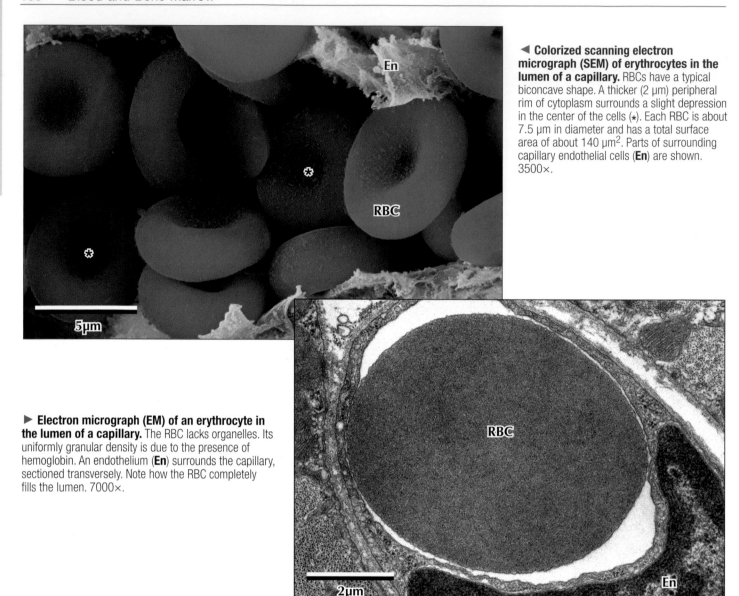

◄ **Colorized scanning electron micrograph (SEM) of erythrocytes in the lumen of a capillary.** RBCs have a typical biconcave shape. A thicker (2 μm) peripheral rim of cytoplasm surrounds a slight depression in the center of the cells (✱). Each RBC is about 7.5 μm in diameter and has a total surface area of about 140 μm². Parts of surrounding capillary endothelial cells (**En**) are shown. 3500×.

▶ **Electron micrograph (EM) of an erythrocyte in the lumen of a capillary.** The RBC lacks organelles. Its uniformly granular density is due to the presence of hemoglobin. An endothelium (**En**) surrounds the capillary, sectioned transversely. Note how the RBC completely fills the lumen. 7000×.

7.3   ULTRASTRUCTURE AND FUNCTION OF ERYTHROCYTES

RBCs are anucleate **biconcave discs** that are highly flexible and malleable as they travel in narrow capillary lumina. They make up 99% of the formed elements of blood and have a lifespan in circulation of about 120 days. Numbers of RBCs per liter of blood usually average 5×10^{12} in men and 4.5×10^{12} in women. In the human embryo, RBCs are initially nucleated, up to 7 weeks of gestation. During final stages of erythropoietic development in bone marrow, RBCs lose the nucleus and almost all organelles except the cytoskeleton and then enter the circulation. Because RBCs lack a nucleus but have a plasma membrane, they are more aptly termed **corpuscles** than true cells. A sticky surface often causes RBCs to adhere to each other in circulating blood and form loose rows known as *rouleaux*. In standard blood smears, the RBC center is a pale area surrounded by a thicker, eosinophilic peripheral zone. A biconcave shape provides a large surface area for primary functions: transporting O_2 from lungs to tissues and returning CO_2 from tissues to lungs for elimination. The iron-

containing protein **hemoglobin** in RBCs accounts for their red color. Hemoglobin rapidly binds to O_2 for transport. It is a conjugated protein containing the pigment *heme* and the protein *globin.* Heme is a porphyrin combined with iron. Normal values of hemoglobin in whole blood are about 14-18 g/dl for males and 12-16 g/dl for females. Several forms of inherited hemoglobin abnormalities, including *anemias* and *thalassemia syndromes,* occur in humans.

CLINICAL POINT

A deficiency of RBCs and/or hemoglobin is **anemia,** many different types of which exist. Correct diagnosis relies on calculating the RBC number in peripheral blood, determining hemoglobin concentration, and examining RBC morphology in blood smears. **Sickle cell anemia** is an autosomal recessive disorder leading to faulty synthesis of the β-globin chain of hemoglobin. Resulting hemoglobin S causes RBC deformities. Instead of biconcave discs, they become crescent-shaped sickle cells, which lose malleability and malfunction. Current treatment alleviates symptoms, but *bone marrow transplants* may provide a cure in some cases.

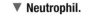

▼ **Neutrophil.**

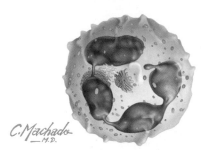

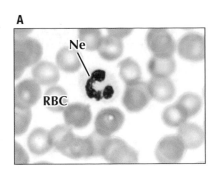

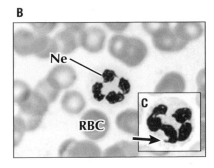

▲ **LMs of neutrophils in blood smears.** The young neutrophil (**Ne**) in **A** has a U-shaped, darkly stained nucleus. The neutrophil in **B** is more mature; its nucleus has four lobes connected by fine strands. The cytoplasm of both cells is pale and finely speckled. Their granules are difficult to distinguish. Surrounding erythrocytes (**RBC**) are smaller than neutrophils, which are 9-12 μm in diameter. 1000×. **C.** The inset shows a Barr body (**arrow**) on the neutrophil nucleus. It has a drumstick shape and appears to be attached to a lobe of the nucleus by a thin strand of chromatin. Present in females, it is inactive heterochromatin of one of the two X chromosomes. 1500×. *Wright's.*

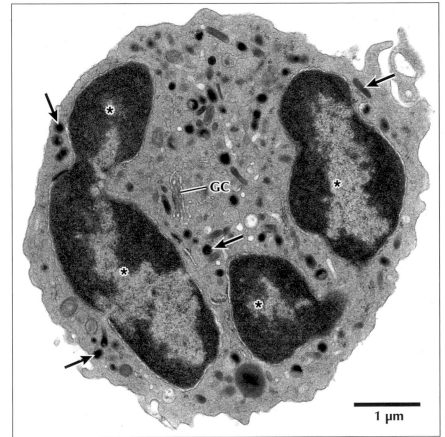

◄ **EM of a neutrophil.** Four lobes (∗) of the nucleus, but not connecting chromatin strands, are in the plane of section. The cytoplasm has a Golgi complex (**GC**) and many electron-dense granules (**arrows**) of various sizes, which are primary (azurophilic) lysosomes and specific granules. Although specific granules are hard to distinguish from each other at this magnification and without special stains, they are usually smaller than nonspecific azurophilic granules. 17,000×.

7.4 STRUCTURE AND FUNCTION OF NEUTROPHILS

Neutrophils are the most numerous leukocytes and constitute 60%-70% of the leukocyte count. The nucleus has a distinctive morphology and many forms (thus the name **polymorphonuclear leukocytes**), with a clump-like pattern and three to five lobes connected by fine chromatin strands. Immature neutrophils show only slight nuclear lobulation; older cells have more, dark-staining lobes. Females often have a small drumstick-shaped lobe—the **Barr body.** It is absent in males and may be useful in determining chromosomal sex. Neutrophil cytoplasm is lightly eosinophilic and, as in other granular leukocytes, contains two types of granules. Many small, membrane-bound **specific granules** are not acidophilic or basophilic but stain faintly with neutral dyes. Occasional large **azurophilic granules** that stain reddish purple are primary lysosomes containing peroxidase and hydrolytic enzymes. A small Golgi complex, a few scattered mitochondria, and some glycogen deposits are also in the cytoplasm. Like all other leuko-cytes, neutrophils are actively motile and function outside the circulation. After they develop in bone marrow, they stay in the bloodstream for 8-12 hours. They then migrate across venule and capillary walls. Their lifespan may be 4 days in connective tissues, where they are avidly phagocytic—scavengers that engulf bacteria, cell debris, and foreign matter. The specific granules contain *bactericidal enzymes* for receptor-mediated *phagocytosis.* Neutrophil numbers increase in *acute bacterial infections.*

CLINICAL POINT

Like all leukocytes, neutrophils circulate in the blood for a short time and migrate across small blood vessel walls to perform functions outside the circulation. **Neutropenia** is an abnormal decrease in neutrophil numbers in peripheral blood so that too few cells are available to defend against bacterial infections. Neutropenia may be caused by genetic, drug-induced, or other factors, but it is often associated with *autoimmune diseases* and is a common feature of *AIDS.*

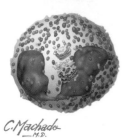

▼ Eosinophil.

C. Machado
—M.D.

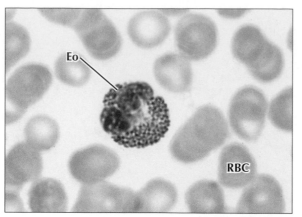

◄ **LM of an eosinophil in a blood smear.**
The distinctive, closely packed eosinophilic granules fill the cytoplasm of the eosinophil (**Eo**). The usually bilobed nucleus has an irregular shape. This granular leukocyte has a larger diameter than that of the erythrocytes (**RBC**). 1350×. *Wright's.*

▶ **EM of part of an eosinophil.** Two nuclear lobes (★) contain euchromatin and a peripheral rim of heterochromatin. Large specific granules (**SG**) with electron-dense crystalloid cores occupy the cytoplasm. A small Golgi complex (**GC**) is between the lobes. 18,000×.

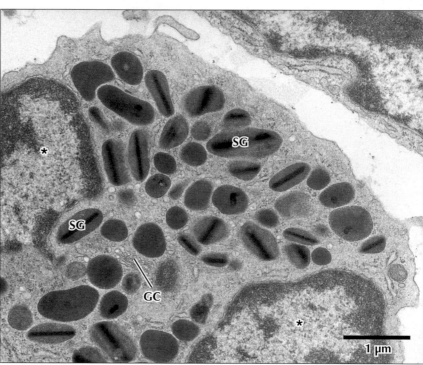

7.5 STRUCTURE AND FUNCTION OF EOSINOPHILS

Eosinophils make up a small proportion of leukocytes in peripheral blood: 1%-4% of the leukocyte count. Eosinophil numbers normally fluctuate and show a diurnal pattern, with larger numbers often at night and lower numbers in daytime. With a diameter of 12-15 μm, they are slightly larger than neutrophils. Their **nucleus** is typically **bilobed,** but multiple lobes are not unusual. Their **specific granules** are distinctive, uniform in size, highly refractile, and have an affinity for acid dyes and thus stain dark pink to crimson. These granules contain various hydrolytic enzymes and secrete histaminase, which inactivates histamine produced by basophils and mast cells. Electron microscopy shows the membrane-bound specific granules to have an irregular shape, ranging from ellipsoid to a football form, and in some species, including humans, to have an internal **crystalloid core.** This core makes them highly refractile by light microscopy. Eosinophils circulate in the bloodstream for 6-8 hours; once they migrate to connective tissues, their lifespan is 8-10 days. Eosinophils are common in mucosal connective tissues in the respiratory and gastrointestinal tracts. The cells release various substances including *major basic protein, peroxidase,* and *eosinophilic cationic protein.* The cells phagocytose antigen-antibody complexes and parasites, and elevated cell numbers occur in *parasitic infections* and *allergic responses* such as hay fever and asthma.

CLINICAL POINT

Eosinophilia—an increased absolute number of circulating eosinophils above normal—occurs in *parasitic infestations, allergic reactions,* and some *malignancies.* Eosinophils play a central role in controlling parasitic diseases such as *schistosomiasis.* They kill parasitic larval helminths by releasing toxic molecules from the specific granules. In *bronchial asthma* and *allergic eczema,* local eosinophil accumulations in tissues may cause severe cell injury and necrosis. These harmful effects are likely related to major basic protein and eosinophil cationic protein, which are components of the specific granules.

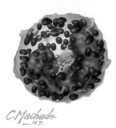

▼ **Basophil.**

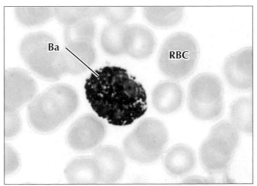

C. Machado
M.D.

◄ **LM of a basophil in a blood smear.**
The easily recognized basophil (**Ba**) has many large basophilic specific granules that are blue. The nucleus, being masked by the granules, is less evident. The erythrocytes (**RBC**) are smaller than the basophil. 1200×. *Wright's.*

► **EM of a basophil.** Its nucleus is bilobed (∗). A peripheral rim of heterochromatin surrounds central euchromatin. The cytoplasm has many prominent, closely packed specific granules (**SG**) that are derived from the Golgi complex (**GC**). These membrane-bound granules vary in size and density. 11,300×.

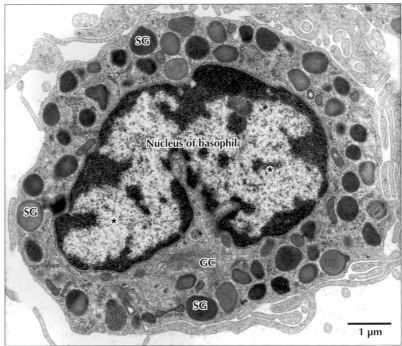

7.6 STRUCTURE AND FUNCTION OF BASOPHILS

Basophils, the least numerous leukocytes, account for less than 1% of the leukocyte count. These **granulocytes**—between neutrophils and eosinophils in size, with a diameter of 10-14 μm—have large, distinctive **specific granules** that are intensely basophilic and fill the cytoplasm. The **nucleus** is often irregular in shape or **bilobed.** In blood smears, the nucleus is usually obscured by many closely packed basophilic granules, which often stain more deeply than nuclear chromatin. Basophils closely resemble mast cells of connective tissue; their granules, like those of mast cells but larger and fewer, have metachromatic staining properties and contain *histamine* and *heparin.* By electron microscopy, the basophil's membrane-bound granules vary in internal appearance, electron density, and size, often reaching a diameter of 1 μm. Basophils also produce *platelet-activating* and *eosinophilic chemotactic factors,* which exert powerful pharmacologic effects outside the circulation. Basophils probably originate in bone marrow from cell precursors different from those of mast cells. In both cell types, histamine released by exocytosis at cell surfaces increases vascular permeability during an inflammatory response. Heparin, the

reason for basophilia of the granules, prevents *blood coagulation.* Both cells also have surface receptors that bind immunoglobulin IgE, which is produced by plasma cells in connective tissue. The motile basophils are involved in *allergic reactions* and increase in number in many clinical conditions such as hay fever, urticaria, chronic sinusitis, and some leukemias.

CLINICAL POINT

Basophilia—an elevated basophil count in peripheral blood—rarely occurs in most benign conditions. Mild basophilia may be part of a general inflammatory response to some infections, for example, *smallpox, chickenpox,* or *influenza.* It also occurs in allergic disorders or autoimmune inflammation such as *rheumatoid arthritis* or *ulcerative colitis.* More often, and for unclear reasons, basophilia is noted in malignant hematologic conditions called *myeloproliferative disorders.* The most common such condition is *chronic myeloid leukemia,* in which basophils are often markedly increased, as are eosinophils, neutrophils, and immature neutrophilic forms such as band cells, metamyelocytes, myelocytes, and promyelocytes. In patients with chronic myeloid leukemia, an increasing basophil count can suggest worsening of disease.

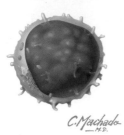

▼ **Lymphocyte.**

C. Machado
_M.D._

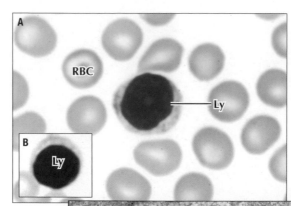

◄ **LMs of lymphocytes in a blood smear. A.** A rim of blue-gray cytoplasm caps a darkly stained round nucleus in a large lymphocyte (**Ly**). Erythrocytes (**RBC**) are also in view. **B.** A small lymphocyte at the same magnification is shown for comparison. 1275×. *Wright's.*

► **EM of a lymphocyte.** The spherical, slightly indented nucleus contains condensed heterochromatin with patches of euchromatin. The cytoplasm shows many free ribosomes (**Ri**), scattered mitochondria (**Mi**), and a few profiles of **RER**. A few short microvilli (**arrows**) are at the cell surface. 16,000×.

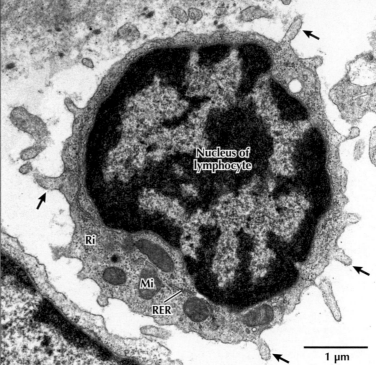

7.7 STRUCTURE AND FUNCTION OF LYMPHOCYTES

At 20%-40% of the leukocyte count, lymphocytes are the most numerous **agranular leukocyte.** They can be classified as small (6-10 μm) and medium to large (11-16 μm), with most circulating lymphocytes in normal blood being small. These spherical cells have a densely stained nucleus and a thin rim of blue-gray cytoplasm. The larger the cell, the more cytoplasm is visible. All lymphocytes derive from bone marrow stem cells; those that differentiate and mature in the thymus are **T cells,** and those that develop in bone marrow where they acquire specific cell surface antigens are **B cells.** B and T cells are indistinguishable in conventional blood smears. In normal peripheral blood, 60%-80% of lymphocytes are T cells, 10%-15% are B cells, and the rest are null cells, which lack both B and T cell markers. T cell subpopulations defined by antigenic markers are *CD4⁺ (helper), CD8⁺ (suppressor), killer (cytotoxic),* and *memory cells.* CD4⁺ cells are depleted in HIV infection and AIDS. B cells express various cell surface makers; when the cells are activated by antigen, they differentiate into plasma cells, which synthesize and secrete immunoglobulins. *Cell-mediated immunity* involves T cells, whereas B cells function in *humoral (antibody) immunity.* The lymphocyte life span ranges from a few days to many years. By electron microscopy, many free ribosomes and scattered profiles of rough endoplasmic reticulum (RER) dominate the cytoplasm. A small Golgi complex, small numbers of mitochondria, and occasional lysosomes are also present.

CLINICAL POINT

Lymphocytosis is an abnormal increase in absolute number of lymphocytes in peripheral blood. It often occurs in infants and adolescents during infections that would likely produce a neutrophil response in adults. Of the many causes, the most common is primary infection with *Epstein-Barr virus* (EBV). The condition, also known as *infectious mononucleosis,* causes a rise in circulating T lymphocyte numbers in response to EBV infection of B cells. Lymphocytes are larger than normal and look atypical. Specific antibodies to EBV nuclear antigen appear in the blood and last for life. Most patients need only symptomatic treatment, as recovery is usually 4-6 weeks after symptoms begin.

▼ Monocyte.

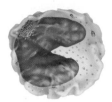

C. Machado
—M.D.—

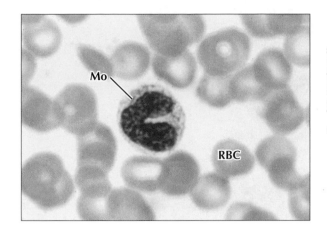

◀ **LM of a monocyte in a blood smear.** A monocyte (**Mo**) nucleus is highly indented and less densely stained than that of lymphocytes. Throughout the light blue cytoplasm are many faintly stained granules, so the cytoplasm looks dusty. The monocyte is twice as large as the erythrocytes (**RBC**). 1350×. *Wright's.*

▶ **Colorized SEM showing a venule lumen.** Surface features of a monocyte (**Mo**) are clear. The cell attaches to the endothelium (**En**) by pseudopodia (**arrows**) as it begins migrating from the lumen on its way to becoming a macrophage. This migratory process— diapedesis—enables leukocytes to leave the circulation for functions in surrounding tissues. 3440×. (*Courtesy of Dr. M. E. Todd*)

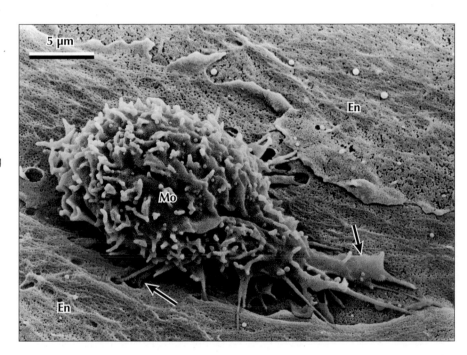

7.8 STRUCTURE AND FUNCTION OF MONOCYTES

Monocytes are **agranular leukocytes** that are immediate precursors to cells of the *monocyte-macrophage system.* They constitute 3%-10% of the total leukocyte count and, with a diameter of 12-20 μm, are the largest leukocytes in blood smears. They usually circulate in the bloodstream for only 1-3 days and perform almost all functions outside the circulation. These actively motile cells enter connective tissues to become **macrophages** (or **phagocytes**). Each cell has a nucleus that varies in form and may have an oval, kidney, or horseshoe shape. In contrast to the coarse, dark-staining nuclear chromatin of lymphocytes, monocyte nuclear chromatin is finely granular and pale stained, and indented. Monocyte cytoplasm has a blue-gray tinge and contains a moderate number of small, scattered **azurophilic granules** but no specific granules. Electron microscopy reveals the granules to be membrane-bound primary lysosomes. A well-formed Golgi complex is near the indentation of the nucleus; the cytoplasm also contains scattered elements of RER, free ribosomes, and a few small mitochondria. Cytoplasmic filaments and many irregular **pseudopodia** are typical of cell surfaces, consistent with motility. Monocytes can cross walls of venules and capillaries to enter and migrate through surrounding connective tissue. Large numbers are found in areas of *inflammation*, where they engage in *phagocytosis* and scavenging of cell debris.

CLINICAL POINT

Monocytosis is an abnormal rise in the monocyte count above 0.8 × 10^9/L. Although monocytosis is rare, many conditions may cause it: chronic bacterial infections, bacterial endocarditis (inflammation of the inner lining of the heart wall), typhoid, malaria, syphilis, and protozoan infections. Monocytes are important in defense against malignancies, and two malignant disorders associated with extremely high monocyte counts are *Hodgkin's lymphoma* and *chronic myelomonocytic leukemia.* **Monocytopenia**—low monocyte count—occurs in *hairy cell leukemia, AIDS,* and *bone marrow failure.*

▼ Platelets.

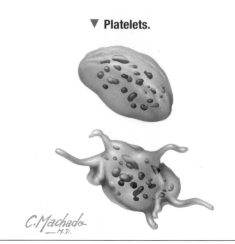

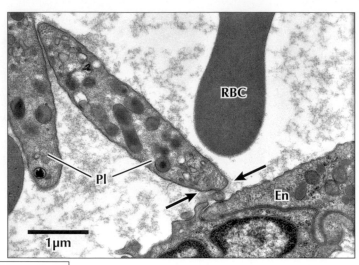

▲ **EM of two platelets and part of an erythrocyte (RBC) in the lumen of a blood vessel.** The platelets (**Pl**) contain several dense, membrane-bound granules. One platelet seems to adhere (**arrows**) to the vessel's endothelium (**En**). 14,000×.

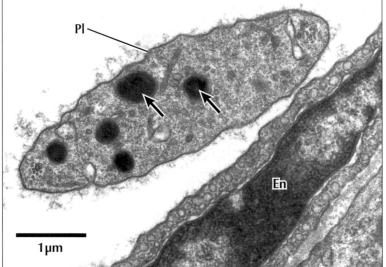

▲ **EM of a platelet in the lumen of a blood vessel.** The platelet (**Pl**), enclosed by a plasma membrane, contains several dense granules (**arrows**) and a dense network of cytoskeletal elements. The endothelium of the blood vessel (**En**) is shown. 19,000×.

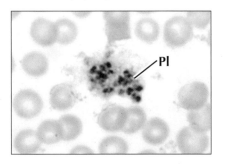

▲ **LM of a clump of platelets in a blood smear.** Platelets (**Pl**) are round to oval discs containing a dark-staining central granulomere surrounded by a homogeneous, pale hyalomere. 900×. *Wright's.*

7.9 STRUCTURE AND FUNCTION OF PLATELETS

Platelets—motile **cytoplasmic fragments** enveloped by a **plasma membrane**—arise from megakaryocytes in bone marrow. These smallest formed elements in peripheral blood, with a diameter of 2-4 μm, appear as plate-like structures without nuclei. They normally range from 150 to 400×10^9/L of blood. Their other name, **thrombocytes,** is a misnomer, as they are not whole cells in humans. Conventional blood smears and stains reveal that they often stick together and aggregate into clumps, and two cytoplasmic regions can be recognized: a central zone, the **granulomere,** is a compact region that stains blue to purple. A peripheral, pale blue homogeneous region that is known as the **hyalomere** (because it looks glassy) surrounds it. By electron microscopy, the hyalomere contains a circumferential bundle of microtubules and cytoplasmic filaments just under the cell membrane. These cytoskeletal elements help maintain platelet shape and are involved in movement. Actin and myosin in this region likely play a role in contraction during *blood clot* formation. Membranous canaliculi invaginate from the cell surface and allow discharge of secretory products during platelet activation. The central granulomere contains a small Golgi complex, elements of RER, a few scattered mitochondria, glycogen deposits, and various membrane-bound granules and lysosomes. **Alpha granules** correspond to azurophilic granules and contain clotting substances. Platelets, which play a major role in *blood coagulation,* produce *von Willebrand factor, thrombospondin,* and *platelet-derived growth factor.*

CLINICAL POINT

Thrombocytopenia is a condition involving abnormal depletion of platelets in blood. It may be caused by failure of bone marrow to produce adequate numbers of platelets or by a greater rate of removal of platelets from blood. Platelets are critical for blood clotting, so an untreated disorder leads to bruising and severe bleeding. Low platelet counts are a common side effect of *radiation treatment* and *chemotherapy* (for lymphoma and other cancers), which destroy cell precursors in bone marrow. *Autoimmune* and *viral diseases,* including systemic lupus and HIV infection, also destroy platelets.

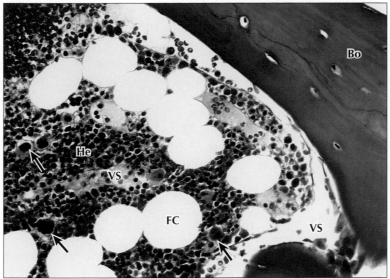

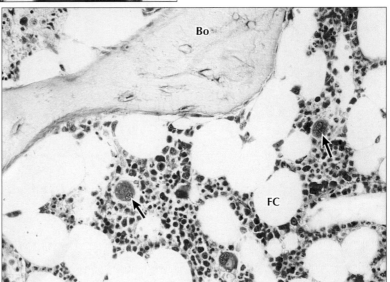

◄ ▼ **LMs showing the architecture of the bone marrow.** Many adipocytes (**FC**), hematopoietic cells (**He**), and venous sinusoids (**VS**) occupy spaces between bony trabeculae (**Bo**). Megakaryocytes (**arrows**), as the largest cells of the marrow, are conspicuous. Both cellularity and the ratio of adipocytes to hematopoietic cells may vary markedly in different parts of the same section. 255×. **Left:** *H&E;* **Below:** *Wright's.*

7.10   HISTOLOGY OF BONE MARROW

Bone marrow is a special type of connective tissue in medullary cavities of bones. It consists of a **stroma** of *loose reticular connective tissue* and a **parenchyma** of **hematopoietic cells** arranged as irregular cellular cords or islands separated by thin-walled **venous sinusoids.** It has a vital role in lifelong production of blood cells and platelets. Two types of bone marrow occur in adults: **red** and **yellow.** Red marrow—the actively hematopoietic tissue—is abundant in prenatal life and in the young. Its red color is due to erythrocytes and their precursors. Until age 20-25 years, progressive fatty replacement of the marrow leads to yellow (or fatty) marrow, which is relatively inactive and is mainly composed of **adipocytes** (fat cells). The two types of marrow are quite labile throughout life, with their relative distribution depending on the need for new blood cells. Venous sinusoids of bone marrow are thin-walled vessels with a diameter of 15-100 μm. They form an extensive, communicating network and are derived from branches of nutrient arteries to the bones. A single layer of extremely attenuated endothelial cells linked by gap and tight junctions lines them. A surrounding basal lamina is either absent or discontinuous. Adventitial *reticular cells,* which are modified fibroblasts, have many branching processes and produce the reticular fiber network that supports hematopoietic cells. Also, many cellular adhesion molecules on surfaces of reticular cells in the stroma attach to developing blood cells. Newly formed blood cells migrate across sinusoid walls to enter the bloodstream and then large veins. Bone marrow contains no lymphatics.

CLINICAL POINT

Aplastic anemia is a hematologic disorder caused by bone marrow failure. It is usually defined as a *pancytopenia,* or a reduced count of all major blood cells of the erythroid and myeloid series. Common clinical signs are bruising or bleeding (low platelet count), infection (lower production of leukocytes), and lethargy (reduced erythrocyte and low hemoglobin values). The disease—congenital or acquired—is probably caused by markedly reduced numbers of hematopoietic stem cells. Diagnosis is confirmed via bone marrow biopsy. In many cases, effective treatment is *bone marrow* (stem cell) *transplantation* in patients who are matched with a donor.

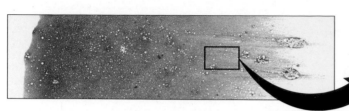

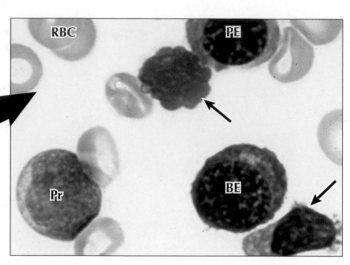

▲ **LM of a bone marrow smear at low (Above) and high (Right) magnifications.** The smear, made from a bone marrow aspirate, shows details of hematopoiesis. Hematopoietic cells of the erythroid lineage at different stages of development in **B** include a proerythroblast (**Pr**), basophilic erythroblast (**BE**), and early polychromatophilic erythroblast (**PE**). Mature erythrocytes (**RBC**) and two unidentifiable cells (**arrows**) are also seen. **Above:** 8×; **Right:** 2000×. *Wright's.*

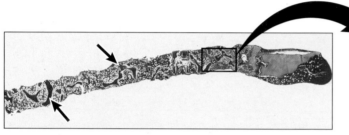

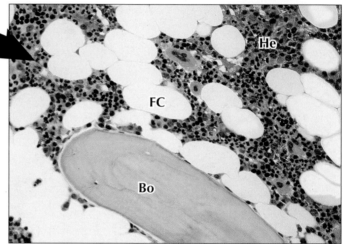

▲ **LM of a bone marrow biopsy specimen at low (Above) and high (Right) magnifications.** The solid core of tissue contains bone marrow and bony trabeculae (**arrows**). Normal bone marrow consists of a heterogeneous population of cells in various stages of differentiation. Clusters of tightly packed hematopoietic cells (**He**) sit between large adipocytes (**FC**) and bony trabeculae (**Bo**). Adipocytes look empty because of lipid extraction during specimen preparation. **Above:** 8×; **Right:** 200×. *H&E.*

7.11 METHODS OF STUDYING BONE MARROW

Smears and **trephine needle biopsy** (for preparation of bone marrow sections) are used to sample and examine bone marrow. The optimal site for both aspiration and trephine biopsies is the posterior iliac crest, other sites being the sternum and tibia. After insertion of a needle into the marrow, a liquid sample is aspirated into a syringe and spread as a smear onto a slide. It is then fixed and stained by hematoxylin and eosin (H&E) or the usual polychrome blood stains and then examined via a microscope. A small amount of aspirated marrow can make several thin smears. Smears are the best preparations for evaluating cell details, studying maturation of **hematopoietic cells,** making *differential counts,* and assessing the ratio of **myeloid** (leukocyte) to **erythroid** (erythrocyte) cells. An advantage is preservation of individual cells so that subtle morphologic changes and infiltration by *malignant cells* in disease can be detected. Smears can also detect *anemias, leukemias,* and *myeloma.* The trephine biopsy entails cutting out a solid core of bone marrow, including some trabecular bone, with a large-bore cutting needle. Fixation in formalin, decalcification, sectioning, and staining the specimen follow. Sections are less valuable than smears for elucidating cell details but provide a panoramic view of bone marrow and its normal architecture. They are also useful for estimating *bone marrow cellularity,* which is an index of the proportion of hematopoietic cells to adipocytes. Bone marrow cellularity is high in young persons, is reduced in the elderly, and may be altered in disease.

CLINICAL POINT

Bone marrow is easily accessible and its hematopoietic stem cells are replaced in many conditions, so **bone marrow transplantation** is a valuable tool in medicine. Stem cell transplants are used to reconstitute marrow after *chemotherapy* or replace primary loss of stem cells in disease. **Autologous transplantation** is used in certain forms of lymphoma in which malignant cells contaminate marrow. It involves harvesting bone marrow stem cells from a patient, followed by high-dose chemotherapy and then intravenous injection of reconstituted marrow. A stem cell transplant from another person is an **allogeneic transplant.** Its success requires donor matching for the major histocompatibility complex (MHC) on chromosome 6.

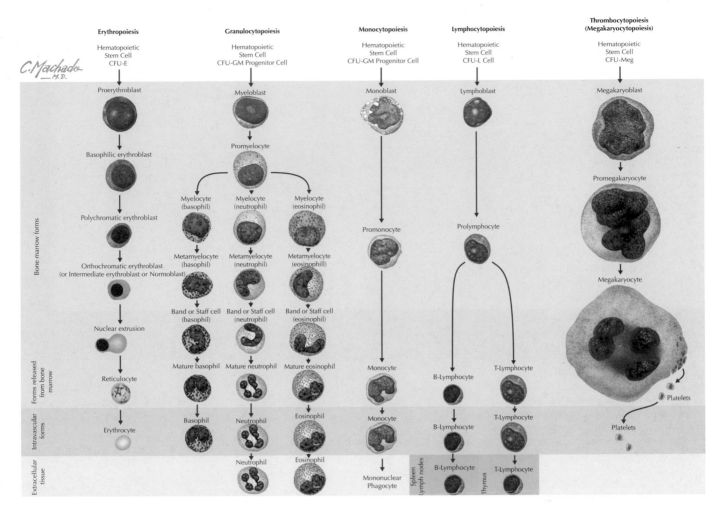

▲ **Schematic showing stages of hematopoiesis.** Although not all cells are included in each sequence, main cell types seen in bone marrow smears are shown in erythropoiesis (**left**), granulocytopoiesis (**center, left**), monocytopoiesis (**center**), lymphocytopoiesis (**center, right**), and megakaryocytopoiesis (**right**). The various CFU cells that arise from the hematopoietic stem cell (not shown) closely resemble lymphocytes. Except for megakaryocytes, cells in erythroid and myeloid series as a rule get smaller during differentiation. Also, nuclear size declines, nuclear density increases, and special features related to cell lineage—such as hemoglobin production and nuclear extrusion in erythropoiesis, and specific granules (eosinophilic, basophilic, or neutrophilic) in granulocytopoiesis—appear. Various growth factors and cytokines mediate cell proliferation rate and survival and maturation of progenitor cells. Some of these are colony-stimulating factors, erythropoietin, thrombopoietin, interleukins (IL-1, IL3, IL-6, IL-11), and stem cell factors.

7.12 HEMATOPOIESIS

Bone marrow is the site of hematopoiesis after birth. Because most blood cells are short-lived, they need continuous replacement. In the normal adult, about 2.5×10^9 erythrocytes, 1×10^9 granulocytes, and 2.5×10^9 platelets per kg of body weight are produced daily in bone marrow. All mature blood cells derive from **pleuri-potential stem cells** in bone marrow, which have a capacity for self-renewal, asymmetric replication, and differentiation. In asymmetric replication, one daughter cell after mitosis retains a self-renewing capability, and the other differentiates into a nondividing population of stem cells. Bone marrow stem cells are small, mono-nucleated, and not easily identified under the microscope, but their existence is inferred from in vitro cell cultures, which generate more mature, recognizable **progenitor cells.** Experimentally, these cells form visible **colony-forming units (CFUs)** when injected into the spleen. Different CFUs form depending on cell of origin; four types of progenitors exist. CFUs committed to **erythroid lineage** production contain progenitor cells known as **colony-forming unit-erythrocytes (CFU-E).** Granulocyte and monocyte cell lines develop from one progenitor cell known as the **colony-forming unit-granulocyte-monocyte (CFU-GM).** As cells mature, progeny become committed to either granulocytes or monocytes. Cells of the **lymphocyte lineage** are generated from **colony-forming unit-lymphocytes (CFU-L).** Progenitor cells for megakaryocytes produce colonies that contain **colony-forming unit-megakaryocytes (CFU-Me).** Later stages in hematopoiesis involve transformation of progenitor cells to precursor (blast) cells, which become recognizable as members of a specific lineage.

▼ **Nuclear extrusion.**

▼ **Reticulocyte.**

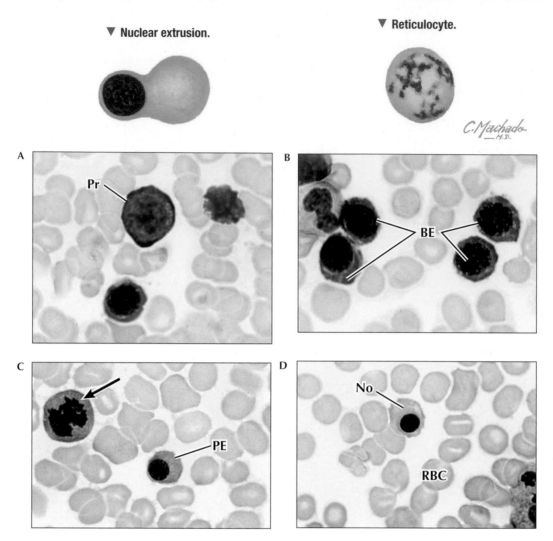

▲ **Bone marrow smears showing different stages of erythropoiesis. A.** Proerythroblast (**Pr**). **B.** Basophilic erythroblasts (**BE**). **C.** Polychromatophilic erythroblast (**PE**), plus a large, unidentifiable cell (**arrow**), which is probably undergoing mitosis. **D.** Orthochromatophilic erythroblast (or late normoblast) (**No**). Mature erythrocytes (**RBC**) are also seen. 1500×. *Wright's.*

7.13 ERYTHROPOIESIS

During maturation of the **erythroid lineage,** large primitive cells become smaller. The nucleus of young cells, which is large in relation to the cytoplasm, also becomes smaller as well as pyknotic and is extruded. The **CFU-erythrocyte** first differentiates into the earliest recognizable cell of this series: a large, round **proerythroblast,** with a diameter of 15-30 μm. Its deep blue cytoplasm is due to abundant ribosomal RNA, which has affinity for basic dyes. Many free cytoplasmic ribosomes begin to synthesize hemoglobin. Nuclear chromatin is euchromatic; one or two nucleoli are prominent. The erythroblast divides into two smaller (10-18 μm) **basophilic erythroblasts,** which have intensely basophilic cytoplasm and a more heterochromatic nucleus. Ribosomes continue to synthesize more hemoglobin. This cell undergoes two or three cell divisions, and progeny form the **polychromatophilic erythroblast,** with a diameter of 10-12 μm. The slate gray tinge of its cytoplasm is due to steady buildup of hemoglobin and decrease in ribosomes. Its nucleus has condensed chromatin but no nucleoli. With higher hemoglobin content, the cytoplasm becomes more eosinophilic, and the cell is now called an **orthochromatophilic erythroblast** (or **late normoblast**). This 8- to 10-μm cell has a small, densely stained, pyknotic nucleus. After extrusion of the nucleus and loss of all organelles, the cell becomes biconcave and has a diameter of 7-10 μm—an **erythrocyte.** Erythrocytes remain in the bone marrow for 2-3 days until fully mature, when they are released into peripheral circulation. About 1%-2% of newly formed erythrocytes contain a few residual ribosomes that give a slight basophilia and reticular staining pattern to the cytoplasm. Named **reticulocytes,** these cells in peripheral blood provide a rough estimate of the rate of erythropoiesis, as the reticulocyte count. They slowly lose ribosomes and become mature erythrocytes. Erythropoiesis is regulated by the glycoprotein hormone *erythropoietin,* which is secreted by interstitial peritubular cells of the kidneys, mostly in response to hypoxia. Erythropoiesis, from the proerythroblast to the mature erythrocyte, takes 7-8 days.

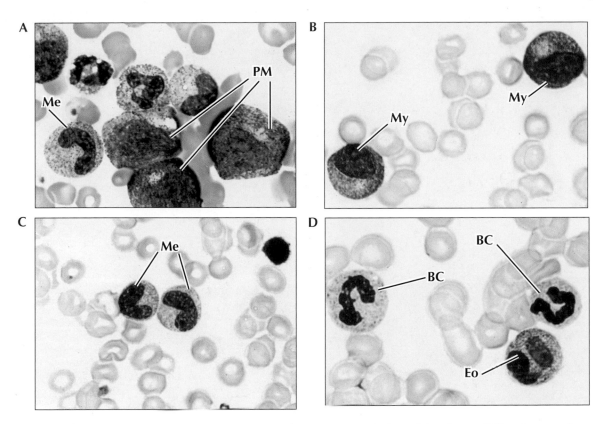

▲ **Bone marrow smears showing different stages of granulocytopoiesis. A.** Promyelocytes (**PM**) and metamyelocytes (**Me**). **B.** Myelocytes (**My**). **C.** Metamyelocytes (**Me**). **D.** Neutrophilic band cells (**BC**) and a mature eosinophil (**Eo**). 1500×. *Wright's.*

7.14 GRANULOCYTOPOIESIS

Granulocytes and monocytes derive from a common precursor, the **CFU-GM,** in bone marrow. The maturation sequence whereby the three types of granulocytes are produced—granulocytopoiesis—takes 14-18 days. Although the maturation continuum is similar to that of erythropoiesis, cells undergo detectable morphologic changes, and the terminology associated with each stage may vary. As a rule, the nucleus first becomes flattened and indented, and then smaller and lobulated; the cytoplasm accumulates nonspecific and specific granules. In the granulocyte series, the CFU-GM gives rise to three cell populations, known as **myeloblasts, promyelocytes,** and **myelocytes,** each with proliferative or mitotic potential. Myeloblasts are large, spherical cells, 12-18 μm in diameter. Their basophilic cytoplasm lacks specific granules but contains abundant ribosomes. A large, round nucleus contains finely dispersed chromatin with several nucleoli. Myeloblasts divide and give rise to promyelocytes, with diameters of 15-25 μm. They have a slightly flattened nucleus and basophilic cytoplasm containing a few nonspecific azurophilic granules. Promyelocytes divide and give rise to myelocytes, which are slightly smaller, at 15-18 μm in

diameter. Myelocytes have a pale, lightly basophilic cytoplasm; their nucleus appears pushed off to the side of the cell and occupies about 50% of the cell area. Specific granules in the cytoplasm first appear at this stage. Three types of cells with distinct specific granules may be described but not readily distinguished: **neutrophilic, basophilic,** and **eosinophilic myelocytes.** Myelocytes of these three cell lines mature into **metamyelocytes,** which have a full complement of specific granules as well as nonspecific granules. These cells, about 12 μm in diameter, have a deeply indented, horseshoe-shaped nucleus. As cells mature, the nucleus becomes more segmented and the cytoplasm less basophilic. At this stage, these **band** (or **stab**) **cells** have a diameter of about 10 μm. Also known as *juvenile granulocytes,* they are immediate precursors to the three kinds of mature granulocytes that are released into circulation. A small percentage (1%-3%) of band cells may normally enter the bloodstream, but a significantly increased number indicates a rise in cell production. Known clinically as a *shift to the left,* this condition may indicate a disorder such as a *granulocytic leukemia.*

▼ **Blood clot or thrombus.**

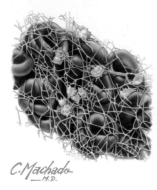

C. Machado — M.D.

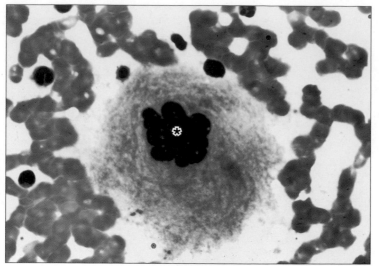

◀ **A bone marrow smear showing a megakaryocyte.** The cell, the largest in bone marrow, has an irregular outline. The single nucleus (✱) is lobulated. The cytoplasm appears foamy and lightly basophilic. One megakaryocyte may produce several thousand platelets. Once platelets are released, the remaining cytoplasm and nucleus degenerate and are then phagocytosed in the marrow. 825×. *Wright's.*

▶ **EM of part of a megakaryocyte in a bone marrow section.** Parts of several lobes (✱) of the polyploid nucleus do not appear connected in this plane. Extensive networks of platelet demarcation channels (**arrows**) are in the cell periphery. These channels arise by fusion of vesicles, which eventually become continuous with each other. They permit regional partitioning of cytoplasm by outlining areas for detachment of separate platelets for release into circulation. Various other organelles, including small electron-dense granules, ribosomes, and mitochondria, are seen in the cytoplasm. 10,000×. *(Courtesy of Dr. W. A. Webber)*

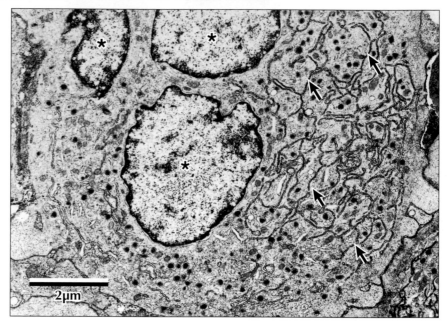

2μm

7.15 MONOCYTOPOIESIS, LYMPHOCYTOPOIESIS, AND THROMBOCYTOPOIESIS

Other forms of **myelopoiesis** in the bone marrow are monocytopoiesis, lymphocytopoiesis, and thrombocytopoiesis (production of monocytes, lymphocytes, and platelets, respectively). **Monocytes** develop from **CFU-GM progenitor cells,** which give rise to **monoblasts.** These cells look similar to myeloblasts, but they are relatively rare and hard to identify. They differentiate into **promonocytes,** which give rise to monocytes. Monocytes in bone marrow rapidly enter the circulation where they mature, after which they migrate to tissues and organs to become **macrophages.** **Lymphocytes** arise from **lymphoblasts,** which derive from a precursor **CFU-L cell.** Large lymphoblasts (15-20 μm in diameter) give rise to smaller **prolymphocytes.** Some prolymphocytes in bone marrow differentiate into **B cells,** which enter the circulation to go to the spleen and lymph nodes. Other prolymphocytes enter the bloodstream during early stages of embryonic and early postnatal life to populate the thymus gland. These cells in the thymus mature into **T cells,** which gain access to the circulation. Thrombocytopoiesis in bone marrow begins with a large precursor known as a **CFU-Me cell.** This unipotential cell differentiates into a **megakaryoblast,** about 50 μm in diameter and with a lobulated nucleus and many nucleoli. This cell is transformed into a large **megakaryocyte,** which varies in diameter from 30 to 100 μm. An irregular outline is due to many pseudopods that project from the cell surface. The highly convoluted lobulated nucleus shows coarse chromatin. The uniquely **polyploid nucleus** is due to multiple replication of nuclear DNA without division of cytoplasm. By light microscopy, the homogeneous cytoplasm is lightly basophilic because of large numbers of free ribosomes and many small azurophilic granules. By electron microscopy, megakaryocytes contain a unique, extensive membranous network of **platelet demarcation channels.** Platelets form by fragmentation of cytoplasm along these demarcation channels. This process is analogous to selective tearing of a sheet of postage stamps, with single stamps removed along perforations that outline them.

II: SYSTEMS

8

CARDIOVASCULAR SYSTEM

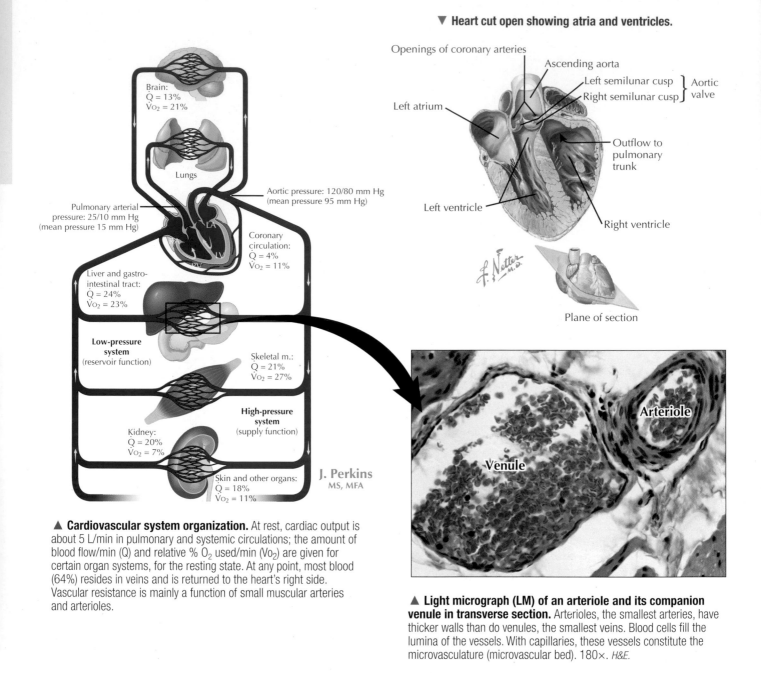

▼ **Heart cut open showing atria and ventricles.**

Openings of coronary arteries

Ascending aorta

Left semilunar cusp
Right semilunar cusp } Aortic valve

Left atrium

Outflow to pulmonary trunk

Left ventricle

Right ventricle

J. Netter M.D.

Plane of section

Brain:
Q̇ = 13%
V̇O₂ = 21%

Lungs

Aortic pressure: 120/80 mm Hg
(mean pressure 95 mm Hg)

Pulmonary arterial pressure: 25/10 mm Hg
(mean pressure 15 mm Hg)

Coronary circulation:
Q̇ = 4%
V̇O₂ = 11%

Liver and gastro-intestinal tract:
Q̇ = 24%
V̇O₂ = 23%

Low-pressure system
(reservoir function)

Skeletal m.:
Q̇ = 21%
V̇O₂ = 27%

High-pressure system
(supply function)

Kidney:
Q̇ = 20%
V̇O₂ = 7%

Skin and other organs:
Q̇ = 18%
V̇O₂ = 11%

J. Perkins
MS, MFA

▲ **Cardiovascular system organization.** At rest, cardiac output is about 5 L/min in pulmonary and systemic circulations; the amount of blood flow/min (Q) and relative % O₂ used/min (Vo₂) are given for certain organ systems, for the resting state. At any point, most blood (64%) resides in veins and is returned to the heart's right side. Vascular resistance is mainly a function of small muscular arteries and arterioles.

Arteriole

Venule

▲ **Light micrograph (LM) of an arteriole and its companion venule in transverse section.** Arterioles, the smallest arteries, have thicker walls than do venules, the smallest veins. Blood cells fill the lumina of the vessels. With capillaries, these vessels constitute the microvasculature (microvascular bed). 180×. *H&E.*

8.1 OVERVIEW

The cardiovascular system consists of the **heart**—a muscular pump—and closed vessels through which blood circulates in the body. **Arteries** leave the heart, branch repeatedly, and have smaller diameters as they course toward the periphery. They deliver blood to **capillaries,** which are the thinnest vessels and are closest to body cells. Blood in capillaries is returned to the heart via **veins.** The blood circulatory system consists of two functional parts: **pulmonary** (which conducts blood to and from lungs for gas exchange) and **systemic** (which delivers blood to and from other parts of the body). Closely associated with this circulatory system is a large network of **lymphatic vessels** that collects excess fluid from body tissues and returns it as **lymph** to the blood circulation. The cardiovascular system consists of tubular structures, the heart itself being a cone-shaped tube with dilated segments reflected on itself. Continuous, simple squamous epithelium known as cardiac and vascular *endothelium* lines the whole system internally. Capillaries are made almost entirely of a single layer of *endothelial cells* and associated cells called *pericytes.* All other vessels have added tissue layers that are arranged concentrically around the endothelium. Arteries operate in a high-pressure system and veins serve a reservoir function under low pressure, so arteries usually have thicker **walls** than veins. Blood vessels differ in size, function, and distribution, but they share a histologic plan, with structural differences reflecting functions in various parts of the system. Walls of blood vessels above the capillary level have three layers, or tunics: inner *tunica intima* (closest to the lumen), middle *tunica media,* and outer *tunica adventitia.*

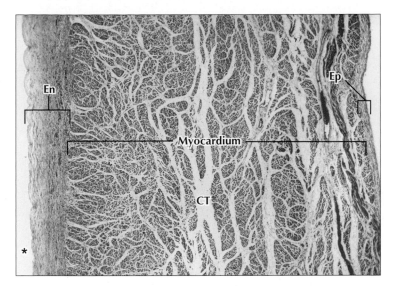

◀ **LM of the atrial wall.** The innermost endocardium (**En**) lines the atrial chamber (✶). This prominent layer is continuous with intima of vessels entering and leaving the heart. The myocardium—the bulk of the heart wall—consists of bundles of cardiac muscle cells, coursing in different directions and separated by loose connective tissue (**CT**). The thin outer epicardium (**Ep**) is fibrous connective tissue covered by thin mesothelium. The small, clear space to the extreme right is the pericardial cavity. 35×. *H&E.*

▶ **LM of the outer part of the ventricular wall.** The epicardium and part of the myocardium can be seen. Nerve fibers (**NF**) and large blood vessels (**BV**), which are branches of coronary arteries and cardiac veins, run through the adipose tissue of the epicardium. 50×. *H&E.*

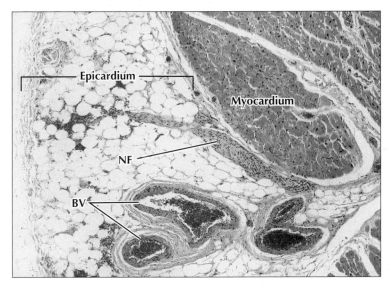

8.2   HISTOLOGY AND FUNCTION OF THE HEART WALL AND PERICARDIUM

The heart develops embryonically from a simple blood vessel and thus retains the three concentric tunics of vessel walls. In the heart wall, the organization and tissue composition of these layers—endocardium, myocardium, and epicardium—are modified to reflect the heart's main function as a *four-chambered muscular pump.* The inner **endocardium,** homologous to the **tunica intima,** is in contact with blood, which fills the heart chambers. This layer consists of an **endothelium** and underlying **connective tissue.** The **myocardium** substitutes for the **tunica media** of vessels. Forming the bulk of the heart wall, it consists mostly of **cardiac muscle.** The outer layer, analogous to the **tunica adventitia,** is the **epicardium.** Unlike the adventitia, the epicardium has two layers: deeper loose, fatty connective tissue is covered externally by **mesothelium.** One layer of squamous to cuboidal mesothelial cells—mainly secretory cells resembling mesothelial cells lining pleural and peritoneal cavities—rests on a basal lamina and makes up the mesothelium, which also forms the visceral layer of the pericardium. The **pericardium,** the fibroelastic, fluid-filled sac that holds the heart, consists of an

outer parietal layer that reflects onto the heart surface as a visceral layer (epicardium). Mesothelial cells lining these two parts of the pericardium secrete a thin film of clear, serous fluid (usually less than 50 mL) into the pericardial sac. The fluid lubricates the heart's surface during contraction to reduce friction. The epicardium contains **adipose tissue** to act as a shock absorber and support branches of **coronary arteries; veins** that drain blood from the heart wall; lymphatics; and many **nerve fascicles** and ganglia.

HISTORICAL POINT
English physician **William Harvey** (1578-1657), considered to be the father of physiology, discovered the circulation. In 1616, he aptly described the heart as a pump and the direction of blood flow in arteries and veins. He graduated from Cambridge University and received his medical degree from the University of Padua. Later that century, **Marcello Malpighi** (1628-1694), the Italian physician and father of histology and embryology, was the first to systematically and fruitfully exploit the microscope in anatomic research. He studied medicine in Padua, was a physician to one of the popes, and was professor of anatomy in Bologna. In 1661, he proved the existence of capillaries and coined the term from the Latin *capillaris,* because of their resemblance to fine hairs.

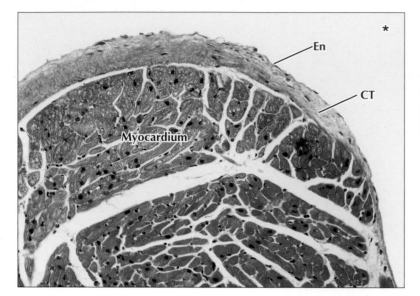

◀ **LM of the inner part of the ventricular wall.** The endocardium consists of an inner layer of endothelium (**En**) and a deeper subendocardial layer of connective tissue (**CT**). Endothelial cell nuclei bulge into the ventricular chamber (⋆), which, in life, is filled with blood. Sheets of cardiac muscle cells separated by connective tissue make up the myocardium. 180×. *H&E.*

▶ **LM of the inner part of the atrial wall.** The atrial endocardium is much thicker than that in the ventricles. Endothelial cells (**En**) here form an internal lining in direct contact with the heart chamber (⋆). Endocardial connective tissue organization ranges from dense fibrous to loose irregular. Adjacent myocardium contains bundles of tightly packed cardiac muscle cells separated by loose connective tissue. 180×. *H&E.*

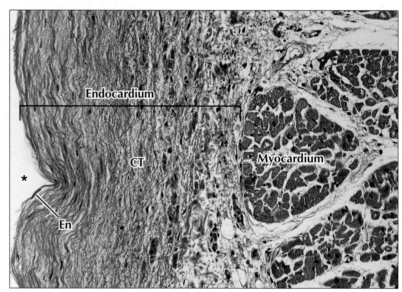

8.3 HISTOLOGY OF THE ENDOCARDIUM AND MYOCARDIUM

The endocardium contains several distinct layers, which may vary histologically in different parts of the heart. An innermost **endothelium,** derived embryonically from mesoderm, is made of one layer of **endothelial cells,** which are a type of simple squamous epithelium. It is continuous with endothelium of veins and arteries that enter and leave the heart. A subendothelial layer of **connective tissue** consists of *collagen fibers, elastic fibers,* and scattered *smooth muscle cells.* In some areas is another layer of loose fibroelastic connective tissue, the **subendocardium.** It may contain elements of the *cardiac conduction system,* such as Purkinje fibers, which are modified **cardiac muscle cells** (see Chapter 4). The endocardium is usually thicker in the **atria** than in the **ventricles.** The inner surface of the ventricles under the endocardium has trabeculae that project into the lumen and are composed of cardiac muscle—called papillary muscles. Although the luminal surface of the atria is relatively smooth, a small auricular appendage is trabeculated internally by muscular bands, or pectinate muscles. The much thicker ventricular myocardium compared with the atrial layer reflects differences in workload of heart chambers. The myocardium consists of interlacing bundles, or sheets, of cardiac muscle cells embedded in richly vascularized, loose connective tissue, which is the *endomysium.* The muscle fibers in each sheet have a complex spiral pattern that winds around the atria and ventricles. Cardiac muscle cells form a three-dimensional anastomosing network whereby intercalated discs link almost all cells and other cells insert into the cardiac skeleton of dense fibrous connective tissue.

CLINICAL POINT

Rheumatic fever is a systemic, immunologically mediated disorder caused by *streptococcal bacterial infection* of the pharynx or upper respiratory tract in children and adolescents. It affects the joints, dermis, and brain and may also lead to **rheumatic heart disease** (RHD). RHD may cause inflammation of all three layers of the heart wall, but its most serious complication is an effect on endocardium covering valves of the left side of the heart, which can become ulcerated and scarred and thereby deformed. Serious, life-threatening consequences, such as *mitral insufficiency* and *aortic stenosis,* may result. Antibiotic therapy has dramatically reduced the incidence of RHD.

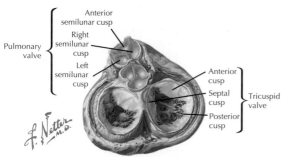

▼ **Heart in diastole (viewed from the base with atria removed)**

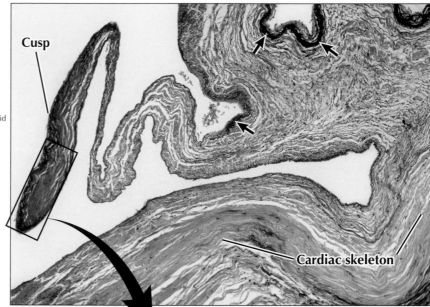

Cusp

Cardiac skeleton

► **LM of part of the aortic (semilunar) valve.** The free edge of the cusp is to the left. The valve core contains mainly collagen fibers (orange-pink). Densely packed collagen that is part of the cardiac skeleton anchors the valve base. A dense network of black elastic fibers (**thick arrows**) lies just under the endothelium at the superior surface of the valve (**top**). 70×. *Verhoeff-van Gieson.*

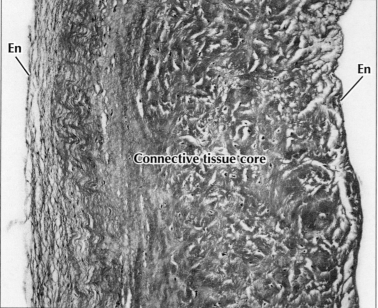

En

En

Connective tissue core

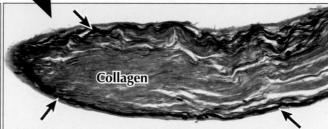

Collagen

▲ **LM of the cusp of the aortic semilunar valve.** A network of elastic fibers (**arrows**) is among densely packed collagen. 240×. *Verhoeff-van Gieson.*

◄ **LM of part of the pulmonary (semilunar) valve.** A core of dense connective tissue, which originates from the annulus fibrosus, forms the bulk of the valve and consists of a tightly packed mixture of collagen and elastic fibers with scattered fibroblasts. Endothelial cells (**En**) cover the valve on both surfaces. The histologic structure of atrioventricular valves closely resembles that of semilunar valves. 100×. *H&E.*

8.4 HISTOLOGY OF HEART VALVES

The four heart valves are attenuated folds of **endocardium** that prevent backflow of blood. Two **atrioventricular (AV) valves** are intake valves for the right and left ventricles. The right AV valve, between right atrium and right ventricle, has three leaflets and is called the **tricuspid valve.** The left AV valve, between left atrium and left ventricle, has two leaflets and is the **bicuspid valve,** or, because it resembles a bishop's miter, the **mitral valve.** The free edges of the AV valves are continuous with thin tendinous cords, the *chordae tendinae,* which attach to papillary muscles associated with ventricles. The two ventricles have outtake valves that guard orifices of the pulmonary artery and aorta: the **pulmonary** and **aortic semilunar valves.** The first, the valve of the right ventricle, is found where the pulmonary artery originates from the right ventricle. The outtake valve of the left ventricle, the aortic valve,

lies where the aorta originates from the left ventricle. Although leaflets of the two semilunar valves are thinner than those of AV valves, all heart valves possess the same basic histologic plan. Each valve leaflet has a central core of **dense fibrous connective tissue,** which is covered externally on both sides by endocardium. In AV valves, the endocardium is thicker on the ventricular side than on the atrial side. The central, avascular connective tissue core of each valve is dominated by a mixture of **collagen** and **elastic fibers** but also contains **fibroblasts** and occasional **smooth muscle cells.** These cells receive nutrients and O_2 from blood in the heart chambers. The heart also has a framework of dense irregular connective tissue—the **cardiac skeleton**—that consists of four *annuli fibrosi,* a *septum membranaceum,* and two *trigona fibrosa.* Annuli fibrosi support heart valves; the other two elements of the cardiac skeleton serve as attachment sites for cardiac muscle.

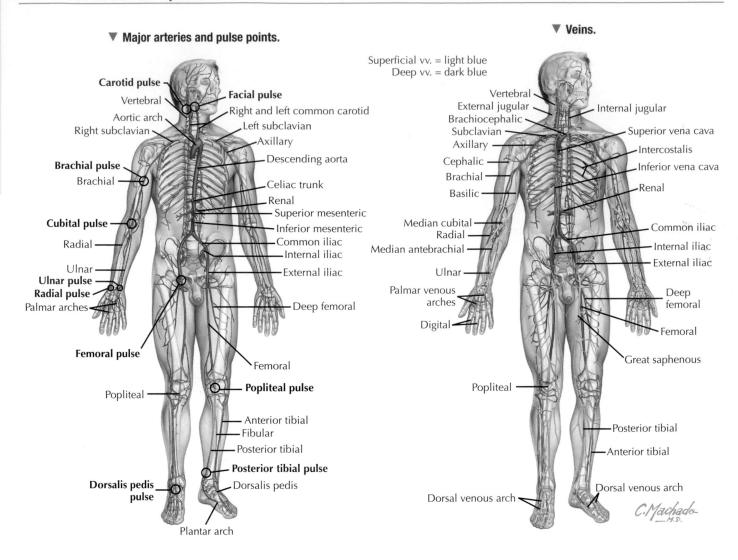

▼ Major arteries and pulse points.

Carotid pulse
Vertebral
Aortic arch
Right subclavian
Facial pulse
Right and left common carotid
Left subclavian
Axillary
Descending aorta
Brachial pulse
Brachial
Celiac trunk
Renal
Superior mesenteric
Cubital pulse
Radial
Inferior mesenteric
Common iliac
Internal iliac
Ulnar
Ulnar pulse
Radial pulse
Palmar arches
External iliac
Deep femoral
Femoral pulse
Femoral
Popliteal pulse
Popliteal
Anterior tibial
Fibular
Posterior tibial
Posterior tibial pulse
Dorsalis pedis pulse
Dorsalis pedis
Plantar arch

▼ Veins.

Superficial vv. = light blue
Deep vv. = dark blue

Vertebral
External jugular
Brachiocephalic
Subclavian
Axillary
Cephalic
Brachial
Basilic
Internal jugular
Superior vena cava
Intercostalis
Inferior vena cava
Renal
Median cubital
Radial
Median antebrachial
Ulnar
Palmar venous arches
Digital
Common iliac
Internal iliac
External iliac
Deep femoral
Femoral
Great saphenous
Popliteal
Posterior tibial
Anterior tibial
Dorsal venous arch
Dorsal venous arch

C. Machado, M.D.

8.5   CLASSIFICATION OF ARTERIES AND VEINS

Arteries are efferent vessels that function in a high-pressure system; **veins** are afferent vessels that function under low pressure. Their histologic organization and tissue composition reflect physiologic conditions under which they operate. Arteries and veins are classified into types that differ mainly in size, microscopic structure, and location; the scheme is arbitrary because gradual histologic changes occur along the length of the vessels. The scheme is useful, however, as these vessels do more than merely transport blood along the circulatory route. Of three types of arteries, *elastic* (*conducting,* or *conduit*) *arteries* are closest to the heart, are the largest, and include the *aorta* and *pulmonary, common carotid, subclavian,* and *common iliac* arteries. With highly elastic walls, they can expand during ventricular contraction (*systole*) and passively recoil during ventricular relaxation (*diastole*) to sustain continuous blood flow despite pulsatile pumping of the heart. *Muscular arteries,* also called *distributing arteries,* regulate blood flow to organs and parts of the body by contraction and relaxation of smooth muscle in their walls. Many bear names such as femoral and brachial arteries. *Arterioles,* the smallest arteries at 100 μm or less in diameter, are small-resistance vessels that mainly regulate systemic blood pressure. Their walls contain one or two layers of circularly arranged smooth muscle. The three

types of veins have thin walls relative to their arterial counterparts and often look collapsed in histologic sections. *Large veins,* such as *superior* and *inferior venae cavae,* are large-capacitance vessels that return blood under low pressure to the heart. *Muscular* (or *medium-sized*) veins commonly travel with muscular arteries. Because of low intraluminal pressure, they often have simple flap-like valves that prevent backflow of blood against gravity as it is returned to the heart. *Venules,* the smallest veins, accompany arterioles and have very thin walls, which are often porous to allow migration of leukocytes from the circulation, especially during an inflammatory response.

CLINICAL POINT

Understanding the histology of the cardiovascular system is functionally and clinically relevant. This system is the first to develop and begin functioning in the embryo, which signifies its importance. By 3 weeks of gestation, a primitive heart is formed and begins pumping blood into new mesenchymally derived blood vessels. Understanding and treatment of cardiovascular disorders also require this histologic knowledge. In North America, more than 50 million people have cardiovascular disease, and more than 2 million people die annually, usually from effects of cell and tissue breakdown in walls of blood vessels or the heart.

▼ **Heart viewed from below and behind.**

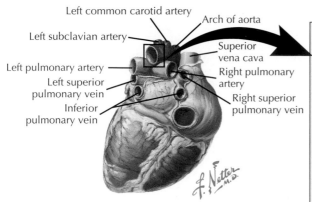

Left common carotid artery
Arch of aorta
Left subclavian artery
Superior vena cava
Left pulmonary artery
Right pulmonary artery
Left superior pulmonary vein
Right superior pulmonary vein
Inferior pulmonary vein

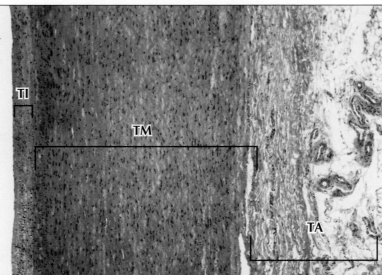

► **LM of part of the aortic wall.** The intima (**TI**) abuts the lumen (left). A thick media (**TM**) and an outer adventitia (**TA**) are also shown. Nuclei in the media at this magnification are mostly those of smooth muscle cells. Elastic laminae are not easily seen with this stain and need special preparative and staining methods for elucidation. 60×. *H&E.*

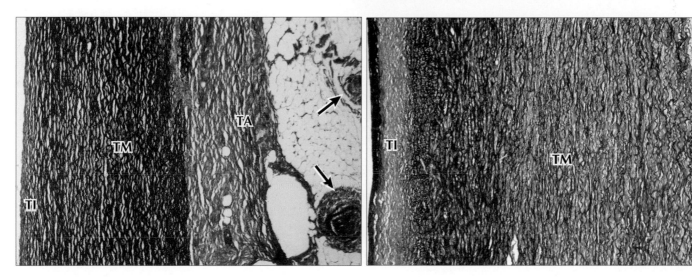

▲ **Comparative LMs of the wall of the aorta of a newborn (Left) and 25-year-old (Right).** In both vessels, a relatively thin tunica intima (**TI**) merges with a prominent tunica media (**TM**). This stain specifically demonstrates elastic tissue, a prominent feature of these arteries. The number of elastic laminae —the dark, wavy bands—increases with age. Vasa vasorum (**arrows**) occupy loose connective tissue of the adventitia (**TA**). 60×. *Gomori aldehyde fuchsin.*

8.6 HISTOLOGY OF ELASTIC ARTERIES

Elastic arteries, with a large lumen relative to wall thickness, conduct blood from the heart to muscular arteries. The **tunica media** in the wall of elastic vessels is the most prominent of three layers. It has abundant **elastic fibers** organized as multiple, concentric, fenestrated **laminae** interspersed with scattered, circularly arranged **smooth muscle cells.** The number and thickness of elastic laminae vary with age: for example, newborn aortas have about 25 concentric laminae, adult aortas, 50-75. Smooth muscle cells in the media synthesize and secrete elastic fibers of the laminae as well as some *collagen* and other elements of extracellular matrix. Collagen confers tensile strength to arterial walls, and elastic fibers impart distensibility, which allows passive recoil under pressure. The **tunica intima,** at up to 20% of wall thickness, is relatively thick, with its luminal surface lined internally by an *endothelium* of flattened cells resting on a **basal lamina.** A deeper, subendothelial layer of **connective tissue** consists mostly of collagen and elastic fibers embedded in ground substance, plus scattered *fibroblasts* and occasional smooth muscle cells. Underneath the intima is a border of an *internal elastic lamina,* which is often difficult to discern as it merges imperceptibly with elastic laminae of the media. The **tunica adventitia** of these arteries consists of loose irregular connective tissue with a predominance of longitudinally oriented collagen fibers and scattered fibroblasts. In most elastic arteries, the adventitia contains small nutritive blood vessels—the **vasa vasorum**—and lymphatic capillaries. This microvasculature extends into the outermost part of the media. The abdominal aorta is an exception; it lacks vasa vasorum, which may explain its susceptibility to *dilation* and *aneurysm* formation.

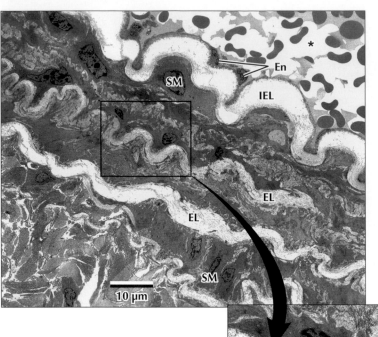

▲ ▼ **Electron micrographs (EMs) of parts of the aortic wall at low (Left) and medium (Below) magnification.** The endothelium (**En**) lining the lumen (⋆) consists of elongated cells, some of which are sectioned at the level of the nuclei. The underlying internal elastic lamina (**IEL**) is thick and electron lucent. The mononucleated smooth muscle cells (**SM**) alternate with multiple, concentric elastic laminae (**EL**) in the media. These muscle cells are branched and touch other muscle cells. The elastic laminae look corrugated because of partial constriction of the vessel at the time of fixation. **Left**: 1100×; **Below**: 4250×.

8.7 ULTRASTRUCTURE OF THE AORTA

The adult aorta has an **intima** that is 100-150 μm thick. *Simple squamous epithelium,* made of one layer of **endothelial cells,** lines the large lumen. In section, these polygonal cells look flattened or rounded, with the one nucleus of each cell protruding slightly into the lumen. The longitudinal axis of each endothelial cell usually parallels the direction of blood flow. Each cell is 15 μm wide and 25-30 μm long. The endothelium rests on an inconspicuous *basal lamina.* The subendothelial layer of *connective tissue* consists of a delicate, interlacing network of *collagen* and *elastic fibers.* This layer also contains small bundles of longitudinally disposed smooth muscle and a few isolated fibroblasts. The **internal elastic lamina** is indistinct because the innermost elastic lamina of the **media** blends with adjacent laminae, without clear distinction between them. The media, 0.5-2 mm thick, contains broad concentric **elastic laminae** that alternate with adjacent, circularly arranged **smooth muscle cells.** Each lamina is 2-3 μm thick and is fenestrated, with a few connecting bundles of elastic fibers in between. The elongated, branched aortic smooth muscle cells are attached to adjoining elastic laminae by types I, II, and IV collagen and are embedded in ground substance rich in chondroitin sulfate. A distinct external elastic lamina is missing. The *adventitia* is loose connective tissue with vasa vasorum, myelinated and unmyelinated nerve fibers, lymphatics, and abundant adipocytes.

CLINICAL POINT

An **aneurysm** is an abnormal localized dilation in the weakened wall of an artery. An aortic aneurysm occurs when the diameter of part of the aorta increases by 50% or more. A true aneurysm is a large bulge in the wall that consists of all three tunics. Rupture may lead to fatal bleeding in only a few minutes. **Atherosclerosis** is a major cause of most aortic aneurysms. Infection, inflammation, syphilis, and the genetic connective tissue disorder Marfan syndrome also weaken arterial walls, and *chronic hypertension* induces susceptibility to aneurysms because elevated arterial pressures place undue stress on vessel walls.

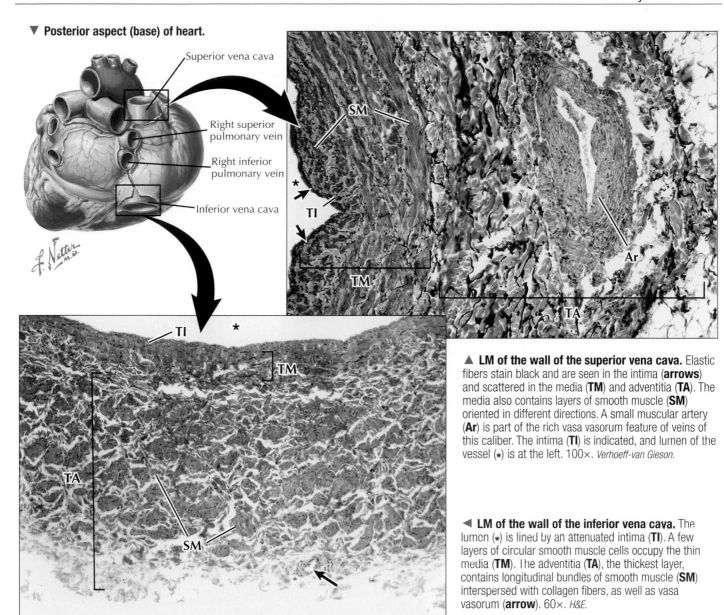

▼ Posterior aspect (base) of heart.

Superior vena cava

Right superior pulmonary vein

Right inferior pulmonary vein

Inferior vena cava

▲ **LM of the wall of the superior vena cava.** Elastic fibers stain black and are seen in the intima (**arrows**) and scattered in the media (**TM**) and adventitia (**TA**). The media also contains layers of smooth muscle (**SM**) oriented in different directions. A small muscular artery (**Ar**) is part of the rich vasa vasorum feature of veins of this caliber. The intima (**TI**) is indicated, and lumen of the vessel (∗) is at the left. 100×. *Verhoeff-van Gieson.*

◄ **LM of the wall of the inferior vena cava.** The lumen (∗) is lined by an attenuated intima (**TI**). A few layers of circular smooth muscle cells occupy the thin media (**TM**). The adventitia (**TA**), the thickest layer, contains longitudinal bundles of smooth muscle (**SM**) interspersed with collagen fibers, as well as vasa vasorum (**arrow**). 60×. *H&E.*

8.8 HISTOLOGY OF LARGE VEINS: THE VENAE CAVAE

The **superior** and **inferior venae cavae** are large veins that deliver deoxygenated blood to the right atrium. Others in this class with similar histologic features are the *portal, pulmonary, azygos, renal, suprarenal, splenic,* and *superior mesenteric veins.* They all have a thin **intima** with one layer of endothelial cells resting on an incomplete basement membrane. Subendothelial connective tissue in these veins contains a network of **elastic fibers** with scattered fibroblasts. The **media** is not well developed, and its content of circularly arranged **smooth muscle** varies greatly according to location; for example, media in uterine veins has several layers of smooth muscle, whereas that in meningeal and retinal veins has no smooth muscle. In contrast, the **adventitia**—the thickest layer in large veins—may contain bundles of longitudinally oriented smooth muscle cells interspersed with collagen and elastic fibers. The abundant **collagen fibers** have either a longitudinal or helical

orientation. At their entrances to the heart, venae cavae and pulmonary veins have a small amount of cardiac muscle in the adventitia. Compared with arterial walls, walls of veins have more extensive **vasa vasorum,** penetrating from the adventitia into deeper regions.

CLINICAL POINT

Varicose veins—abnormally dilated, tortuous veins—result from increased intraluminal pressure or decreased support in vein walls. Most commonly affected veins are superficial ones in the upper and lower parts of the legs. Varicose veins may also develop in the esophagus as a result of *cirrhosis* of the liver or in the hemorrhoidal venous plexus at the rectoanal junction. Such varicose dilations usually occur when valves become weakened and incompetent. Venous congestion, painful ulcerations, edema, and thrombosis may also arise. Varicose vein rupture may cause *hemorrhage.* Another serious complication is *deep vein thrombosis,* which may lead to *pulmonary embolism.*

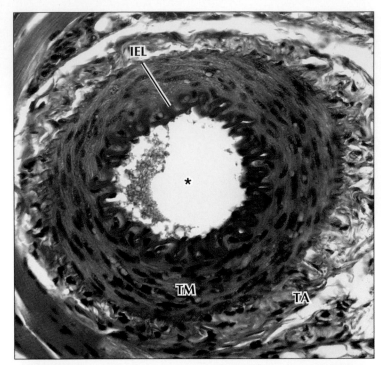

◀ **LM of the wall of a muscular artery.** In this partly constricted artery, the lumen (*) caliber is small relative to the muscular wall thickness. A prominent internal elastic lamina (**IEL**) looks corrugated. Several layers of circular smooth muscle occupy the media (**TM**); loose connective tissue, the adventitia (**TA**). 320×. *H&E.*

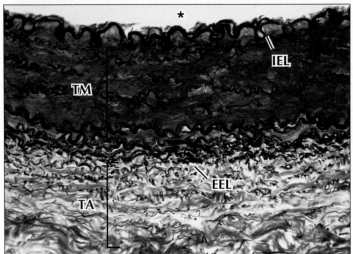
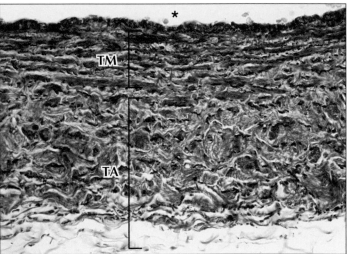

▲ **LMs of the wall of a muscular artery (Left) and muscular vein (Right).** The arterial wall has more elastic fibers (in black), whereas the vein has more collagen (in orange). Smooth muscle in the artery imparts an intense eosinophilia to the media (**TM**). Internal elastic lamina (**IEL**), external elastic lamina (**EEL**), adventitia (**TA**), and lumen (*) are indicated. 320×. *Gomori aldehyde fuchsin.*

8.9 HISTOLOGY OF MUSCULAR ARTERIES AND VEINS

At 0.3-10 mm in diameter, muscular arteries vary greatly in size and can change their size markedly in response to functional demands. They often travel with muscular veins. Walls of both muscular arteries and veins have three tunics, each structurally different according to vessel type. Relative to lumen caliber, these arteries have thick walls. **Smooth muscle** dominates the **tunica media,** which is the thickest layer of the arteries. The number of smooth muscle layers varies with artery size: from 3-4 in small arteries to 20-40 in larger ones. In the media, smooth muscle cells are circularly or helically disposed and communicate with neighboring muscle cells via *gap junctions.* Between smooth muscle layers are variable numbers of **elastic fibers** mixed with **collagen fibers** and occasional fibroblasts. Larger arteries have elastic fibers arranged concentrically in **laminae,** which form a conspicuous

internal elastic lamina at the border with the intima and an **external elastic lamina** at the interface with the adventitia. As muscular arteries become smaller, the number of elastic fibers and layers of smooth muscle gradually decrease. The **tunica adventitia—loose connective tissue** containing helically or longitudinally oriented collagen and elastic fibers—usually blends imperceptibly with surrounding connective tissue. Muscular vein diameters are 1-9 mm. A thin intima is adjacent to a deeper media, which contains small bundles of circularly arranged smooth muscle cells. Walls of veins usually have more collagen, which imparts great tensile strength, than elastic fibers. The adventitia is prominent, with longitudinally oriented smooth muscle interposed with large amounts of collagen. Veins have well-developed *vasa vasorum* in their walls, and many veins have valves, which are folds of intima with a connective tissue core covered on both sides by *endothelium.*

▼ **Sternocostal surface of the heart showing coronary vessels.**

▼ **Structure of the coronary artery.**

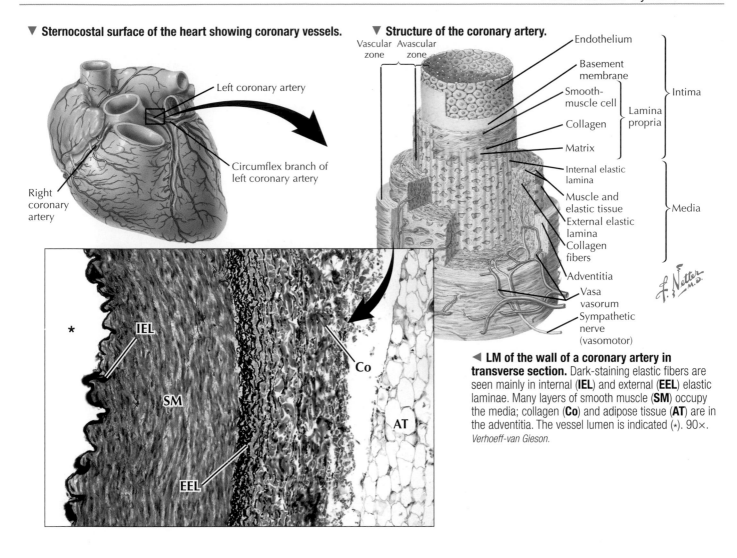

LM of the wall of a coronary artery in transverse section. Dark-staining elastic fibers are seen mainly in internal (**IEL**) and external (**EEL**) elastic laminae. Many layers of smooth muscle (**SM**) occupy the media; collagen (**Co**) and adipose tissue (**AT**) are in the adventitia. The vessel lumen is indicated (∗). 90×. *Verhoeff-van Gieson.*

8.10 STRUCTURE AND FUNCTION OF CORONARY ARTERIES

Coronary arteries supply oxygenated blood to cardiac muscle in the myocardium. These arteries are often involved in *atherosclerosis* and *coronary artery disease,* so knowledge of their normal histology is important. Like other arteries, coronary arteries consist of three concentric tunics with a histologic structure similar to that of other muscular arteries, plus unique features. The adventitia, for example, is quite thick relative to that of other muscular arteries; it consists of loosely packed **collagen, adipose tissue,** and some **elastic fibers.** Bundles of **smooth muscle cells** in the media have exceptionally rich innervation. Because coronary arteries bend repeatedly during systole and diastole, both media and adventitia contain bundles of longitudinally oriented smooth muscle as well as circularly arranged bundles. Coronary arteries are also unique in their high collagen-to-elastic fiber ratio, which reflects high tensile strength and relatively low stretchability. Branching sites of these arteries show normal, periodic thickenings of the intima, called *musculoelastic cushions.* These focal areas may contribute to development of atherosclerosis (via accumulation of *low-density lipoproteins* and rapid lesion formation). From their epicardial location, coronary arteries give rise to arterioles that supply blood to a large network of myocardial capillaries. Collateral connections between arterioles form in response to disease-induced obstruction of a coronary artery. Compared with men, women usually have coronary arteries with smaller diameters, so coronary artery surgery is often more difficult and may contribute to a poorer outcome.

CLINICAL POINT

Atherosclerosis, a form of **arteriosclerosis,** is a thickening and hardening of both muscular and elastic arteries. Involvement of coronary arteries may result in **ischemic heart disease** and life-threatening **myocardial infarction.** High circulating levels of low-density lipoproteins damage arterial endothelium, which usually leads to formation of atherosclerotic *plaques.* These induce inflammation of the intima accompanied by fatty necrotic debris. Blood monocytes migrate across the endothelium to become macrophages, which accumulate lipids. Smooth muscle cells in the media also migrate to affected intimal sites and become cholesterol-laden foam cells. These changes may trigger formation of a *thrombus,* which can obstruct lumina of affected arteries.

▼ **Structure of arterioles.**

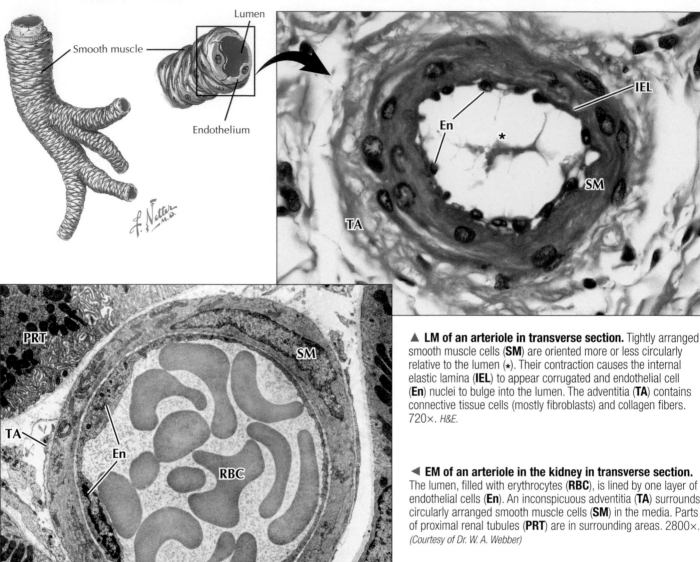

▲ **LM of an arteriole in transverse section.** Tightly arranged smooth muscle cells (**SM**) are oriented more or less circularly relative to the lumen (∗). Their contraction causes the internal elastic lamina (**IEL**) to appear corrugated and endothelial cell (**En**) nuclei to bulge into the lumen. The adventitia (**TA**) contains connective tissue cells (mostly fibroblasts) and collagen fibers. 720×. *H&E.*

◀ **EM of an arteriole in the kidney in transverse section.** The lumen, filled with erythrocytes (**RBC**), is lined by one layer of endothelial cells (**En**). An inconspicuous adventitia (**TA**) surrounds circularly arranged smooth muscle cells (**SM**) in the media. Parts of proximal renal tubules (**PRT**) are in surrounding areas. 2800×. *(Courtesy of Dr. W. A. Webber)*

8.11   STRUCTURE AND FUNCTION OF ARTERIOLES

Arterioles, the smallest arteries, are often seen in tissue sections to travel closely with venules. Arterioles, which branch repeatedly and become smaller, are easily distinguished from larger muscular arteries via diameter—outer diameters of ≤100 μm and inner diameters of about 30 μm—and the number of **smooth muscle cells** in the walls. Arteriole walls are thick relative to the lumen, with the **media,** the most prominent tunic, consisting of one or two layers of closely packed, helically arranged smooth muscle cells. Physiologically, arterioles are *resistance vessels* and can undergo *vasoconstriction* or *vasodilation* in response to neural and nonneural stimuli. Smooth muscle action in the media controls *systemic blood pressure.* The intima, similar to that of other blood vessels, consists of flattened **endothelial cells** resting on a **basal lamina** that is seen only with electron microscopy. Deep to the intima is an **internal elastic lamina,** which is prominent in larger arterioles but either extremely thin or absent in the smallest arterioles; in sections this lamina often looks corrugated, depending on the state of vessel constriction at fixation. Arteriolar adventitia consists mostly of loosely arranged **collagen** and **elastic fibers.** Arterioles receive blood from larger muscular arteries and deliver blood to capillaries. Terminal segments of arterioles, or *metarterioles,* consist of a single layer of smooth muscle and, by vasoconstriction, control the amount of blood entering capillaries.

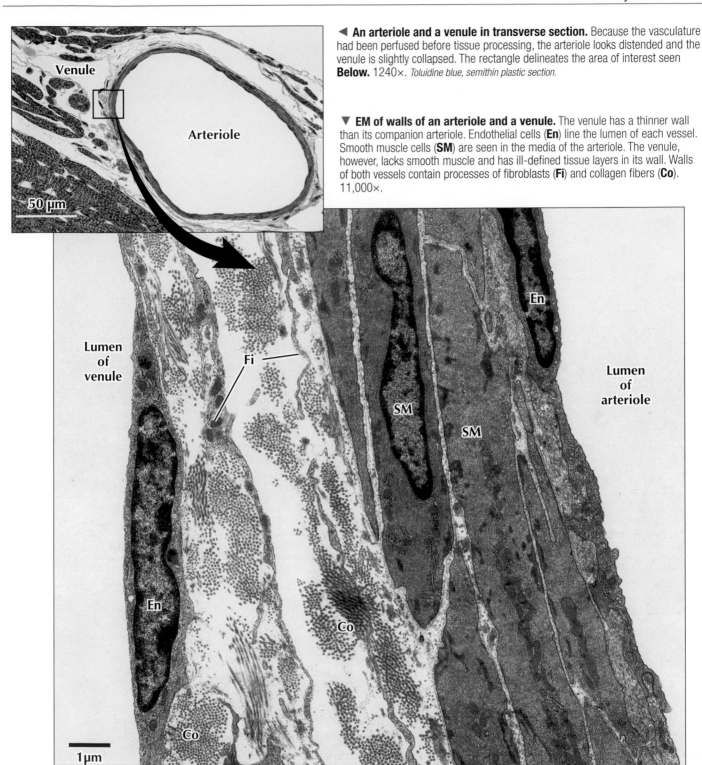

◄ **An arteriole and a venule in transverse section.** Because the vasculature had been perfused before tissue processing, the arteriole looks distended and the venule is slightly collapsed. The rectangle delineates the area of interest seen **Below.** 1240×. *Toluidine blue, semithin plastic section.*

▼ **EM of walls of an arteriole and a venule.** The venule has a thinner wall than its companion arteriole. Endothelial cells (**En**) line the lumen of each vessel. Smooth muscle cells (**SM**) are seen in the media of the arteriole. The venule, however, lacks smooth muscle and has ill-defined tissue layers in its wall. Walls of both vessels contain processes of fibroblasts (**Fi**) and collagen fibers (**Co**). 11,000×.

8.12 ULTRASTRUCTURE AND FUNCTION OF ARTERIOLES AND VENULES

Arterioles and venules travel close together, so views of them in the same section and field of view and with identical fixation conditions permit direct comparisons. Many structural features reflect their different functions. Both vessels are lined by continuous **endothelium,** although that of venules is usually looser than that of arterioles. Venule **walls** are also thinner than walls of companion arterioles. Intraluminal pressure differences often cause venules to appear collapsed in section and with an irregular contour; arterioles usually have circular profiles because of a relatively high elastin content in the walls. **Smooth muscle** distinguishes arterioles. Its coordinated contraction enables blood flow and distribution to be regulated before entering capillaries. The thin venule wall is adapted to functions in fluid exchange and as common sites of transendothelial leukocyte migration, known as *diapedesis.*

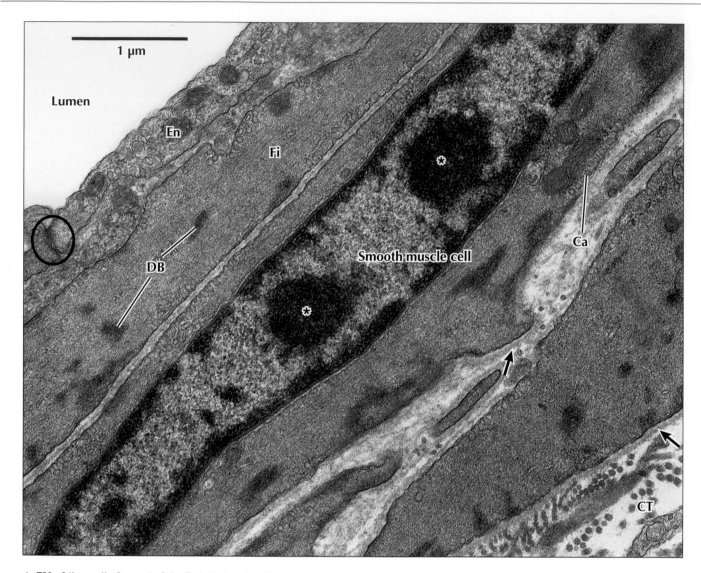

▲ **EM of the wall of an arteriole.** Endothelium (**En**) lines the lumen, and an intercellular junction (**circle**) lies between two endothelial cells. Cytoplasm of several smooth muscle cells, sectioned longitudinally, shows filaments (**Fi**), dense bodies (**DB**), and caveolae (**Ca**). A basal lamina (**arrows**) surrounds each cell. The elongated nucleus of one muscle cell contains two nucleoli (∗). Connective tissue (**CT**) occupies intervening areas. 31,000×.

8.13 ULTRASTRUCTURE AND FUNCTION OF VASCULAR SMOOTH MUSCLE

All blood vessels except true capillaries contain vascular smooth muscle cells, which have two basic functions in vessel walls. By contracting, they regulate the lumen caliber by *vasoconstriction.* As *secretory cells,* they produce large amounts of *elastic tissue* in arterial walls and other connective tissue components of *extracellular matrix,* such as *collagen fibers* and *ground substance.* These cells, usually arranged in helical or circular layers, are linked to adjacent smooth muscle cells by many **gap junctions.** These intercellular specializations are sites of electrical coupling that allow cells to act synchronously, especially during narrowing of the vessel lumen. A **basal lamina** surrounds each muscle cell, and collagen fibrils in extracellular matrix also bind cells together. Smooth muscle cells in walls of muscular arteries and arterioles are small and spindle shaped, but those in walls of elastic arteries have irregular shapes and many branched processes (see Chapter 4). The **nucleus** of each muscle cell is large and centrally placed, with a shape conforming to cell shape; a contracted cell has an irregular, corrugated nucleus, and a relaxed cell has an elongated nucleus. **Thin (actin), thick (myosin),** and **intermediate (desmin** and **vimentin) filaments** dominate the cytoplasm. Actin filaments are in small parallel bundles and are arranged hexagonally; myosin filaments surround actin filament bundles. The actin-to-myosin ratio is usually 12:1. **Dense bodies** that contain the protein α-actinin are either scattered in the cytoplasm or attached to the **sarcolemma.** Thin filaments with opposite polarity insert into dense bodies. Near the cell periphery are scattered profiles of sarcoplasmic reticulum and small invaginations of the sarcolemma, or **caveolae,** that play a role in calcium regulation during contraction. The cytoplasm next to the nucleus contains a Golgi complex, numerous elongated mitochondria, free ribosomes, and profiles of rough endoplasmic reticulum.

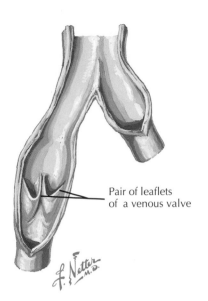

Pair of leaflets
of a venous valve

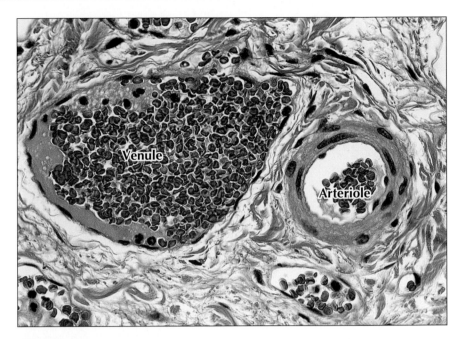

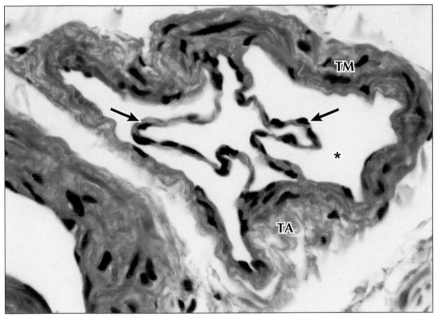

▲ **LM of a venule and arteriole in transverse section.** The venule has a thin wall and a relatively larger lumen than the arteriole. The lumen of each vessel holds many erythrocytes, but the venule lumen also has many white blood cells, a feature often seen in sections of venules. Venules have thin walls and are thus the main site of migration of leukocytes from the bloodstream to tissues. Via contraction, smooth muscle in arterioles regulates pressure in the arterial system. 450×. *H&E.*

◀ **LM of a small vein and its valve in transverse section.** Two leaflets (**arrows**) of the valve project into the lumen (✱). Endothelium covering each leaflet is continuous with that lining the vessel lumen. An indistinct tunica media (**TM**) consists of circularly arranged smooth muscle cells; a prominent adventitia (**TA**) is made of connective tissue. 700×. *H&E.*

8.14   HISTOLOGY AND FUNCTION OF VENULES, VEINS, AND VENOUS VALVES

Venules—the smallest veins that receive blood from converging capillaries—begin as *postcapillary venules,* which are 50-650 μm long with 10- to 50-μm diameters. Attenuated **endothelium** that is 0.2-0.4 μm wide lines these venules. These vessels are preferred sites for exchange of blood cells and tissue exudate from the circulation to surrounding tissues, especially during acute inflammation. A few intercellular junctions link adjacent endothelial cells of venules, but the endothelium, usually resting on a thin basal lamina, is loosely organized and relatively leaky compared with other parts of the vascular system. The smallest postcapillary venule walls have an incomplete layer of pericytes; larger venules and small to medium sized veins have one or two layers of **smooth muscle cells** in the media. Small and medium-sized veins are 1-9 mm in diameter. Walls of these veins have three **tunics,** whose boundaries are less distinct than those of arteries. The **media** of the veins, made of up to three layers of circumferentially oriented smooth muscle cells, is relatively thinner than that of arteries of the same size. The **adventitia,** usually the thickest layer, consists mostly of longitudinally oriented **collagen fibers. Valves** are characteristic of small and medium sized veins, especially those in lower extremities, and are usually found in pairs, or **bicuspid leaflets.** These local infoldings of tunica intima form **semilunar folds** that project into a lumen in the direction of blood flow and prevent backflow of blood as it returns to the heart against the force of gravity. They are often found just distal to where minor venous branches join to form larger veins. A thin endothelium covers each valve externally, which is reinforced internally by a core of **connective tissue**—a mixture of collagen and **elastic fibers.**

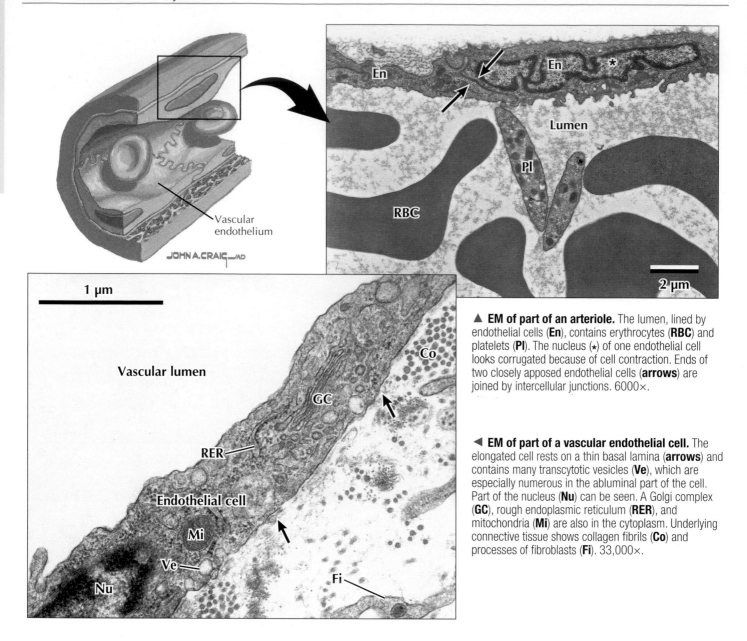

▲ **EM of part of an arteriole.** The lumen, lined by endothelial cells (**En**), contains erythrocytes (**RBC**) and platelets (**Pl**). The nucleus (★) of one endothelial cell looks corrugated because of cell contraction. Ends of two closely apposed endothelial cells (**arrows**) are joined by intercellular junctions. 6000×.

◀ **EM of part of a vascular endothelial cell.** The elongated cell rests on a thin basal lamina (**arrows**) and contains many transcytotic vesicles (**Ve**), which are especially numerous in the abluminal part of the cell. Part of the nucleus (**Nu**) can be seen. A Golgi complex (**GC**), rough endoplasmic reticulum (**RER**), and mitochondria (**Mi**) are also in the cytoplasm. Underlying connective tissue shows collagen fibrils (**Co**) and processes of fibroblasts (**Fi**). 33,000×.

8.15 ULTRASTRUCTURE AND FUNCTION OF THE ENDOTHELIUM

One layer of **simple squamous epithelial cells**—the endothelium—lines the entire cardiovascular system; its total surface area is about 1000 m². Its strategic location between the circulation and surrounding tissues allows a dynamic interface between blood and vessels or the heart wall. The endothelium has active roles in many physiologic processes, including metabolic and secretory functions. The cells are linked by **intercellular junctions,** which allow them to act synchronously and to serve as a selective *permeability barrier.* Cells regulate *hemostasis,* they secrete prostaglandins and release nitric oxide (first called endothelium-derived relaxing factor), and they actively mediate *leukocyte adhesion* and *transmigration.* These mononucleated cells rest on a thin **basal lamina,** which they secrete and which separates them from surrounding tissues. Their attenuated cytoplasm contains a small **Golgi complex,** scattered free **ribosomes,** a few **mitochondria,** and sparse **rough endoplasmic reticulum.** Many membrane-bound **vesicles** and **caveolae,** 70-90 nm in diameter, engage in transendothelial transport of water-soluble molecules. *Weibel-Palade bodies,* unique to endothelial cells, are 3-μm diameter membrane-bound organelles that contain parallel tubular arrays and store von Willebrand protein, a procoagulant secreted by the cells. *Lysosomes* in the cells digest both foreign debris and metabolic products. The cytoskeleton consists of microtubules and a network of actin and intermediate filaments. These organelles provide structural support and a mechanism for changes in cell shape during endothelial contraction. A negatively charged glycocalyx rich in proteoglycans and glycoproteins coats the luminal surface of each cell. Immunocytochemistry showed that endothelial cells are heterogeneous cells that express various antigens. Abnormalities in endothelium may play a role in development of diseases (e.g., *thrombosis* and *atherosclerosis*), so knowledge of its structure and function is important for treatment design.

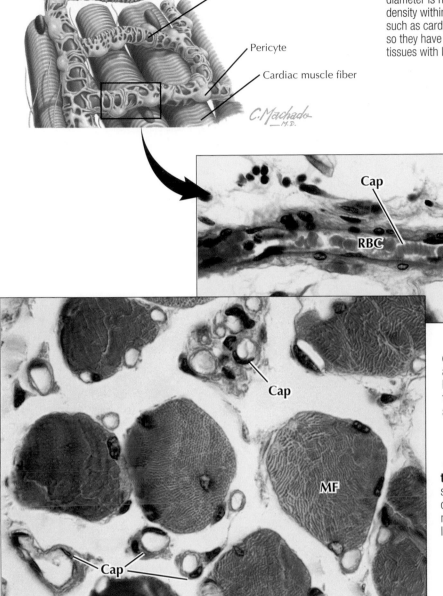

Endothelial cell
Capillary
Pericyte
Cardiac muscle fiber

C. Machado
_M.D._

◀ **Branching network of capillaries in the myocardium.**
Endothelial cells and pericytes form walls of capillaries, whose
diameter is no greater than that of an erythrocyte. Capillary
density within organs and tissues varies with function. Tissues
such as cardiac muscle in the heart have high energy requirements
so they have a dense, highly branched capillary network. Other
tissues with low metabolic activity typically have fewer capillaries.

Cap   CT   En
RBC

▲ **LM of a capillary in longitudinal section.** The
capillary (**Cap**) has a uniform caliber and runs through
adipose connective tissue (**CT**). Endothelial cells (**En**)
have elongated nuclei that align along the long axis of
the capillary. The lumen shows erythrocytes (**RBC**)
stacked in single file. 800×. *H&E.*

Cap
MF
Cap

◀ **LM of capillaries in skeletal muscle in
transverse section.** Some capillaries (**Cap**) are
sectioned through the nucleus of an endothelial cell;
others appear as a thin ring without a nucleus. In skeletal
muscles, capillaries are close to muscle fibers (**MF**) or
lie in intervening connective tissue. 800×. *H&E.*

8.16 STRUCTURE AND FUNCTION OF CAPILLARIES

Abundant anastomoses characterize capillaries—simple tubes
with very thin walls—which constitute more than 90% of all
blood vessels in the body. Their total cross-sectional surface area
is about 800 times that of the aorta, and the rate of blood flow
through them is about 0.4 mm/s versus 320 mm/s in the aorta.
These smallest blood vessels usually have a luminal diameter of
5-10 μm, which is barely large enough for blood cells to squeeze
along them. With *arterioles* and *venules,* they make up the **micro-
circulation,** or **microvascular bed.** They function in exchange of
O_2, CO_2, nutrients, and hormones between the bloodstream and
the tissues. In adults, about 20 L of fluid is exchanged daily across

capillary walls. Each capillary consists of an **endothelium,** an
underlying basal lamina, and a few randomly scattered **pericytes**
covered by a loose network of **collagen** and **reticular fibers.** Pericytes are pale-stained, relatively undifferentiated cells that are
intimately associated with the abluminal aspect of the endothelium. Endothelial cells and pericytes, derived embryonically from
mesenchyme, can still undergo mitosis. Although true capillaries
lack smooth muscle and conform to a basic structural plan, three
types that vary in ultrastructure and permeability exist in the
body: **continuous** (or **tight**), **fenestrated,** and **sinusoidal.** Their
morphologic features are adapted to functional demands of specific organs and tissues.

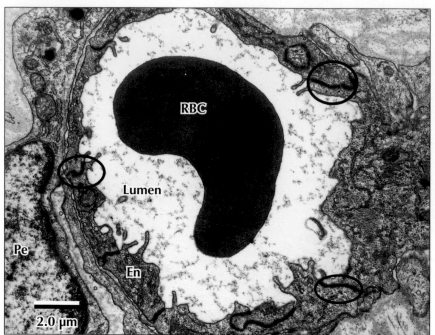

◄ **EM of a tight capillary in the central nervous system.** The lumen contains an erythrocyte (**RBC**); endothelial cells (**En**) form an uninterrupted, complete lining (parts of several cells are seen). Endothelial cells are linked by intercellular junctions, most of which are tight junctions (**circles**) that are linear densities between adjacent cells. A grazing section through one endothelial cell (to the right) reveals abundant, tightly packed organelles in the cytoplasm. A pericyte (**Pe**) surrounds the endothelium on its abluminal aspect and shares the same basal lamina. Unlike endothelial cells, pericytes do not completely encircle the capillary lumen. 6000×.

► **EM of a skeletal muscle tight capillary sectioned transversely.** The vessel has a signet ring appearance. Parts of two endothelial cells line the lumen and are held together by tight junctions (**circles**). One cell is sectioned at the level of its euchromatic nucleus, which has an irregular contour. Cytoplasm of both cells contains abundant organelles, including many spherical transcytotic vesicles (**arrows**). In contrast to more numerous transcytotic vesicles, the less common coated vesicles (**CV**) are usually on the luminal side of the endothelium. The process of a pericyte (**Pe**) adheres to the outer aspect of the endothelium, with which it shares a basal lamina. 12,000×.

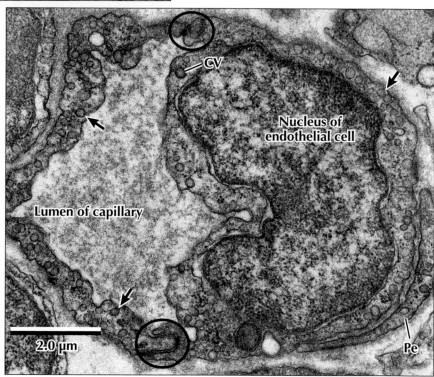

8.17 ULTRASTRUCTURE AND FUNCTION OF TIGHT CAPILLARIES

Tight capillaries, the most common type, are found in all muscle tissues and in areas with a *blood-tissue barrier,* such as the *blood-brain barrier* (central nervous system), *blood-air barrier* (lungs), and *blood-thymus, blood-ocular,* and *blood-testis barriers.* Tight capillaries have uninterrupted **endothelium.** Their reduced permeability restricts indiscriminate passage of material from capillary lumen to surrounding tissues. Many **tight junctions, desmosomes,** and **gap junctions** link endothelial cells in these capillaries. Lipids and lipid-soluble molecules, including gases, diffuse freely across the endothelium, but larger water-soluble molecules are moved across the cells by small spherical **trans-**cytotic vesicles that are either free in the cytoplasm or open to the cell periphery. These 60- to 80-nm diameter vesicles engage in bidirectional *transcytosis* by pinching off from endothelial surface membranes, moving across the cytoplasm, and discharging contents on the opposite surface. Low-density lipoproteins, however, travel across the endothelium in **clathrin-coated pits** and **vesicles** via receptor-mediated endocytosis. An overlying **basal lamina** (20-50 nm thick) encloses the endothelium and surrounds occasional **pericytes,** or *Rouget cells,* and their branching processes. Pericytes are mesenchymally derived pleuripotential stem cells that can give rise to endothelial cells, fibroblasts, or smooth muscle cells in blood vessel walls, depending on the type of vessel, especially in response to injury or stimulation by growth factors.

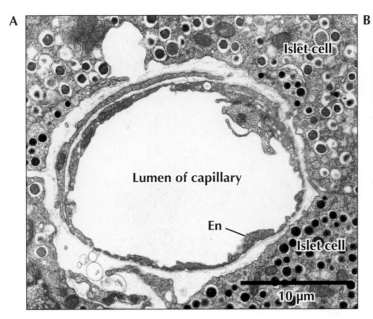

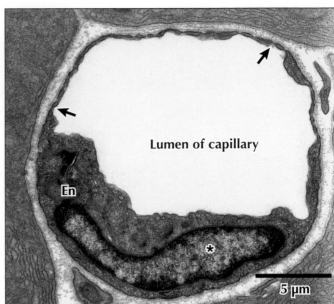

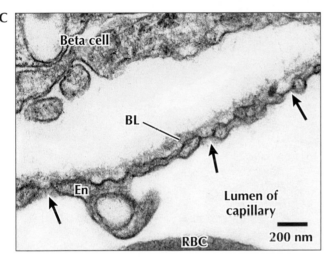

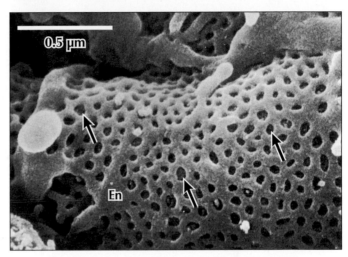

▲ **EMs of fenestrated capillaries in the endocrine pancreas in transverse section.** Thin endothelium (**En**) lines wide capillary lumina. The endothelium of one capillary is close to islet cells (**A**) and an endothelial cell nucleus (*) is in the plane of section of another (**B**). Higher magnification (**C**) better shows endothelium and several fenestrae (**arrows**), each spanned by a thin diaphragm. A surrounding basal lamina (**BL**) and a beta cell are also seen. **A:** 3000×; **B:** 4000×; **C:** 40,000×.

▲ **High-resolution scanning EM of a glomerular capillary in the renal corpuscle.** This surface view of endothelium (**En**), from inside the lumen, shows circular fenestrae (**arrows**). 50,000×. *(Courtesy of Dr. M. J. Hollenberg)*

8.18 ULTRASTRUCTURE AND FUNCTION OF FENESTRATED CAPILLARIES

Fenestrated capillaries are highly permeable, so they occur in areas engaged in fluid transport—mainly in the lamina propria of the intestines, glomeruli of the renal corpuscles, choroid plexus of the brain, choriocapillaris of the eye, and all endocrine organs. Their **endothelial cells** resemble those of tight capillaries (in content of transcytotic vesicles and other cytoplasmic organelles), but the **endothelium** is quite thin, often 0.1 μm or less. Endothelial cells, held together by *tight junctions* and *gap junctions,* usually rest on a thin **basal lamina.** Pericytes are less numerous than in tight capillaries. A unique feature is the presence of minute, circular transcellular openings—**fenestrae**—in endothelial cells. They are 60-80 nm in diameter and perforate the endothelium like round

windows in walls of a building. A thin **diaphragm,** 6-8 nm wide, usually closes each fenestra. Diaphragms have a high net negative charge and contain heparan sulfate-rich proteoglycans. Renal glomerular capillaries lack diaphragms but are surrounded by a thick basal lamina. **Sinusoidal capillaries** are a highly specialized type of capillary with a relatively wide (diameter of 15-20 μm) and irregular lumen. They are found in bone marrow, spleen, liver, adenohypophysis, and adrenal cortex. Ends of their endothelial cells are separated by wide gaps through which fluid, large molecules, and blood cells may pass. At certain sites, such as sinusoids of liver and spleen, phagocytes project into the lumen and are closely associated with sinusoidal endothelial cells. A basal lamina is either absent or incomplete.

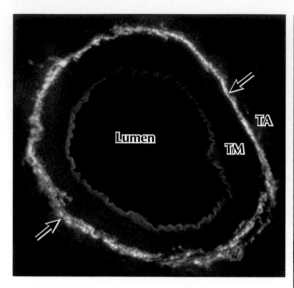

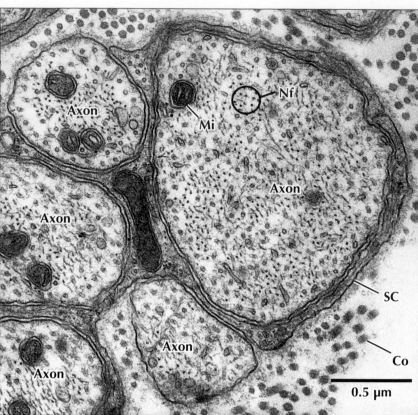

▲ **LM of a muscular artery treated histochemically to demonstrate innervation.** Unmyelinated axons of adrenergic nerves (**arrows**) are at the border between the adventitia (**TA**) and media (**TM**). Although not normally visible in H&E-stained sections, axons can be seen via fluorescence microscopy after norepinephrine in storage vesicles is converted to a fluorescent isoquinoline. 300×. *Glyoxylic acid. (Courtesy of Dr. V. Palaty)*

▲ **EM of conducting segments of unmyelinated axons in the adventitia of an artery.** Axons (in transverse section) are completely or partly enclosed by projections of a non-myelinating Schwann cell (**SC**). Axons contain a few mitochondria (**Mi**) and many neurofilaments (**Nf**) and microtubules. Collagen fibrils (**Co**) are in surrounding areas. 42,000×.

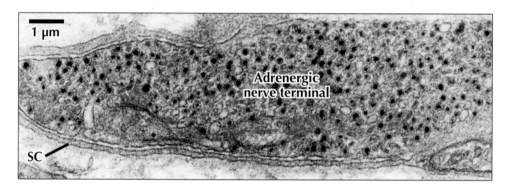

▲ **EM of an adrenergic nerve terminal at the border between adventitia and media.** At this site of neurotransmitter release, norepinephrine in small membrane-bound storage vesicles was converted to an electron-dense precipitate by a chromaffin reaction. The thin process of a non-myelinating Schwann cell (**SC**) partly covers the nerve terminal, but not at the upper surface of the axon (at the top), which faces the media. This design facilitates release of neurotransmitters, which can diffuse toward smooth muscle in the media. 9000×. *(Courtesy of Dr. V. Palaty)*

8.19　INNERVATION OF BLOOD VESSELS

Blood vessels have a rich supply of **nerves,** most of which are vasomotor, keep vessels partly constricted, and control lumen calibers. These nerves, derived from the *sympathetic autonomic nervous system,* are primarily **unmyelinated adrenergic nerve fibers** originating from postganglionic sympathetic ganglia. They form a plexus in the **adventitia** and end in the outer parts of the **media,** close to **smooth muscle cells.** The **nerve terminals** are small knob-like endings that are best seen by techniques using silver staining, fluorescence histochemistry, immunocytochemistry, or electron microscopy. These nerve terminals have spherical, membrane-bound **storage vesicles** containing the **neurotrans**mitter **norepinephrine.** Neurotransmitter released from nerve terminals diffuses to the surface of a smooth muscle cell to activate receptor sites on the sarcolemma and mediate contraction. Gap junctions linking smooth muscle cells permit contraction stimuli to reach other cells and to elicit vessel wall constriction. Distribution of *cholinergic nerves* from the *parasympathetic nervous system* is less common. When present, these nerves use the neurotransmitter *acetylcholine,* which causes mainly smooth muscle relaxation and vasodilation. *Myelinated nerve fibers,* which are sensory, also supply adventitia of blood vessels. They end freely as unmyelinated sensory nerve terminals.

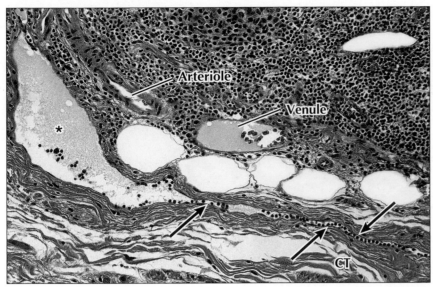

◀ **LM of a lymphatic capillary in longitudinal section.** This narrow, thin-walled vessel (**arrows**) has a uniform caliber, and its lumen contains a row of lymphocytes. It courses through connective tissue (**CT**), gradually increases in size, and drains into a larger lymphatic channel (✱), which has an irregular contour and a lumen filled with flocculent precipitate and scattered lymphocytes. An arteriole and venule are close to the lymphatic channel. Smooth muscle cells make up the arteriole wall; erythrocytes are in the lumen of the venule. 280×. *H&E.*

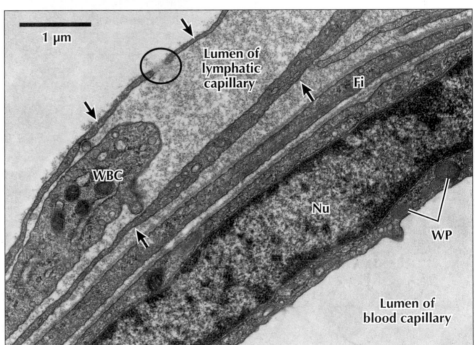

▶ **EM contrasting endothelium of lymphatic and blood capillaries.** Note the proximity of the two vessels. The highly attenuated endothelium of the lymphatic (**arrows**) encloses its lumen, which holds a white blood cell (**WBC**). A wide intercellular gap (**circle**) separates ends of two endothelial cells of the lymphatic. The cells have many vesicles and filaments. The thicker endothelium of the blood capillary is sectioned at the level of a nucleus (**Nu**). The cytoplasm contains Weibel-Palade bodies (**WP**), which are unique to those cells, are close to the surface, and face the lumen. The process of a fibroblast (**Fi**) is in interstitial connective tissue between the two vessels. 19,000×. *(Courtesy of Dr. A. W. Vogl)*

8.20 ULTRASTRUCTURE AND FUNCTION OF LYMPHATIC CAPILLARIES

Lymphatic capillaries, which begin as blind-ended dilations (10-50 µm wide), are delicate anastomosing channels that constitute a drainage system. They often lie close to **blood capillaries.** They absorb *lymph,* which is a protein-rich exudate of blood, as well as electrolytes and water, from blood capillaries, with lymph being moved mainly by contraction of surrounding skeletal muscles. This fluid normally fills extracellular **connective tissue** spaces, and some is reabsorbed back into the venous end of blood capillaries. Lymphatic capillaries continually take up excess fluid, plus wandering **lymphocytes** and other cells, and eventually add them back to the systemic circulation. They thus play a role in *homeostasis* by regulating interstitial fluid pressure and maintaining plasma volume. Each day, lymphatics return about 40% of total plasma protein to veins and permit entry of chylomicrons and immuno-globulins into circulation. Lymphatics also remove foreign substances from tissues and aid in clearance of debris after tissue injury. They consist of one layer of flat **endothelial cells,** which are thinner and slightly larger than those of blood capillaries, but no pericytes. **Gaps** between endothelial cells may approach 10 µm. An absent or incomplete basal lamina facilitates permeability of these vessels to large molecules and cells. The endothelium features transcytotic vesicles, which engage in transport, and actin filaments, which are contractile. Lymphatic capillaries coalesce into larger vessels that resemble veins and transport lymph via large **lymphatic channels** and ducts to the venous circulation. Like veins, lymphatic channels have three concentric tunics, although they are not as clearly delineated as they are in veins of similar size. They also have valves, which are often more numerous than valves in veins.

9

LYMPHOID SYSTEM

▼ **Organization of lymphatic system.**

▼ **Gut-associated lymphoid tissue in the intestine.**

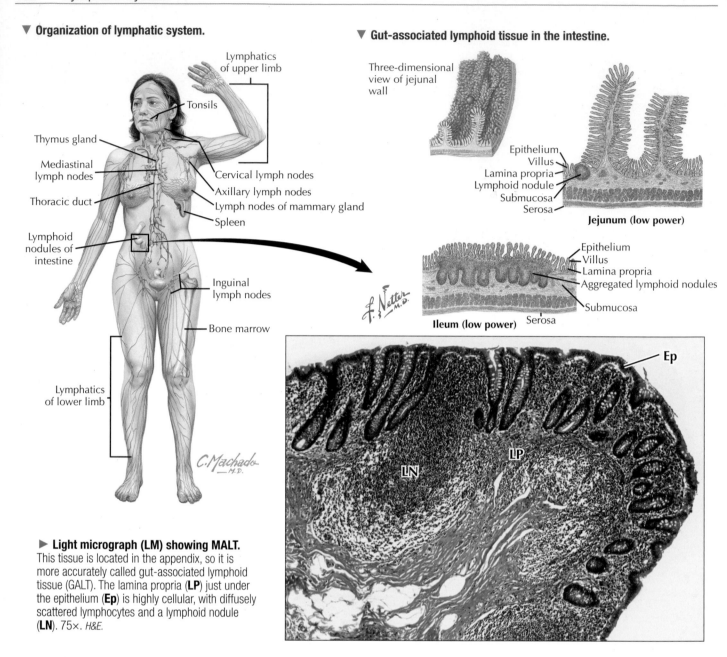

Lymphatics of upper limb

Tonsils

Thymus gland

Mediastinal lymph nodes

Thoracic duct

Lymphoid nodules of intestine

Cervical lymph nodes

Axillary lymph nodes

Lymph nodes of mammary gland

Spleen

Inguinal lymph nodes

Bone marrow

Lymphatics of lower limb

Three-dimensional view of jejunal wall

Epithelium
Villus
Lamina propria
Lymphoid nodule
Submucosa
Serosa

Jejunum (low power)

Epithelium
Villus
Lamina propria
Aggregated lymphoid nodules
Submucosa
Serosa

Ileum (low power)

Ep

LN

LP

▶ **Light micrograph (LM) showing MALT.**
This tissue is located in the appendix, so it is more accurately called gut-associated lymphoid tissue (GALT). The lamina propria (**LP**) just under the epithelium (**Ep**) is highly cellular, with diffusely scattered lymphocytes and a lymphoid nodule (**LN**). 75×. *H&E.*

9.1 OVERVIEW

The extensive **lymphoid**—or **immune**—**system** protects the body against potentially harmful effects of pathogens, foreign substances, infectious agents (bacteria and viruses), and abnormal cells. Its major functions are thus to serve as a source of immunocompetent cells that can react with and neutralize antigens and to distinguish self from nonself. The system comprises **lymphoid tissues** and **organs** whose main constituents are aggregates of **lymphocytes** and other cells of the mononuclear phagocyte system. These cells are enmeshed in a supportive framework (stroma) of reticular cells and fibers, so lymphoid tissue is classified as a specialized *reticular connective tissue*. **Lymphatic vessels** are also part of the system. Components of the system have different arrangements: diffuse subepithelial lymphocyte aggregates are the most ubiquitous and occur throughout gastrointestinal, respiratory, and genitourinary tracts as **mucosa-associated lymphoid tissue (MALT)**. More densely packed, spherical clusters of lymphocytes called **lymphoid nodules** (or **follicles**) may also be found in these and other sites. The nodules may appear as single collections of lymphocytes or as more permanent, multiple aggregates, such as *tonsils* and *Peyer's patches*. Discrete lymphoid organs may be encapsulated (*lymph nodes, thymus,* and *spleen*) or unencapsulated (*bone marrow*). Lymphoid organs are classified in functional terms as primary or secondary. *Primary lymphoid organs*—major sites of lymphocyte production and maturation—include bone marrow, where B lymphocytes are produced, and thymus, where T lymphocytes mature. B cells mediate humoral immunity by giving rise to plasma cells, which synthesize antibodies (or immunoglobulins) that inactivate foreign antigens. T cells, in contrast, mediate cellular immunity against microorganisms. Immune responses occur in *secondary lymphoid organs,* such as lymph nodes and spleen. All lymphoid tissue derives embryonically from mesoderm, except for the thymus, which arises from mesoderm and endoderm.

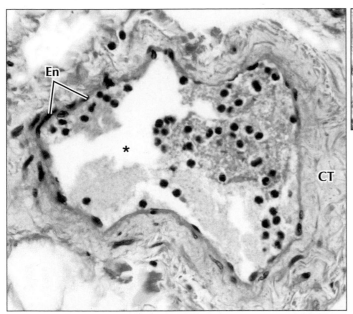

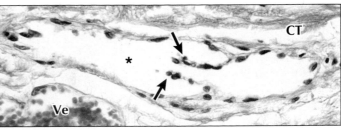

▲ **LM of a small lymphatic capillary in connective tissue (CT).** Its lumen (✶) appears empty. A valve (**arrows**) facilitates movement of lymph in one direction by preventing backflow. Part of a small systemic venule (**Ve**) filled with erythrocytes is seen. 376×. *H&E.*

◀ **LM of a lymphatic capillary in transverse section.** An attenuated wall lined by endothelium (**En**) typifies this vessel. The lumen (✶) contains nucleated blood cells, mostly lymphocytes, and a flocculent precipitate, which corresponds to the lightly eosinophilic protein of lymph. Connective tissue (**CT**) invests the outer aspect of the vessel. 350×. *H&E.*

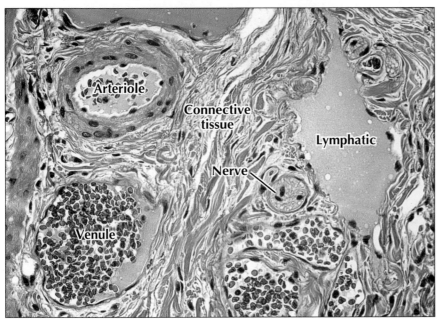

◀ **LM of an arteriole, venule, and lymphatic in transverse section.** These vessels, which travel together in connective tissue, can be compared. The arteriole has the thickest wall with two layers of smooth muscle in its media. The venule has a thinner wall and relatively larger lumen, which is filled with erythrocytes. The lymphatic channel has a very attenuated wall, which is lined by endothelium. The lumen, filled with flocculent precipitate, is irregular and almost collapsed. A small nerve fascicle is next to the lymphatic. 320×. *H&E.*

9.2 HISTOLOGY AND FUNCTION OF LYMPHATIC VESSELS

Cells of the lymphoid system are found in connective tissues throughout the body and can travel in the bloodstream or in **lymphatic vessels**—the lymph—draining part of the circulatory system. Because lymphatic vessels are hard to see in conventional tissue sections, they are probably the least appreciated body structures histologically. By light microscopy, they are similar to capillaries and veins. Lymphatic vessels have wide distribution in many, but not all, body regions. Originating as blind-ended channels in connective tissue spaces, they are then thin-walled **lymphatic capillaries** (100 μm in diameter) that anastomose and become larger. Lymphatic capillaries look similar to blood capillaries except that they lack a basal lamina. Small anchoring fila-

ments connect **endothelial cells** to adjacent collagen fibers and help prevent vessel collapse. Lymphatic capillaries are most abundant in connective tissue of the skin (dermis); beneath mucous membranes of the respiratory, gastrointestinal, and genitourinary tracts; and in connective tissue spaces of the liver. These vessels absorb **interstitial fluid,** which fills the extracellular connective tissue matrix. This fluid and **wandering lymphocytes** are taken up and added back to the circulation. Like veins, lymphatic vessels have **valves** and thin **walls;** contraction of surrounding skeletal muscles causes lymph to move. Lymphatic vessels combine to form the thoracic duct. The large lymphatic ducts drain into the subclavian veins, right at the angle junction where the jugular vein and subclavian vein join together.

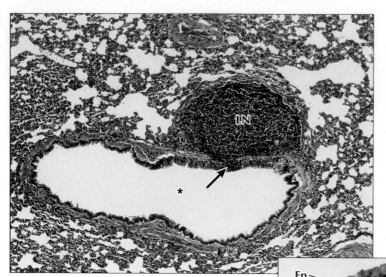

◄ **LM of the lung showing BALT.** A bronchiole (∗) has a prominent lymphoid nodule (**LN**) in its wall. This primary nodule lacks a germinal center but contains a densely packed, spherical cluster of lymphocytes. Some lymphocytes (**arrows**) seem to be infiltrating the bronchiole epithelium. 70×. *H&E.*

► **LM of the mucosa of the appendix showing GALT.** Diffuse infiltration of lymphocytes characterizes the lamina propria (**LP**) just under the epithelium (**Ep**). Lymphocytes usually migrate from the lamina propria and cross the epithelium on their way to the lumen. Small round nuclei of these lymphocytes (**arrows**) are seen in the epithelium. 250×. *H&E.*

9.3   HISTOLOGY AND FUNCTION OF MUCOSA-ASSOCIATED LYMPHOID TISSUE

Mucous membranes of the gastrointestinal, respiratory, and genitourinary tracts are open to the external environment, so they harbor the body's largest, most diverse populations of microorganisms and pathogens. Extensive mucosal surfaces lead to vulnerability to infection. The diffuse lymphoid tissue common in the connective tissue—**lamina propria**—of these membranes is known as **MALT**. MALT may be subdivided, on the basis of location, into **gut-associated (GALT)**, **bronchus-associated (BALT)**, **nose-associated (NALT)**, and **vulvovaginal-associated (VALT) lymphoid tissue.** GALT includes tonsils, Peyer's patches, appendix, and less organized lymphocyte infiltrations scattered along the gastrointestinal tract. MALT is characterized by lymphocyte infiltrations, which are not sharply delineated from surrounding connective tissue but are supported by a loose framework of reticular fibers. Lymphocytes in these areas may also form **lymphoid nodules** (or **follicles**), which are dense aggregations of lymphocytes arranged as spherical, unencapsulated clusters. There are two types, primary and secondary: a **primary nodule** contains small, immature B lymphocytes. In response to antigen exposure, primary nodules become *secondary nodules,* which contain pale-stained *germinal centers.* They are sites of extensive B lymphocyte proliferation and differentiation into *plasma cells* for antibody

production. The major antibody (or immunoglobulin) formed in MALT is *secretory IgA,* which, after being produced by plasma cells, is actively transported via mucosal epithelial cells to the mucosal lumen. Although MALT contains both B and T cells, B cells predominate in nodules and T cells are abundant in adjacent areas. Also, specialized epithelial cells called *M cells* are abundant in the dome epithelium of Peyer's patches. They take up small particles, such as bacteria and viruses, which are then engulfed by submucosal macrophages that process material and present it to B and T cells.

CLINICAL POINT

Infectious diseases caused by various microorganisms—bacteria, viruses, fungi, and parasites—develop when defense mechanisms of the host immune system cannot combat continual exposure to the pathogens. *Rubella,* commonly called *German measles,* is a contagious illness caused by *rubella virus;* its hallmark is an erythematous *maculopapular rash* plus fever and swollen lymph nodes. The portal of entry for the virus is the upper respiratory tract (NALT) through lymphoid tissue, where it reproduces intracellularly in a susceptible host. Rubella occurs mainly in children and young adults; in pregnant women it poses a serious risk to a fetus. A vaccine has greatly reduced the incidence of the disease.

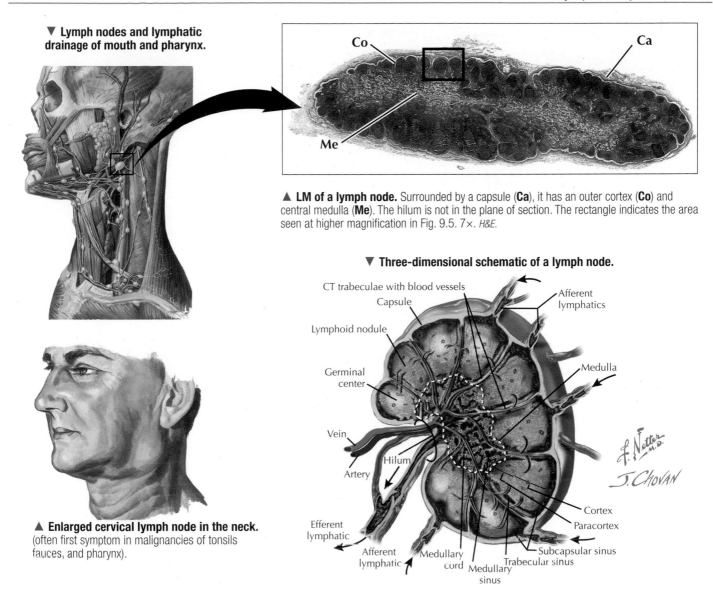

▼ **Lymph nodes and lymphatic drainage of mouth and pharynx.**

Co ── ── Ca

Me

▲ **LM of a lymph node.** Surrounded by a capsule (**Ca**), it has an outer cortex (**Co**) and central medulla (**Me**). The hilum is not in the plane of section. The rectangle indicates the area seen at higher magnification in Fig. 9.5. 7×. *H&E.*

▼ **Three-dimensional schematic of a lymph node.**

CT trabeculae with blood vessels
Capsule
Lymphoid nodule
Germinal center
Vein
Artery
Hilum
Efferent lymphatic
Afferent lymphatic
Medullary cord
Medullary sinus
Trabecular sinus
Subcapsular sinus
Paracortex
Cortex
Medulla
Afferent lymphatics

f. Netter M.D.
J. CHOVAN

▲ **Enlarged cervical lymph node in the neck.** (often first symptom in malignancies of tonsils fauces, and pharynx).

9.4 STRUCTURE AND FUNCTION OF LYMPH NODES

Lymph nodes are bean- or kidney-shaped lymphoid organs, 2-20 mm in diameter; 500-600 nodes are found in the body. They are seen along **lymphatic vessels,** and **lymph** percolates through them. They occur, often as chains or groups, in strategic regions such as the neck, groin, mesenteries, axillae, and abdomen. Lymph nodes derive originally from mesenchyme. During development, specific regions of each node are seeded with **B lymphocytes** from the bone marrow and **T lymphocytes** from the thymus. Main functions of lymph nodes are filtration of lymph before its return to the thoracic duct; production of lymphocytes that are added to lymph; synthesis of antibodies (mainly IgG); and recirculation of lymphocytes by their selective reentry from blood to lymph across walls of specialized efferent lymphatics. An outer **capsule** of dense fibrous connective tissue that typically merges with surrounding tissues and fat invests each node. It sends delicate, radiating partitions called **trabeculae** into the interior of the nodes. These beam-like structures of collagen fibers provide support and serve as

conduits for blood vessels supplying the nodes. Between trabeculae is an internal stroma of *reticular fibers* organized three-dimensionally in which mainly lymphocytes are suspended. Specialized fibroblast-like cells *(reticular cells),* fixed macrophages, and *dendritic (antigen-presenting) cells* are also associated with the reticular fiber network.

CLINICAL POINT

Lymph nodes can undergo hypertrophy and histologic change in response to many clinical conditions. Abnormal enlargement of lymph nodes, or **lymphadenopathy,** may be due to increased numbers of lymphocytes and macrophages in the node during antigenic stimulation in a bacterial or viral infection. It may also be caused by *metastasis,* whereby neoplastic cells spread from a local site of development to distant locations. Such cells are often carried by lymphatics to the nearest lymph node. Surgical biopsy and microscopic examination of a lymph node are used for diagnosis and staging of many malignancies and may provide useful prognostic information.

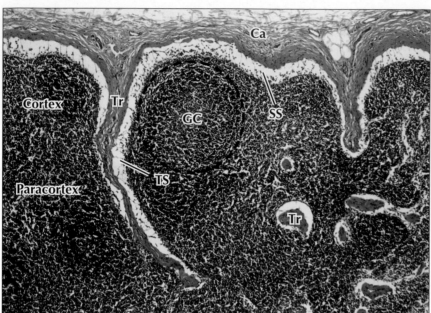

◀ **LM of the outer part of a lymph node.** A fibrous connective tissue capsule (**Ca**) sends in trabeculae (**Tr**) that extend deeply into the node. A prominent subcapsular sinus (**SS**) is continuous with trabecular sinuses (**TS**). The outer cortex consists mostly of B lymphocytes. Deeper parts of the cortex—the paracortex—contain mostly T lymphocytes. A lymphoid nodule (**broken line**) in the cortex contains a germinal center (**GC**). 60×. *H&E.*

▶ **Higher magnification LM of part of a lymph node cortex.** Collagen fibers of the capsule (**Ca**) and trabecula (**Tr**) are seen clearly. A broad subcapsular sinus (**SS**) drains lymph into smaller trabecular sinuses (**arrows**). Aside from lymph and lymphocytes, sinuses contain reticular fibers and macrophages, which cannot be seen at this magnification. The lymphoid nodule has a peripheral rim of closely packed lymphocytes around a pale central zone—a germinal center (**GC**)—that contains mainly activated B lymphocytes. 180×. *H&E.*

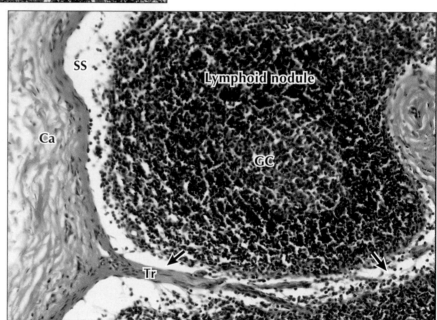

9.5 HISTOLOGY OF LYMPH NODES: CORTEX AND PARACORTEX

Lymph nodes contain aggregates of **lymphocytes** organized into an outer cortex, a paracortex, and an inner medulla. The darkly stained cortex just under the capsule consists of **lymphoid nodules.** In highly characteristic positions in the node, **B cells** occupy lymphoid nodules in the cortex, and **T cells** are in the paracortex, or thymus-dependent region. B cells in the nodules are those that originated from bone marrow (equal to the bursa of Fabricius in chickens). The cortex has two types of nodules. *Primary nodules* are spherical aggregates of tightly packed B cells in a meshwork of reticular fibers. After antigenic stimulation, primary nodules develop into *secondary nodules,* which have a **germinal center** surrounded by a *mantle zone.* Germinal centers are major sites of B cell proliferation and contain small and large lymphocytes, *lym-*

phoblasts, and *follicular dendritic cells.* The surrounding mantle zone contains small lymphocytes. Antigen-dependent T cell differentiation and proliferation occur in the paracortex, beneath and between nodules.

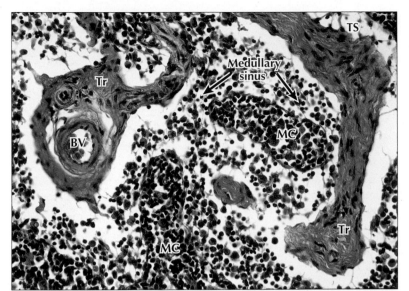

◄ ▼ **LMs of the medulla of a lymph node at medium (Left) and high (Below) magnifications.**
Trabeculae (**Tr**) of dense irregular connective tissue contain fibroblasts, collagen fibers, and blood vessels (**BV**). Parts of two medullary cords (**MC**) are in view (**A**). The term *cord* is a misnomer: when viewed under the microscope, each medullary cord looks more like an irregular sheet of various cells, the most abundant being lymphocytes, plasma cells (**PC**), and macrophages (**Ma**). Medullary sinuses, through which lymph percolates, are continuations of trabecular sinuses (**TS**). Lying between medullary cords, they form a labyrinth of fluid-filled channels lined by a discontinuous layer of endothelial cells and macrophages. They drain into larger efferent lymphatics that leave at the hilum. The sinuses contain a three-dimensional cobweb-like network of reticular fibers and reticular cells that bridge the lumen.
Left: 250×; **Below:** 400×. *H&E.*

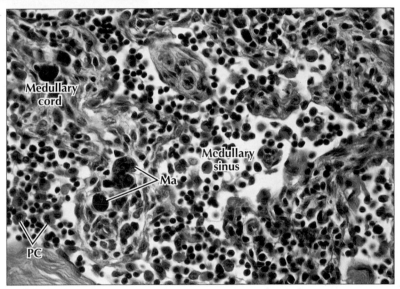

9.6 HISTOLOGY OF LYMPH NODES: MEDULLA AND SINUSES

The lymph node medulla is a pale-staining area that varies in width and abuts the *hilum,* or concave surface, of the node. It contains irregular strands of loosely arranged lymphoid tissue, the **medullary cords,** which consist mainly of **lymphocytes, macrophages,** and **plasma cells.** These highly branched cords anastomose freely and lie near lymph-filled **medullary sinuses** to facilitate immunoglobulin secretion into the sinuses. Irregularly arranged **trabeculae** also occupy the medulla. Lymph enters the node via afferent lymphatics that pierce the capsule on its convex surface. These vessels contain *valves* that control the direction of lymph flow into the node; valves in efferent lymphatics force lymph to flow out. Lymph circulating in the node slowly diffuses through a series of spaces or sinuses. Lymph is first delivered to a narrow channel just under the capsule—the **subcapsular (or marginal) sinus.** Lymph then moves into **trabecular sinuses** that accompany trabeculae. These sinuses converge into larger, more tortuous medullary sinuses that become continuous with efferent lymphatics, which leave the node at the hilum, where **blood vessels** supplying the node also enter and leave it. The lymph node is the only lymphoid structure that has both *afferent* and *efferent lymphatics.* An attenuated, discontinuous layer of endothelial cells lines the sinuses. The sinuses contain, in addition to lymph and lymphocytes, a crisscrossing network of reticular fibers interspersed with reticular cells. Macrophages in the cords project pseudopods between endothelial cells lining the sinuses and phagocytose antigens and foreign material, thus filtering lymph.

CLINICAL POINT
Graft-versus-host disease (GVHD) may occur after allogeneic bone marrow transplantation. It is caused by a mismatch of histocompatibility antigens of donor and recipient. GVHD develops when graft immunocompetent T cells see epithelial target tissue of the host as foreign. An induced inflammatory response is followed by apoptosis of target tissue. Hepatitis, dermatitis, and enteritis (intestinal bleeding and diarrhea) are common. *Immunosuppressive treatments* with corticosteroids and cyclosporine lower the incidence of GVHD. Using the *umbilical cord* as a source of donor cells reduces the risk of developing GVHD.

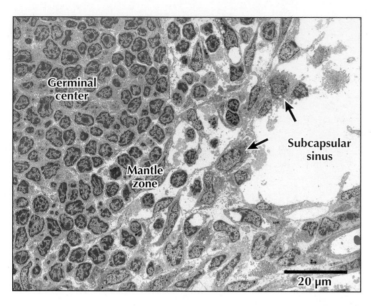

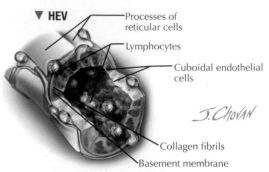

▲ **HEV**
Processes of reticular cells
Lymphocytes
Cuboidal endothelial cells
Collagen fibrils
Basement membrane

J. Chovan

◄ **Low-magnification EM of part of a lymphoid nodule in the cortex of a lymph node.** A mantle zone of small lymphocytes surrounds a more central germinal center. A few macrophages (**arrows**) are in the subcapsular sinus to the right. 800×.

▼ **EM showing key features of a high endothelial venule in the paracortex of a lymph node.** Erythrocytes (**RBC**) are in the vessel lumen. The endothelium is made of cuboidal cells (**En**) with rounded, euchromatic nuclei. Several small lymphocytes (**Ly**) are in the wall and next to the vessel. A plasma cell (**PC**) is also seen. 3000×.

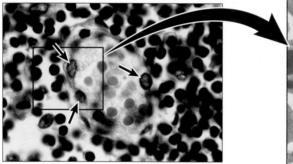

▲ **LM of a high endothelial venule in the paracortex of a lymph node**. Plump nuclei (**arrows**) of endothelial cells bulge into the lumen of this thin-walled vessel. Dark-staining nuclei of lymphocytes are next to the venule. 535×. *H&E.*

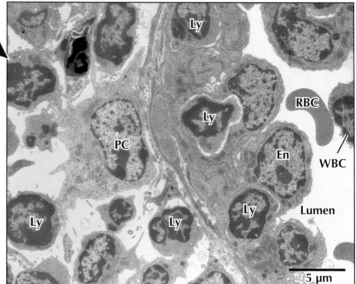

9.7   STRUCTURE AND FUNCTION OF HIGH ENDOTHELIAL VENULES

Continuous **lymphocyte** circulation between the bloodstream and lymph occurs by way of **lymph nodes** and other secondary lymphoid organs including tonsils, Peyer's patches, and spleen. Circulating B and T cells enter lymph nodes via incoming arteries. Lymphocytes are intrinsically mobile, so they can leave the bloodstream by preferential migration across walls of specialized blood vessels called high endothelial venules (HEVs). These thin-walled vessels, with diameters of 30-50 µm, are in the **paracortex** of a lymph node. They are specialized for passage, by selective *diapedesis,* of B and T cells from the blood into perivascular areas. **Endothelial cells** in HEVs have *cell adhesion molecules* that facilitate highly specific transmigration of T and B cells. These cells squeeze between adjacent HEV endothelial cells and penetrate the basement membrane. After gaining access to surrounding lym-

phoid parenchyma, T cells usually stay in the paracortex, but B cells migrate to **lymphoid nodules.** Lymphocytes can leave the lymph node by entering efferent lymphatics to travel in lymph; eventually they reenter the systemic circulation. HEVs have a unique morphology: cuboidal endothelial cells, a prominent perivascular sheath, and a thick basal lamina. Movement of B and T cells across HEVs into lymph nodes and other sites is called *homing.* It is determined by specific cell adhesion molecules on lymphocyte surfaces; the molecules bind to complementary *cytokines* (adhesion molecules) on endothelial cells. This pathway permits circulation of lymphocytes from blood to lymph nodes to lymph and then to other lymph nodes. HEVs are found in other sites in mucosa-associated lymphoid tissue, such as interfollicular areas of tonsils and Peyer's patches. The spleen lacks HEVs, but its capillaries have similar transmigratory functions.

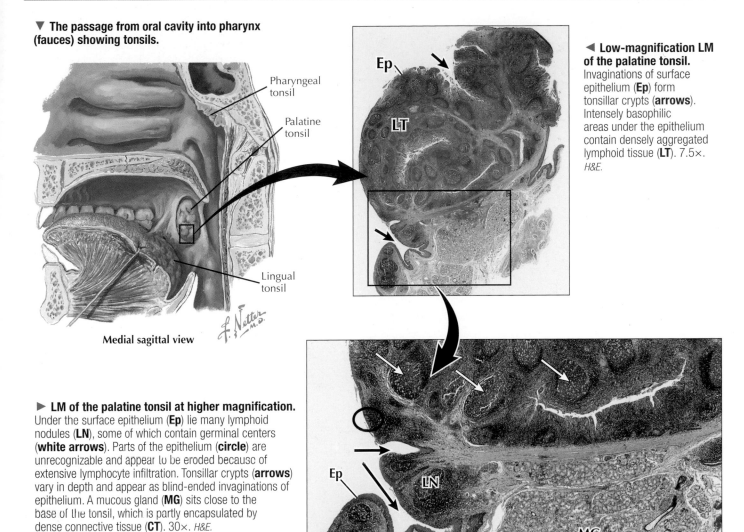

▼ The passage from oral cavity into pharynx (fauces) showing tonsils.

Pharyngeal tonsil

Palatine tonsil

Lingual tonsil

Medial sagittal view

◄ Low-magnification LM of the palatine tonsil. Invaginations of surface epithelium (**Ep**) form tonsillar crypts (**arrows**). Intensely basophilic areas under the epithelium contain densely aggregated lymphoid tissue (**LT**). 7.5×. *H&E.*

► LM of the palatine tonsil at higher magnification. Under the surface epithelium (**Ep**) lie many lymphoid nodules (**LN**), some of which contain germinal centers (**white arrows**). Parts of the epithelium (**circle**) are unrecognizable and appear to be eroded because of extensive lymphocyte infiltration. Tonsillar crypts (**arrows**) vary in depth and appear as blind-ended invaginations of epithelium. A mucous gland (**MG**) sits close to the base of the tonsil, which is partly encapsulated by dense connective tissue (**CT**). 30×. *H&E.*

9.8   STRUCTURE AND FUNCTION OF TONSILS

Tonsils are discrete aggregates of lymphoid nodules under the epithelium lining entrances to the digestive and respiratory tracts. Part of MALT, they can be seen with the naked eye as groups of separate masses. In the wall of the oropharynx lies a bilateral pair of **palatine tonsils.** At the base of the tongue sit two **lingual tonsils,** and one **pharyngeal tonsil** is in the posterior part of the nasopharynx. These tonsils together form a prominent, broken ring of strategically located lymphoid tissue called *Waldeyer's ring.* The tonsils are partly encapsulated structures that lack afferent lymphatic vessels but are drained by efferent lymphatic channels. They do share a common histologic plan but show some variations in microscopic structure depending on location. Their major role is defense against bacterial and viral infections via production of immunoglobulins by B cell–derived plasma cells. Hypertrophy and chronic inflammation of the pharyngeal tonsil are common in children. This condition, called *adenoiditis,* may obstruct breathing.

CLINICAL POINT

Tonsillitis, or inflammation of tonsils, is especially common in children and often accompanies *pharyngitis* (inflammation of mucous membrane and underlying parts of the pharynx). It results from infection with bacteria such as *Streptococcus* or viruses such as *Epstein-Barr virus.* Sore throat (painful discomfort in the throat) and fever are symptoms. Surgical removal of the tonsil, or *tonsillectomy,* was the standard treatment more than 20 years ago. However, it is no longer advised for most children and is now used only when swallowing and breathing are compromised or when repeated episodes occur in a year.

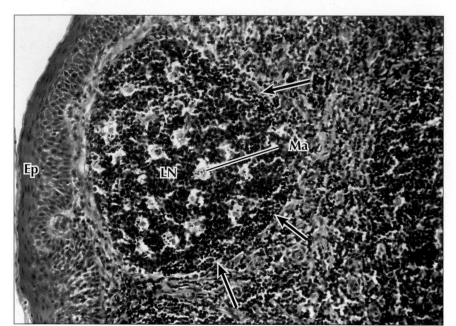

◄ LM of a lymphoid nodule in the palatine tonsil.
Under the stratified squamous epithelium (**Ep**) that covers the tonsil surface is a profusion of dark-staining, closely packed lymphocytes. A spherical lymphoid nodule (**LN**) in the lamina propria is capped externally by a mantle zone of similar lymphocytes (**arrows**). The germinal center of this nodule is not seen. Tonsillar nodules also contain many macrophages (**Ma**), known as tingible (or stainable) macrophages. Their presence among the smaller, darker lymphocytes produces a unique "starry night" pattern in the nodule, which is a useful distinguishing feature of this tonsil. These macrophages phagocytose developing B lymphocytes in the nodule that are either apoptotic or undergoing degeneration. 160×. *H&E.*

► LM of a mucous gland in the palatine tonsil.
Like clusters of grapes attached to stems, groups of secretory cells of the mucous gland (**MG**), organized as acini, are connected to a branched excretory duct (∗). Epithelium lines this duct. The secretory cells appear washed out because of a preparation artifact. Surrounding connective tissue stroma (**CT**) contains loosely arranged lymphocytes and plasma cells. Although the full excretory duct is not seen in this section, it conveys mucus to the epithelial surface of the tonsil. This secretion normally cleanses the crypts and keeps them free of bacteria and cell debris. 140×. *H&E.*

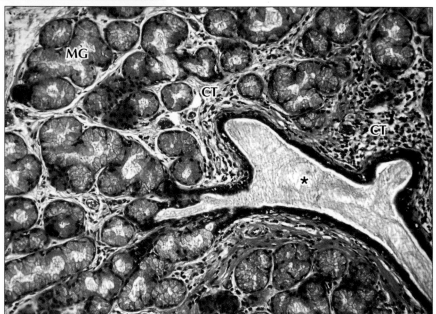

9.9 HISTOLOGY AND FUNCTION OF TONSILS

Palatine tonsils are almond-shaped masses, 1-2.5 cm in diameter. Their free surfaces are covered by **nonkeratinized stratified squamous epithelium** heavily infiltrated by **lymphocytes.** The surface epithelium forms 10-20 deep invaginations, or **tonsillar crypts,** which increase surface area and enhance interaction of antigens with underlying immunocompetent cells. The **lamina propria** around the crypts contains many **lymphoid nodules.** Some may have **germinal centers** with lightly stained central regions of primarily large proliferating B cells and macrophages surrounded by more closely packed, small resting cells. B cells are found mostly in nodules; T cells, in the periphery of each nodule or between nodules. **Macrophages** are also abundant in nodules, and their numbers increase after intense antigenic stimulation. These macrophages are less basophilic than are surrounding lymphocytes. Also, shrinkage and preparation artifact make them seem to reside in small clear areas within nodules, which produces a distinct pattern. In some areas, epithelium lacks a basement membrane, which aids lymphocyte infiltration. An incomplete capsule of dense, fibrous **connective tissue** separates palatine tonsils from tissues below. The capsule sends occasional connective tissue trabeculae into lymphoid tissue to partly separate the tonsil into lobules, thereby providing a plane of section for surgical removal, or *tonsillectomy,* to treat *tonsillitis.* External to the capsule are **mucous glands** with ducts that drain at the surface or into crypts. The secretions usually keep crypts clean, but crypts may become clogged or obstructed with bacteria or debris, the result being infected and enlarged tonsils. The **pharyngeal tonsil** has histologic features similar to those of palatine tonsils, except that pseudostratified (respiratory) epithelium covers its outer (free) surface. The smaller **lingual tonsils** are buried under stratified squamous epithelium of the base of the tongue.

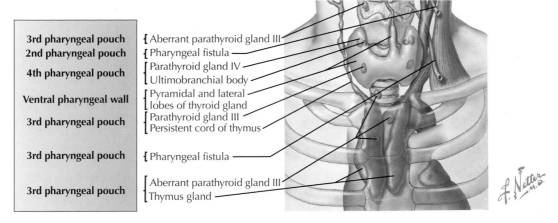

3rd pharyngeal pouch	{ Aberrant parathyroid gland III
2nd pharyngeal pouch	{ Pharyngeal fistula
4th pharyngeal pouch	[Parathyroid gland IV
	[Ultimobranchial body
Ventral pharyngeal wall	[Pyramidal and lateral
	[lobes of thyroid gland
3rd pharyngeal pouch	[Parathyroid gland III
	[Persistent cord of thymus
3rd pharyngeal pouch	{ Pharyngeal fistula
3rd pharyngeal pouch	[Aberrant parathyroid gland III
	[Thymus gland

▲ **Location of thymus gland and surrounding structures.**

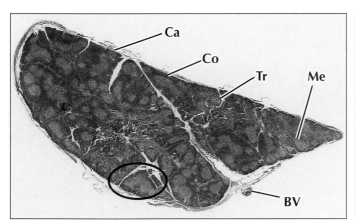

▲ **LM of part of a child's thymus.** A thin outer capsule (**Ca**) sends thin connective tissue trabeculae (**Tr**) into the lobe to form lobules. Each lobule (one is **encircled**) has a dark-staining peripheral cortex (**Co**) and a pale-staining central medulla (**Me**). Medullary areas of adjacent lobules often look confluent. Blood vessels (**BV**) travel in trabeculae to the organ's interior. Unlike other lymphoid organs, the thymus usually lacks lymphoid nodules. 4×. *H&E.*

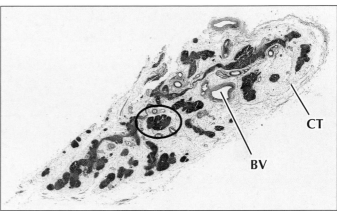

▲ **LM of part of an adult thymus showing partial involution.** Adipose connective tissue (**CT**), made mostly of fat cells, predominates at this stage because of a gradual loss of lymphocytes with age. Remnants of lymphoid parenchyma (**circle**) have a round to irregular shape. They may contain areas of cortex and medulla, but the boundary between these areas becomes indistinct. Blood vessels (**BV**) are prominent in the connective tissue of the involuting thymus. 4×. *H&E.*

9.10   DEVELOPMENT AND FUNCTION OF THE THYMUS

The thymus gland is a flat, bilobed primary lymphoid organ found in the anterior mediastinum of the thorax, behind the upper part of the sternum. It weighs 12-15 g at birth and reaches maximal size, up to 30-40 g, at puberty. It then undergoes involution (or atrophy) with slow replacement of its **lymphoid parenchyma** by **adipose connective tissue.** This *lymphoepithelial organ* is derived from two primary germ layers. The endoderm of the third and fourth *pharyngeal pouches* gives rise to specialized *epithelial reticular cells,* which form the supportive framework (or stroma). Surrounding mesenchyme, derived from mesoderm, gives rise to a thin outer **capsule** and **trabeculae** that originate from it and extend into the substance of the gland. During fetal development, immature lymphocytes from mesenchyme-derived bone marrow migrate among epithelial reticular cells in the outer cortex of the thymus to become pre-T lymphocytes that make up thymic parenchyma. The **cortex** contains mainly small lymphocytes that are so densely and uniformly packed that they often obscure the epithelial reticular cells.

The main function of the thymus is antigen-independent maturation of **T lymphocytes** (also called *thymocytes*). Several classes of these cells with specific receptors that recognize foreign antigens differentiate from precursor T lymphocytes. As T cells mature, they are discharged into the circulation to go to secondary lymphoid tissues and organs. Epithelial reticular cells secrete the hormones *thymosin* and *thymopoietin,* which induce T cell maturation and maintain cell-mediated immunity.

CLINICAL POINT

DiGeorge syndrome, also known as **thymic aplasia,** is a rare congenital disorder involving failure of the thymus to develop properly. The syndrome is due to a defect on chromosome 22 produced by a recombination error at meiosis, which causes faulty development of the third and fourth pharyngeal pouches in the early embryo. Its selective T cell deficiency leads to *immunodeficiency* with recurrent *opportunistic infections.* Malformations of the heart, esophagus, great vessels, and parathyroid glands also occur. Maternal alcohol consumption in the first trimester of pregnancy may be an environmental factor responsible for this disorder.

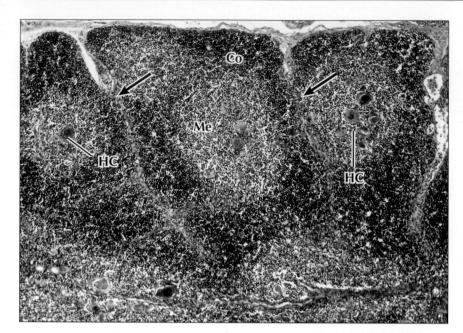

◄ **LM of part of a child's thymus.** A delicate connective tissue capsule (at the top) sends in thin trabeculae (**arrows**) to form irregular lobules, three of which are seen here. Lymphocytes are more densely packed in the cortex (**Co**) than in the medulla (**Me**). The plane of section determines the appearance of the lightly stained regions of medulla: either closed compartments surrounded by cortex or a confluent central region continuous between lobules. The medulla contains loosely packed lymphocytes and many Hassall's corpuscles (**HC**), which are recognizable at this magnification. 85×. *H&E.*

► **LM of part of the cortex of a child's thymus at high magnification.** Many closely packed lymphocytes (**Ly**) with small, round, densely stained nuclei predominate. Epithelial reticular cells (**ERC**) have large, round euchromatic nuclei, with prominent nucleoli. Their cytoplasm is eosinophilic. Processes of these cells (**arrows**) appear to invest capillaries (**Cap**), many of which are seen in transverse section. This pattern in the cortex constitutes the blood-thymus barrier, which limits access of blood-borne antigens to immature lymphocytes. 820×. *H&E.*

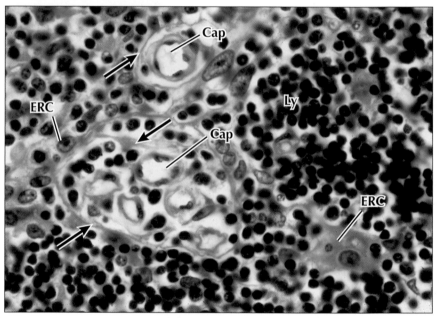

9.11 HISTOLOGY OF THE THYMUS

Each **lobe** of the thymus is organized into smaller **lobules** that are incompletely separated from each other by **connective tissue trabeculae** made of collagen and elastic fibers. Each lobule contains an outer, dark-staining lymphocyte-dense **cortex** and an inner **medulla** that stains more lightly; medullary areas of adjacent lobules may be confluent. Trabeculae derive from the thin, fibrous outer **capsule** that invests the organ and extend perpendicularly from the capsule into the cortex. **Blood vessels** enter and exit the thymus via trabeculae. The thymus lacks afferent lymphatics, but it does have *efferent lymphatics* and nerves, which also course in trabeculae. **Lymphocytes** in the cortex divide often, migrate into the medulla as they mature, and then exit the thymus. Lymphocytes in the medulla are less numerous and compact but larger than those in the cortex. Part of the general circulating population

of lymphocytes, they are eventually released into efferent lymphatics of the circulatory and lymphatic systems and migrate to T cell-dependent areas of other lymphoid tissues, including paracortex of lymph nodes, periarteriolar lymphatic sheaths in the spleen, and interfollicular regions of Peyer's patches. *Macrophages* and *dendritic cells*, both originating in bone marrow, are also seen among lymphocytes in the thymic cortex and medulla. Macrophages are most abundant in a poorly defined boundary, called the *corticomedullary junction*, which separates cortex from medulla. **Epithelial reticular cells** form a loose intercommunicating network that supports the entire lymphoid parenchyma. These cells are either flattened or stellate, with many tapering processes. They are hard to see by conventional microscopy but do have intensely eosinophilic cytoplasm and an ovoid, pale-staining nucleus with distinct nucleoli.

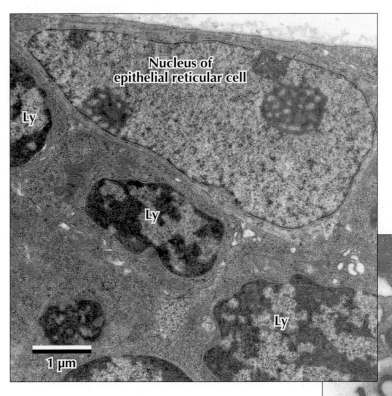

◄ **Electron micrograph (EM) of the cortex of the thymus.** An epithelial reticular cell has a large euchromatic nucleus with several nucleoli. Called a thymic nurse cell in this area of the thymus, which is directly under the capsule, it is closely associated with small, tightly packed lymphocytes (**Ly**) that are maturing. Although not well seen at this magnification, the epithelial reticular cell cytoplasm contains abundant tonofilaments. 19,300×.

► **EM showing key features of the blood-thymus barrier in the cortex.** Capillary endothelial cells in this area are usually linked by desmosomes (**circle**). A thick basement membrane (**BM**) surrounds the endothelium and also invests the thin cytoplasmic processes (**arrows**) of adjacent epithelial reticular cells. Part of a macrophage seen is recognizable by the numerous lysosomes (**L**). 17,700×.

9.12 STRUCTURE AND FUNCTION OF THE BLOOD-THYMUS BARRIER

In the thymus, **epithelial reticular cells** perform many functions. These reticular cells, called **thymic nurse cells,** are invested by a basal lamina and form part of the blood-thymus barrier in the **cortex.** Their **cytoplasmic processes,** which are linked by **desmosomes,** support clusters of maturing **lymphocytes** in the subjacent, intervening spaces of the cortex. The thin processes partially invest the **endothelium** of **continuous (nonfenestrated) capillaries** in the cortex. The basal lamina of these reticular cells is often fused with the thick basal lamina of the capillary endothelium. Together, these cellular and extracellular structures create a physical barrier that protects immature lymphocytes from foreign blood-borne antigens. This barrier prevents premature exposure of lymphocytes to foreign and self-antigens so that an immune reaction does not occur. By electron microscopy, epithelial reticular cells contain lysosomes, electron-dense granules, and abundant intermediate filaments, or **tonofilaments. Macrophages** are

found close to these perivascular areas and may enhance the barrier's effectiveness by engulfing *antigens* before they can enter the cortex. Thymic macrophages are also involved in lymphocyte phagocytosis because most of them undergo *apoptosis* during differentiation and are destroyed, so only a relatively small number is released into circulation.

CLINICAL POINT

Human immunodeficiency virus (HIV) is an RNA retrovirus that can infect CD4⁺ helper T cells and macrophages expressing CD4 surface marker. HIV infection, a chronic *infectious disease,* can cause a broad spectrum of clinical manifestations, ranging from an asymptomatic carrier state to **AIDS,** or *acquired immunodeficiency syndrome.* No cure is available, but treatments with a combination of antiretroviral agents reduce the level of HIV in the bloodstream. Prolonged suppression of HIV levels (measured by a viral load blood test) plus a CD4⁺ T cell count higher than 200/μL (normally 500-1600/μL) significantly improves quality of life and reduces mortality.

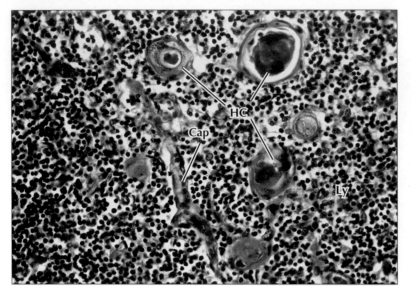

◀ **LM of part of the medulla of a child's thymus.** Eosinophilic Hassall's corpuscles (**HC**) are in view; their sizes vary (20-150 µm). Some show concentric epithelial reticular cells and others, hyalinization or degeneration. Capillaries (**Cap**) are seen among the lymphocytes (**Ly**). 310×. *H&E.*

▶ **LM of Hassall's corpuscle at higher magnification.** This spherical body is characteristic of the thymus and is unique to the medulla. Its central area of degenerated or necrotic cells is surrounded by flattened or polygonal cells. Around the corpuscle are epithelial reticular cells (**ERC**) and lymphocytes (**Ly**). 750×. *H&E.*

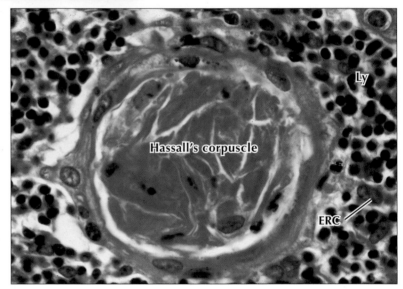

9.13 HISTOLOGY AND FUNCTION OF THE THYMIC MEDULLA AND HASSALL'S CORPUSCLES

The medulla contains many **epithelial reticular cells** (ERCs), macrophages, and occasional plasma cells, as well as **lymphocytes,** which are fewer in the medulla than in the cortex. These ERCs are less branched than are ERCs in the cortex. **Capillaries** that enter the medulla from the cortex at the corticomedullary junction immediately drain into postcapillary venules that are not ensheathed by barrier components. The venules are thus more permeable than are capillaries in the cortex, and the medulla has no blood-thymus barrier. Lymphocytes that proliferate in the cortex enter the blood vascular system by passing through walls of these vessels. Medullary venules drain into larger veins that course in interlobular trabeculae before leaving the thymus. A unique feature of the medulla is the presence of spherical bodies with lamellar centers—**Hassall's** (or **thymic**) **corpuscles**—which help differentiate the thymus from other lymphoid organs. They vary in diameter from 20 to 150 µm and have a central hyaline core that is eosinophilic and may show signs of keratinization. They

appear to contain clusters of degenerating ERCs arranged concentrically and rich in *cytokeratins.* The English physician A. H. Hassall first described these bodies in the 1840s. Their function is not well understood, but they express the cytokine *thymic stromal thymopoietin,* which instructs dendritic cells in the human thymus to induce CD4+ regulatory T cell development. They may also play a role in removing apoptotic thymocytes. Their size and number increase in the elderly, and they often calcify with advancing age.

CLINICAL POINT

Systemic lupus erythematosus (SLE) is a generalized *autoimmune disorder* associated with many cellular and humoral immunologic abnormalities. This chronic noninfectious disease, which is most common in women of childbearing age, may affect many organs. Although its cause is unknown, tissue injury is mediated by immune complexes that initiate an inflammatory response when deposited on tissues. Evidence exists that reduced suppressor T cell function in SLE accounts for overproduction of autoantibodies that combine with autoantigens, such as in DNA-anti-DNA complexes. As with most autoimmune diseases, severity of SLE varies markedly among patients.

▼ **Views of the spleen.**

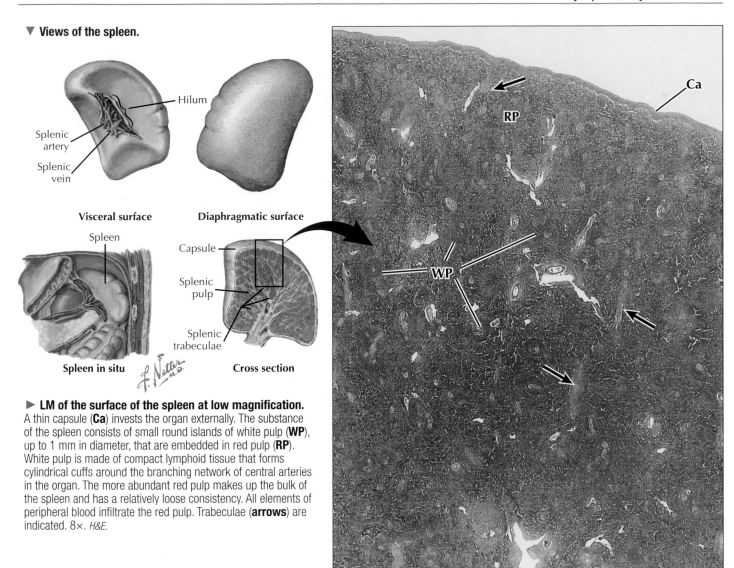

Visceral surface | Diaphragmatic surface

Spleen

Spleen in situ | Cross section

Hilum
Splenic artery
Splenic vein

Capsule
Splenic pulp
Splenic trabeculae

▶ **LM of the surface of the spleen at low magnification.**
A thin capsule (**Ca**) invests the organ externally. The substance of the spleen consists of small round islands of white pulp (**WP**), up to 1 mm in diameter, that are embedded in red pulp (**RP**). White pulp is made of compact lymphoid tissue that forms cylindrical cuffs around the branching network of central arteries in the organ. The more abundant red pulp makes up the bulk of the spleen and has a relatively loose consistency. All elements of peripheral blood infiltrate the red pulp. Trabeculae (**arrows**) are indicated. 8×. *H&E.*

9.14 STRUCTURE AND FUNCTION OF THE SPLEEN

The spleen lies in the upper left quadrant of the abdomen, behind the stomach and just below the diaphragm. In adults, this largest **lymphoid organ** is the size of a clenched fist and weighs 180-250 g. At the **hilum** (an indentation on the medial surface), the **splenic artery** and nerves enter and the **splenic vein** and lymphatics leave. The spleen derives embryonically from a condensation of mesenchyme in the dorsal mesogastrium. During early fetal development, it is temporarily an organ of *hematopoiesis;* this role is taken over by the liver and then bone marrow. However, in severe cases of anemia in children and adults, the spleen may produce new blood cells. The spleen is a major repository for *mononuclear phagocytic cells,* accounts for 25% of the total number of lymphocytes, and stores about a third of the body's platelets. The organ filters blood by clearing particulate matter, infectious organisms, and aged or defective erythrocytes and platelets. It recycles iron from worn out erythrocytes. Primarily macrophages

perform these functions. The spleen is also a secondary lymphoid organ: lymphocytes respond to blood-borne antigens by initiating an immune reaction that activates T and B cells. The spleen also produces lymphocytes, plasma cells, and both IgM and IgG.

CLINICAL POINT
Many clinical conditions can produce **splenomegaly,** or enlargement of the spleen. A common cause is *portal hypertension* resulting from cirrhosis of the liver. The spleen of affected patients is modestly enlarged, weighing 300-800 g, and the capsule becomes thick and fibrotic. Histologic study of the red pulp shows dilated venous sinusoids and increased macrophage numbers; the white pulp is usually atrophic. *Splenectomy,* or removal of the spleen, is used as therapy for some chronic disorders or an emergency procedure for traumatic rupture of the spleen. Splenectomy in adults usually has no clinical consequence, but in children it leads to increased occurrence and severity of infections.

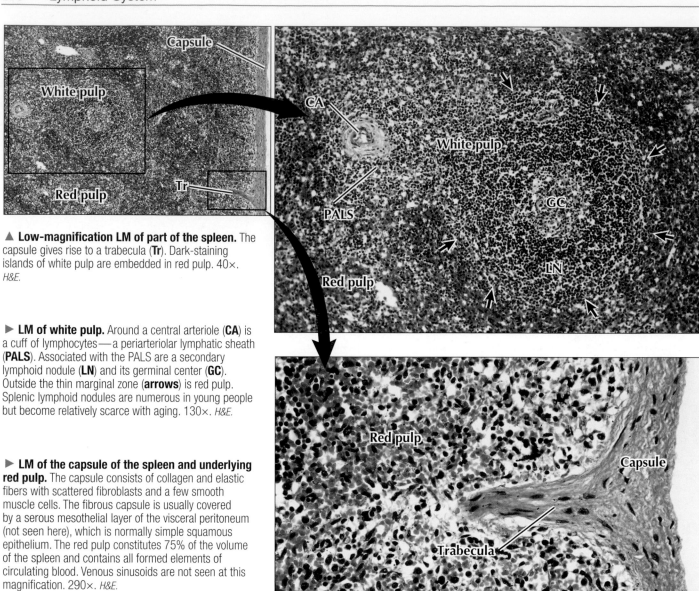

▲ **Low-magnification LM of part of the spleen.** The capsule gives rise to a trabecula (**Tr**). Dark-staining islands of white pulp are embedded in red pulp. 40×. *H&E.*

▶ **LM of white pulp.** Around a central arteriole (**CA**) is a cuff of lymphocytes—a periarteriolar lymphatic sheath (**PALS**). Associated with the PALS are a secondary lymphoid nodule (**LN**) and its germinal center (**GC**). Outside the thin marginal zone (**arrows**) is red pulp. Splenic lymphoid nodules are numerous in young people but become relatively scarce with aging. 130×. *H&E.*

▶ **LM of the capsule of the spleen and underlying red pulp.** The capsule consists of collagen and elastic fibers with scattered fibroblasts and a few smooth muscle cells. The fibrous capsule is usually covered by a serous mesothelial layer of the visceral peritoneum (not seen here), which is normally simple squamous epithelium. The red pulp constitutes 75% of the volume of the spleen and contains all formed elements of circulating blood. Venous sinusoids are not seen at this magnification. 290×. *H&E.*

9.15 HISTOLOGY OF THE SPLEEN

The spleen is covered by an outer dense irregular connective tissue **capsule,** which sends radiating **trabeculae** into the organ's interior. Suspended between trabeculae is a communicating network of *reticular fibers,* with many attached *macrophages* and *reticular cells.* Unlike other lymphoid organs, the spleen does not have a cortex and medulla. It consists of **white pulp** and **red pulp,** so named because of their color in the fresh state. White pulp is made of grayish white islands of lymphoid tissue, most surrounding a **central arteriole** to form **periarteriolar lymphatic sheaths** (PALS). T cells are found mainly in PALS around the central arteriole, which is derived from the splenic artery after many tree-like branchings. **Lymphoid nodules** lie in more peripheral white pulp relative to the arterioles. As in lymph nodes, B cells may be found in primary (unstimulated) lymphoid nodules or secondary (stimulated) nodules with germinal centers. Surrounding white pulp is a shell of sparsely cellular lymphoid tissue—the *marginal zone*—that contains many macrophages and some B lymphocytes. This zone is not as well defined in humans as in animals, and its demonstration requires special staining methods. Red pulp makes up most of the spleen, its color being due mostly to abundant erythrocytes. Found around white pulp, it consists of many thin-walled **venous sinusoids** and intervening *cellular,* or *splenic, cords* (of *Billroth*). The term *splenic cords* is misleading, in that these are labyrinthine spaces between sinuses containing a scaffold of reticular fibers. Many closely packed fixed or wandering cells—reticular cells, lymphocytes, plasma cells, macrophages, and all formed elements of circulating blood—occupy these spaces.

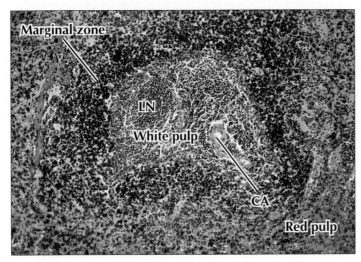

▲ **LM of rat spleen showing white and red pulp after injection of India ink.** Macrophages are often difficult to discern in conventional histologic sections. Injection of India ink into an experimental animal, followed by removal of the spleen and then its microscopic examination, allows reaction product in macrophages to be seen. This section, so prepared, shows a high concentration of macrophages in the marginal zone of white pulp after cells ingested black carbon particles of ink. Other areas of white pulp seen are a central arteriole (**CA**), which is surrounded by PALS, and a lymphoid nodule (**LN**). 70×. *H&E.*

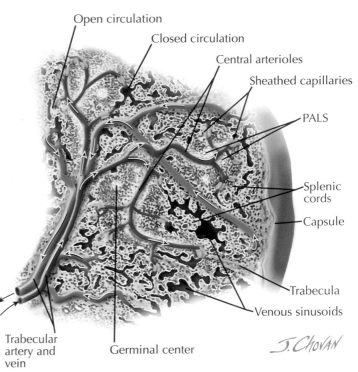

▲ **Blood circulation in the spleen.**

▶ **EM of part of a central arteriole (CA) in white pulp.** Flattened endothelial cells (**En**) line the vessel lumen. Two layers of smooth muscle cells make up the tunica media. Between the endothelium and smooth muscle is a prominent layer of elastic tissue, the internal elastic lamina (**arrows**). The outermost adventitia of the vessel consists mainly of connective tissue (**CT**). Lymphocytes of the PALS are also seen. 3800×.

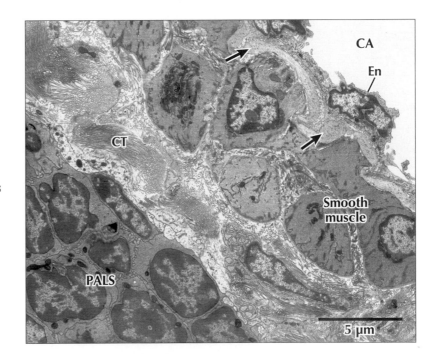

9.16   BLOOD SUPPLY TO WHITE PULP

Functions of the spleen are best understood in relation to its blood supply. The *splenic artery* enters at the *hilum* and divides into several smaller *trabecular arteries,* so named because they travel in trabeculae. These arteries branch repeatedly and enter white pulp to become **arterioles.** They are known collectively as **central arterioles,** which is a misnomer as these vessels are usually in an eccentric position in white pulp. They also have two layers of **smooth muscle cells** in their walls, which is a feature of arterioles.

A cuff of **lymphocytes** that constitutes a PALS surrounds central arterioles. Associated with PALS are occasional **lymphoid nodules** with **germinal centers** that seem to push arterioles to an eccentric site. Some branches of the central arteriole end as marginal sinuses that supply the **marginal zone** of the white pulp. Other arterial branches enter the **red pulp** as short straight *penicillar arterioles.* These drain into *sheathed capillaries,* which have an external sheath of *reticular fibers* and many **macrophages.**

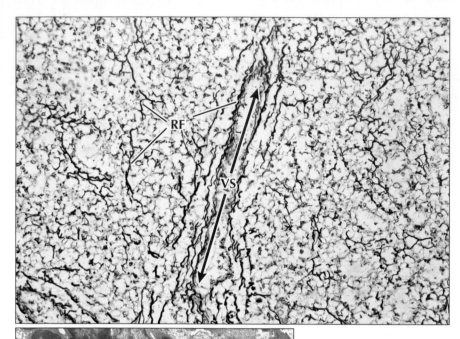

◄ LM of the stroma of red pulp. Like the stroma of other lymphoid organs, the spleen's stroma consists of an extensive network of reticular fibers (**RF**) for internal support. In red pulp, they accommodate many lymphocytes, macrophages, and other cells in splenic cords. They also support the sinusoids. A venous sinusoid (**VS, arrows**) is seen in longitudinal section. With silver stains, reticular fibers are black fibrous strands that form an interweaving network in the organ. 280×. *Reticulin.*

▼ Higher power LM of red pulp. Venous sinusoids (**VS**), seen in transverse and longitudinal (**arrows**) views, form a tortuous, anastomosing vascular network. Each sinusoid has a wide lumen and is lined by cuboidal endothelial cells. Macrophages closely associated with sinusoid walls often require special techniques for detection. Splenic cords (**SC**) are in intervening areas of red pulp. 500×. *H&E.*

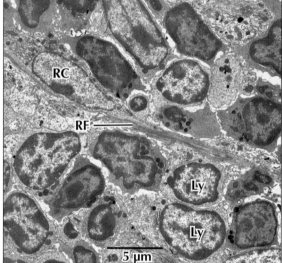

▲ EM of a splenic cord. Various closely packed cells, including lymphocytes (**Ly**), make up splenic cords. Reticular cells (**RC**), which are modified fibroblasts, produce reticular fibers (**RF**) of the stroma. 3000×.

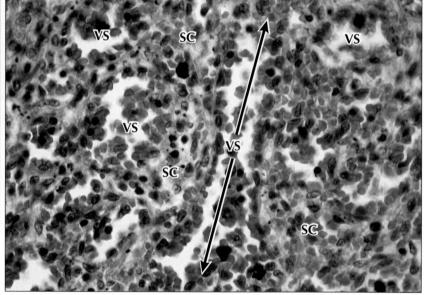

9.17 BLOOD SUPPLY TO RED PULP

Whether circulation in red pulp is a closed or open circuit is debatable. In the closed system, about 90% of capillaries supplying red pulp drain directly into **venous sinusoids,** such as normally occurs elsewhere in the body. An alternative is an open system: remaining open-ended capillaries discharge blood freely into the intersinusoidal meshwork, so blood seeps out and percolates slowly between **splenic cords** before regaining access to sinusoids. Both open and closed patterns likely operate at different times, according to physiologic conditions. Venous sinusoids are a tortuous network of thin-walled vessels with irregular lumina. With diameters of 30-50 μm, they have a unique structure related to high permeability. They are made of spindle-shaped, longitudi-

nally oriented **endothelial cells.** Although adjacent endothelial cells lack junctions, they are separated by slit-like spaces, 1-5 μm wide. A thin, discontinuous *basal lamina* forms circular bands around the endothelial cells, like hoops around staves of a leaky barrel. Formed elements of blood can thus traverse the highly porous walls of venous sinusoids by squeezing through the slits. However, worn out or fragile erythrocytes, which have lost pliability, cannot reenter the circulation and are phagocytosed by macrophages. Sinusoids drain into larger venules, which empty into trabecular veins. These merge to form the splenic vein, which leaves the organ at the hilum. The spleen lacks *afferent lymphatics,* but *efferent lymphatics* beginning in white pulp exit at the hilum.

10

ENDOCRINE SYSTEM

▼ **Organization of the endocrine system.**

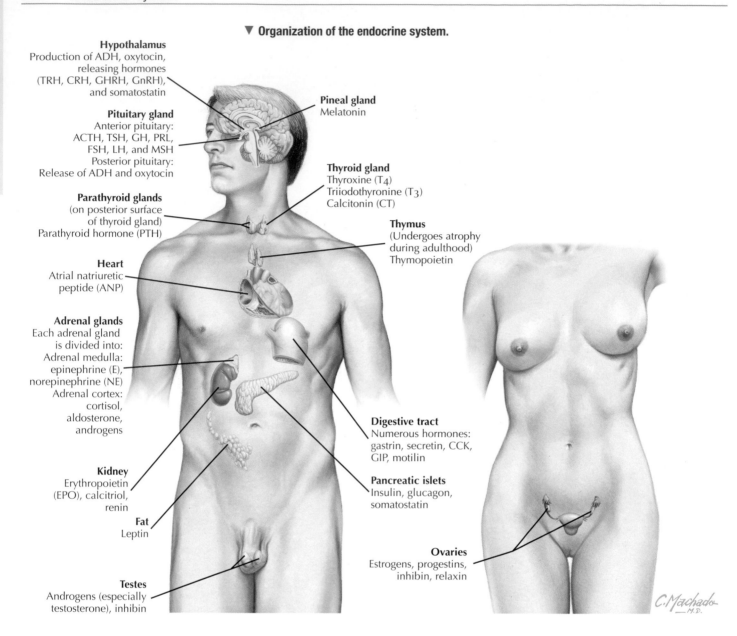

Hypothalamus
Production of ADH, oxytocin,
releasing hormones
(TRH, CRH, GHRH, GnRH),
and somatostatin

Pituitary gland
Anterior pituitary:
ACTH, TSH, GH, PRL,
FSH, LH, and MSH
Posterior pituitary:
Release of ADH and oxytocin

Parathyroid glands
(on posterior surface
of thyroid gland)
Parathyroid hormone (PTH)

Heart
Atrial natriuretic
peptide (ANP)

Adrenal glands
Each adrenal gland
is divided into:
Adrenal medulla:
epinephrine (E),
norepinephrine (NE)
Adrenal cortex:
cortisol,
aldosterone,
androgens

Kidney
Erythropoietin
(EPO), calcitriol,
renin

Fat
Leptin

Testes
Androgens (especially
testosterone), inhibin

Pineal gland
Melatonin

Thyroid gland
Thyroxine (T_4)
Triiodothyronine (T_3)
Calcitonin (CT)

Thymus
(Undergoes atrophy
during adulthood)
Thymopoietin

Digestive tract
Numerous hormones:
gastrin, secretin, CCK,
GIP, motilin

Pancreatic islets
Insulin, glucagon,
somatostatin

Ovaries
Estrogens, progestins,
inhibin, relaxin

C.Machado
M.D.

10.1 OVERVIEW

The **endocrine system** comprises glands and tissues composed of parenchymal cells, which synthesize and secrete products called **hormones.** The term *hormone* derives from a Greek word meaning to set in motion. Like the nervous system, the endocrine system has diverse regulatory functions that control and coordinate activities of many other organs and tissues. Because the two systems have integrally linked functions, they are often termed the **neuroendocrine system.** The major **endocrine glands**—or ductless glands—are the **pituitary** (or **hypophysis**), **hypothalamus, thyroid, parathyroids, adrenals, islets of Langerhans,** and **pineal.** The **placenta,** which exists only during pregnancy, also elaborates several hormones, and other organs such as the *heart, kidneys, thymus, gonads* (*testis* and *ovary*), and *intestines* have isolated single cells or groups of cells with endocrine functions. Unlike exocrine glands that deliver secretions to a surface by ducts, endo-

crine glands lack ducts and release hormones into interstitial connective tissue. Hormones then pass to the blood or lymphatic circulation, their secretion usually being controlled by feedback mechanisms. Hormones are chemically diverse molecules—modified amino acids, peptides, glycoproteins, steroids, or biogenic amines—that typically affect target cells at sites distant from the site of release. Hormones usually bind target receptors either on cell membranes or within cells. Most endocrine glands consist of cords of parenchymal cells closely associated with a very rich vascular supply composed of a network of fenestrated capillaries and a relatively small amount of stroma. Hormone-secreting cells are usually, but not always, epithelial cells that abut walls of blood or lymphatic vessels. Nonepithelial cells that perform endocrine functions include **atrial myocardial cells** in the heart, **smooth muscle cells** in the **juxtaglomerular apparatus** of the kidney, and **fat cells** in adipose tissue.

▼ Anatomy and relations of the pituitary gland.

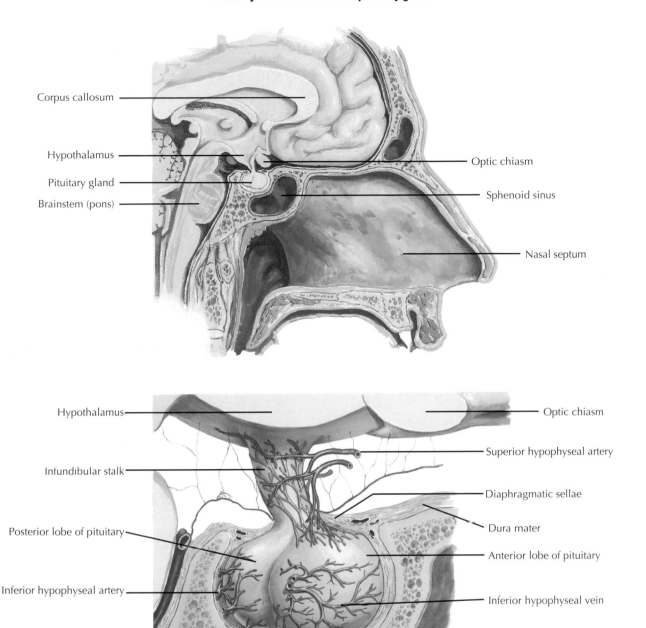

Corpus callosum

Hypothalamus

Pituitary gland

Brainstem (pons)

Optic chiasm

Sphenoid sinus

Nasal septum

Hypothalamus

Infundibular stalk

Posterior lobe of pituitary

Inferior hypophyseal artery

Optic chiasm

Superior hypophyseal artery

Diaphragmatic sellae

Dura mater

Anterior lobe of pituitary

Inferior hypophyseal vein

Sella turcica of sphenoid bone

10.2 ANATOMY OF THE PITUITARY

The pituitary, or hypophysis, is often called the *master* endocrine gland because its hormones regulate physiologic activities of many other endocrine glands and tissues. It affects the growth, differentiation, and functions of many parts of the body, either directly by its own hormones or indirectly via secretions of other glands under its control. The size of a slightly flat grape or pea, it weighs 500-900 mg in adults; it is slightly larger in women, especially during pregnancy. The pituitary is strategically located at the base of the brain, at the **hypothalamus,** where the **pituitary** (or **infundibular**) **stalk,** to which it has extensive vascular and neural connections, suspends it. It lies in the midline in a depression of the sphenoid bone, the **sella**

turcica, and is thus well protected. It has several important gross anatomic relationships. It is close anterolaterally to the **optic chiasm** and **optic nerves,** so pituitary lesions or tumors impinging on these structures can cause significant visual deficits. The **sphenoid air sinus** lies inferiorly to the gland, which allows relatively easy transsphenoidal surgical access to it. The superior aspect is covered by a thickened extension of the **dura mater,** named the **diaphragmatic sellae,** and is surrounded by a thin connective tissue capsule. It releases secretions into the bloodstream and is thus richly vascularized. The pituitary and the hypothalamus together make up a complex *neuroendocrine circuit* whose functions are closely linked. Despite its small size, the pituitary is essential to life.

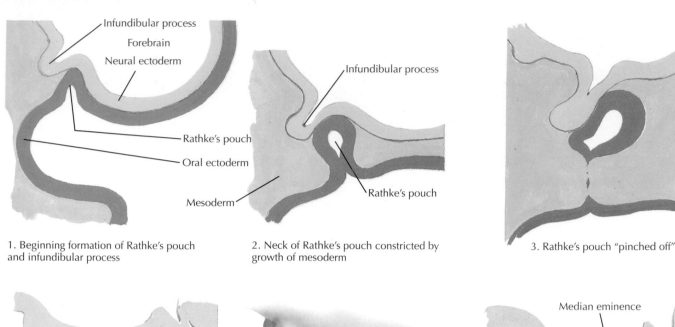

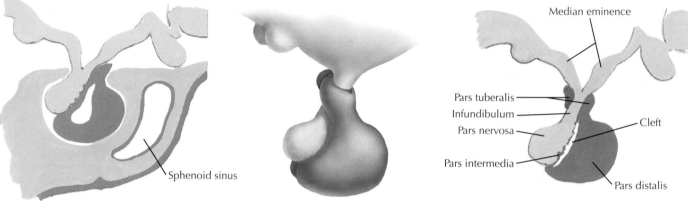

1. Beginning formation of Rathke's pouch and infundibular process

2. Neck of Rathke's pouch constricted by growth of mesoderm

3. Rathke's pouch "pinched off"

4. "Pinched off" segment conforms to neural process, forming pars distalis, pars intermedia and pars tuberalis

5. Pars tuberalis encircles infundibular stalk (lateral surface view)

6. Mature form

10.3 DEVELOPMENT OF THE PITUITARY

The pituitary has a dual embryonic origin, a combination of two distinct tissues. Early in gestation, the **adenohypophysis**—or **anterior pituitary**—arises as a dorsal outpocketing of thickened **oral ectoderm** called **Rathke's pouch.** By week 6 of gestation, it pinches off from the roof of the oral cavity and migrates to a site just anterior to a simultaneous downgrowth of **neural ectoderm** called the **infundibular process.** Cell proliferation in the anterior wall of Rathke's pouch then gives rise to the main part of the anterior lobe, which is the **pars distalis.** The terminal end of the ventral downgrowth of neural ectoderm becomes solid. Its cells give rise to the **pars nervosa (posterior lobe)** of the **neurohypophysis (posterior pituitary),** which keeps its neural connection to the brain. The two tissues become closely apposed but their microscopic structure remains different, reflecting the developmental dichotomy. Remnants of Rathke's pouch may persist as either a vestigial cleft or colloid-filled cysts at the anterior border with the neurohypophysis. The dorsal wall of the cleft fuses with

the adjoining part of the posterior lobe to make up the small **pars intermedia.** In adults, the gland measures 1.2-1.5 cm in the transverse plane and about 1 cm in the sagittal plane. Its size varies greatly throughout life, however, depending on physiologic states.

CLINICAL POINT

About 10%-15% of *intracranial tumors* are usually benign **pituitary adenomas** of the adenohypophysis. Rarely malignant, they may be secretory or nonsecretory. They may arise from multiple oncogene abnormalities, such as G-protein and *ras* gene mutations, *p53* gene deletions, and mutations that lead to *multiple endocrine neoplasia.* One type of secretory adenoma that usually requires surgery causes *acromegaly* in adults and *gigantism* in children. It is due to overproduction of growth hormone. Another type causes *Cushing's disease*—an excess of corticotropin (ACTH)—which leads to overproduction of cortisol by adrenal glands.

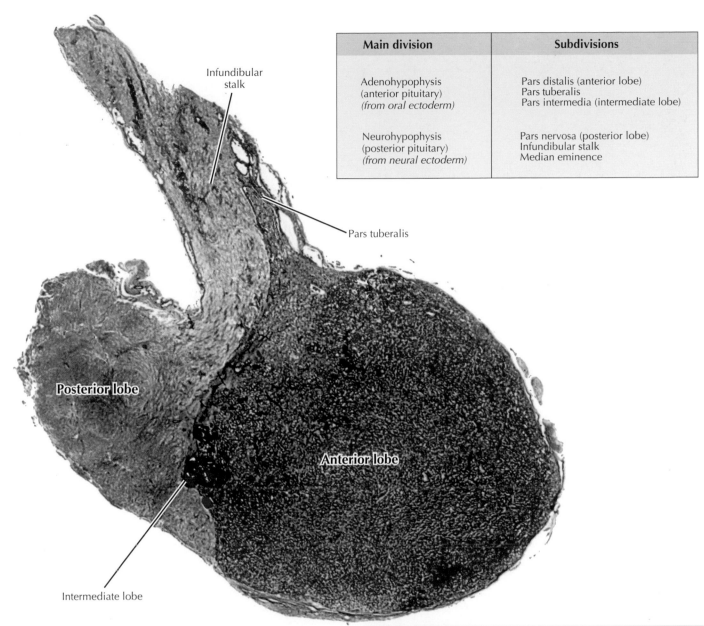

Main division	Subdivisions
Adenohypophysis (anterior pituitary) *(from oral ectoderm)*	Pars distalis (anterior lobe) Pars tuberalis Pars intermedia (intermediate lobe)
Neurohypophysis (posterior pituitary) *(from neural ectoderm)*	Pars nervosa (posterior lobe) Infundibular stalk Median eminence

Infundibular stalk

Pars tuberalis

Posterior lobe

Anterior lobe

Intermediate lobe

▲ **Light micrograph (LM) of the pituitary in sagittal section.** This panoramic view of general topography and main parts shows a darkly stained anterior lobe with a lightly stained posterior lobe. The intermediate lobe contains small vestigial clefts. The pars tuberalis, a thin strip of tissue that extends upward from the anterior lobe, incompletely surrounds the infundibular stalk. 15×. *Masson trichrome.*

Pituitary Hormones	
Anterior lobe	**Posterior lobe**
Growth hormone (GH) Prolactin (PRL) Corticotropin (ACTH) Follicle-stimulating hormone (FSH) Luteinizing hormone (LH) Thyrotropin TSH	Oxytocin (OXY) Antidiuretic hormone (ADH)
	Intermediate lobe
	Melanocyte-stimulating hormone (MSH) β-endorphin

10.4 DIVISIONS AND FUNCTIONS OF THE PITUITARY

The adult **adenohypophysis** and **neurohypophysis** are each divided into three parts. The adenohypophysis, made of glandular epithelium, consists of the **anterior lobe (pars distalis),** the largest part; **pars tuberalis,** a thin collar of tissue surrounding the infundibular stalk; and **pars intermedia** (intermediate lobe), a narrow rudimentary band just posterior to the vestigial cleft and in contact with the posterior lobe. The neurohypophysis, made of neural tissue, comprises the **posterior lobe,** the main, most expanded part; **median eminence,** the upper part that attaches the gland to the hypothalamus; and connecting **infundibular stalk.** The median eminence is partly encircled by the pars tuberalis, which links it via a network of many capillaries to the anterior lobe. The adenohypophysis synthesizes and secretes several polypeptide and glycoprotein hormones; the neurohypophysis (by way of modified neurons from the hypothalamus) secretes two peptide hormones. All hormones enter the systemic circulation and are taken to distant target tissues to regulate functions.

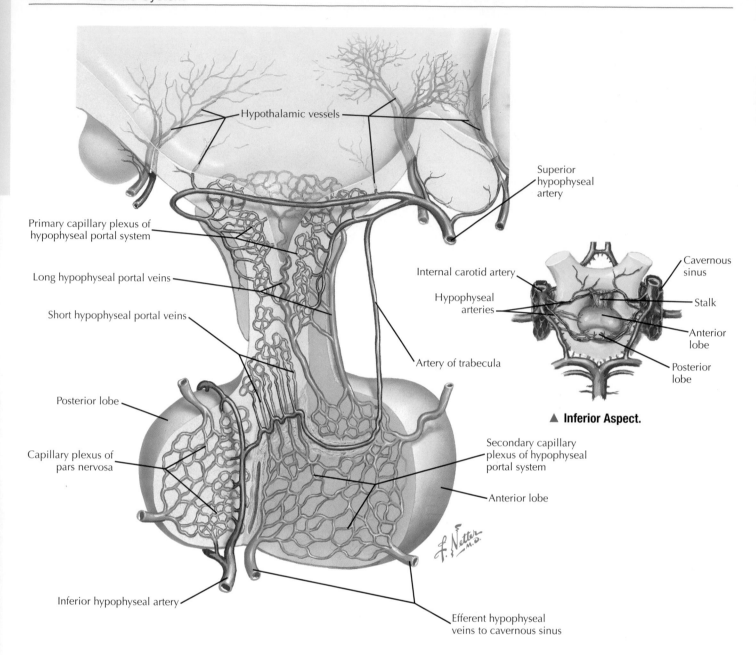

Primary capillary plexus of hypophyseal portal system

Long hypophyseal portal veins

Short hypophyseal portal veins

Posterior lobe

Capillary plexus of pars nervosa

Inferior hypophyseal artery

Hypothalamic vessels

Superior hypophyseal artery

Internal carotid artery

Hypophyseal arteries

Artery of trabecula

Cavernous sinus

Stalk

Anterior lobe

Posterior lobe

▲ **Inferior Aspect.**

Secondary capillary plexus of hypophyseal portal system

Anterior lobe

Efferent hypophyseal veins to cavernous sinus

10.5 BLOOD SUPPLY OF THE PITUITARY

Two paired hypophyseal arteries—branches of **internal carotids**—have profuse anastomoses on the gland's surface. The **superior hypophyseal arteries,** from above, bring blood to the anterior lobe by first forming a **primary capillary plexus** made of vascular loops in the area of the median eminence and pars tuberalis. These vessels give rise to a network of **portal venules**—the **hypophyseal portal system**—which crosses the ventral aspect of the pituitary stalk to drain into a **secondary plexus** of **sinusoidal fenestrated capillaries** in the anterior lobe. This portal system is critical for control of the adenohypophysis by neurosecretions from hypothalamic neurons that convey releasing and inhibiting hormones to the primary plexus. Neurosecretions reach the secondary plexus to regulate release of specific adenohypophysis hormones, which are also secreted into the secondary capillary plexus. Small **efferent veins,** in turn, drain into **cavernous sinuses** surrounding the gland. **Inferior hypophyseal arteries,** below, carry arterial blood to the posterior lobe. They drain into a plexus of sinusoidal fenestrated capillaries that take blood via efferent hypophyseal veins to the cavernous sinus. An important branch of the superior hypophyseal artery, the **artery of the trabecula,** bypasses the portal circulation and forms small capillary loops in the pars intermedia, which anastomose with capillaries in the anterior lobe. The anterior and posterior lobes are richly vascularized, but the pars intermedia is not.

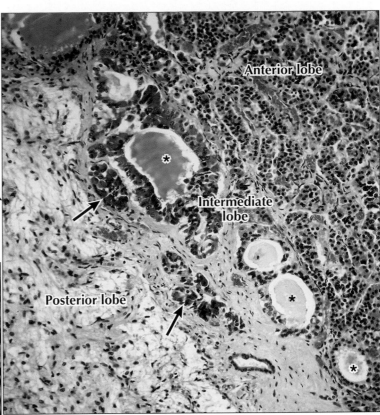

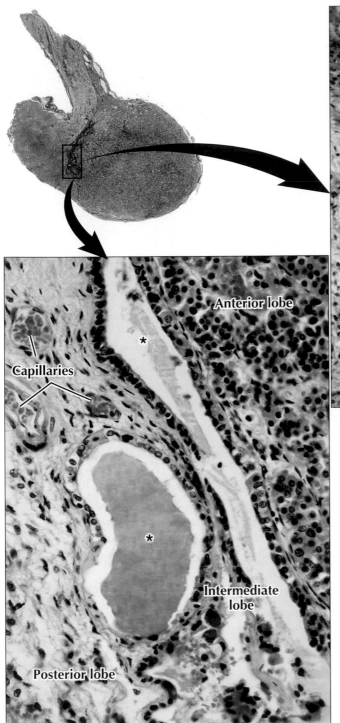

▲ **LM showing the three pituitary lobes at low magnification.** The anterior lobe consists of typical glandular epithelium; the posterior lobe resembles nervous tissue seen in the central nervous system. Colloid-filled cysts (∗) and scattered groups of basophilic cells (**arrows**) are in the intermediate lobe. 160×. *H&E.*

◀ **LM showing details of the junction between the anterior and posterior lobes.** The intermediate lobe lies between the other lobes. A few small basophilic cells are scattered in that lobe, and others line colloid-filled cysts (∗). Several sinusoidal capillaries are in the posterior lobe. 320×. *H&E.*

10.6 HISTOLOGY AND FUNCTION OF THE PITUITARY LOBES

Low magnification resolves the contrasting histologic structure between the pars distalis of the **anterior lobe** and pars nervosa of the **posterior lobe.** The anterior lobe is **glandular epithelium,** which stains dark because of its many, tightly packed nucleated parenchymal cells. The posterior lobe is more lightly stained because it is typically made of **nervous tissue.** In the **intermediate lobe,** at the border with the posterior lobe, rudiments of *Rathke's pouch* persist as accumulations of small **colloid-filled cysts.**

Showing great size variation among species, the intermediate lobe constitutes less than 2% of the adult human pituitary. This lobe is rudimentary in humans and its function in adults is uncertain, but it consists of either isolated groups of low columnar epithelial cells or a discontinuous epithelial layer, which often surrounds colloid-filled follicles, and contains **basophilic parenchymal cells** and a few scattered, lightly stained polygonal cells. Cells in this lobe produce *melanocyte-stimulating hormone* and the opiate peptide *β-endorphin*. Basophilic cells from the intermediate lobe often invade the posterior lobe.

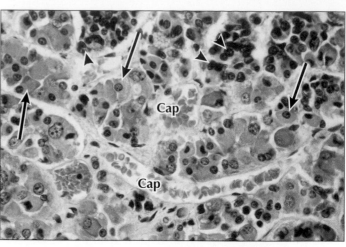

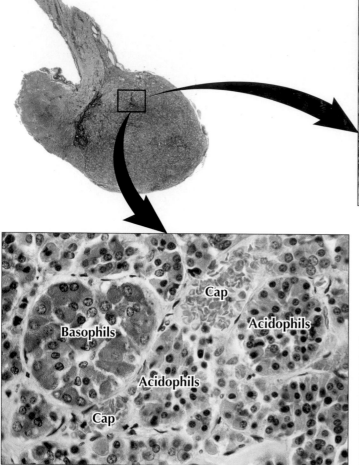

▲ **LM of chromophils and chromophobes in the anterior lobe.** Cytoplasm of chromophils (**arrows**) is stained; that of smaller chromophobes is not, but their nuclei (**arrowheads**) are. Cells are interspersed with sinusoidal capillaries (**Cap**) and delicate connective tissue stroma. Parenchymal cells are round to polygonal. Chromophobes usually have small, heterochromatic nuclei; chromophils have larger, euchromatic nuclei with prominent nucleoli. 420×. *H&E.*

▲ **LM of the anterior lobe.** The different staining pattern of the small acidophils and larger basophils reflects their granule content. A large network of sinusoidal capillaries (**Cap**) is between the clumps of parenchymal cells. The vessels receive hormones released by these cells and deliver releasing or inhibiting factors from the hypothalamohypophyseal portal system to affect cells of the anterior lobe. 420×. *H&E.*

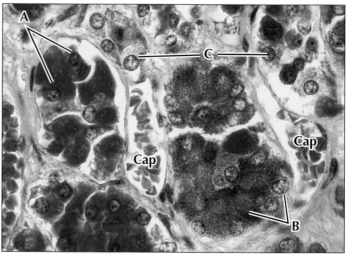

▲ **LM showing tinctorial differences between chromophobes and the two kinds of chromophils in the anterior lobe.** Acidophils (**A**) have intensely eosinophilic cytoplasm (red), basophils (**B**) are dark (green), and chromophobes (**C**) stain poorly. Capillaries (**Cap**) are also seen. 635×. *Masson's trichrome.*

10.7 HISTOLOGY OF THE ANTERIOR LOBE: CHROMOPHILS AND CHROMOPHOBES

About 75% of the *adenohypophysis* is anterior lobe. It consists of clumps or cords of **glandular epithelial cells** in close relation to a network of **sinusoidal capillaries** with large and irregular lumina. Scant loose connective tissue is made of delicate reticular fiber stroma, which supports glandular cells and sinusoid walls. Hematoxylin and eosin (H&E) reveals two distinct parenchymal cell types: chromophils (large, have secretory granules, stain intensely) and chromophobes (smaller, have few or no secretory granules, stain faintly). Chromophobes have less cytoplasm than do chromophils and may be quiescent, degranulated, or undifferentiated cells. Chromophils can be distinguished as **acidophils** or **basophils** on the basis of their cytoplasmic affinity for acid or basic dyes and on the tinctorial properties of their secretory granules. Acidophils, typically smaller cells with smoothly refractive cytoplasm, secrete two polypeptide hormones. The larger basophils are more granular and secrete four major polypeptide hormones. Via routine stains, proportions of glandular cell types are about 40% acidophils, 10% basophils, and 50% chromophobes. Their distribution differs regionally and varies locally. Immunocytochemistry with specific antibodies has allowed more precise identification of these cells and their hormone content. A functional nomenclature is now routinely used to designate cell types according to the secreted hormone or target organ.

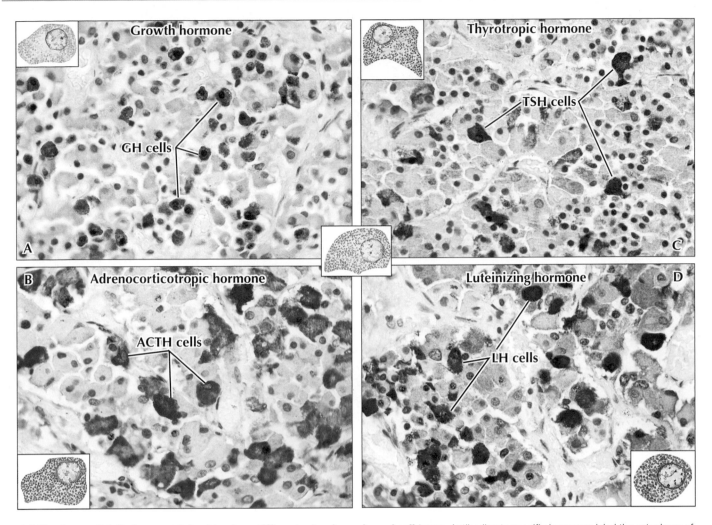

▲ **LMs of pars distalis immunostained to show different adenohypophyseal cell types.** Antibodies to specific hormones label the cytoplasm of specific cells brown. **A.** GH cells are small and intensely stained. **B.** Large, polygonal ACTH cells are arranged in clusters. **C.** TSH cells are medium sized and angular. **D.** LH cells are medium sized and polyhedral. 350×. *Diaminobenzidine, immunoperoxidase. (Courtesy of Dr. K. Dorovini Zis)* Inset drawings show cells stained with aldehyde thionine-PAS; center drawing is a PRL cell.

10.8 IMMUNOCYTOCHEMISTRY OF CELLS OF THE PARS DISTALIS

Immunocytochemistry uses **antibodies** to protein secretory products and allows identification of five adenohypophyseal cell types on the basis of intracellular localization of one or more *hormones*. Use of immunocytochemistry helps clarify the normal regional distribution of cells, correlates structure to function, and aids tumor diagnosis. Small, ovoid **somatotrophs** (GH [growth hormone] **cells**) are mostly in lateral wings of the anterior lobe. Their abundant secretory granules produce intense immunostaining. **Corticotrophs** (ACTH [**adrenocorticotropic hormone, or corticotropin**] **cells**) are most numerous in middle and posterior parts of the gland, typically in clusters. These polygonal, medium to large cells stain for corticotropin, melanocyte-stimulating hormone, endorphin, and enkephalin. Many cells have an unstained area near the nucleus, which indicates a large lysosome. Medium-sized, angular **thyrotrophs** (TSH [**thyroid-stimulating hormone, or thyrotropin**] **cells**) are found in small groups in an anterior wedge part of the gland. **Gonadotrophs** (FSH [**follicle-stimulating hormone**] and **LH** [**luteinizing hormone**] **cells**) are

evenly distributed throughout the anterior lobe. The same or different cells may produce the two hormones. Large, polyhedral **mammotrophs** (known as either **PRL** [**prolactin**] or **LTH** [**lactogenic hormone**] **cells**) are in posterior parts of the lateral wings. They are densely or sparsely granulated. In pregnant or lactating women, PRL cells usually undergo significant hyperplasia and hypertrophy.

CLINICAL POINT

Immunocytochemistry helps detect **pituitary adenomas** and allows diagnosis on the basis of hormones produced by neoplastic cells. **Prolactinoma,** accounting for 30% of all neoplastic pituitary tumors, is the most common type. A tumor of mammotrophs, it leads to amenorrhea, infertility, osteopenia, and galactorrhea in women and erectile dysfunction and loss of libido in men. *Amyloid* deposits and calcified spherites (or *psammoma bodies*) accompany excessive synthesis and secretion of prolactin. Treatment with the dopamine agonist bromocriptine reduces tumor size and inhibits prolactin secretion. Tumors larger than 10 mm in diameter (*macroadenomas*) require surgery or radiation.

Cell Type	Hormone	Principal Action	% of Cells
Acidophils			
Somatotroph	Growth hormone (GH)	Stimulates growth of bones, muscles, organs	40–50
Mammotroph	Prolactin (PRL)	Stimulates milk secretion	15–20
Basophils			
Corticotroph	Adrenocorticotropic hormone (ACTH)	Stimulates hormone release from adrenal cortex	15–20
Gonadotroph	Follicle-stimulating hormone (FSH), luteinizing hormone (LH)	Stimulates ovarian follicle development in females and spermatogenesis in males	10
Thyrotroph	Thyroid-stimulating hormone (TSH)	Stimulates thyroid hormone synthesis and secretion	5

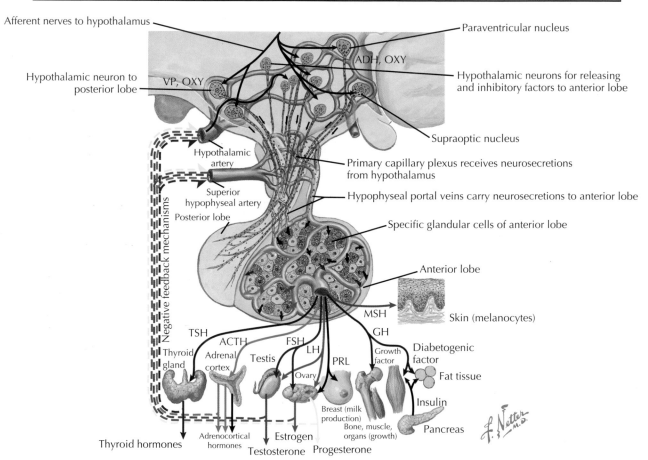

10.9 FUNCTIONS OF THE ADENOHYPOPHYSIS

The *hypothalamohypophyseal portal system* carries hypothalamic releasing and inhibiting factors secreted by modified neurons from two hypothalamic nuclei (*paraventricular* and *supraoptic*). Epithelial parenchymal cells in the adenohypophysis respond to these factors by secreting their own hormones, which, in turn, affect distant target organs. Target organ hormones then act on the hypothalamus and anterior lobe by *negative feedback* mecha-nisms. The anterior lobe contains two types of acidophils—**somatotrophs** and **mammotrophs**—that are best visualized by immunocytochemistry. They synthesize *growth hormone* and *pro-lactin*, respectively. Three types of basophils in the anterior lobe are also best seen via special stains. They are named **corticotrophs, gonadotrophs,** and **thyrotrophs** on the basis of the hormone that they secrete and their target organ. A subtype of basophil in the pars intermedia synthesizes *melanocyte-stimulating hormone.*

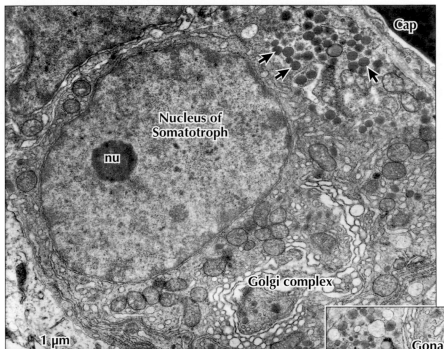

◀ **Electron micrograph (EM) of a somatotroph in the anterior lobe.** These ultrastructural features are typical of those of a protein-secreting endocrine cell. Many organelles such as a well-developed Golgi complex needed for hormone synthesis and clustered round to ovoid secretory vesicles (**arrows**) with a moderately dense core are close to the cell membrane. The oval euchromatic nucleus has a prominent nucleolus (**nu**). The cell abuts a fenestrated capillary (**Cap**), which contains an erythrocyte. 12,000×.

▶ **EM showing the varied appearance of secretory vesicles of two cell types in the anterior lobe.** The somatotroph has larger, more densely stained secretory vesicles than does the gonadotroph. In the interstices lie stellate fibroblast-like cells (**F**) with conspicuous cytoskeletal elements such as microtubules and filaments. Intercellular junctions, which are better seen at higher magnification, link these supportive cells. 10,000×.

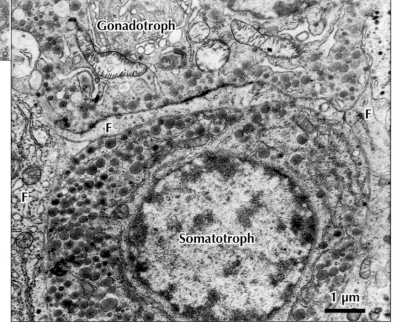

10.10   ULTRASTRUCTURE OF THE ANTERIOR LOBE

Electron microscopy has helped reveal the cytologic architecture of the adenohypophysis. The ultrastructure of its **parenchymal cells** closely resembles that of glandular epithelial cells of most other endocrine glands that synthesize and secrete protein hormones. These cells are round to polygonal, with organelles needed for synthesis, packaging, storage, and release of secretory products. Active cells have a prominent **Golgi complex,** many *mitochondria,* an extensive *rough endoplasmic reticulum,* and typical membrane-bound **secretory granules (vesicles).** The one nucleus is round to irregular in shape and has one or more prominent nucleoli. Secretory vesicles scattered in the cytoplasm or near the cell surface discharge by *exocytosis* close to thin-walled and highly permeable **fenestrated capillaries** with *diaphragms.* Rapid delivery of hormones and regulatory factors to and from the anterior lobe and bloodstream thus occurs. Electron microscopy used with immunocytochemistry can reveal the types of secretory cells in the anterior lobe. Correlation of size and morphology of secretory granules—which vary in size, shape, and staining properties—with immunocytochemical localization of antibodies to specific hormones permitted ultrastructural identification of cell types. Specific cell type/hormone associations include **somatotrophs/** *GH;* **mammotrophs/***PRL;* **thyrotrophs/***TSH;* **gonadotrophs/***LH* and *FSH,* and **corticotrophs/***ACTH.* An attenuated *basal lamina* covers cells externally. Also, stellate fibroblast-like cells with pale cytoplasm and prominent cytoskeleton form a supportive framework in the gland.

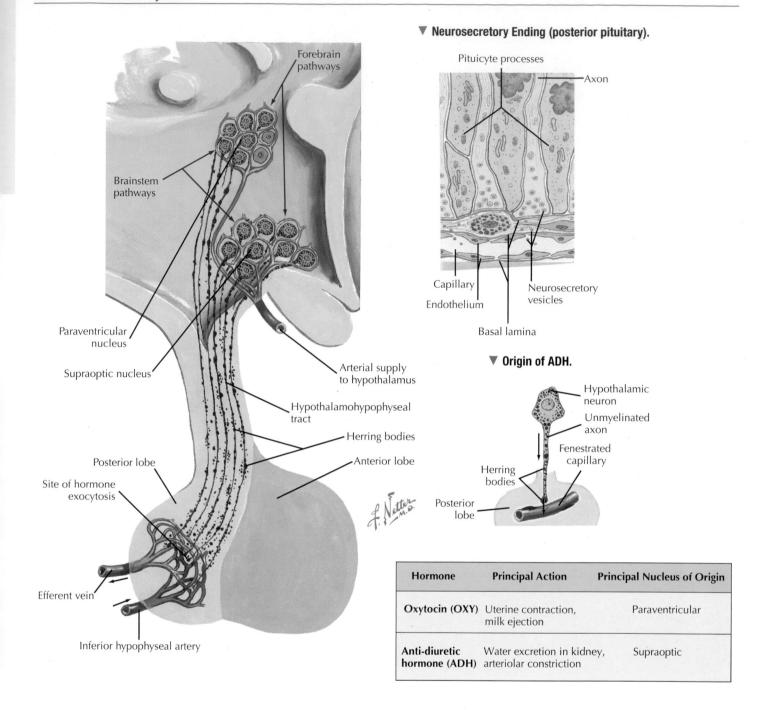

▼ Neurosecretory Ending (posterior pituitary).

Pituicyte processes

Axon

Capillary

Endothelium

Neurosecretory vesicles

Basal lamina

▼ Origin of ADH.

Hypothalamic neuron

Unmyelinated axon

Fenestrated capillary

Herring bodies

Posterior lobe

Forebrain pathways

Brainstem pathways

Paraventricular nucleus

Supraoptic nucleus

Arterial supply to hypothalamus

Hypothalamohypophyseal tract

Herring bodies

Anterior lobe

Posterior lobe

Site of hormone exocytosis

Efferent vein

Inferior hypophyseal artery

Hormone	Principal Action	Principal Nucleus of Origin
Oxytocin (OXY)	Uterine contraction, milk ejection	Paraventricular
Anti-diuretic hormone (ADH)	Water excretion in kidney, arteriolar constriction	Supraoptic

10.11 FUNCTIONS OF THE NEUROHYPOPHYSIS

The two peptide hormones released in the neurohypophysis are *oxytocin* and *antidiuretic hormone* (ADH, also known as vasopressin). Synthesized in **supraoptic** and **paraventricular nuclei** of the **hypothalamus,** they are taken via axoplasmic transport in the **hypothalamohypophyseal tract** to the posterior lobe. Then, in response to an action potential, they are discharged by exocytosis of *neurosecretory granules* directly to thin-walled sinusoidal fenestrated capillaries. Main actions of ADH are water excretion in the kidney and arteriolar constriction. Oxytocin stimulates uterine contraction during late stages of pregnancy and contraction of myoepithelial cells in the breast for milk ejection.

CLINICAL POINT
ADH promotes urinary concentration in the kidney. It increases absorption of glomerular filtrate in renal collecting ducts and distal convoluted tubules, thereby conserving water. Damage to supraoptic and paraventricular nuclei of the hypothalamus or destruction of the hypothalamohypophyseal tract may interfere with ADH production and lead to the rare **diabetes insipidus.** Symptoms are *polyuria,* with great amounts (15-20 L) of hypotonic urine produced daily, and *polydipsia* (extreme thirst), with a tendency to drink large quantities of fluid.

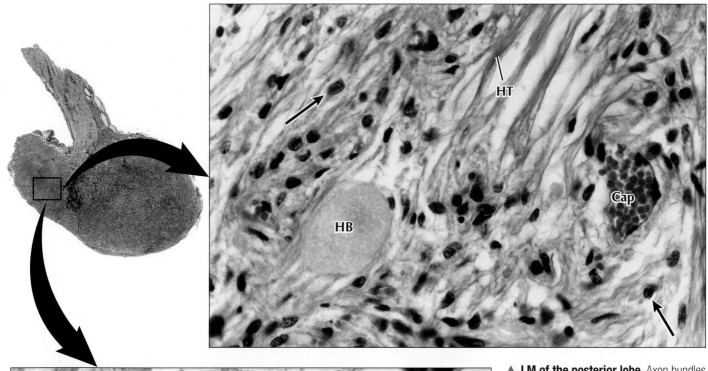

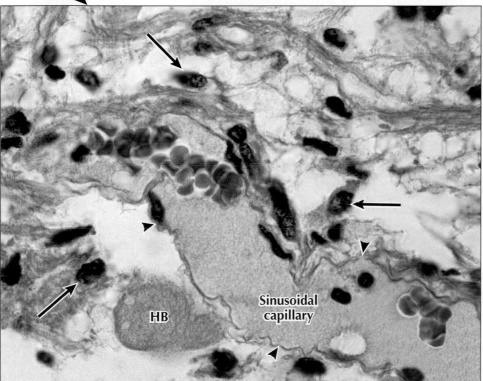

▲ **LM of the posterior lobe.** Axon bundles of the hypothalamohypophyseal tract (**HT**) mingle with many pituicytes with pleomorphic nuclei (**arrows**). A sinusoidal capillary (**Cap**), sectioned transversely, holds erythrocytes. A round Herring body (**HB**) can be recognized by its smooth, homogeneous, lightly stained appearance. 530×. *H&E.*

◀ **Higher magnification LM showing the intimate relation of a Herring body (HB) with a sinusoidal capillary.** The vessel has an attenuated wall (**arrowheads**), which is lined by endothelial cells. Its lumen contains erythrocytes and a few nucleated leukocytes. This relation allows rapid diffusion of stored neurosecretory material across the thin vessel wall and directly into the bloodstream. Many pituicytes (**arrows**) in nearby areas contain plump nuclei. 790×. *H&E.*

10.12   HISTOLOGY OF THE POSTERIOR LOBE

Most of the neurohypophysis consists largely of bundles of **unmyelinated axons** of **neurosecretory neurons** whose cell bodies are in the hypothalamic paraventricular and supraoptic nuclei. Mingled with about 100,000 axons of the **hypothalamohypophyseal tract** are distinctive irregularly shaped cells with oval nuclei—**pituicytes**—and a rich network of sinusoidal fenestrated capillaries. Like *astrocytes* of the central nervous system, pituicytes and their processes ensheath and support axons. Often difficult to see with the light microscope are **Herring bodies,** a unique feature of the neurohypophysis. These dilated terminal expansions of the axons contain aggregates of neurosecretory material, which are stored before release. By light microscopy, these bodies appear as amorphous, lightly eosinophilic amorphous areas in close contact with capillaries.

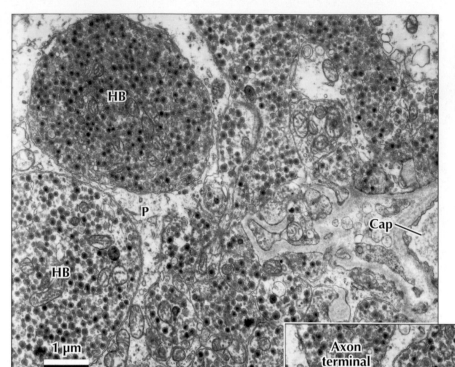

◀ **EM of the posterior lobe.** Many dilated axonal processes, filled with dense-core neurosecretory granules, are the ultrastructural equivalent of Herring bodies (**HB**). Part of a fenestrated capillary (**Cap**) is seen. The process of a pituicyte (**P**) is closely associated with axonal processes. 12,000×.

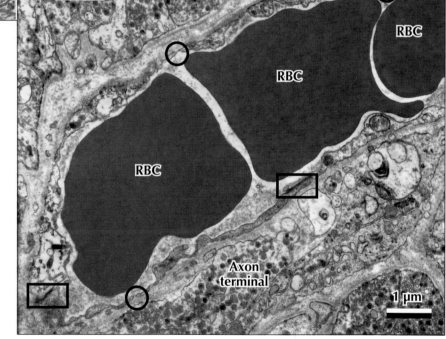

▶ **EM of part of a sinusoidal fenestrated capillary in the posterior lobe.** It is in close relation to many tightly packed axon terminals with abundant dense-core vesicles. Endothelial cells forming this capillary wall are very attenuated and are linked by intercellular junctions (**rectangles**). The many fenestrae (**circles**) enhance permeability. The capillary lumen shows three erythrocytes (**RBC**). 12,000×.

10.13 ULTRASTRUCTURE AND FUNCTION OF THE POSTERIOR LOBE

Electron microscopy best resolves neurohypophysis **neurosecretory granules** in **unmyelinated axons** and their terminal swellings in the neurohypophysis. These small membrane-bound **secretory vesicles** (120-200 nm in diameter) contain oxytocin or ADH, each combined with specific neurophysins. Axonal swellings have prominent *mitochondria* and many *microtubules* for axoplasmic transport. Nearby **pituicyte** processes appear as elongated, pleomorphic profiles with scanty cytoplasm. Adhering closely to surfaces of axonal varicosities, they provide an intimate spatial relationship like that seen between astrocytes and neuronal elements in the central nervous system. Abundant **sinusoidal capillaries** in the posterior lobe have walls with attenuated **endothelial cells** with numerous **fenestrae,** which have *diaphragms* covered externally by a thin perivascular *basal lamina.* Axon terminals are mainly filled with dense-core secretory vesicles, which are close to the sinusoidal endothelium. This facilitates axonal discharge of hormones and rapid diffusion of contents into the circulation. Oxytocin and ADH released from neurosecretory axons by *exocytosis* travel a short distance to cross the fenestrated endothelium and enter the bloodstream. Vesicle features vary within one axonal process, as between different axons. Clear axonal vesicles also accumulate in close relation to capillaries.

▼ **Anatomy of the thyroid and parathyroid glands.**

▼ **Development.**

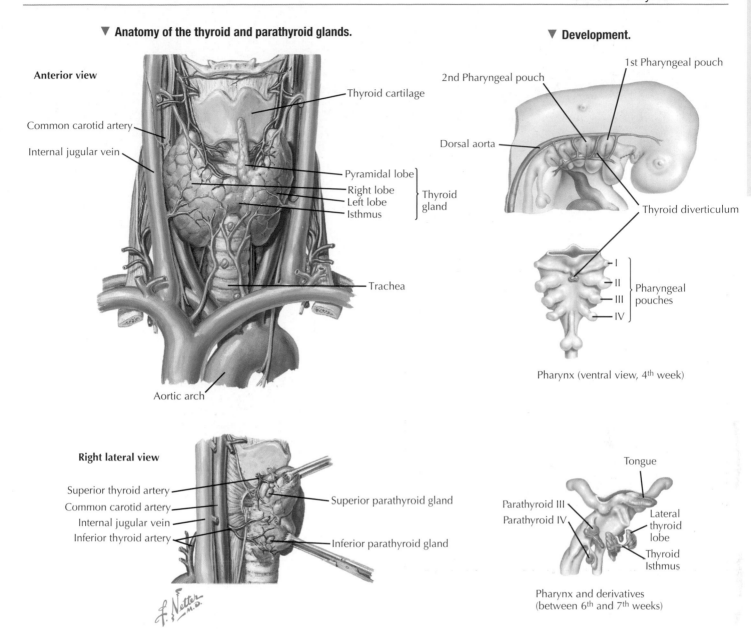

Anterior view

Common carotid artery

Internal jugular vein

Thyroid cartilage

Pyramidal lobe
Right lobe
Left lobe } Thyroid gland
Isthmus

Trachea

Aortic arch

2nd Pharyngeal pouch

1st Pharyngeal pouch

Dorsal aorta

Thyroid diverticulum

I
II } Pharyngeal pouches
III
IV

Pharynx (ventral view, 4th week)

Right lateral view

Superior thyroid artery
Common carotid artery
Internal jugular vein
Inferior thyroid artery

Superior parathyroid gland

Inferior parathyroid gland

Tongue

Parathyroid III
Parathyroid IV

Lateral thyroid lobe
Thyroid Isthmus

Pharynx and derivatives
(between 6th and 7th weeks)

10.14 OVERVIEW OF THE THYROID AND PARATHYROID

The thyroid lies in the lower part of the front of the neck in contact with the upper trachea. A **connective tissue capsule** derived from cervical fascia encloses the two **lobes** and a connecting **isthmus.** The normal gland is asymmetric, with the right lobe often twice as large as the left. Each is the size of a flattened chestnut. A small pyramidal lobe, a vestige of embryonic **thyroglossal duct,** persists in about 15% of the population. Adults typically have four small ovoid parathyroid glands, each about the size of an apple seed—3 by 6 mm. They are embedded on the thyroid's posterior surface, close to branching **superior** and **inferior thyroid arteries,** which

provide a rich vascular supply. A thin fibrous connective tissue capsule surrounding each gland separates it from the thyroid. In the 4-week embryo, the thyroid develops at the level of the first and second **pharyngeal pouches** from an endodermal sac-like ventral diverticulum of the pharynx. First connected to the pharynx floor by the thyroglossal duct, the sac migrates caudally, losing its connection to the surface to give rise to thyroid parenchyma. Surrounding **mesenchyme** becomes its stroma. By 6 weeks of gestation, parathyroids develop bilaterally from **endoderm** of the third and fourth pharyngeal pouches, which lose their connection to the pharyngeal surface.

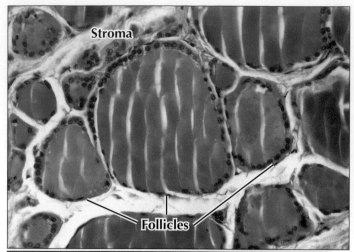

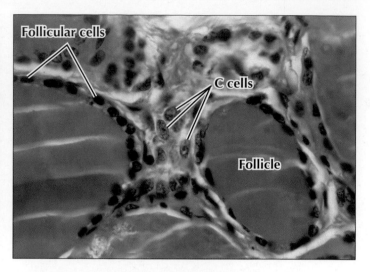

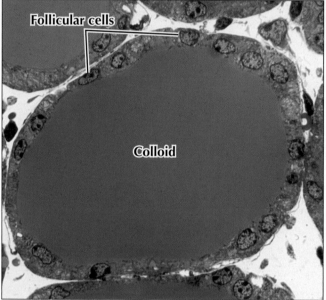

▲ **LM of the thyroid at higher magnification.** A small clump of parafollicular (**C**) cells is in the stroma between follicles. Large size and clear, lightly stained cytoplasm identify these cells. Each contains a spherical euchromatic nucleus. Follicular cells around each follicle are low to high cuboidal and have darkly stained nuclei. They are fairly small compared with the parafollicular cells. 550×. *H&E.*

▲ **LM of the thyroid at low magnification.** Closely packed follicles—functioning units of the gland—have varied sizes and shapes. One layer of flattened to cuboidal epithelial cells lines each one. Lumina contain thyroglobulin, which appears homogeneous and eosinophilic, with some crack-like fixation artifacts. Loose connective tissue makes up the delicate stroma that contains a network of capillaries, which are hard to see. 240×. *H&E.*

◀ **LM of a thyroid follicle.** The gelatinous colloid in this mouse thyroid follicle lacks fixation artifacts and looks homogeneous. A continuous layer of follicular cells lines the follicular lumen. The cells have euchromatic nuclei because they are functionally active. 640×. *Plastic section, toluidine blue.*

10.15 HISTOLOGY AND FUNCTION OF THE THYROID

Trabeculae of the *capsule* penetrate the gland to provide internal support and a pathway for a large vascular and nervous supply. **Glandular parenchyma** consists of spherical **follicles** of various sizes (50-500 μm in diameter) whose total number may exceed 20 million. Follicle lumina are filled with gelatinous **colloid** made of *thyroglobulin.* This iodinated glycoprotein is the temporary storage form and precursor to main thyroid hormones before release as *triiodothyronine* (T_3) and *tetraiodothyronine* (*thyroxine;* T_4). They increase oxygen consumption and metabolic rates of most body tissues and are essential for normal growth, maturation, and mental activity. Follicles are lined by simple cuboidal epithelium, which consists of thyroid **follicular cells** that rest on an inconspicuous *basement membrane.* The height of the epithelium varies with function: usually low cuboidal in an underactive gland and high in an overactive one. A large network of **fenestrated capillaries** is in delicate reticular **connective tissue** between follicles. Also, small numbers of larger and paler **parafollicular** (or **C**) **cells** lie, as single cells or small groups, between the basement mem-

brane of the follicles and follicular cells, or in an interfollicular position. These *neural crest*-derived parenchymal cells secrete *calcitonin,* which lowers blood calcium levels and counterbalances actions of parathyroid hormone. Hard to see in routine histologic sections, they are best revealed by immunocytochemical methods or electron microscopy.

CLINICAL POINT

Goiter, a nonspecific term for chronic enlargement of the thyroid, may occur in various disorders of this organ. *Hyperthyroidism* leads to many thyroid diseases, the most common being **exophthalmic goiter (Graves disease).** This *autoimmune disorder* is caused by antibodies to the TSH receptor on follicular cells. Histologically, the enlarged gland contains highly infolded follicles lined by high cuboidal epithelium. Thyroid hormone production increases markedly, colloid volume is reduced, and TSH production by the adenohypophysis is suppressed. Lymphocyte infiltration of surrounding stroma accompanies lymphoid follicles with germinal centers.

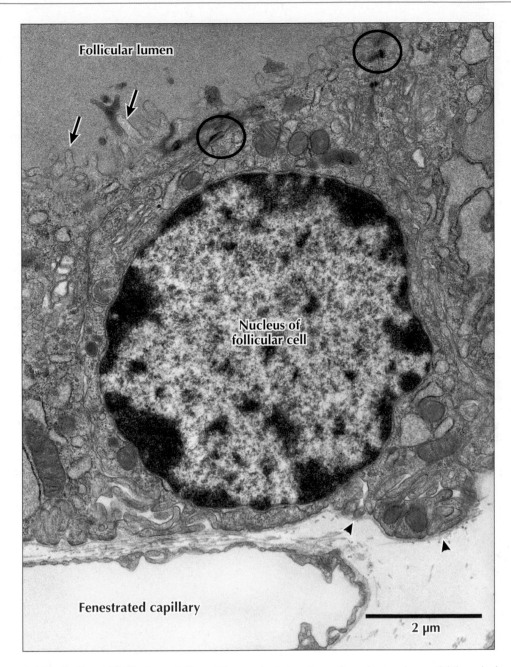

Follicular lumen

Nucleus of
follicular cell

Fenestrated capillary

2 μm

▲ **EM of a thyroid follicular cell.** The cell has a spherical euchromatic nucleus and many tightly packed organelles. Its basal aspect is close to a fenestrated capillary. Short stubby microvilli (**arrows**) project from its apical surface into a colloid-filled follicular lumen. Intercellular junctions (**circles**) link lateral borders of the cells, whose basal surfaces rest on an inconspicuous basal lamina (**arrowheads**). 15,000×.

10.16 ULTRASTRUCTURE AND FUNCTION OF THYROID FOLLICULAR CELLS

The thyroid differs from other endocrine glands by storing an intermediate secretory product—*thyroglobulin*—extracellularly as **colloid** rather than internally in cytoplasmic vesicles. Pituitary *TSH* stimulates synthesis and storage of thyroglobulin. Amino acids are taken up from the bloodstream at the base of **follicular cells.** This tyrosine-rich protein is synthesized on the *rough endoplasmic reticulum* (RER), followed by glycosylation in the RER and *Golgi complex,* and packaging in vesicles. Fusion of vesicles with apical *plasma membrane* leads to *exocytosis* of thyroglobulin into follicle lumina. Uptake of circulating iodide at the cell basal membrane is followed by oxidation by peroxidase and transfer to cell apices. Enzymes in apical **microvilli** that project into colloid catalyze iodination of tyrosine residues in thyroglobulin. Stimulation by TSH causes follicular cells to pinocytose portions of colloid and form vesicles containing iodinated thyroglobulin. They fuse with lysosomes that cleave thyroglobulin. Resultant T_3 and T_4 diffuse out of *secondary lysosomes* and cross the basal plasma membrane to reach the bloodstream in **fenestrated capillaries.** T_3 and T_4 act on cells in the body to increase basal metabolic rate, promote cell growth, increase heart rate, raise body temperature, and enhance energy-requiring cell functions. They also act on *thyrotrophs* in the adenohypophysis to reduce TSH secretion by negative feedback.

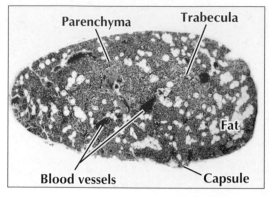

Parenchyma   Trabecula

Blood vessels   Capsule

Fat

▲ **LM of the parathyroid in the midsagittal plane.**
A delicate connective tissue capsule sends in trabeculae
to penetrate the parenchyma and divide it into irregular
lobules. Blood vessels are abundant. With age,
numerous fat cells intermingle with parenchyma.
20×. *H&E.*

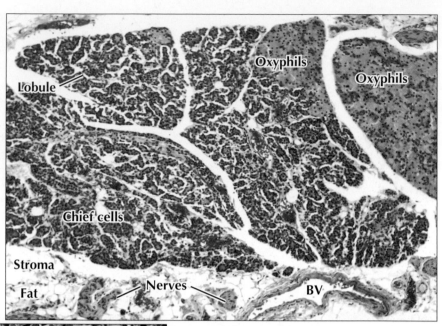

Oxyphils

Oxyphils

Lobule

Chief cells

Stroma

Fat   Nerves   BV

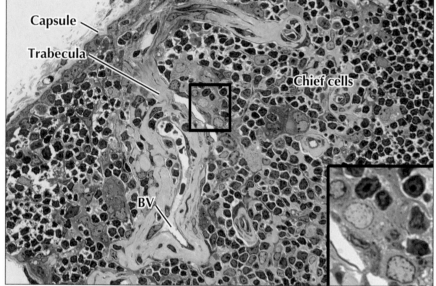

Capsule

Trabecula

Chief cells

BV

▲ **LM of part of the parathyroid.** Organization of the
parenchyma and stroma is seen. Blood vessels (**BV**),
nerves, and fat cells occupy the stroma. Parenchymal
cells form irregular, poorly defined lobules. Chief cells
predominate and are arranged in cords; nests of oxyphils
either mingle with chief cells or are in separate lobules.
80×. *H&E.*

◀ **LM of the outer part of the parathyroid.** A
capsule surrounding the organ sends in a trabecula
that conveys blood vessels (**BV**) to the interior. Most
of the parenchyma consists of tightly packed chief
cells (shown at higher magnification in the inset).
400×; inset: 650×. *Plastic section, toluidine blue.*

10.17 HISTOLOGY AND FUNCTION OF THE PARATHYROID

The outer fibrous **capsule** gives rise to delicate **trabeculae** that convey **blood vessels**, lymphatics, and **nerves** to the interior of the gland and divide it into poorly defined **lobules**. The parathyroid synthesizes and secretes *parathyroid hormone* (PTH), which maintains blood calcium levels by increasing the rate of osteoclastic activity, thus mobilizing calcium from bone. The adult **parenchyma** consists of two types of cells—**chief cells** and **oxyphils.** The polyhedral, slightly eosinophilic chief cells are more numerous and form irregular, anastomosing **cords** supported by delicate connective issue. The source of PTH, they have features of other endocrine secretory cells and are close to an extensive network of **capillaries.** Oxyphils, which appear after the first decade of life, are larger, more acidophilic cells that are irregularly distributed and occur singly or in clumps. By electron microscopy, oxyphils are packed with *mitochondria* but, unlike chief cells, lack *secretory*

vesicles; they are thought to be nonsecretory. **Fat cells** may also be found in the **stroma** and increase in number with age. Parathyroid glands are essential for life.

CLINICAL POINT

Primary hyperparathyroidism is usually due to an *adenoma* of one or more parathyroid glands. Histologically, these tumors are made of tightly packed sheets of mostly chief cells, interspersed with multinuclear giant cells. Excessive production of PTH in this disorder leads to *hypercalcemia* (high serum calcium levels) because of increased osteoclastic activity of bone. Enhanced reabsorption of calcium in renal tubules may lead to *nephrolithiasis*, or formation of renal stones, rich in calcium oxalate and calcium phosphate. A rare form of primary hyperparathyroidism is due to *carcinoma* of the parathyroid, which typically has a poor prognosis because of a high incidence of recurrence and tendency to metastasize to distant sites.

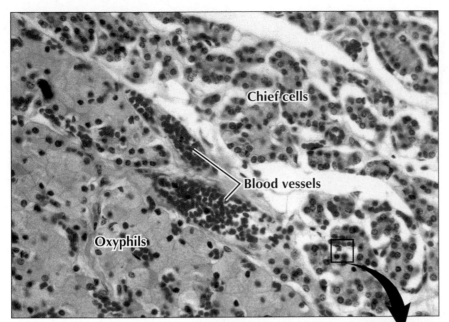

◀ **LM of part of the parathyroid at high magnification.** Features of the two main types of parenchymal cells are seen. Chief cells are spherical and have pale cytoplasm with a central, round nucleus. Oxyphils are larger and more eosinophilic, each with a small dark nucleus. The stroma contains abundant blood vessels, most being sinusoidal capillaries that are in close contact with parenchymal cells and many being filled with erythrocytes. 300×. *H&E.*

▼ **Ultrastructure of parathyroid gland.**

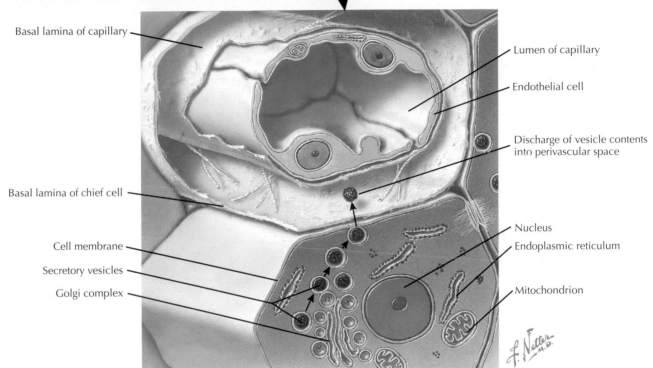

10.18 HISTOLOGY AND ULTRASTRUCTURE OF PARATHYROID CHIEF CELLS

Ultrastructure of parathyroid chief cells and the mode of secretion are typical of those of other polypeptide-secreting endocrine cells. These features correlate with the cells' functional activity. These polyhedral cells, 5-8 μm in diameter, are linked to neighboring cells by **desmosomes**. A prominent **nucleolus** occupies the nucleus. In active cells, cytoplasm around the small **euchromatic nucleus** contains a prominent juxtanuclear **Golgi complex**. Numerous flat cisternae of RER, scattered free **ribosomes,** a few **mitochondria,** occasional **lysosomes,** and small **glycogen** deposits are also present. Many small (200-400 nm in diameter) **secretory vesicles** are a prominent feature of these cells. Membrane-bound, the vesicles have a dense core surrounded by a clear halo. They contain the polypeptide PTH, and many are seen near the **plasma membrane** where it abuts the perivascular space, which surrounds the attenuated **endothelium** of **fenestrated capillaries.** Thin **basal laminae** surround plasma membranes of chief cells and capillary endothelial cells. A few **collagen fibrils** occupy the intervening perivascular space. As in other endocrine cells, fusion of secretory vesicles with the plasma membrane facilitates discharge of hormone to the bloodstream (*exocytosis*). This occurs in response to *hypocalcemia* (low blood calcium levels).

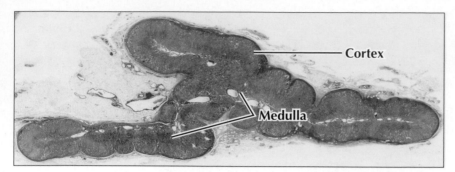

◄ LM of the whole adrenal in the midsagittal plane. Its triangular, flattened shape resembles a cocked hat. The gland is divided into an outer cortex and an inner medulla which contains large vascular channels. 6×. *H&E.*

▼ Histology of the adrenal gland.

▼ Anatomy and blood supply of the adrenal (suprarenal) glands.

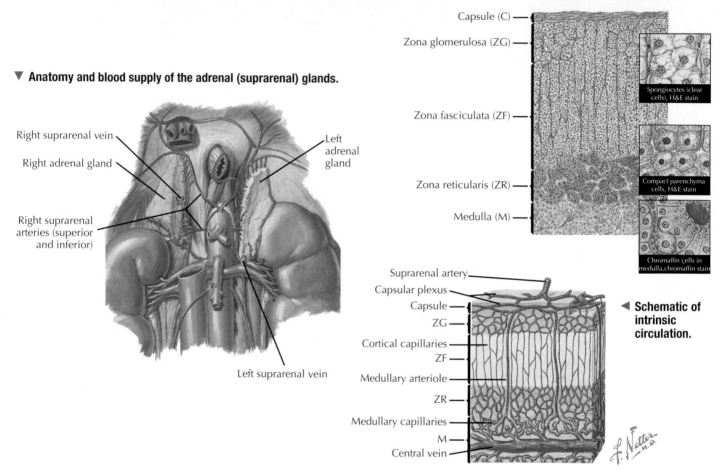

◄ Schematic of intrinsic circulation.

10.19 OVERVIEW OF THE ADRENAL AND ITS BLOOD SUPPLY

The paired **adrenal,** or **suprarenal, glands** lie on the superior pole of each kidney. Roughly triangular, flattened glands, they are about 7 cm long, 3 cm high, and 1 cm thick, with a combined weight of about 10 g. Each is an organ composed of two distinct parts—**cortex** and **medulla**—with separate functions, and all-enclosed in a common **connective tissue capsule.** Adrenals have a rich vascular supply. The cortex receives blood from many arterioles in the capsule that enter the gland and break up into **sinusoidal capillaries,** which pass downward in close association with

parenchymal cells in the cortex. The capillaries, with thin endothelium and many fenestrations, pass through all three layers of the cortex. At the corticomedullary junction, they drain into veins, which enter the medulla. Some arterioles from the capsule do not supply the cortex but go directly into the medulla. There, they drain into sinusoidal fenestrated capillaries, which lead into collecting veins. The medulla thus has a dual blood supply. Venous blood from both cortex and medulla is drained by a large **central vein,** which exits at the *hilum* of the gland as the *adrenal (or suprarenal) vein.*

Embryonic origin and development of the adrenal gland

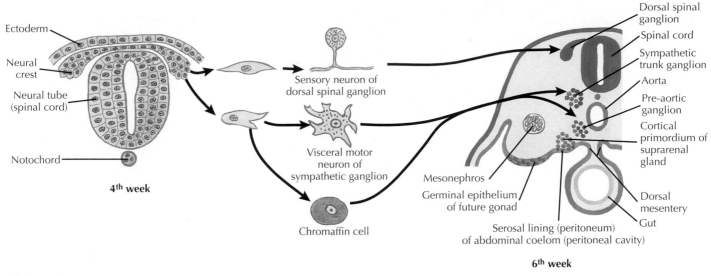

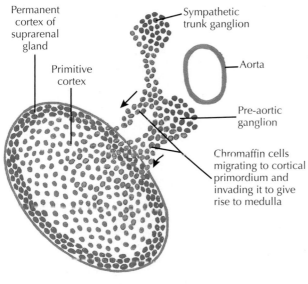

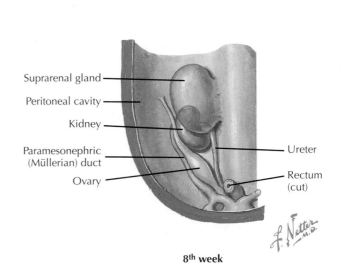

10.20 DEVELOPMENT OF THE ADRENAL

The adrenal arises from two distinct embryonic tissues: **meso-derm** (which develops into the **cortex**) and **neural crest ectoderm** (which develops into the **medulla**). During development, they become a single gland and are enveloped by a common *connective tissue capsule.* Early in gestation, the *fetal (or provisional) cortex* of each gland arises from proliferating mesodermal cells of **peritoneal epithelium.** These cells are near the root of the dorsal mesentery and next to the cranial end of the primitive kidney, called the *mesonephros.* This close anatomic relation to the kidney remains throughout life, so the gland is named the adrenal (or suprarenal) gland. The first group of mesodermal cells is then surrounded by a second mass of tightly packed mesodermal cells that will become the *permanent (or adult) cortex.* The fetal cortex,

active during fetal life, produces corticosteroids and at birth makes up about 80% of the gland. It then undergoes rapid involution and within the first few months after birth, the permanent cortex replaces it. It differentiates in the next 3 years into three distinct zones: *glomerulosa, fasciculata,* and *reticularis.* The medulla derives from neural crest cells that migrated in the early fetus to form the **celiac ganglia** of the *sympathetic* part of the *autonomic nervous system.* These cells migrate to the cortex and invade it to form the inner medulla. Their content of epinephrine causes these cells to stain yellow-brown when exposed to chrome salts, thus the name *chromaffin cells.* They form synapses with preganglionic sympathetic nerve fibers, but rather than becoming ganglion cells, they form *secretory epithelial cells* that produce the two hormones of the medulla.

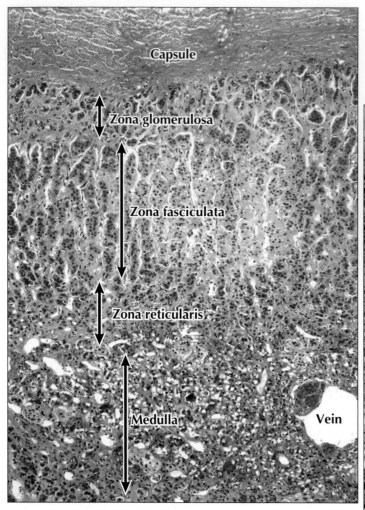

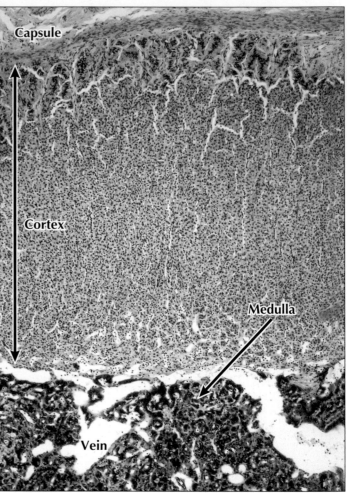

◀ **LM of the adrenal at low magnification.** The outer capsule is made of dense fibrous connective tissue. The cortex has three distinct zones with cells arranged in cords perpendicular to the capsule. The inner medulla has an irregular network of cells in close association with many capillaries and thin-walled veins. 95×. *H&E.*

▶ **LM of the adrenal fixed in a potassium dichromate solution.** With this method, parenchymal cells in the medulla undergo a histochemical reaction that readily separates them from parenchymal cells in the cortex. The medullary cells, named chromaffin cells, have brown cytoplasm. 80×. *Chromaffin.*

10.21   HISTOLOGY AND HISTOCHEMISTRY OF THE ADRENAL

The outer **cortex** and inner **medulla** of the adrenal differ structurally, functionally, and developmentally. The cortex is essential to life, but the medulla is not. The cortex, yellow to the naked eye, makes up 90% of the gland. Its secretory cells produce three classes of *steroid hormones.* The medulla makes up 10% of the gland and in life is reddish-brown. Its secretory cells are called **chromaffin cells** because of a characteristic *chromaffin reaction* in response to oxidation by salts of chromic acid. These cells are the source of the catecholamines *epinephrine* and *norepinephrine,* which are stored in secretory granules. The reaction occurs after fixation with potassium dichromate, which results in oxidation of the catecholamine precursors and a brown stain. The outer **capsule** is made of dense fibrous **connective tissue,** which consists mostly of collagen interspersed with fibroblasts. The capsule sends

thin *trabeculae* into the gland interior; these give rise to a delicate *stroma* made mostly of reticular fibers and forming a supportive network for parenchymal cells in both cortex and medulla.

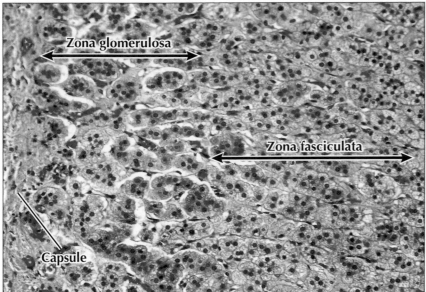

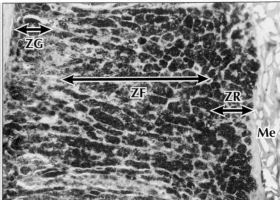

▲ **LM of the adrenal stained to show lipid.** Lipid droplets in cells of zonae glomerulosa (**ZG**), fasciculata (**ZF**), and reticularis (**ZR**) stain red; cells in the medulla (**Me**), without fat, are unstained. 60×. *Oil red O, hematoxylin.*

▲ **LM of the adrenal cortex.** Note the distinctive arrangements and morphology of darker parenchymal cells of the zona glomerulosa under the capsule and pale, lipid-laden spongiocytes of the zona fasciculata. Spongiocytes in this area form radial cords, usually one or two cells thick. A network of thin-walled, fenestrated capillaries occupies intervening spaces. 175×. *H&E.*

▶ **LM of the adrenal medulla showing the irregular, anastomosing arrangement of its polyhedral parenchymal cells.** Cords or clusters of these chromaffin cells are in close relation to a large network of vascular elements, mostly sinusoidal capillaries. Lightly basophilic cytoplasm and one round euchromatic nucleus typify each cell. Delicate connective tissue stroma supports the parenchyma. 285×. *H&E.*

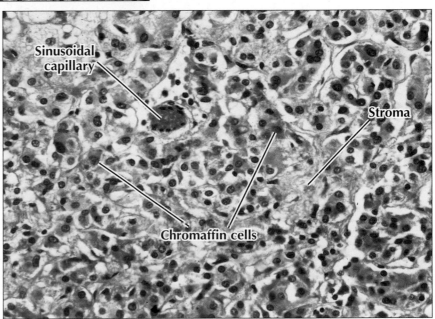

10.22 HISTOLOGY AND FUNCTION OF THE ADRENAL CORTEX AND MEDULLA

Three concentric zones characterize the cortex. The **zona glomerulosa,** just under the capsule, represents 10%-15% of the cortex and is made of closely packed, rounded clusters of parenchymal cells that produce *mineralocorticoids,* mainly *aldosterone.* The middle **zona fasciculata,** forming up to 75% of the cortex, consists mainly of radially oriented cords of polyhedral cells in close relation to **sinusoidal fenestrated capillaries.** These cells contain many lipid droplets, so they appear washed out and are called **spongiocytes.** The main source of *steroid hormones* such as cortisol, they also produce *androgens.* The thin innermost **zona reticularis** makes up 5%-10% of the cortex. Its smaller, more acidophilic parenchymal cells are arranged as an anastomosing network of short cords with intervening sinusoidal capillaries.

These cells synthesize androgens. The medulla contains cords or nests of polyhedral **chromaffin cells** surrounded by fenestrated capillaries. Developmentally, they are modified postganglionic sympathetic neurons that produce two classes of *catecholamines.*

CLINICAL POINT

Pheochromocytoma and **neuroblastoma** are tumors of the adrenal medulla. Occurring mostly in adults, pheochromocytoma is a *neoplasm* that arises from catecholamine-producing cells. Ensuing elevated levels of epinephrine and norepinephrine released into the blood lead to sustained or intermittent hypertension. In contrast, neuroblastoma is a *malignant tumor* of infancy and childhood. It derives from embryonic neural crest cells that normally migrate to give rise to either chromaffin cells of the medulla or postganglionic nerve cells in peripheral ganglia. Tumors arising from these cells retain embryonic migratory features.

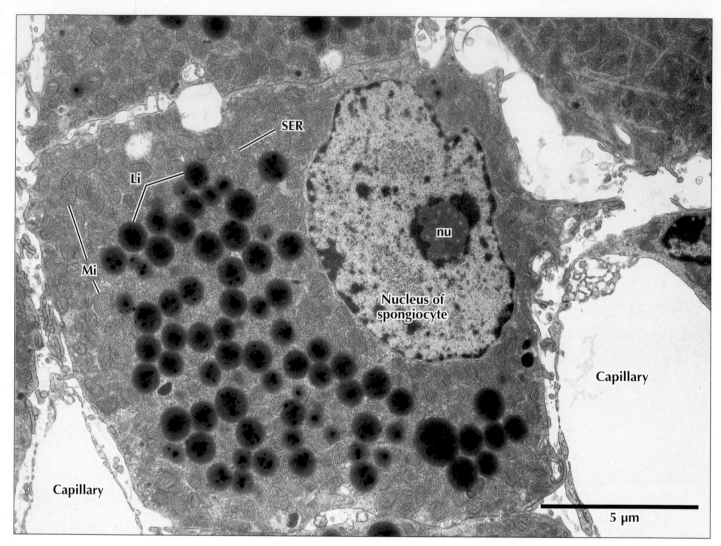

▲ **EM of a spongiocyte in the adrenal cortex.** The cell is associated with two closely apposed fenestrated capillaries and abuts two other spongiocytes. Many round, electron-dense lipid droplets (**Li**) are in the cytoplasm, which also shows smooth endoplasmic reticulum (**SER**) and mitochondria (**Mi**) with tubulovesicular cristae. A euchromatic nucleus with a prominent nucleolus (**nu**) is typical of this active cell. The endothelium in the capillary walls is quite thin and fenestrated. 8200×.

10.23 ULTRASTRUCTURE OF SPONGIOCYTES IN THE ZONA FASCICULATA

The ultrastructure of spongiocytes in this zone is consistent with a role in synthesis and secretion of *steroid hormones.* As in other steroid-secreting cells, abundant **smooth endoplasmic reticulum** (SER) and **tubulovesicular mitochondria** are hallmark features of the cytoplasm. Non-membrane-bound **lipid droplets,** also abundant, are storage sites for *cholesterol,* a precursor to cortico-steroid hormones. Cholesterol is taken to mitochondria, where it is processed and modified by cleavage. Mitochondria here have an increased surface area of internal cristae to accommodate cata-lytic enzymes involved in the cleavage. SER membranes also contain enzymes involved in hormone modification and synthe-sis. As a rule, these steroid-secreting cells do not store secretory products but synthesize them only when needed. Lipid-soluble hormones are released into the bloodstream via adjacent **fenes-trated capillaries.** Spongiocyte *plasma membranes* often bear short, stubby *microvilli,* which amplify surface area for secretion. Next to the perivascular space, these membranes are in contact with a thin, intervening *basal lamina* of the attenuated, fenestrated endothelium of adjacent capillaries. Ultrastructural features of secretory cells in zonae glomerulosa and reticularis are similar to those of spongiocytes in the fasciculata, but usually fewer lipid droplets are found. *Lipofuscin,* a wear-and-tear pigment associated with *tertiary lysosomes,* is often more abundant in the zona reticu-laris than in other cortical layers.

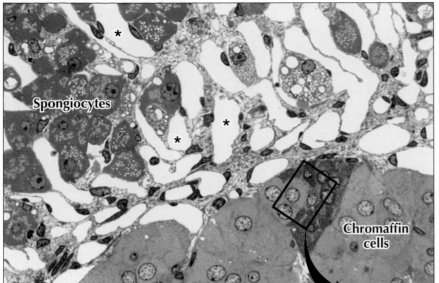

◀ **LM of the junction between adrenal cortex and medulla.** Part of the zona reticularis (left) shows spongiocytes and a closely associated network of sinusoidal capillaries (∗). Light and dark chromaffin cells are in the medulla (lower right). 1000×. *Toluidine blue, plastic section.*

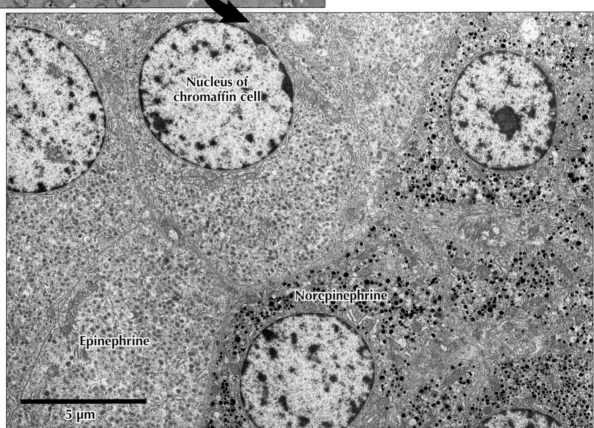

▲ **EM of the adrenal medulla at low magnification.** Closely packed chromaffin cells have round euchromatic nuclei and cytoplasm filled with many dense-core secretory vesicles. Norepinephrine vesicles are relatively large and quite electron dense. Vesicles storing epinephrine are usually smaller with a light or moderately dense core. 6600×.

10.24 ULTRASTRUCTURE OF CHROMAFFIN CELLS IN THE ADRENAL MEDULLA

The distinguishing ultrastructural feature of medullary chromaffin cells is the presence of membrane-bound, electron-dense **secretory vesicles.** These Golgi-derived cytoplasmic organelles, 150-350 nm in diameter, are storage sites for the two main peptide hormones of the medulla. As a rule, **epinephrine** is stored in smaller vesicles with a light or moderately dense core; **norepi-**nephrine is in larger vesicles with very high density content. Mammals such as rodents have two types of chromaffin cells—one with only epinephrine vesicles and one with entirely norepinephrine vesicles. In humans, however, most vesicles contain norepinephrine, and the same chromaffin cell typically includes both hormones. *Preganglionic sympathetic neurons,* which innervate these cells, regulate their secretion.

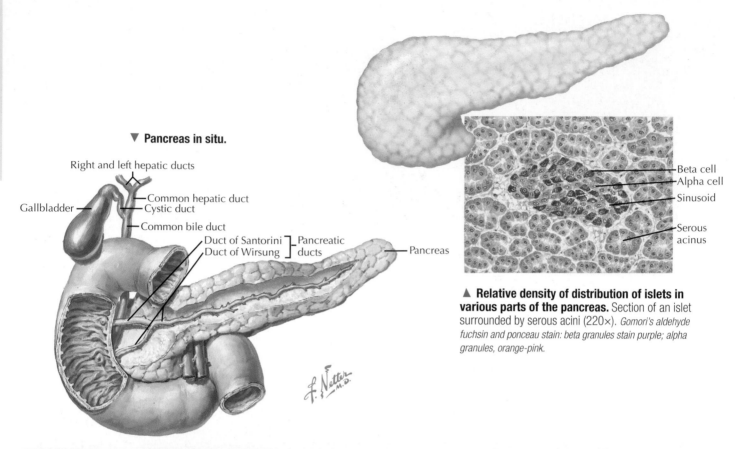

▼ **Pancreas in situ.**

Right and left hepatic ducts

Common hepatic duct
Cystic duct

Gallbladder

Common bile duct

Duct of Santorini ⎤ Pancreatic
Duct of Wirsung ⎦ ducts

Pancreas

f. Netter M.D.

Beta cell
Alpha cell
Sinusoid
Serous acinus

▲ **Relative density of distribution of islets in various parts of the pancreas.** Section of an islet surrounded by serous acini (220×). *Gomori's aldehyde fuchsin and ponceau stain: beta granules stain purple; alpha granules, orange-pink.*

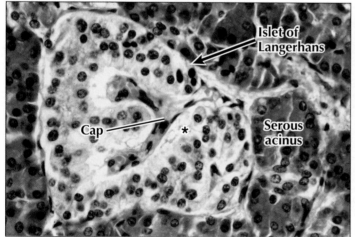

Islet of Langerhans

Cap

*

Serous acinus

▲ **LM of the pancreas.** Dark serous acini surround a richly vascularized islet of Langerhans. Delicate loose connective tissue (*) invests a compact aggregate of pale islet cells. A capillary (**Cap**) ramifies in the islet center. Precise identification of individual cells requires either electron microscopy or more specialized immunocytochemistry. 470×. *H&E.*

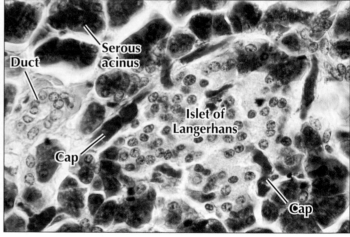

Serous acinus

Duct

Islet of Langerhans

Cap

Cap

▲ **LM of an islet of Langerhans in the pancreas.** Many closely packed, pale cells make up the islet. These spherical cells contain one euchromatic nucleus. Several capillaries (**Cap**) supply blood to the islet. Surrounding exocrine pancreas contains serous acini and a small duct. 390×. *Masson's trichrome.*

10.25 OVERVIEW AND HISTOLOGY OF ISLETS OF LANGERHANS

The **pancreas** is a major *exocrine gland* of the digestive tract with a well-developed acinar and duct system. Early in embryonic development, groups of cells arise from ends of endodermally derived ducts and then lose connection with them. These cells form small spherical clumps and become the **endocrine** parts of the pancreas—islets of Langerhans. Individual islets are scattered throughout the pancreas, but they are twice as numerous in the tail of the gland as in other parts. About 1 million exist in the normal human pancreas and together weigh only about 1.5 g. Islet diameters are 300 μm or less. Richly vascularized, islets are incompletely separated from the exocrine pancreas by scanty investment of delicate reticular **connective tissue. Islet cells** make up compact, cord-like clusters and in H&E sections appear as closely packed, pale-stained polygonal cells. Distinguishing different types of islet cells requires special stains.

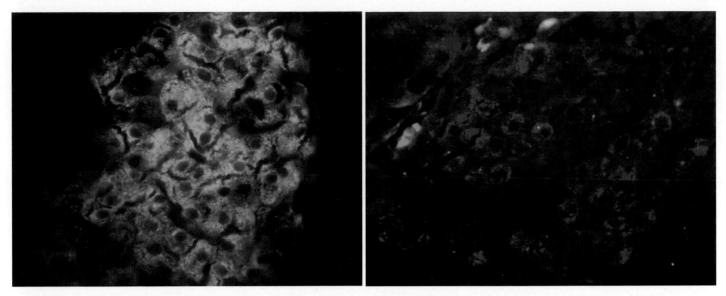

▲ **Companion frozen section LMs of islets of the normal (Left) and type 1 diabetic (Right) mouse pancreas.** Immunofluorescent treatment localizes antibodies to insulin in beta cells (green) and glucagon in alpha cells (red). In the normal islet, alpha cells are mostly at the periphery with a few isolated cells in the interior; beta cells, the predominant cell type, occupy the central area. In the type 1 diabetic islet, beta cells are almost absent and alpha cells predominate. This form of diabetes is caused by autoimmune destruction of beta cells. 585×. *Alexa Fluor and Texas Red. (Courtesy of Dr. B. Verchere)*

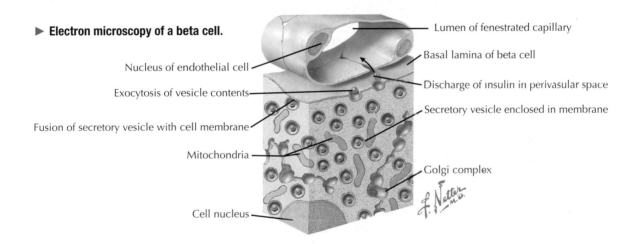

▶ **Electron microscopy of a beta cell.**

- Lumen of fenestrated capillary
- Nucleus of endothelial cell
- Basal lamina of beta cell
- Exocytosis of vesicle contents
- Discharge of insulin in perivasular space
- Fusion of secretory vesicle with cell membrane
- Secretory vesicle enclosed in membrane
- Mitochondria
- Golgi complex
- Cell nucleus

10.26 IMMUNOCYTOCHEMISTRY AND ULTRASTRUCTURE OF PANCREATIC BETA CELLS

Immunocytochemistry utilizing antibodies conjugated to fluorescent markers for insulin and other hormones, which are produced by **islet cells,** provides precise means to selectively stain various cell types in islets. This powerful tool can show how certain diseases such as *diabetes* affect islet cell morphology. Electron microscopy is also useful for determining normal beta cell ultrastructure. It helps elucidate intracellular pathways in synthesis and secretion of insulin, and discharge of this peptide hormone by *exocytosis* into circulation. Beta cell cytoplasm contains a prominent juxtanuclear **Golgi complex,** moderate amounts of RER, scattered free *ribosomes,* and few, small **mitochondria.** Distinctive membrane-bound **secretory vesicles,** which derive from the Golgi complex, dominate the cytoplasm, usually between the ovoid **nucleus** of the cell and the **plasma membrane,** which abuts a **fenestrated capillary.** Vesicle morphology differs markedly among species and among other islet cell types, but secretory vesicles in human beta cells, about 200-250 nm in diameter, typically have an electron-dense crystalloid composed of an insulin-zinc complex, surrounded by pale matrix, and enclosed by a loosely fitting membrane.

CLINICAL POINT

Diabetes mellitus is a disorder of the endocrine pancreas with high morbidity and mortality in humans. Two main clinical types have different causes. *Type 1—insulin-dependent diabetes—*is caused by autoimmune destruction of islet beta cells. In early stages, lymphocytes infiltrate islets; islets later fail to produce insulin, show fibrosis, and accumulate amyloid. In *type 2—non-insulin-dependent diabetes—*islets usually appear normal but produce inadequate amounts of insulin, and target cell receptors for insulin are abnormal.

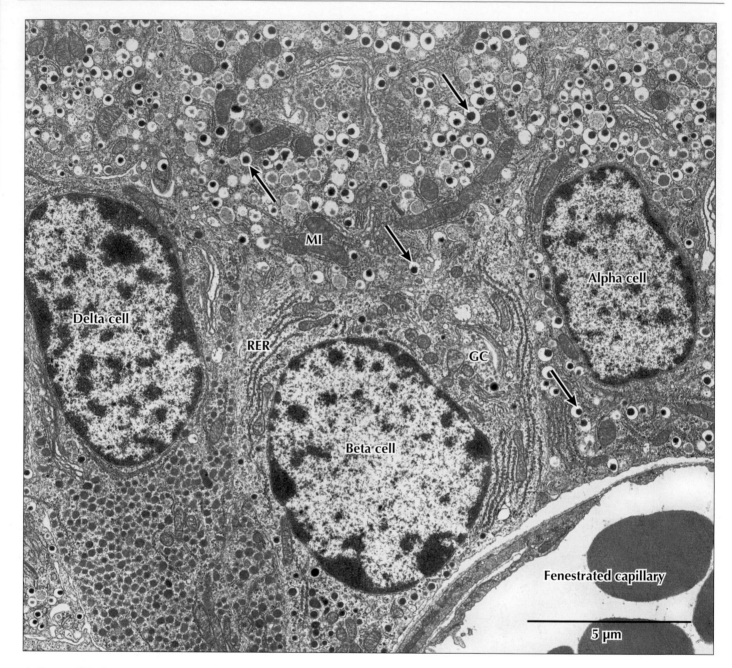

▲ **Survey EM of a mouse pancreatic islet.** Parts of several tightly packed polyhedral islet cells are close to a fenestrated capillary. A dominant feature of these cells is dense-core secretory vesicles (**arrows**) whose size and appearance (i.e., internal density) vary among species. Beta cell vesicles in the mouse are relatively small. Bounded externally by a membrane, they have an electron-dense homogeneous core surrounded by an electron-lucent area. Profiles of rough endoplasmic reticulum (**RER**), well-developed Golgi complexes (**GC**), and scattered mitochondria (**Mi**) also occupy the cytoplasm. 8600×.

10.27   ULTRASTRUCTURE OF ISLETS OF LANGERHANS

Electron microscopy reveals that **islet cells** are arranged in cords and are linked to neighboring cells by *intercellular junctions.* Their free surfaces are close to **fenestrated capillaries.** Their ultrastructure is consistent with a role in synthesis and secretion of peptide hormones. The predominant feature of their cytoplasm is the many membrane-bound **secretory vesicles** of various sizes and internal density. The protein hormones involved in regulation of carbohydrate metabolism are *insulin,* which lowers blood glucose by promoting its entry into cells, and *glucagon,* which raises blood glucose levels. Their location in the islet, size, and internal morphology of secretory vesicles permit islet cells to be separated into at least four main types with specific hormone associations: **alpha cells:** *glucagon;* **beta cells:** *insulin;* **delta (D) cells:** *somatostatin;* and **F-cells:** *pancreatic polypeptide.*

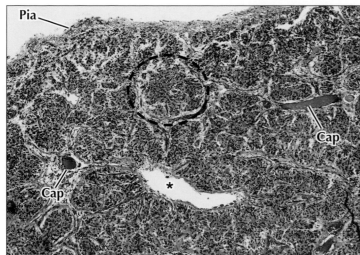

◀ **LM of the pineal at low magnification.** Glandular architecture shows many closely packed parenchymal cells arranged in ill-defined lobules (**dashed circle**). Intervening stroma, which supports the parenchyma, contains several enlarged, thin-walled capillaries (**Cap**) and a venule (∗). Loose connective tissue, which derives from pia mater, covers the gland's outer surface. 55×. *H&E.*

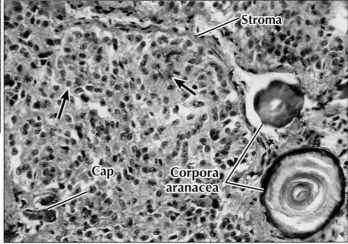

▲ **LM of the pineal at higher magnification.** Groups of pinealocytes (**arrows**) with euchromatic nuclei and prominent nucleoli are mingled with smaller, dark glial cells. Intervening areas contain delicate connective tissue stroma and a network of capillaries (**Cap**). Two round corpora aranacea with concentric lamellae are seen. 275×. *H&E.*

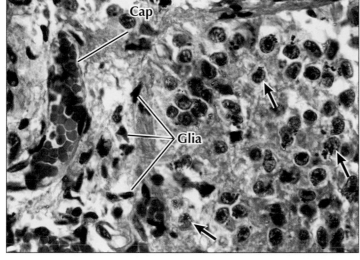

◀ **LM of the pineal at high magnification.** Many closely packed pinealocytes (**arrows**) occupy the organ. These round cells with pale nuclei have accumulations of golden brown pigment—lipofuscin—in the cytoplasm. Glial cells with elongated, heterochromatic nuclei serve a supportive role. A sinusoidal capillary (**Cap**) is in view. 635×. *H&E.*

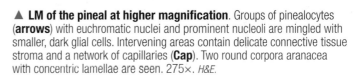

10.28 HISTOLOGY OF THE PINEAL

The pineal is a small, cone-shaped, richly vascularized neuroendocrine organ. About 7 mm long and weighing less than 0.2 g, it projects from the roof of the third ventricle in front of the midbrain and is supplied by both *sympathetic* and *parasympathetic nerves.* It is divided into poorly defined **lobules** by delicate **connective tissue septa** that extend inward from the capsule formed around the gland by **pia mater.** The pineal has a mostly glandular architecture and consists mainly of closely packed, pale cells—**pinealocytes**—forming cords or clusters. They derive embryonically from *neural ectoderm.* Each cell has a pale pleomorphic nucleus with one or more nucleoli. Pinealocytes are the source of the hormone *melatonin,* which is released from long terminal cell expansions into closely associated **fenestrated capillaries.** This hormone exerts powerful effects on circadian rhythms and in some species regulates reproduction. After puberty, mineralized extracellular concretions, called **corpora aranacea** (brain sand),

are a salient feature. They increase with age and, because of radiopacity, are a useful radiologic midline marker for clinicians. Smaller, darker cells, which resemble *astrocytes,* also occupy the interstitium. They are supportive and are best seen by immunocytochemistry with antibodies to *glial fibrillary acidic protein* (GFAP).

CLINICAL POINT

In 1629, French philosopher René Descartes proposed that the pineal is the seat of the soul. The precise functions of the human pineal remain unclear, but evidence exists that fluctuations in **melatonin** secretion regulate the diurnal rhythm, related to darkness and light, of other endocrine glands. The pineal may also control gonadal development before puberty via the hypothalamic-pituitary axis by suppressing growth hormone and gonadotropin. Childhood pineal tumors lead to gonadal hypertrophy and precocious puberty. Also, use of melatonin may help counteract drowsiness and disorientation related to jet lag.

11

INTEGUMENTARY SYSTEM

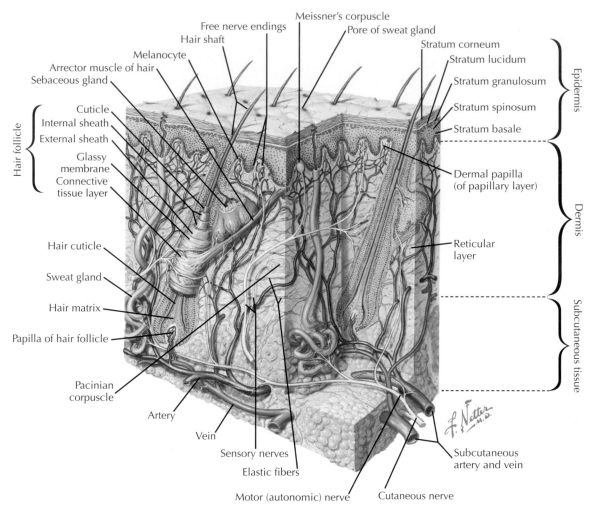

Free nerve endings
Hair shaft
Melanocyte
Arrector muscle of hair
Sebaceous gland

Meissner's corpuscle
Pore of sweat gland
Stratum corneum
Stratum lucidum
Stratum granulosum
Stratum spinosum
Stratum basale

Epidermis

Hair follicle
Cuticle
Internal sheath
External sheath
Glassy membrane
Connective tissue layer

Dermal papilla
(of papillary layer)

Dermis

Hair cuticle
Sweat gland
Hair matrix
Papilla of hair follicle

Reticular layer

Subcutaneous tissue

Pacinian corpuscle
Artery
Vein
Sensory nerves
Elastic fibers
Motor (autonomic) nerve

Subcutaneous artery and vein

Cutaneous nerve

▲ Schematic of skin and its appendages that shows the epidermis, dermis, and subcutaneous tissue.

11.1 OVERVIEW

The **integument,** the largest organ of the body, is composed of **skin** and skin **appendages—nails, hair, sweat glands,** and **sebaceous glands.** The total weight and overall surface area of skin in the adult are 3-5 kg and 1.5-2 m², respectively. Skin thickness, between 0.5 and 3 mm, varies regionally; skin is thickest on the back and thinnest on the eyelid. At mucocutaneous junctions, skin is continuous with mucous membranes lining digestive, respiratory, and urogenital tracts. As well as serving as a protective barrier against injury (e.g., abrasions, cuts, burns), infectious pathogens, and ultraviolet radiation, skin assists in body temperature regulation, vitamin D synthesis, ion excretion, and sensory reception (touch and pain), and it has a remarkable regenerative capacity. It consists of **stratified squamous keratinized epithelium** on its outer part, called the **epidermis,** and an inner layer of **fibrous connective tissue,** called the **dermis.** A loose layer of **subcutaneous connective tissue,** the **hypodermis,** attaches skin to underlying structures and permits movement over most body parts. Skin has a dual embryologic origin: epidermis and its appendages derive mostly from surface ectoderm; dermis originates from mesoderm. The epidermis consists primarily of cells called keratinocytes, which make up more than 90% of the cell population. Other epidermal cells are **melanocytes** and Merkel cells, which derive from neural crest, and Langerhans cells, which have a monocytic origin. During embryonic development, skin appendages deriving from the epidermis grow down into the dermis.

CLINICAL POINT

Skin diseases, especially of **pigmentation,** are common and can result from a change in number of melanocytes or a decrease or increase in their activity. **Leukoderma** associated with inflammatory disorders of the skin, such as atopic dermatitis, and **vitiligo** are two more common *hypopigmentation* disorders. One of the most common *hyperpigmentation* disorders is **melasma.** It is seen primarily, but not only, in women; its onset may be during pregnancy, so it is also called mask of pregnancy. Exposure to the sun is important in induction and maintenance of hyperpigmented areas on the face.

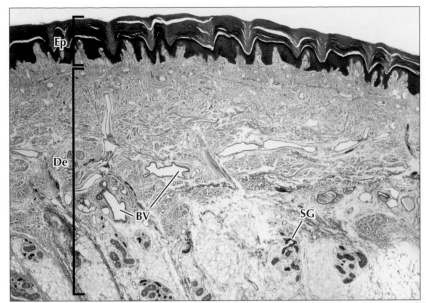

◄ **Light micrograph (LM) of thick skin showing its architectural organization in vertical section at low power.** The epidermis (**Ep**) and dermis (**De**) are clearly shown. The interface between the thick, keratinized epidermis and underlying, lightly stained dermis is highly convoluted. Deeper layers of dermis contain sweat glands (**SG**) but lack hair and pilosebaceous units, which consist of hair, hair follicles, arrector pili muscles, and sebaceous glands. Blood vessels (**BV**) also appear in the dermis and hypodermis. 25×. *H&E.*

► **LM of thin skin at the same magnification.** A thinner epidermis (**Ep**) overlies the dermis (**De**), which consists of strands of dense connective tissue fibers. Epidermal ridges are shallow, and the keratin layer is relatively thin. The dermis contains hair follicles (**HF**), sebaceous glands (**Seb**), and sweat glands (**SG**). 25×. *H&E.*

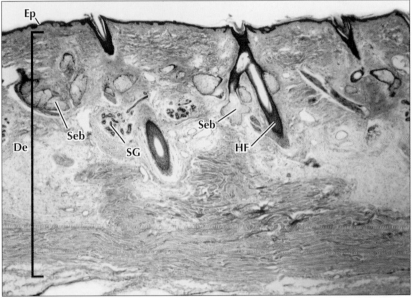

11.2 HISTOLOGY OF THICK AND THIN SKIN

On the basis of the structural complexity and thickness of the **epidermis,** skin is classified into **thick** or **thin.** Thick skin, which is **glabrous,** is found on palms of the hands and soles of the feet; thin skin covers most of the remaining body surface. Whereas the multilayered epidermis of thick skin is 0.8-1.5 mm thick, the epidermis of thin skin is 0.07-0.15 mm thick, with fewer cellular layers. The junction between the avascular epidermis and richly vascularized **dermis**—the dermoepidermal border—is usually highly corrugated and has many downward, ridge-like extensions of epidermis, called **epidermal,** or **rete, ridges** that project between alternating, upward projections of dermis, the dermal papillae. The contour of this border resembles the undersurface of an egg carton and is more complex in thick than in thin skin. A basement membrane separates epidermis from dermis. The thick dermis is divided into two layers: a superficial papillary layer of loose **connective tissue** containing type I and III collagen fibers interspersed with elastic fibers, connective tissue cells, and rich network of capillaries; and a deeper reticular layer of dense irregular connective tissue consisting of coarse, interlacing bundles of collagen fibers, mostly type I. Aside from fibroblasts, other connective tissue cells in the dermis include macrophages, mast cells, adipocytes, plasma cells, and lymphocytes.

CLINICAL POINT

Skin cancer is the most common malignant disease in North America. The three major types are **basal cell carcinoma** and **squamous cell carcinoma** (arise from keratinocytes) and **melanoma** (originates from melanocytes). Basal cell carcinoma accounts for more than 90% of all skin cancers; it grows slowly and seldom spreads to other parts of the body. Squamous cell carcinoma is associated with long-term exposure to sun and has a greater likelihood of metastasis. Malignant melanoma causes more than 75% of all deaths from skin cancer. If it is diagnosed early, treatment is usually effective; melanoma diagnosed at a late stage is more likely to metastasize and cause death.

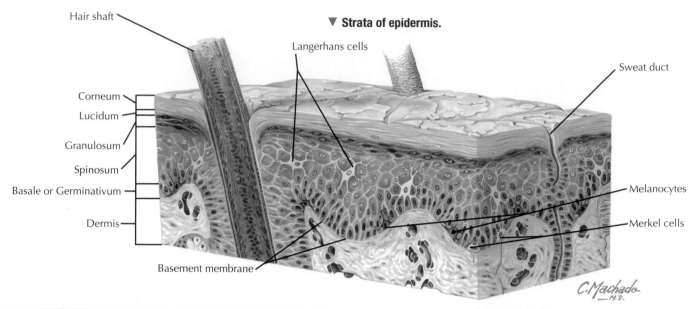

▼ **Strata of epidermis.**

Hair shaft

Langerhans cells

Sweat duct

Corneum
Lucidum
Granulosum
Spinosum
Basale or Germinativum
Dermis

Melanocytes

Merkel cells

Basement membrane

C. Machado
—M.D.

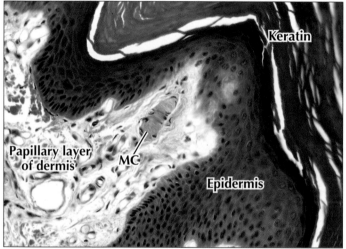

▲ **LM of thick skin at the dermoepidermal junction.** A thick keratin layer characterizes the outermost stratum corneum. A dermal papilla that projects superficially into the epidermal region consists of loose connective tissue of the papillary layer. This layer contains many small blood vessels and a Meissner corpuscle (**MC**), which is an encapsulated touch receptor. 240×. *H&E.*

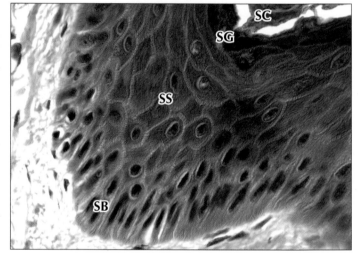

▲ **Higher magnification LM of the epidermis of thick skin.** The epidermis, a continually renewing epithelium, shows progressive differentiation and keratinization in a basal to superficial direction. Main features of its layers—strata basale (**SB**), spinosum (**SS**) (note prickle cells), granulosum (**SG**), and a small part of the corneum (**SC**)—are seen here. Part of the underlying dermis appears at the bottom. 575×. *H&E.*

11.3 HISTOLOGY OF THE EPIDERMIS

The epidermis consists of cells that undergo *mitosis, differentiation, maturation,* and *keratinization* as they are displaced outward toward the skin surface to be shed. Four or five distinct layers, or strata, constitute the epidermis. The **stratum basale, or germinativum,** is the deepest; it consists of a single layer of closely packed, basophilic cuboidal to columnar epithelial cells, known as keratinocytes, resting on a basement membrane. These cells have oval nuclei that often show mitotic figures; they continuously undergo cell division to replace cells that move outward through the epidermis. The next layer, the **stratum spinosum,** is several cells thick and has polyhedral cells that become progressively flatter toward the surface. Processes of adjacent cells are attached by desmosomes. Cell shrinkage caused by a fixation artifact accentu-

ates the processes and creates spines or prickles—thus the name prickle cells. The next layer, the **stratum granulosum,** consists of three to five layers of flattened cells, their axes aligned parallel to the epidermal surface. They contain numerous basophilic granules, the keratohyalin granules. Superficial to this layer is a thin, translucent, lightly eosinophilic layer, known as the *stratum lucidum.* Absent in thin skin but present in thick skin, it consists of a few layers of tightly packed squamous cells that lack organelles and nuclei. The outermost layer, the **stratum corneum,** is made of dead, anucleate cornified cells; its thickness varies regionally. The protein *keratin* replaces cytoplasm in its cells. The most superficial cells are continuously shed in a process known as *desquamation.*

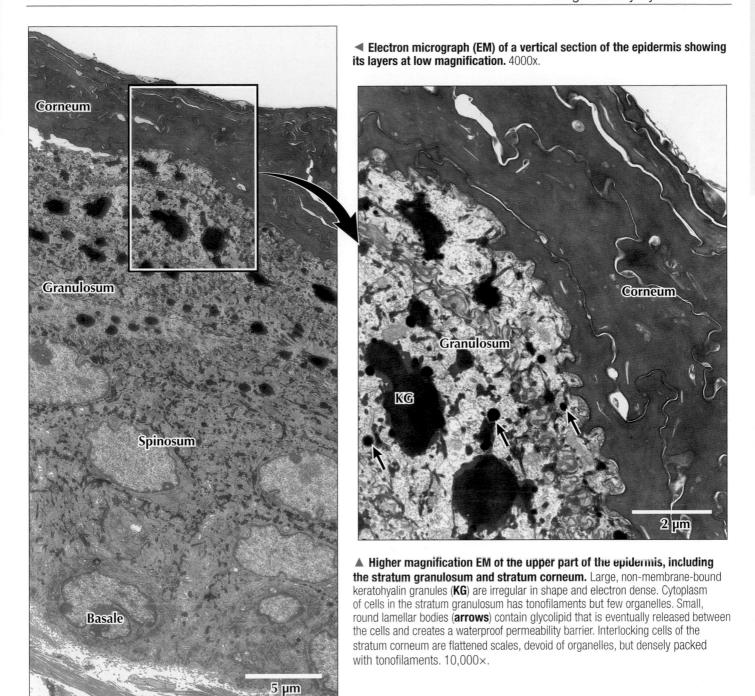

◀ **Electron micrograph (EM) of a vertical section of the epidermis showing its layers at low magnification.** 4000x.

▲ **Higher magnification EM of the upper part of the epidermis, including the stratum granulosum and stratum corneum.** Large, non-membrane-bound keratohyalin granules (**KG**) are irregular in shape and electron dense. Cytoplasm of cells in the stratum granulosum has tonofilaments but few organelles. Small, round lamellar bodies (**arrows**) contain glycolipid that is eventually released between the cells and creates a waterproof permeability barrier. Interlocking cells of the stratum corneum are flattened scales, devoid of organelles, but densely packed with tonofilaments. 10,000×.

11.4 ULTRASTRUCTURE OF THE EPIDERMIS

In upper layers of the **stratum spinosum,** keratinocytes contain irregular, non-membrane-bound, electron-dense **keratohyalin granules** with diameters of 100-150 nm. These granules consist of the protein filaggrin, which cross-links with keratin. In the **stratum granulosum,** almost all cytoplasmic organelles and nuclei disappear because of lysosomal enzyme activity. The residual cellular profiles are filled with tightly packed filaments and are enclosed by a thickened cell membrane—the **horny cell membrane.** The protein **involucrin** binds to the inner cell membrane. Round to oval membrane-bound granules in keratinocytes in upper layers—the **lamellar bodies**—are 300-500 nm in diameter, are derived from Golgi complex, and are rich in **glycolipids.** They are eventually released from and deposited between keratinocytes, most likely forming an intercellular barrier to water. Unique keratin packing probably accounts for the presence of a stratum lucidum in plantar and palmar skin. The **stratum corneum** is made of interlocking cells arranged in orderly vertical stacks. These cells have thickened cell membranes and lack desmosomes, which allows cells to dissociate and desquamate easily. The normal time for turnover of keratinocytes from stratum basale to uppermost stratum corneum varies from 20 to 75 days. Turnover and transit times may be even more rapid in some diseases, such as *psoriasis*, in which transit time is about 8 days.

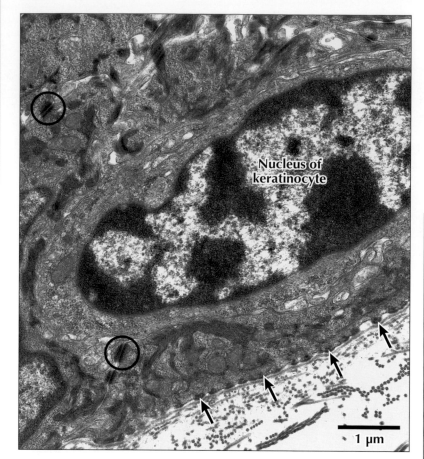

◄ **Low-magnification EM of the dermoepidermal junction.** A keratinocyte in the stratum basale contains an elongated nucleus with euchromatin and heterochromatin. Keratin-containing tonofilaments, organized into tightly packed bundles, are seen throughout the cytoplasm and insert into desmosomes (**circles**) linking adjacent keratinocytes. Basal aspects of the cells contain numerous hemidesmosomes (**arrows**) that attach to underlying basement membrane. Part of the papillary dermis appears at the bottom. 16,500×.

Nucleus of keratinocyte

1 μm

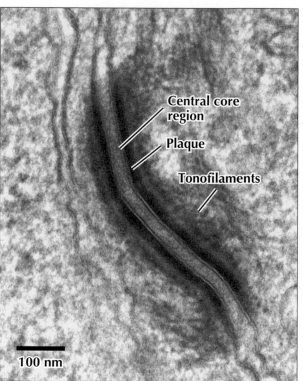

Central core region

Plaque

Tonofilaments

100 nm

► **High-magnification EM showing details of a desmosome between adjacent keratinocytes.** A central core region that bridges the gap between cells separates two identical electron-dense plaques. Tonofilaments (keratin) of the cytoskeleton are associated with these cytoplasmic plaque regions. 125,000×.

11.5 ULTRASTRUCTURE OF KERATINOCYTES

Cells of the stratum basale have relatively **euchromatic nuclei** compared with those of more superficial layers. Their cytoplasm contains many ribosomes, mitochondria, and an extensive **cytoskeleton** of 10-nm intermediate filaments known as **tonofilaments.** These are made of the **keratin** family of intermediate filament proteins. All epithelial cells contain keratins, and almost 50 different types of keratins are found in skin. **Keratinocytes** of the strata basale and spinosum are connected by **desmosomes.** These complex intercellular junctions mediate and enhance cell adhesion by anchoring keratin filaments to keratinocyte plasma membranes. By linking tonofilament bundles of adjacent cells, desmosomes provide the epidermis with structural continuity and mechanical strength. To further counteract mechanical forces, basal aspects of keratinocytes are firmly attached to underlying **basement membrane** by **hemidesmosomes.** Hemidesmosomes have only one intracytoplasmic attachment **plaque** to which tonofilaments from the cell interior attach. Fine anchoring filaments radiate from the outer aspect of the plasma membrane into the basal lamina. The basement membrane at the **dermoepidermal junction** usually requires special light microscopic techniques to be visible. This specialized supporting zone of extracellular matrix consists of several layers. A lamina lucida and lamina densa together constitute the basal lamina, which contains type IV collagen, laminin, fibronectin, and proteoglycans. A deeper reticular lamina, made mainly of type I collagen fibers, merges with underlying connective tissue.

CLINICAL POINT

Some debilitating **blistering disorders** of skin result from disrupted epidermal adhesion and attachment. Antigens for these diseases are components of either desmosomes or hemidesmosomes and belong to three genetic families—cadherin, armadillo, and plakin. Autoantibodies may react with the keratinocyte cell surface or epidermal basement membrane, which induces separation of epidermal keratinocytes or dermoepidermal junctions. **Pemphigus** is the most common disease with anti-keratinocyte cell surface antibodies; the related **bullous pemphigoid** causes subepidermal blisters. In these diseases, mutations in genes encoding desmosomal components have been identified, which may lead to novel, efficient treatment strategies.

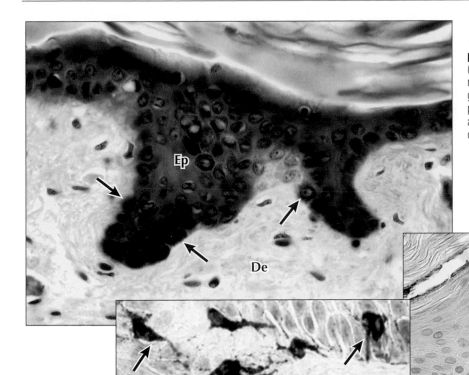

◄ **LM of the epidermis and dermis of heavily pigmented thick skin.** Numerous melanocytes (**arrows**) occupy basal layers of epidermis (**Ep**). They are recognizable by an intrinsic color and content of brown granular deposits of melanin. In most routine tissue preparations and in paler skin, however, melanocytes are usually clear cells in the basal epidermis. Underlying dermis (**De**) is loose connective tissue. 465×. *H&E.*

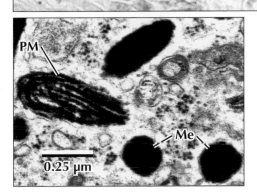

▲ **Immunostained LMs of thick skin showing melanocytes in the epidermis.** Above, Melan-A, an antibody to melanin, is immunolocalized in melanocytes (**arrows**) and reveals their dendritic processes. The darkly stained melanocytes lie in the basal layer of the epidermis (**Ep**). Nuclei of surrounding keratinocytes are blue; the lighter dermis (**De**) is below. Middle left LM shows the branching pattern of melanocytes (**arrows**) at high magnification. **Middle left**: 275×; **Above**: 630×. *Immunoperoxidase and toluidine blue.*

▲ **EM of pigment granules.** Membrane-bound premelanosomes (**PM**) are elliptical organelles derived from Golgi complex. They have concentric internal lamellae and give rise to round melanosomes (**Me**), which contain melanin. 60,000×. *(Courtesy of Dr. B. J. Crawford)*

11.6 HISTOLOGY AND FUNCTION OF EPIDERMAL MELANOCYTES

Melanocytes are **melanin** pigment-producing cells that determine color of skin and hair. The major determinant of color is not melanocyte number but activity, which is affected by corticotropin from the pituitary. Derived from the neural crest, melanocytes migrate to the basal layer of the **epidermis** and hair matrices as early as 8 weeks in the embryo, and to eyes, ears, and brain meninges. Typically, 1000-2000 melanocytes occur per 1 mm^2 of epidermis. Instead of being linked by desmosomes, each melanocyte establishes contact via **dendritic processes** with about 30 nearby **keratinocytes.** Melanin is produced in membrane-bound organelles known as *melanosomes.* They rearrange themselves within cells in response to external cues such as ultraviolet (UV) rays;

they usually cluster near cell centers and can rapidly redistribute along microtubules to ends of dendritic processes. Keratinocytes then phagocytose the dendritic tips. Melanosomes are pinched off into keratinocyte cytoplasm, where they are often packaged in secondary lysosomes. Darkly pigmented skin, hair, and eyes have melanosomes that contain more melanin. Two major forms of melanin are found in humans, *eumelanin,* which is brown to black, and *pheomelanin,* which is yellow to red; both are derived from tyrosine. *Tanning* of the skin caused by UV exposure represents an increased eumelanin content of the epidermis. Its major purpose is enhanced protection against damaging effects of UV radiation on DNA. With aging, melanocyte numbers decline significantly in skin and hair.

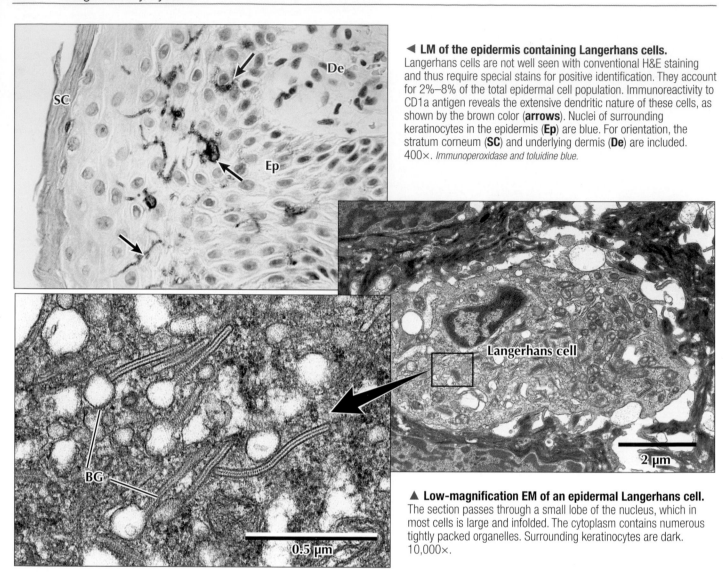

◀ **LM of the epidermis containing Langerhans cells.**
Langerhans cells are not well seen with conventional H&E staining and thus require special stains for positive identification. They account for 2%–8% of the total epidermal cell population. Immunoreactivity to CD1a antigen reveals the extensive dendritic nature of these cells, as shown by the brown color (**arrows**). Nuclei of surrounding keratinocytes in the epidermis (**Ep**) are blue. For orientation, the stratum corneum (**SC**) and underlying dermis (**De**) are included. 400×. *Immunoperoxidase and toluidine blue.*

▲ **Low-magnification EM of an epidermal Langerhans cell.**
The section passes through a small lobe of the nucleus, which in most cells is large and infolded. The cytoplasm contains numerous tightly packed organelles. Surrounding keratinocytes are dark. 10,000×.

▲ **Higher magnification EM of a Langerhans cell.** Several Birbeck granules (**BG**) occupy the cytoplasm. Each has a pentalaminar rod-shaped region attached to a clear vesicle at one or both ends. The precise function of Birbeck granules remains obscure but may be related to receptor-mediated endocytosis. 70,000×.

11.7 STRUCTURE AND FUNCTION OF EPIDERMAL LANGERHANS CELLS

Langerhans cells are **monocyte-derived dendritic cells** that reside in the epidermis after migration from bone marrow. Phagocytic and antigen-processing and -presenting cells of the *immune system,* they express **CD1a cell surface antigen.** They are most common in superficial layers of the stratum spinosum and stratum granulosum. Like melanocytes, they are not linked by desmosomes to adjacent keratinocytes and possess slender dendritic processes emanating from a spherical cell body. They typically have a single, **indented nucleus.** Their cytoplasm contains the usual organelles including a well-developed Golgi complex and lysosomes. They also have unique cytoplasmic inclusions known as **Birbeck granules,** which look like tennis rackets and are best resolved by electron microscopy. These consist of superimposed, zippered pentalaminar membranes that contain a protein called *langerin* and are thought to be infoldings of cell membrane, possibly a result of antigen processing. They also contain clathrin, similar to that in coated pits of other cells, which suggests a role in receptor-mediated processing and recognition. The number of these cells increases in various *inflammatory conditions,* such as contact dermatitis. The rare autoimmune *histiocytosis X,* or **Langerhans cell histiocytosis,** also involves Langerhans cells. These cells, in which HIV particles are found, are depleted in late stages of *AIDS.*

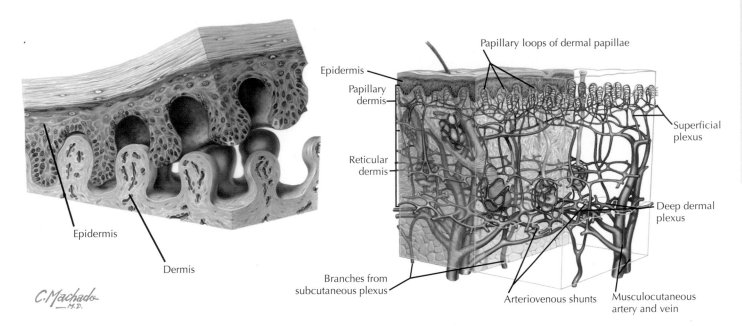

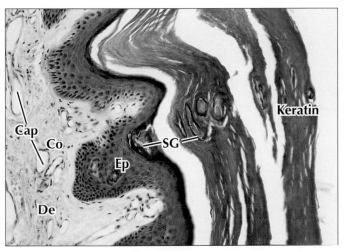

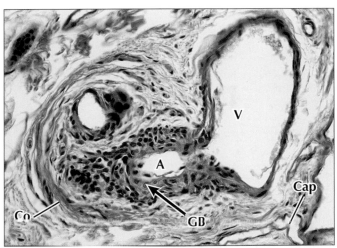

▲ **LM of the dermoepidermal junction.** The dermis (**De**) is less cellular than the epidermis (**Ep**). The papillary dermis is loose connective tissue with collagen fibers (**Co**) interspersed with mononuclear cells. Capillaries (**Cap**) form loops that extend into dermal papillae and are derived from the horizontal superficial plexus of arterioles. The three-dimensional organization of the papillae has been likened to a candelabra, with the loops representing candles. The fortuitously sectioned duct of a sweat gland (**SG**) courses through epidermis on its way to the skin surface. 150×. *H&E.*

▲ **LM of an arteriovenous anastomosis in the reticular dermis.** This short, coiled vascular shunt consists of the terminal segment of an arteriole (**A**) directly connected to a venule (**V**) with no intervening capillary network. The tunica media of the arteriole is thickened with multiple layers of modified smooth muscle cells making up a glomus body (**GB**), the cells thus known as glomus cells. Condensed connective tissue with bundles of collagen fibers (**Co**) encapsulates the glomus body. Capillaries (**Cap**) are in other areas of the dermis. 245×. *H&E.*

11.8   HISTOLOGY AND VASCULATURE OF THE DERMIS

The dermis, a richly vascularized **connective tissue,** provides mechanical support, pliability, and tensile strength to skin. Blood vessels furnish nutrients and are involved in *thermoregulation.* Large muscular **arteries** that supply skin are found in subcutaneous connective tissue and are accompanied by muscular **veins.** They branch, anastomose, and form a network that runs parallel with the skin surface. Smaller arteries, veins, and capillaries constitute the main vasculature in the dermis. Networks of these small vessels form deep plexuses in the **reticular dermis** and superficial plexuses in the **papillary dermis,** which are connected by communicating vessels. A subepidermal network of **arterioles** immediately under **dermal papillae** supplies blood to capillary loops in each papilla. An exten-sive network of **capillaries** immediately under the **epidermis** supplies nutrients to the avascular epithelium. Capillaries also surround the matrix of hair follicles and are closely associated with sweat and sebaceous glands. Many **arteriovenous anastomoses** in deeper layers of the dermis, especially in the dermis of fingers, lips, and toes, are direct connections between arterioles and **venules** and lack an intervening capillary network. At the arteriole end, these vascular shunts are coiled and surrounded by a row of modified **smooth muscle cells** serving as sphincters. These specialized structures, known as **glomus bodies,** play a role in peripheral temperature regulation. They are under autonomic vasomotor control and divert blood from the superficial to the deep plexus to reduce heat loss. Lymphatics of skin accompany venules and are also located in deep and superficial plexuses.

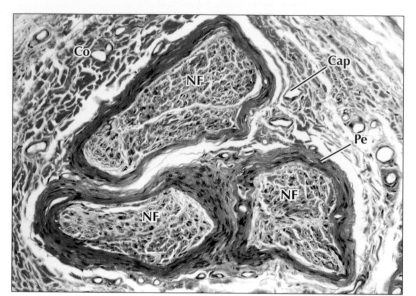

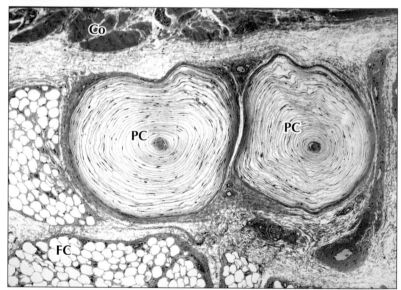

◀ **LM showing several peripheral nerve fascicles in the dermis.** Each fascicle (**NF**) contains many nerve fibers surrounded by a thick outer capsule of perineurium (**Pe**). Surrounding dermal connective tissue contains irregular coarse bundles of collagen fibers (**Co**) interspersed with many small blood vessels and capillaries (**Cap**). Intervening spaces contain amorphous extracellular matrix that is rich in glycosaminoglycans and dermatan sulfate. 170×. *H&E.*

▶ **LM showing the junction of the reticular dermis and the hypodermis.** In each Pacinian corpuscle (**PC**), shown in transverse section, a central axon is surrounded by multiple capsular lamellae. The dermis (**at top**) contains intensely eosinophilic bundles of collagen (**Co**); hypodermis (**at bottom**) is a loose connective tissue with many tightly packed fat cells (**FC**), or adipocytes. 70×. *H&E.*

11.9 HISTOLOGY AND INNERVATION OF THE DERMIS

Skin is the largest sensory organ in the body. A rich nerve supply throughout the dermis includes a complex network of **sensory nerves** and efferent sympathetic innervation to sweat glands, vascular smooth muscles, and arrector pili muscles. Branching **nerve fascicles** containing myelinated and unmyelinated **nerve fibers** make up extensive subpapillary dermal plexuses. Myelinated nerve fibers supply nerve endings to the epidermis and encapsulated sensory receptors in the dermis including Meissner and Pacinian corpuscles. Nerve fibers entering epidermis lose myelin sheaths and end between epidermal cells either as free nerve endings or are closely associated to Merkel cells, where they serve as tactile receptors. Located in dermal papillae, Meissner corpuscles are mechanoreceptors that mediate touch. Abundant in palms and soles, they have a characteristic elongated shape, like that of a pinecone, an average diameter of 30-80 μm, and a capsule of modified, flattened Schwann cells that are arranged perpendicularly to the long axis of the receptor. Each Meissner corpuscle receives a myelinated nerve fiber that loses its myelin sheath as it ends within it. **Pacinian corpuscles** are larger encapsulated receptors in deeper regions of dermis and subcutaneous tissue. Deep pressure receptors, they are up to 1 mm long; they are ovoid and often flattened spheres. They consist of multiple layers of loosely arranged concentric **lamellae** that, on cross section, resemble layers of an onion. A single myelinated nerve fiber supplies each corpuscle and loses its myelin sheath as it enters the receptor.

CLINICAL POINT

Scleroderma is a rare, progressive chronic disorder of dermal connective tissue characterized by tightening of skin with extensive deposition of types I and III collagen. It may also affect other organs. The initial, localized cutaneous lesions begin in the papillary layer; eventually lesions extend into the entire reticular dermis. Its histologic picture includes enlarged collagen fiber bundles, occluded microvasculature, and patchy lymphocyte infiltration extending into subcutaneous connective tissue. Production of autoantibodies, accompanied by abnormal T and B cell activation, points to an *autoimmune etiology.*

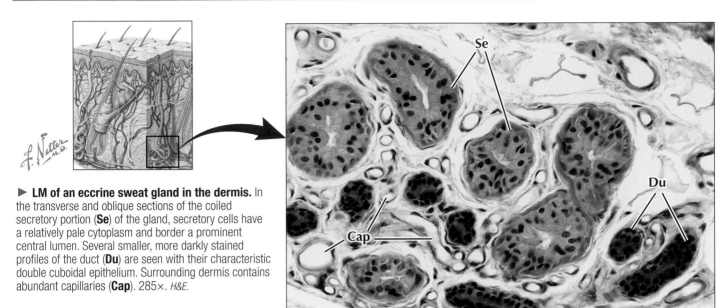

▶ **LM of an eccrine sweat gland in the dermis.** In the transverse and oblique sections of the coiled secretory portion (**Se**) of the gland, secretory cells have a relatively pale cytoplasm and border a prominent central lumen. Several smaller, more darkly stained profiles of the duct (**Du**) are seen with their characteristic double cuboidal epithelium. Surrounding dermis contains abundant capillaries (**Cap**). 285×. *H&E.*

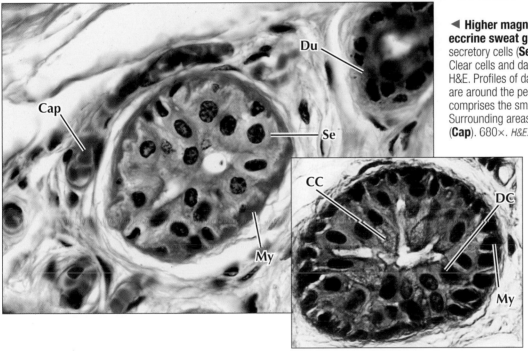

◀ **Higher magnification LM showing details of an eccrine sweat gland.** Light-staining, pyramidal secretory cells (**Se**) line the lumen of a secretory acinus. Clear cells and dark cells are not readily distinguished by H&E. Profiles of darkly stained myoepithelial cells (**My**) are around the periphery. The double cuboidal epithelium comprises the small duct (**Du**) in the upper right. Surrounding areas contain a rich network of capillaries (**Cap**). 680×. *H&E.*

◀ **LM of an acinus of a sweat gland.** This staining method distinguishes dark cells (**DC**) from clear cells (**CC**) in the secretory acinus. Surrounding myoepithelial cells (**My**) at the base of the acinus share a basement membrane with secretory cells. 800×. *Masson trichrome.*

11.10 HISTOLOGY AND FUNCTION OF ECCRINE SWEAT GLANDS

Eccrine sweat glands are simple, coiled tubular glands consisting of **secretory** and narrower **excretory duct** portions. With cholinergic innervation, they mainly serve a *thermoregulatory* role and maintain body temperature by evaporative heat loss. They also aid ion excretion and may, under normal conditions, produce 500–750 mL or more of sweat daily in response to thermal and emotional stimuli. They occur throughout the body but are absent on the glans penis, clitoris, and labia minora. They develop in the embryo as invaginations of epidermis, independent from pilosebaceous units, into underlying **dermis.** They appear first in palms and soles in the fourth gestational month. The tightly convoluted secretory part of a gland deep in the dermis consists of two types of cuboidal to pyramidal **secretory cells—clear cells** and **dark cells.** Clear cells primarily secrete water and electrolytes; dark cells elaborate macromolecular substances in sweat. Smaller, intensely eosinophilic **myoepithelial cells,** which share the same basement membrane but do not reach the lumen of the secretory **acinus,** border them. Myoepithelial cells are mainly contractile and help expel sweat into the lumen of an acinus. The spiraling duct is made of two layers of dark-staining **cuboidal epithelial cells.** The duct has a smaller diameter than does the secretory acinus and lacks myoepithelial cells. As it nears the surface, the duct becomes continuous with a corkscrew-shaped cleft between epidermal cells, which opens at the surface via a round aperture.

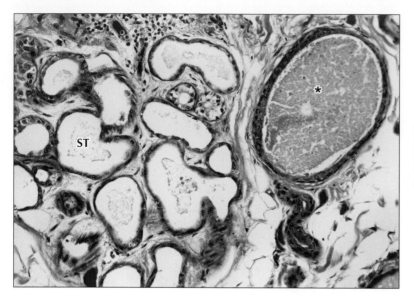

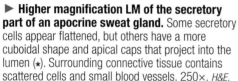

◄ **LM of an apocrine sweat gland in axillary skin.** These glands store secretions, and secretory product (∗) fills this dilated secretory coil. Neighboring secretory tubules (**ST**) appear relatively empty. Loose connective tissue surrounds the gland. 145×. *H&E.*

► **Higher magnification LM of the secretory part of an apocrine sweat gland.** Some secretory cells appear flattened, but others have a more cuboidal shape and apical caps that project into the lumen (∗). Surrounding connective tissue contains scattered cells and small blood vessels. 250×. *H&E.*

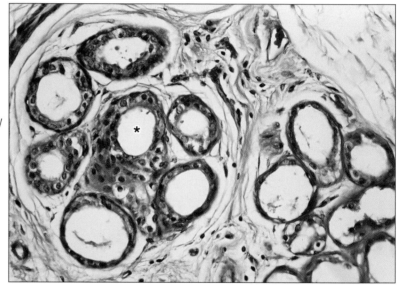

11.11 HISTOLOGY AND FUNCTION OF APOCRINE SWEAT GLANDS

Apocrine sweat glands, also known as *odoriferous sweat glands,* are large, branched glands found in axillae, scrotum, prepuce, labia minora, nipples, and perianal regions. They are less coiled than eccrine sweat glands, and many coils anastomose to form an intertwining tubular network. The sac-like **lumen** of the **secretory tubules** is lined by **simple cuboidal epithelium** and, compared with the eccrine glands, has a wider diameter and larger, more numerous myoepithelial cells that share a basement membrane with secretory epithelium. The height of **secretory cells** varies according to their state of secretion. Their yellow, viscous, oily secretion has an acrid or musky odor in response to *bacterial decomposition.* Secretion formation that was originally thought to be the result of a pinching off of the apical region of a cell is actually an artifact, the mode of secretion most likely being similar to that of eccrine sweat glands, and of the merocrine type. Simple cuboidal epithelium lines gland ducts, which usually open into hair follicles, just above openings of sebaceous glands. Apocrine sweat glands, innervated by adrenergic sympathetic nerve fibers, start to function at puberty and are controlled by sex hormones. Modified apocrine glands include ceruminous glands in the skin of the external auditory meatus (secrete earwax) and Moll glands associated with free margins of eyelids.

CLINICAL POINT

Under the influence of the adrenal hormone aldosterone, ductal epithelium of sweat glands normally reabsorbs sodium and chloride ions so that sweat is hypotonic. Defective chloride ion reabsorption by excretory ducts of eccrine sweat glands occurs in **cystic fibrosis** (CF), an autosomal recessive congenital disease. The gene responsible for CF encodes a membrane-associated protein, *cystic fibrosis transmembrane regulator* (CFTR), which usually resides in apical membranes of epithelial cells. Sweat glands in patients with CF look histologically normal but secrete excessive sodium and chloride ions. Although the exact function of CFTR is unknown, CFTR seems to be part of a cAMP-regulated chloride ion channel and thus controls ion transport.

▼ **Schematic of a pilosebaceous unit and innervation of skin.**

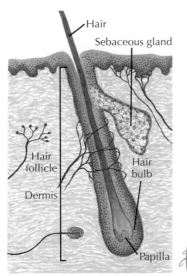

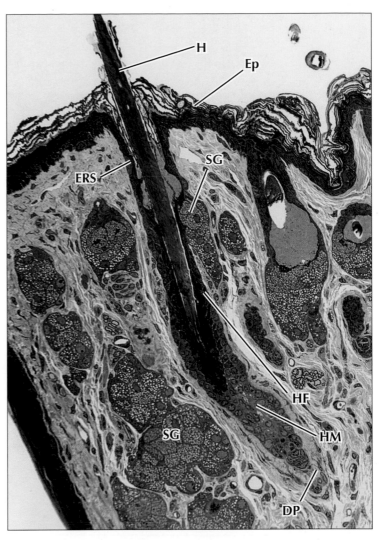

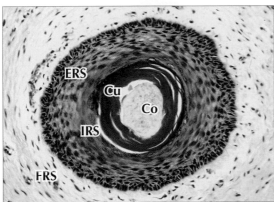

▲ **LM of a hair and its follicle near the epidermis in transverse section.** The cortex of the hair (**Co**) and internal root sheath (**IRS**), external root sheath (**ERS**), and fibrous root sheath (**FRS**) of the hair follicle are shown. The medulla of the hair shaft is not present at this level. The intensely eosinophilic cuticle (**Cu**) is made of overlapping keratinized scales of the cuticle that interlock with cells of the inner root sheath. The fibrous root sheath consists of regularly arranged dermal connective tissue. 220×. *H&E.*

▲ **LM of thin skin of the eyelid.** A hair (**H**) and its follicle (**HF**) are seen in longitudinal section. The hair shaft emerges from an invagination of the epidermis (**Ep**); its root extends into underlying dermis. The external root sheath (**ERS**) of the follicle is continuous with epidermis. One of the sebaceous glands (**SG**) in the dermis opens into the upper part of the hair follicle. The hair matrix (**HM**) at the base of the follicle and part of the dermal papilla (**DP**) are sectioned tangentially. 250×. *Toluidine blue, plastic section.*

11.12 HISTOLOGY OF PILOSEBACEOUS UNITS: HAIR

The pilosebaceous unit consists of the hair, **hair follicle,** an associated arrector pili muscle, and a **sebaceous gland.** An apocrine sweat gland may be associated with a hair follicle. Except for lips, palms, soles, and a few other sites, hairs cover most of the body surface. They develop from **epidermis,** cross the **dermis,** and often extend into subcutaneous connective tissue. Each hair comprises a free **shaft** and a **root,** which is enclosed at its lower end by a tubular hair follicle, composed of epidermal (epithelial) and dermal (connective tissue) parts. In transverse section, a shaft is round to oval. The long axis of each follicle usually lies oblique to the plane of the epidermal surface. Hairs are keratinized threads that vary in thickness and length depending on body region. Each hair is made of three concentric layers of epithelium. The central axis of the hair is the **medulla**—two or three layers of shrunken, keratinized cuboidal cells—which rarely extends the entire length of the hair. Their nuclei are shrunken or lost, and keratin in the medulla is soft. Peripheral to the medulla is the **cortex,** which in colored hair contains flattened keratinized cells with pigment granules between cells. Loss of pigment and the presence of air in the cortex causes hair to be gray to white. The outermost **cuticle** is made of one layer of scale-like cells, which are nucleated in the lower part of the root and shaft but are clear, enucleate squamous cells after keratinization.

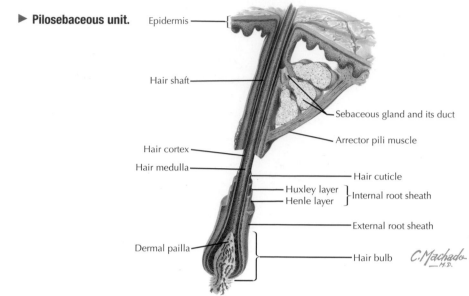

▶ **Pilosebaceous unit.**

Epidermis

Hair shaft

Sebaceous gland and its duct

Arrector pili muscle

Hair cortex

Hair medulla

Hair cuticle

Huxley layer ⎱ Internal root sheath
Henle layer ⎰

External root sheath

Dermal pailla

Hair bulb

C. Machado ___M.D.

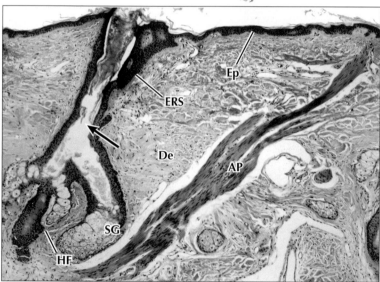

◀ **LM of thin skin close to the epidermis.** An arrector pili muscle (**AP**) and an associated pilosebaceous unit are shown sectioned tangentially. Because of the section level, the hair shaft is not seen. A sebaceous gland (**SG**) and its duct (**arrow**) open into the upper end of a hair follicle (**HF**). The external root sheath (**ERS**) is continuous with the epidermis (**Ep**) on the surface. The arrector pili muscle in the underlying dermis (**De**) extends obliquely from the base of the hair follicle to the papillary dermis. 60×. *H&E.*

11.13   HISTOLOGY AND FUNCTION OF PILOSEBACEOUS UNITS: HAIR FOLLICLES AND HAIR GROWTH

Hair follicles are responsible for production of hair. They arise in the embryo as thickenings of **epidermis** that proliferate as cords and penetrate the **dermis.** The lowest part of this epithelium becomes the expanded, knob-like hair bulb, which consists of a matrix of proliferating cells (similar to the stratum basale of the epidermis). Indented on its inner surface are highly vascularized, finger-like dermal papillae containing clusters of inductive mesenchymal cells for hair follicle growth. Hair matrix is made of mitotically active pleuripotential keratinocytes, interspersed with a few melanocytes and Langerhans cells, that multiply, move outward in columns, and form characteristic layers. The innermost layer keratinizes and forms the hair shaft. The hair follicle consists of three segments: the upper infundibulum and middle isthmus, which are permanent, and the deepest, inferior segment, which germinates hair. Hair growth occurs in cycles, with the histologic appearance of follicles varying according to growth phase. The active growth period, the *anagen* stage, lasts about 3 years. During a 3-week period of regression, the *catagen* phase, hair growth ceases and the follicle undergoes involution. A resting period, the *telogen* phase, lasts about 12 weeks, during which the lower part of the follicle is absent. This cycle ensures that entirely new hair shafts continue to be produced. Baldness occurs in both sexes when follicles cease to be formed and hair cannot be replaced.

CLINICAL POINT

Acne vulgaris is a chronic inflammatory disease of the pilosebaceous unit. In adolescents, it often results from physiologic hormonal variations accompanied by altered maturation of hair follicles and increased sebum production. It is associated with changes in keratinization of follicular epithelium and development of keratin plugs that block sebum outflow to the skin surface and distend follicles. Neutrophils, attracted to the area by chemotactic factors, release hydrolytic enzymes that form a follicular abscess. Acne affects both sexes, but males tend to have more severe disease. Systemic *antibiotics* and temporary use of *topical steroids* are treatments.

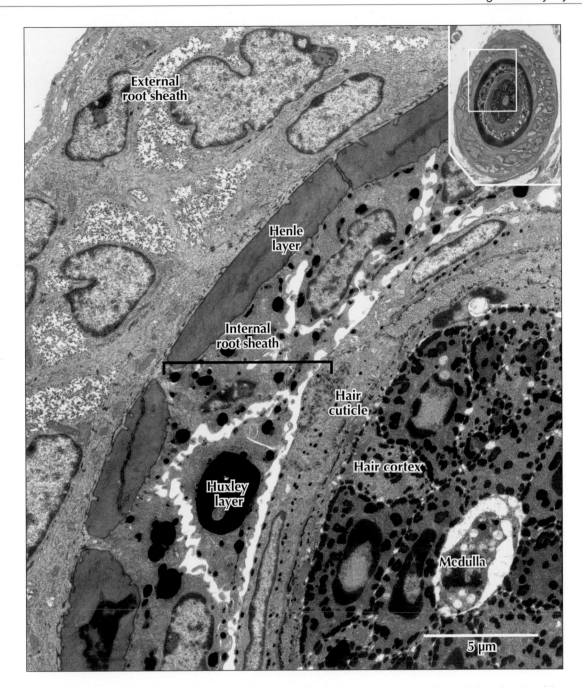

▲ **EM of part of a hair and its follicle in transverse section.** A thin cuticle surrounds the medulla and cortex of the hair shaft. The internal root sheath contains the cuticle, Huxley layer with prominent trichohyalin granules, and Henle layer with clear, flattened cells. The external root sheath is a multilayered epithelium. 6000×. The inset is a semithin plastic section stained with toluidine blue (area in the rectangle seen in the EM). 800×.

11.14 ULTRASTRUCTURE OF HAIR AND ITS FOLLICLES

Cylindrical hair follicles are made of an epithelial root sheath originating from epidermis and an outer connective tissue sheath derived from dermis. The epithelial root sheath, in turn, consists of the **external root sheath** corresponding to the epidermal strata basale and spinosum and the **internal root sheath** corresponding to the strata granulosum and corneum. The latter, in turn, comprises three layers that help secure hair within a follicle: an outer **Henle layer** of clear squamous to cuboidal cells; a **Huxley layer** of two or three layers of flattened keratinized cells with modified keratohyalin granules, known as **trichohyalin granules;** and a **cuticle.** The epithelial root sheath is separated from the connective tissue sheath of the follicle by a homogeneous modified basement membrane, the glassy membrane. Connective tissue condenses around epithelial root sheaths to form dermal fibrous root sheaths and, along with capillaries, pushes into the bottom of follicles to reach hair matrix and form dermal papillae. The dermal root sheath is found around the lower part of the follicle. Sensory nerves, mostly related to cutaneous touch, innervate each hair follicle.

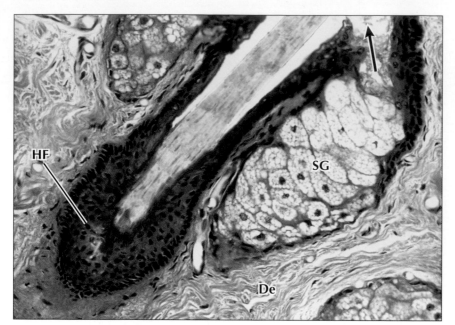

◀ **LM of a pilosebaceous unit.** The base of the hair follicle (**HF**) has a terminal expansion—the hair bulb. An associated sebaceous gland (**SG**) contains pale cells that show progressive enlargement and disintegration as they empty into a duct (**arrow**) at the upper end of the follicle. An optical artifact causes the hair shaft emanating from the hair follicle matrix to appear yellow. Surrounding dermis (**De**) is dense irregular connective tissue. 265×. *H&E.*

▶ **LM of a sebaceous gland and an arrector pili muscle in the dermis.** Peripheral cells of the sebaceous gland (**SG**) are small and flattened; center cells are larger and appear foamy because of lipid. A delicate capsule (**arrows**) surrounds the gland. A bundle of closely packed smooth muscle cells makes up the arrector pili muscle (**AP**). A small nerve fascicle (**NF**) lies nearby. The arrector muscles are innervated by postganglionic sympathetic nerve fibers. Contraction of smooth muscle causes slight erection of the associated hair, which produces goose bumps on the skin surface. Because the arrector muscles are closely associated with sebaceous glands, they also help expel sebum onto the hair. 295×. *H&E.*

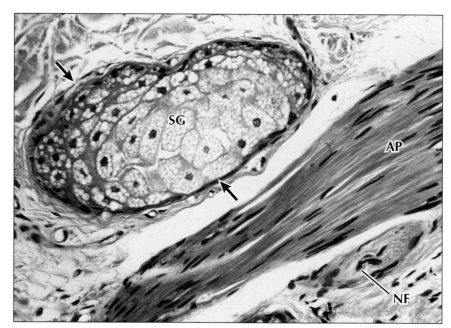

11.15 HISTOLOGY OF SEBACEOUS GLANDS AND ARRECTOR PILI MUSCLES

Sebaceous glands are usually associated with hair and are located between a **hair follicle** and its **arrector pili muscle** in the dermis. They are holocrine glands in which part of the secretory product, known as **sebum,** is made of lipid-rich decomposed cells. Most sebaceous glands empty secretions by a **duct** into the upper part of the hair follicle near the hair shaft. These simple or branched alveolar glands are pale staining and ovoid. A thin connective tissue **capsule** surrounds each alveolus, several of which typically open into a common duct that is lined by stratified squamous epithelium, which is continuous with the outer epithelial root sheath of the hair follicle. Each gland contains a peripheral layer of cuboidal cells (analogous to epidermal basal cells) with spheri-

cal nuclei resting on a thin basement membrane. These mitotically active cells give rise to the larger sebum-producing cells in the center of the gland. The larger cells are polyhedral and accumulate large amounts of **lipid** in the cytoplasm. Their nuclei become pyknotic, and cells gradually disintegrate, the debris becoming part of the secretory product. Sebaceous glands are under hormonal control and enlarge during puberty, when they produce a substantial amount of sebum, which may lead to development of acne in adolescents. Sebaceous glands lack myoepithelial cells, but attached to their capsule is a small bundle of obliquely arranged **smooth muscle** known as the *arrector pili muscle.* Contraction of this muscle compresses the gland and helps expel sebum into the follicle neck.

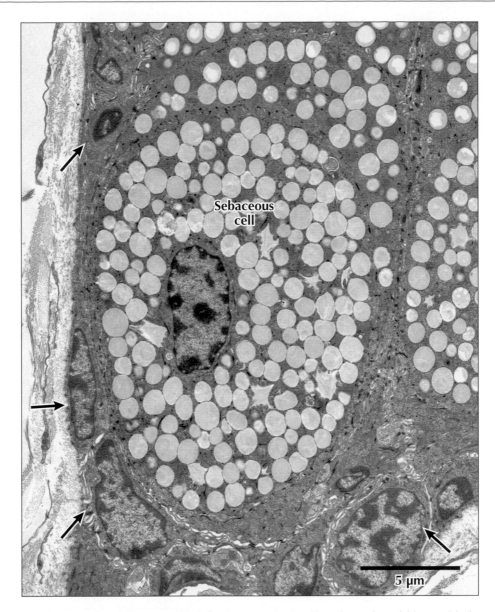

▲ **EM of part of a sebaceous gland**. Small nucleated cells with euchromatic nuclei (**arrows**) in the periphery of the gland serve as proliferating stem cells. A thin basement membrane covers them externally. A large sebaceous cell in the center contains many prominent lipid droplets, which surround a central nucleus. The cells ultimately break down and add their contents to oily secretory product. Sebum reduces water loss from the skin surface and lubricates hair. It may also protect skin from infection with bacteria. 5000×.

11.16 ULTRASTRUCTURE AND FUNCTION OF SEBACEOUS GLANDS

Preservation of sebaceous gland integrity by conventional methods is difficult, so electron microscopy has helped clarify the ultrastructural basis for gland function and unique method of holocrine secretion. The flattened to cuboidal **peripheral cells** of the gland appear relatively undifferentiated and are similar to basal cells of the epidermis, which contain large numbers of tonofilaments. They have a high nucleus-to-cytoplasm ratio and contain numerous free ribosomes and mitochondria. In contrast, central **sebaceous cells** are larger, with cytoplasm filled with lipid vacuoles and occasional lysosomes. **Sebum** is a complex oily mixture of lipids including glycerides, free fatty acids, and cholesterol. The lipid is synthesized in abundant smooth endoplasmic reticulum

and aggregates as **lipid droplets** in well-developed Golgi complex. In mature cells, enlarged lipid droplets become uniform in size and may ultimately fuse. These cells show a distorted shape, pyknotic nuclei, and sparse cytoplasm with few organelles. Sebaceous cells are attached by desmosomes to neighboring cells. Holocrine secretion involves breakdown of the entire sebaceous cell; lysosomal enzymes are responsible for this *autolysis*. The number of lysosomes increases as the sebaceous cell fills with more lipid. Cell breakdown occurs as the final step in the differentiation and enlargement process. Propelled by continuing proliferation of the basal cell layer, cells move to the center of the acinus. The renewal rate of sebaceous gland lobules is 21-25 days; the time from cellular synthesis to excretion is about 8 days.

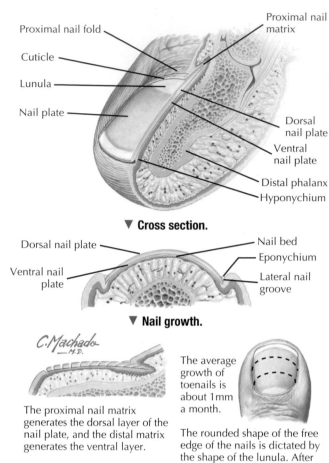

▼ **Sagittal section.**

Proximal nail fold
Cuticle
Lunula
Nail plate
Proximal nail matrix
Dorsal nail plate
Ventral nail plate
Distal phalanx
Hyponychium

▼ **Cross section.**

Dorsal nail plate
Ventral nail plate
Nail bed
Eponychium
Lateral nail groove

▼ **Nail growth.**

C. Machado M.D.

The proximal nail matrix generates the dorsal layer of the nail plate, and the distal matrix generates the ventral layer.

The average growth of toenails is about 1 mm a month.

The rounded shape of the free edge of the nails is dictated by the shape of the lunula. After avulsion of a nail, the free edge of the new one grows parallel to the lunula.

◀ **LM of part of a fetal phalanx in longitudinal section.** The nail (**arrow**) develops similarly to the hair follicle, as a thickened invagination of epidermis. 9×. *H&E.*

EP
NM
NP
De
Hy

▲ **LM of a fetal nail in longitudinal section.** The eponychium (**Ep**) is a superficial layer of epidermis that eventually degenerates, except at the base where it persists as the cuticle. The nail plate (**NP**) consists of intensely eosinophilic keratin and is derived from germinative cells in the nail matrix (**NM**). The nail bed, or hyponychium (**Hy**), underlies the nail plate. It is similar to the epidermis except that its dermal papillae are parallel to the nail surface. This longitudinal orientation allows the plate to move outward. The underlying dermis (**De**) is highly cellular. 35×. *H&E.*

11.17 ANATOMY AND HISTOLOGY OF NAILS

Nails are modifications of the stratum corneum of the **epidermis** on the dorsal aspect of terminal phalanges of fingers and toes. The slightly convex, semitransparent **nail plate** is composed of multiple layers of squamous-shaped, keratinized cells that are firmly held together. These cells contain hard keratin and do not desquamate. The undersurface of both exposed and concealed parts of the nail plate is the **nail bed.** It consists of stratum germinativum of the epidermis and underlying dense **dermis,** which lacks subcutaneous tissue but is firmly attached to periosteum of terminal phalanges. The nail is rooted in a **nail groove,** which is an invagination of the skin surrounded by a crescent-shaped rim of skin, the **nail fold.** The stratum germinativum and stratum corneum of the proximal nail fold continue back above the root of the nail into the groove, but the stratum germinativum alone returns along the underside of the root. The **eponychium,** or **cuticle,** is the projecting crescentic fold of stratum corneum; the **hyponychium** is the epidermal thickening under the free edge of the nail plate. The stratum germinativum of the nail bed is thickened under the proximal portion of the nail plate and becomes the **nail**

matrix—the site of active cellular proliferation. Mitosis of cells in the matrix causes nails to grow outward; dividing cells move outward and distally. They become keratinized, with no interposition of keratohyalin granules, and part of the nail. The **lunula** is the white crescent-shaped area of nail matrix. The average growth rate of nails is 1-2 mm per month. Unlike hair, nails grow continuously, not cyclically, throughout life, with fingernails growing faster than toenails.

CLINICAL POINT

The cuticle normally protects the nail matrix from infections. **Onychomycosis** is a fungal infection of the nail plate that causes fingernails and toenails to thicken, discolor, disfigure, and split. It is difficult to treat because nails grow slowly and receive very little blood supply. People with diabetes commonly develop the disorder because of poor blood circulation in extremities and a compromised ability to fight infections. The prevalence of onychomycosis is higher in males than in females, the incidence increasing with age. Although not life-threatening, it can lead to pain and secondary infection. Treatment options include oral and topical medications.

▼ **Psoriasis: typical distribution.**

Scalp
Sacrum
Intergluteal cleft
Elbow
Hand and nails

Groin and genitalia
Knee
Nail

◄ **Typical appearance of cutaneous lesions (plaque lesion).**

▼ **Section of skin lesion: histopathologic features.**

Surface "silver" scale

Erythematous base

Microabscess

Persistence of nuclei stratum corneum (parakeratosis)

Increased mitotic activity indicative of high cell turnover rate

Elongated rete pegs and dermal papillae

Dilation and tortuosity of papillary vessels

Edema and inflammation of dermis

Increased number of Langerhans cells

C.Machado _M.D._

11.18 HISTOLOGY OF PSORIASIS

Psoriasis is a chronic relapsing disorder of skin affecting 1%-3% of the population, most often at elbows, knees, scalp, and lumbosacral regions. In 80% of patients, nails are also involved. Sharply demarcated and elevated reddish **plaques** covered by silver to white **scales** are characteristic. Linked cellular changes include hyperplasia of keratinocytes, growth and dilation of superficial blood vessels, **chronic inflammation,** and infiltration of T lymphocytes and other leukocytes in affected skin. Excessive keratinocyte turnover causes marked epidermal thickening and downward elongation of epidermal ridges into dermis. Dermal papillae contain tortuous and dilated capillaries, which lie close to adjacent hyperkeratinic surface. Small abscesses of polymorphonuclear leukocytes appear under the hyperkeratotic areas; bleeding occurs when scales are forcibly removed. Mitotic figures are often seen in keratinocytes well above the stratum basale, and the stratum granulosum is often absent or greatly diminished. Neutrophils appear in the stratum corneum, and increased numbers of T cells and **Langerhans cells** are interspersed between keratinocytes throughout the epidermis and in the dermis. Psoriasis is regarded as a T lymphocyte autoimmune disease in which genetic and environmental factors play a role. In addition, *inflammatory cytokines* such as tumor necrosis factor are likely to be major pathogenic factors. Standard treatments include topical and systemic medications or ultraviolet light; novel biologic therapies, such as use of specific antibodies that target T cells, may prove beneficial.

12

UPPER DIGESTIVE SYSTEM

▼ **Organization of the digestive system.**

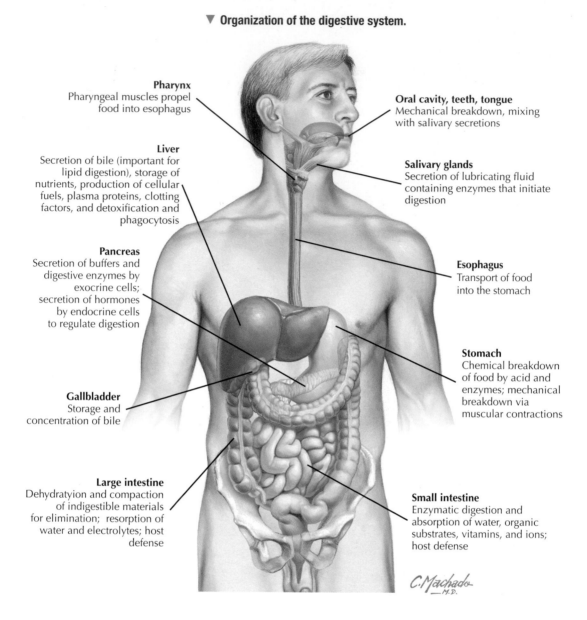

Pharynx
Pharyngeal muscles propel food into esophagus

Liver
Secretion of bile (important for lipid digestion), storage of nutrients, production of cellular fuels, plasma proteins, clotting factors, and detoxification and phagocytosis

Pancreas
Secretion of buffers and digestive enzymes by exocrine cells; secretion of hormones by endocrine cells to regulate digestion

Gallbladder
Storage and concentration of bile

Large intestine
Dehydratyion and compaction of indigestible materials for elimination; resorption of water and electrolytes; host defense

Oral cavity, teeth, tongue
Mechanical breakdown, mixing with salivary secretions

Salivary glands
Secretion of lubricating fluid containing enzymes that initiate digestion

Esophagus
Transport of food into the stomach

Stomach
Chemical breakdown of food by acid and enzymes; mechanical breakdown via muscular contractions

Small intestine
Enzymatic digestion and absorption of water, organic substrates, vitamins, and ions; host defense

C.Machado
_M.D._

12.1   OVERVIEW

The digestive system—a long, tortuous, hollow tube—comprises the *mouth* (or *oral cavity*), *pharynx*, and *digestive tube* or *tract* (also called the *alimentary canal*). Associated with this tract are accessory glands of digestion: **salivary glands, liver, gallbladder,** and **pancreas,** which lie outside the wall of the tube but are connected to it via ducts. The digestive system engages in many functions such as *propulsion, secretion, absorption, excretion, immunologic protection,* and *hormone production.* For convenience, this system can be divided into upper and lower tracts. The **upper digestive tract** facilitates ingestion and initial phases of digestion. It includes the **oral cavity** and associated structures (**lips, teeth, palate, tongue, cheeks**), **pharynx,** and **esophagus.** The lower tract deals mostly with digestion, absorption, and excretion. It includes the **stomach, small** and **large intestines,** and **anal canal.** The microscopic structure of each part of the tract, which is lined internally by mucous membrane, is adapted to reflect functional changes. Mucosa forming the inner lining of the mouth and pharynx is mostly nonkeratinized stratified squamous epithelium and an underlying lamina propria. Submucosa and a subjacent supporting wall, which attaches superficial tissues to skeletal muscle or bone, lie deep to the mucosa. Other parts of the upper and lower tracts conform to a common histologic plan involving four concentric layers (or tunics). A mucosa (or mucous membrane) is adjacent to the lumen. Underlying submucosa is made mostly of highly distensible connective tissue. A prominent muscularis externa consists mainly of smooth muscle oriented in different directions. An outer tunic, the adventitia, is fibrous connective tissue and is known as a serosa in areas in the peritoneal cavity, where this outer tunic is covered externally by peritoneal mesothelium.

▼ **Section through the upper lip.**

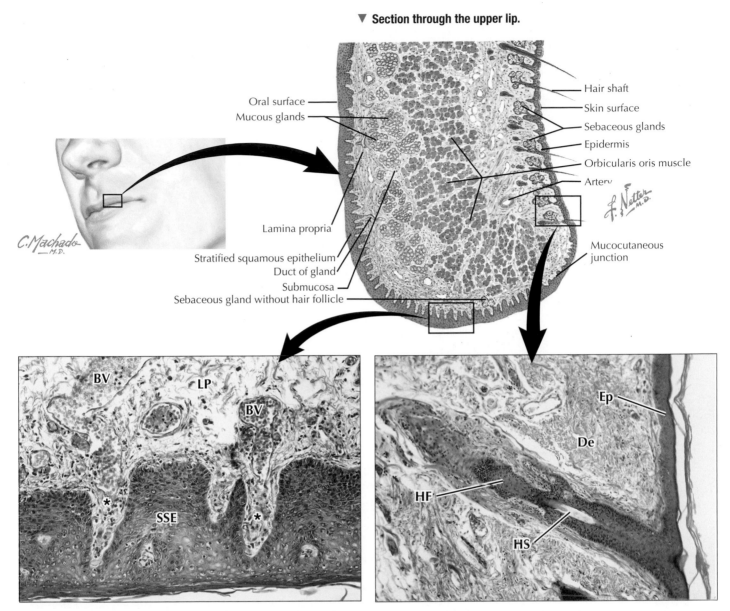

Oral surface
Mucous glands

Hair shaft
Skin surface
Sebaceous glands
Epidermis
Orbicularis oris muscle
Artery

Lamina propria

Stratified squamous epithelium
Duct of gland
Submucosa
Sebaceous gland without hair follicle

Mucocutaneous junction

BV | LP | BV | SSE | * | *

Ep | De | HF | HS

▲ **Light micrographs (LMs) of parts of the lip. Left,** The vermillion border is stratified squamous epithelium (**SSE**) with a thin layer of surface keratin, below. Underlying connective tissue—lamina propria (**LP**)—contains many blood vessels (**BV**). The highly corrugated interface between epithelium and connective tissue shows tall papillae (⋆) penetrating the epithelium to take capillaries close to the surface. **Right,** The external cutaneous surface, of typical thin skin, consists of epidermis (**Ep**) and underlying dermis (**De**). A hair follicle (**HF**) and associated hair shaft (**HS**) are seen. **Left**: 130×; **Right**: 85×. *H&E.*

12.2 HISTOLOGY OF THE LIPS: SKIN AND VERMILLION BORDER

Lips guard the entrance to the digestive tract as a **mucocutaneous junction** between the body exterior and digestive system. Each lip has three surfaces: an outer **cutaneous** part, red (**vermillion**) border, and inner **oral mucosa.** The outer **thin skin** is richly innervated with sensory nerves. Like thin skin in other parts of the body, it consists of an **epidermis** and an underlying **dermis** with **hair follicles, sebaceous glands,** and *sweat glands.* A transitional zone between skin and oral mucosa is the free edge, or vermillion border. Its **stratified squamous epithelium** is thick and either lacks a superficial layer of **keratin** or is lightly keratinized. Under the epithelium are tall **connective tissue papillae** that are close to the surface. The vermillion border is pinkish-red because of the relatively translucent epithelium and the blood in **capillaries** in the papillae. This border lacks hair follicles and, because it has no glands, is dry.

CLINICAL POINT

Carcinoma of the lip is the most common oral cavity malignancy, with almost 95% of cases being **squamous cell carcinoma.** The lower lip is prone to these neoplasms, usually caused by chronic sun exposure, and middle-aged and elderly men are more susceptible to them than women. Compared with other head and neck cancers, lip carcinoma is readily curable, but sometimes regional metastasis, local recurrence, and death may occur. Treatment involves equally effective surgical excision or radiation therapy, the choice depending on tumor size.

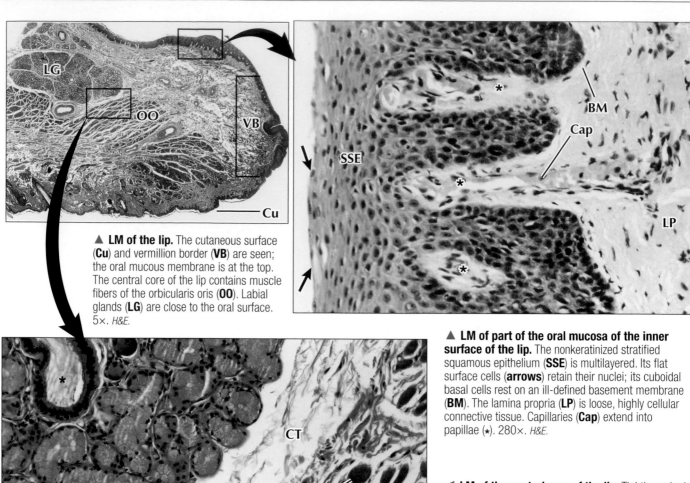

▲ **LM of the lip.** The cutaneous surface (**Cu**) and vermillion border (**VB**) are seen; the oral mucous membrane is at the top. The central core of the lip contains muscle fibers of the orbicularis oris (**OO**). Labial glands (**LG**) are close to the oral surface. 5×. *H&E.*

▲ **LM of part of the oral mucosa of the inner surface of the lip.** The nonkeratinized stratified squamous epithelium (**SSE**) is multilayered. Its flat surface cells (**arrows**) retain their nuclei; its cuboidal basal cells rest on an ill-defined basement membrane (**BM**). The lamina propria (**LP**) is loose, highly cellular connective tissue. Capillaries (**Cap**) extend into papillae (∗). 280×. *H&E.*

◀ **LM of the central core of the lip.** Tightly packed mucous acini of a labial gland (**LG**)—a tubuloacinar minor salivary gland—surround a small duct (∗). Low simple columnar epithelium lines the duct. The connection of the duct is not seen in the plane of section, but it opens onto the oral surface. Adjacent skeletal muscle fibers of the orbicularis oris (**OO**) are organized into fascicles. The pale area between the gland and muscle is fibroelastic connective tissue (**CT**). 125×. *H&E.*

12.3 HISTOLOGY OF THE LIPS: ORAL MUCOSA AND CENTRAL CORE

The inner side of the lip is lined by an **oral mucous membrane** consisting of thick **nonkeratinized stratified squamous epithelium** and underlying **lamina propria** of loose, richly vascularized connective tissue that indents the epithelium with papillae. These papillae resemble those under the epidermis but are thinner and more delicate. The highly corrugated interface between epithelium and lamina propria firmly anchors these tissues against mechanical forces such as friction. The lamina propria contains collagen and elastic fibers, which permit distensibility over underlying tissues. It also harbors capillaries and lymphatics plus many lymphocytes and other cells, which aid in immunologic defense against pathogens and irritants in the external environment. Sensory nerve fibers (branches of cranial nerve V) are also abundant. The mucous membrane forms part of the wall of the oral cavity. Surface cells of the epithelium are continuously shed into the oral cavity lumen, the renewal rate of these cells being 12-14 days. As in other epithelia, a basement membrane separates its basal aspect from the lamina propria. Small groups of **minor salivary glands,** the **labial glands,** are deep to the lamina propria in the submucosa. Secretions of these mainly mucus-secreting exocrine glands drain onto the oral surface via small **ducts,** thereby providing moisture and lubrication. The bulk of the lip is made of a central core of **skeletal muscle,** the **orbicularis oris muscle,** whose fibers are surrounded by fibroelastic connective tissue.

▼ **Oral cavity.**

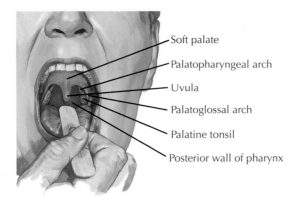

Soft palate

Palatopharyngeal arch

Uvula

Palatoglossal arch

Palatine tonsil

Posterior wall of pharynx

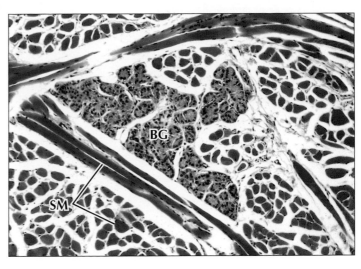

▲ **LM of part of the cheek.** Skeletal muscle fibers (**SM**) of the buccinator are sectioned longitudinally and transversely. Parenchyma of a minor salivary (buccal) gland (**BG**) is in intervening connective tissue. 60×. *H&E.*

▼ **Marginal gingivitis.**

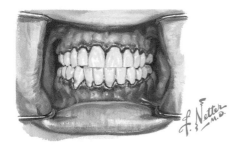

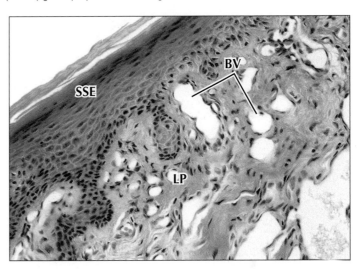

▶ **LM of the gingiva.** Lightly keratinized stratified squamous epithelium (**SSE**) and richly vascularized lamina propria (**LP**) form the masticatory oral mucosa on the surface. Many small, thin-walled blood vessels (**BV**) are in the connective tissue. 250×. *H&E.*

12.4 HISTOLOGY OF THE ORAL CAVITY: CHEEK AND GINGIVA

The **oral mucosa** is regionally modified to reflect differences in function and ability to withstand friction and is classified into three types. *Lining mucosa* forms the inner lining of the lips, cheeks, soft palate, floor of the mouth, and undersurface of the tongue. It is mainly **nonkeratinized stratified squamous epithelium** with underlying, supportive **lamina propria.** *Masticatory mucosa* consists of stratified squamous epithelium that is lightly *keratinized* (cells in the stratum corneum retain nuclei). This relatively immobile mucosa is found in gingivae (gums) and hard palate. *Specialized mucosa* on the dorsal surface of the tongue has many papillae and taste buds. The cheek resembles the lip in histologic features. Stratified squamous epithelium of its mucosa is nonkeratinized. The lamina propria, with short papillae and abundant elastic fibers, attaches at intervals to underlying **skeletal muscle fibers** of the **buccinator.** These fibers are arranged into fascicles that mix with **minor salivary (buccal) glands.** The gingiva, a mucous membrane that lacks glands, covers outer and inner surfaces of the alveolar processes of the maxilla and mandible and surrounds each tooth. Its stratified squamous epithelium

overlying a thick, fibrous lamina propria is lightly keratinized on its surface and lacks a stratum granulosum. The lamina propria is firmly anchored to underlying periosteum of the bone, which makes the mucosa immobile and inelastic. The lamina propria extends into deep papillary projections into the base of the epithelium. As in other areas of the oral cavity, papillae contain a large network of capillaries. The epithelium may also be lightly keratinized. It is subject to abrasion during mastication.

CLINICAL POINT

Poor or inadequate oral hygiene may lead to inflammation of the gums called **gingivitis,** the most common dental pathology in children and adults. Gingivitis is usually caused by accumulation of *plaque* or *calculus (tartar),* containing large numbers of bacteria. Bacterial invasion of the oral mucosa leads to swelling, irritation, bleeding, and redness of gums. Features of chronic gingivitis include accumulation of plasma cells and B lymphocytes in the lamina propria, plus destruction of collagen. Untreated, gingivitis may lead to more serious complications such as **periodontitis.** This often involves destruction of the periodontal ligament and alveolar bone, and ultimately tooth loss.

▼ **Dorsum of tongue.**

Epiglottis
Palatine tonsil
Lingual tonsil
Foramen cecum
Root
Circumvallate
Foliate   } papillae
Filiform
Body
Fungiform

Fungiform papilla

▼ **Schematic stereogram of area indicated above.**

Filiform papillae
Lingual tonsil
papilla
Duct of gland
Crypt
Mucous glands
Circumvallate papilla
Taste buds
Serous glands of von Ebner

Intrinsic muscle

▼ **Section of taste bud.**

Sustentacular cell
Sensory cell
Taste pore

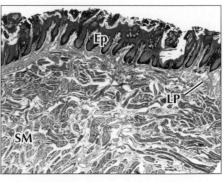

▲ **LM of the dorsum of the tongue at low magnification.** Many lingual papillae give the epithelial surface (**Ep**) an irregular contour. Stratified epithelium rests on a lamina propria (**LP**). Deep in underlying connective tissue are fascicles of skeletal muscle fibers (**SM**) sectioned in different planes. 7×. *H&E.*

◀ **LM of the undersurface of the tongue.** The smooth mucosa has a relatively simple contour. The nonkeratinized stratified squamous epithelium (**Ep**) consists of many layers of cells and rests on a lamina propria (**LP**) of loose connective tissue. Upward projections of lamina propria into the epithelium form connective tissue papillae (*). 120×. *H&E.*

◀ **LM of the dorsal surface of the tongue.** A deep trench-like furrow (*) surrounds the circumvallate papilla (**CVP**) on the mucosal surface. Serous glands of von Ebner (**SG**) drain into the base of each furrow via small ducts (**arrows**). Deep to the lamina propria (**LP**) are bundles of skeletal muscle fibers (**SM**). 20×. *H&E.*

12.5 STRUCTURE AND FUNCTION OF THE TONGUE

The tongue sits in the floor of the **oral cavity.** This mobile, muscular organ covered externally by a **mucous membrane** is divided into two parts. An anterior (oral) two-thirds is separated from a posterior (pharyngeal) one-third by a V-shaped groove called the **sulcus terminalis.** The epithelium of the anterior part derives from oral ectoderm, and that of the posterior part, from foregut endoderm. The tongue engages in mastication, swallowing, speech, and taste. Innervation is by four cranial nerves (V, VII, IX, and XII). Smooth **nonkeratinized stratified squamous epithelium** covers its undersurface and dorsum, except over filiform papillae on the dorsum, where epithelium is parakeratinized. A central mass of intrinsic and extrinsic **skeletal muscle** consists of interlacing bundles of muscle fibers oriented in three planes. A roughened dorsal surface characterizes the anterior two-thirds of the tongue. Three main types of surface vertical projections—**lingual papillae**—are seen, called **filiform, fungiform,** and **circumvallate**

papillae because of differences in form. A fourth type—**foliate papillae**—is not well developed in humans. When present, they are found posteriorly on lateral tongue borders. The posterior third of the tongue lacks lingual papillae, but its dorsal surface is studded by 35-100 irregular mucosal bulges that correspond to **lingual tonsils** and thus has a cobblestone appearance.

CLINICAL POINT

The oral mucosa is the point of entry for pathogens and irritants from the outside into the digestive and respiratory tracts. The clinician must recognize its normal appearance because changes in it are often related to systemic diseases, hormonal states, nutritional deficiencies, and immunologic disorders. **Oral candidiasis,** presenting as white plaque-like lesions, is a fungal infection in healthy adults. Epstein-Barr virus causes **hairy leukoplakia,** which consists of white mucosal lesions on the tongue. HIV-positive patients often have these lesions. Repair of oral mucosa in response to disease or infection is much more efficient than that of skin, as there is almost no scar formation after injury.

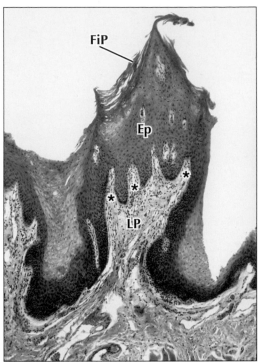

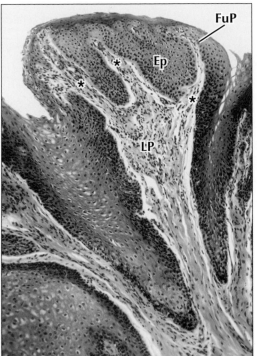

◄ **LMs of filiform (Left) and fungiform (Right) papillae. Left,** A layer of keratin covers the pointed end of the filiform papilla (**FiP**). Underlying stratified squamous epithelium (**Ep**) is a core of lamina propria (**LP**) with secondary connective tissue papillae (✶). **Right,** The mushroom-shaped fungiform papilla (**FuP**) has parakeratinized epithelium (**Ep**). Small secondary connective tissue papillae (✶) emanate from a central core of lamina propria (**LP**). **Left:** 75×; **Right:** 80×. *H&E.*

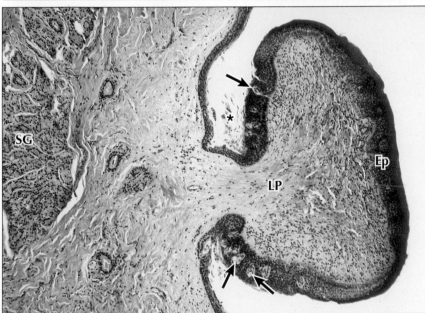

◄ **LM of a circumvallate papilla.** Nonkeratinized stratified squamous epithelium (**Ep**), which has several taste buds embedded in the lateral margins (**arrows**), covers the papilla, and a deep furrow (✶) encircles it. Underlying lamina propria (**LP**) is loose, richly cellular connective tissue. Serous glands of von Ebner (**SG**) are in deeper areas of the connective tissue. Their watery secretions help flush cellular debris from the furrow, to better expose taste buds to gustatory stimuli. 70×. *H&E.*

12.6 HISTOLOGY AND FUNCTION OF LINGUAL PAPILLAE

Cone-shaped **filiform papillae,** the most numerous papillae, are 2-3 mm long and help manipulate food and increase friction with it during mastication. **Keratin** that covers their pointed ends makes the tongue gray. The primary **connective tissue** core in each papilla may have small **secondary connective tissue papillae.** Less numerous, mushroom-shaped **fungiform papillae** are poorly keratinized and are scattered singly or in small groups between filiform papillae. Most are near the tip of the tongue. Fungiform papillae have connective tissue cores with primary and secondary branches, which are richly vascularized, thus appearing as red spots (visible macroscopically) on the tongue surface. One row of 8-12 **circumvallate papillae** lies just anterior to the sulcus termi-

nalis. These largest papillae have a diameter of up to 3 mm and are either nonkeratinized or incompletely keratinized. Each is countersunk beneath the surface and is surrounded by a trench-like circular furrow. **Serous glands of von Ebner** deep in the **lamina propria** drain via ducts into the base of each furrow, their watery secretions clearing it of debris. **Taste buds**—small intraepithelial organs—are embedded on lateral surfaces of the epithelium of fungiform and circumvallate papillae (up to 5 and 250 taste buds on one of each type, respectively). Humans have about 5000 taste buds on the tongue plus about 2500 on the soft palate, 900 on the epiglottis, and 600 in the larynx and pharynx. These special sensory receptors transduce chemical stimuli into nerve impulses, which the brain perceives as gustatory sensations.

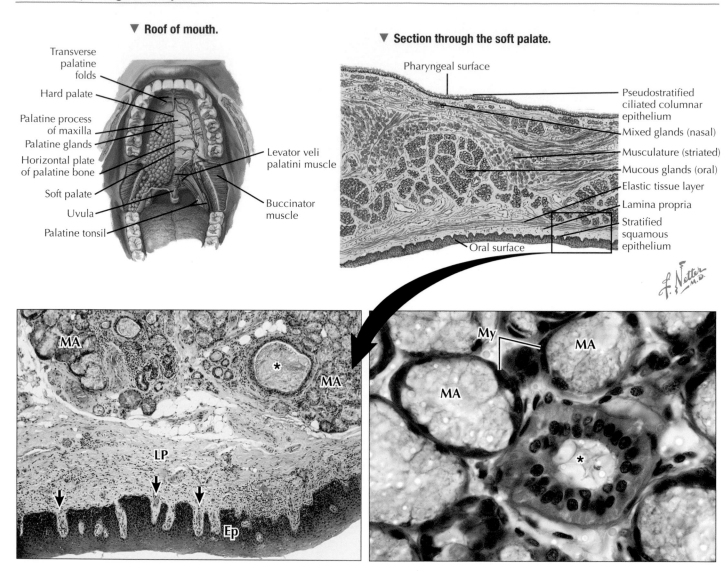

▼ **Roof of mouth.**

Transverse palatine folds
Hard palate
Palatine process of maxilla
Palatine glands
Horizontal plate of palatine bone
Soft palate
Uvula
Palatine tonsil
Levator veli palatini muscle
Buccinator muscle

▼ **Section through the soft palate.**

Pharyngeal surface
Pseudostratified ciliated columnar epithelium
Mixed glands (nasal)
Musculature (striated)
Mucous glands (oral)
Elastic tissue layer
Lamina propria
Stratified squamous epithelium
Oral surface

▲ **LM of the oral surface of the hard palate.** Stratified squamous epithelium (**Ep**) of the mucosa is orthokeratinized. Lymphocytes infiltrate the richly vascularized lamina propria (**LP**). Conical connective tissue papillae (**arrows**) protrude into the epithelium. Part of a palatine gland—consisting of collections of pale mucous acini (**MA**) and a duct (*)—is in the submucosa. 60×. *H&E.*

▲ **LM of part of a palatine gland.** Pale mucous cells make up each mucous acinus (**MA**). More deeply eosinophilic, flat myoepithelial cells (**My**) are associated with the base of each acinus. A duct (*), sectioned transversely, consists of one row of columnar epithelial cells around a central lumen. 560×. *H&E.*

12.7 STRUCTURE AND FUNCTION OF THE PALATE

The palate forms the roof of the mouth and separates oral and nasal cavities. The anterior part is the **hard palate;** the posterior, the **soft palate.** The rigid hard palate is made of horizontal bony processes covered by **masticatory mucosa** that serves as a working surface for the tongue as it presses against the palate during mastication and swallowing. The mucosa adheres firmly to the periosteum of bone and is thus immovable. Its *keratinized* or *orthokeratinized* **stratified squamous epithelium** has underlying connective tissue papillae. These extensions of the **lamina propria** also contain many capillaries and infiltrated lymphocytes. **Ducts** connect small mucus-secreting **palatine glands** in the **submucosa** in the very posterior part to the epithelial surface. The soft palate—a mobile fold with a conical posterior projection called the **uvula**—closes off the nasopharynx from the oropharynx during swallowing. Rich vascularity makes its mucosa red. On the oral side, the epithelium is **nonkeratinized stratified squamous;** the nasopharyngeal side has a respiratory epithelium-ciliated pseudostratified columnar epithelium with goblet cells. Unlike the hard palate, the soft palate lacks bone, but its core contains a support sheet of palatine **skeletal muscle.** Submucosal **mucous glands** are near the oral surface; mixed seromucous glands, the nasopharyngeal side.

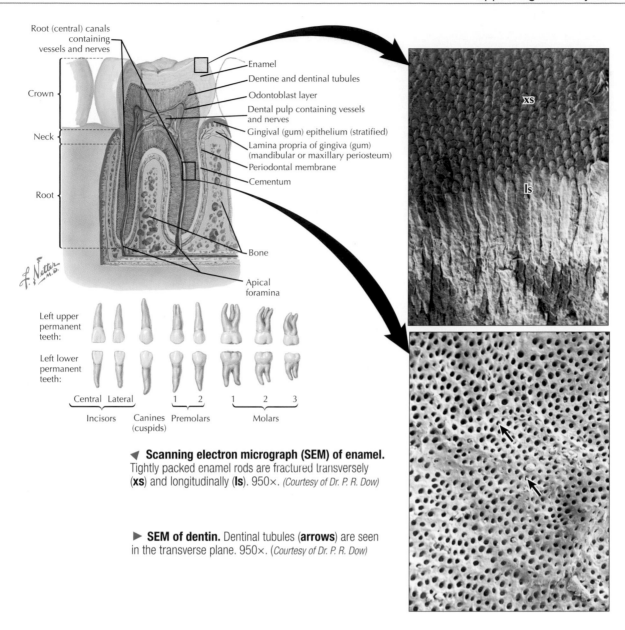

Root (central) canals containing vessels and nerves

Crown

Neck

Root

f. Netter m.d.

Enamel
Dentine and dentinal tubules
Odontoblast layer
Dental pulp containing vessels and nerves
Gingival (gum) epithelium (stratified)
Lamina propria of gingiva (gum) (mandibular or maxillary periosteum)
Periodontal membrane
Cementum

Bone

Apical foramina

Left upper permanent teeth:

Left lower permanent teeth:

Central Lateral   1   2   1   2   3

Incisors Canines Premolars   Molars
          (cuspids)

◀ **Scanning electron micrograph (SEM) of enamel.** Tightly packed enamel rods are fractured transversely (**xs**) and longitudinally (**ls**). 950×. *(Courtesy of Dr. P. R. Dow)*

▶ **SEM of dentin.** Dentinal tubules (**arrows**) are seen in the transverse plane. 950×. *(Courtesy of Dr. P. R. Dow)*

12.8 STRUCTURE AND FUNCTION OF TEETH

Humans have two sets of teeth. The *primary* (or *deciduous*) teeth erupt at about 7 months of age, form a complete set of 20 teeth by about 2 years, and are shed between ages 6 and 12 years. They are replaced by 32 **permanent teeth,** 16 of which are in the maxilla and 16 in the mandible. Each jaw has 4 **incisors,** mostly for cutting during mastication; 2 **canines,** for puncturing and grasping; and 10 **molars/premolars,** for crushing and grinding. Each tooth consists of a free **crown** projecting above the **gingiva,** and one or more **roots** embedded in a **bony socket** (or **alveolus**) of the jaws. Despite different forms and functions, all teeth share the same histologic plan. Each root is attached to **bone** by densely packed collagen fibers, which form the **periodontal membrane.** A central pulp chamber extends into **root canals.** These communicate via **apical foramina,** at root tips, with a periodontal membrane and the tooth exterior. The pulp chamber contains a core of loose connective tissue—soft, gelatinous **dental pulp.** Pulp contains blood vessels, lymphatics, and nerves that enter and leave via apical foramina. Three mineralized tissues—**dentin, enamel,** and **cementum**—make up tooth walls. Dentin surrounds the pulp cavity and is the bulk of the tooth. Enamel forms a cap over the outer dentin surface in the area of the crown and may be 2.5 mm thick in some teeth. On roots, cementum covers dentin.

CLINICAL POINT

Acid-forming bacteria that dissolve enamel cause **tooth decay,** or **dental caries.** The bacteria may penetrate deeper layers of teeth, into the pulp, leading to pain, local infection, and tooth loss. *Fluoridation* has dramatically reduced the incidence of caries. Fluoride-containing compounds are added to drinking water or commercial oral hygiene products or are used in prescribed treatments. Fluoride ions replace hydroxyl ions in hydroxyapatite crystals of enamel to form fluorapatite, which strengthens enamel by making it chemically more stable, less soluble, and more resistant to breakdown by acid bacteria in *plaque.*

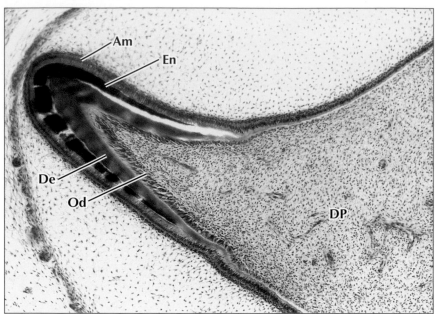

◀ **LM of an enamel organ at the bell stage of odontogenesis.** Outside, one layer of ameloblasts (**Am**) is closely apposed to newly formed, darker enamel (**En**). Deeper in the organ, odontoblasts (**Od**), which are differentiated from mesenchymal cells, are at the outer margin of the dental papilla (**DP**). They form one row of cells, next to newly formed dentin (**De**). At this stage of tooth development, the papilla is a mass of primitive mesenchymal cells, which later become dental pulp. 90×. *H&E.*

▶ **LM of part of an enamel organ with details of the dentinoenamel junction.** Tall columnar ameloblasts (**Am**) form one row on the outer aspect of the enamel organ. They have basally located nuclei and thin apical projections called Tomes' processes (**TP**) that extend toward a thin layer of lightly stained preenamel (**PE**), which is the organic matrix of newly formed enamel. A thicker layer of fully mineralized enamel (**En**), more darkly stained, borders the preenamel. On the opposite side, a layer of differentiating odontoblasts (**Od**) is apposed to a thin, lightly stained layer of predentin (**PD**). Thin apical processes of odontoblasts project across predentin into dentin (**De**), which appears darker and radially striate. A thin, clear artifactual space (**arrows**) marks the dentinoenamel junction. 250×. *H&E.*

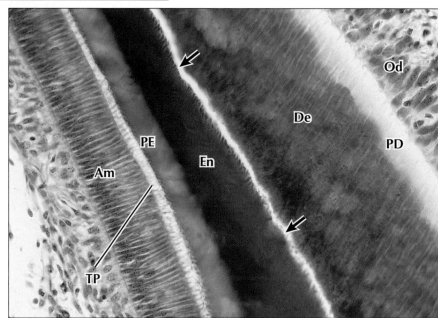

12.9   DEVELOPMENT AND HISTOLOGY OF TEETH: AMELOBLASTS AND ODONTOBLASTS

Teeth develop by a complex process called **odontogenesis** and derive from two embryonic sources. **Enamel** arises from **oral ectoderm; dentin, pulp, cementum,** and **periodontal membrane** originate from **mesenchyme.** Interactions between oral ectoderm and underlying mesenchyme of the developing fetal jaw lead to tooth formation. A bud-like thickening of oral ectoderm first forms a curved *dental lamina*, which invaginates the mesenchyme. The originally cap-shaped dental lamina becomes a bell-shaped **enamel organ** over condensed underlying mesenchyme known as **dental papilla.** The enamel organ wall first consists of outer and inner layers of epithelial cells. Cells of the inner layer become columnar and differentiate into **ameloblasts.** These polarized cells have apical projections called **Tomes' processes.** Outer mesenchymal cells of the papilla enlarge and form a layer of tall columnar

cells, the **odontoblasts.** Ameloblasts and odontoblasts are close to each other. Extracellular deposition of enamel by ameloblasts follows that of dentin by odontoblasts, and the two extracellular tissues lie between the two cell layers. Surrounding mesenchyme in the area of a developing root gives rise to cells called *cementoblasts.* These modified osteoblasts produce cementum that covers dentin in this area. Other mesenchymal cells give rise to the periodontal membrane. Ameloblasts and the enamel organ are lost at tooth eruption, but odontoblasts persist throughout life. **Dental pulp**—loose, highly vascularized and innervated connective tissue—also develops from condensed mesenchyme of the dental papilla. Odontoblasts are highly polarized cells with basal nuclei and cytoplasm that contains organelles engaged in synthesis and secretion of dentin matrix. Apical processes of odontoblasts are eventually trapped in narrow channels in dentin called *dentinal tubules.*

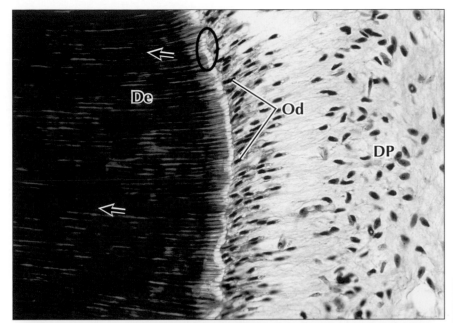

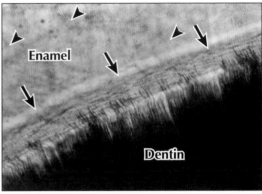

◀ **LM of part of a developing tooth showing details of dentin.** Odontoblasts (**Od**) are close to dentin (**De**), which is intensely eosinophilic because of collagen in its matrix. These cells have thin apical processes (**encircled**) that enter dentin in dentinal tubules (**arrows**), which appear as linear strands running through the dentin. Mesenchymal cells in the dental papilla (**DP**) will later form dental pulp. 340×. *H&E.*

▼ **Part of a mature human tooth.** Enamel covers dentin at the crown of the tooth. The dentinoenamel junction (**arrows**) looks scalloped, and firm attachment of enamel to dentin at this interface is required for tooth function in mastication. Obliquely oriented, ill-defined lines (**arrowheads**) in enamel are enamel rods. Their arrangement contrasts with relatively dark, parallel dentinal tubules in dentin. 300×. *Ground unstained section.*

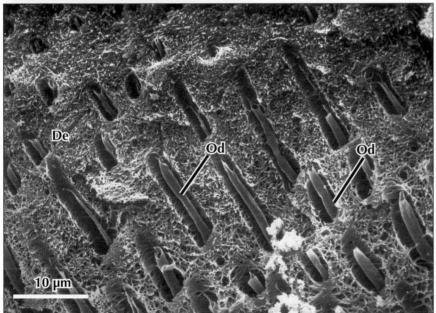

◀ **High-resolution SEM of dentinal tubules.** Many dentinal tubules run through the dentin (**De**) matrix. The 3- to 4-μm-diameter processes of odontoblasts (**Od**) are in the tubules. 2000×. *(Courtesy of Dr. P. R. Dow)*

12.10 HISTOLOGY OF TEETH: DENTIN AND ENAMEL

Dentin, a hard yet resilient tissue, has a chemical composition like that of bone but with a higher calcium content. About 70% of its matrix is inorganic and consists mostly of **hydroxyapatite crystals.** About 18% of the matrix is organic—mostly **type I collagen fibers**—and the rest (12%) is water. **Odontoblasts** produce the organic matrix, and this secretory process closely resembles that by which osteoblasts produce osteoid during bone development. Odontoblasts produce dentin throughout life and have good reparative capacity. They first elaborate predentin, which is mineralized with hydroxyapatite and becomes adult dentin. Dentin appears radially striated because of **dentinal tubules** that are 3-5 μm in diameter and up to 5 mm long. These are organized perpendicularly to the pulp cavity and have an S-shaped course. The lumen of a dentinal tubule contains the apical cytoplasmic process of an odontoblast. **Enamel** is the hardest substance in the body, is brittle, and fractures easily. About 96% of it is hydroxyapatite, the rest (4%) being inorganic matrix made of unique glycoproteins called *amelogenins* and *enamelins;* it lacks collagen. Enamel is composed of tightly packed rods (or prisms), 4-8 μm in diameter, that resemble fish scales. One ameloblast produces each enamel rod. Ameloblasts degenerate after tooth eruption; enamel lasts throughout life, is not static, and is influenced by salivary secretions. Destroyed enamel is repaired only by restorative procedures that use fillings or inlays. *Cementum* is most similar to bone but is avascular and lacks osteons. It is the mineralized tissue into which collagen fibers—*Sharpey fibers*—of the periodontal membrane insert.

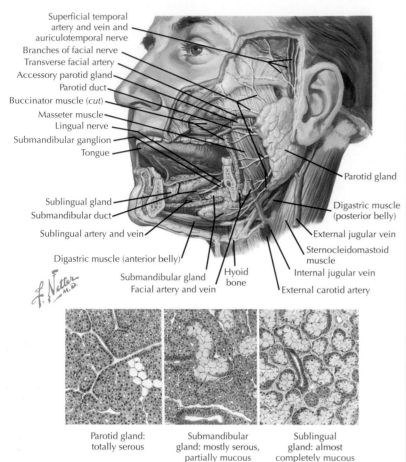

Superficial temporal artery and vein and auriculotemporal nerve
Branches of facial nerve
Transverse facial artery
Accessory parotid gland
Parotid duct
Buccinator muscle (*cut*)
Masseter muscle
Lingual nerve
Submandibular ganglion
Tongue

Parotid gland

Sublingual gland
Submandibular duct

Digastric muscle (posterior belly)

Sublingual artery and vein

External jugular vein
Sternocleidomastoid muscle
Internal jugular vein

Digastric muscle (anterior belly)

F. Netter

Submandibular gland
Facial artery and vein

Hyoid bone

External carotid artery

Parotid gland: totally serous

Submandibular gland: mostly serous, partially mucous

Sublingual gland: almost completely mucous

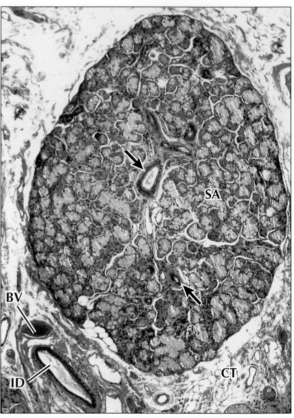

▲ **LM of a lobule of a sublingual gland.** All three major salivary glands are organized into lobules similar to this, with tightly packed parenchyma surrounded by loose connective tissue stroma (**CT**). Grape-like clusters of secretory acini (**SA**) and a few intralobular ducts (**arrows**) are in the lobule; larger interlobular ducts (**ID**) and blood vessels (**BV**) are in the stroma. 60×. *H&E.*

12.11 STRUCTURE AND FUNCTION OF SALIVARY GLANDS

Three pairs of **major salivary glands**—**parotid, submandibular,** and **sublingual**—and several minor salivary glands produce **saliva** and empty secretory products via **ducts** in the oral cavity. About 750-1200 ml of saliva (a watery, viscous suspension of mucus, enzymes, inorganic ions, and antibodies, pH 6.7-7.4) is produced daily. It lubricates and protects oral tissues, is an aqueous solvent for taste, and as a masticatory wetting agent, aids swallowing. It starts digestion of carbohydrates by secreting *α-amylase (ptyalin).* It also contains *bacterial lysozyme,* which inhibits dental caries, and immunoglobulins (e.g., IgA, IgM, IgG), which aid control of microbial flora in the oral cavity. Major salivary glands are **compound tubuloacinar glands.** The parotid, the largest, weighs 15-30 g in adults and is roughly pyramidal; its major duct is *Stensen's duct.* This exclusively serous exocrine gland produces about 30% of saliva. The egg-shaped submandibular gland, the second largest,

weighs 10-15 g and lies in the floor of the oral cavity. Its watery secretion accounts for about 60% of saliva. Most of its secretory units are serous, but it also has **mucous acini.** Its main excretory duct is Wharton's duct. The sublingual gland, the smallest major gland, usually weighs 2 g or less. This flat, almond-shaped organ sits beneath the mucous membrane in the floor of the mouth. This mixed, mostly mucous gland produces about 5% of saliva. *Minor salivary glands* are small, isolated glands in the lips, cheeks, tongue, and palate. They are mainly *mixed seromucous glands,* but purely serous or mucous glands are found in isolated sites. These glands have a **parenchyma** (of glandular epithelium) and **connective tissue stroma.** The parenchyma derives from oral cavity ectoderm: at about 6 weeks of gestation, solid buds form from oropharyngeal epithelium. The buds acquire a lumen and develop into tubuloacinar secretory end pieces and a branching duct system. Mesenchyme around the parenchyma gives rise to the stroma and capsule of the glands.

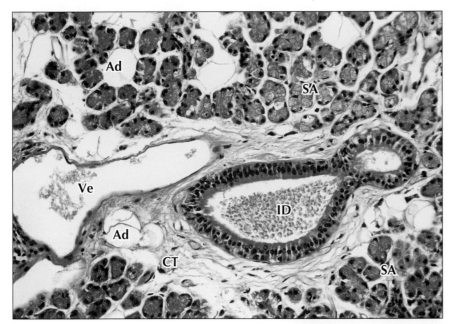

◄ **LM of a parotid gland.** Closely packed clusters of purely serous acini (**SA**) and a branching interlobular duct (**ID**) are visible. Pseudostratified epithelium lines the duct, which is between parts of two lobules, is surrounded by dense irregular connective tissue (**CT**), and accompanies a venule (**Ve**). Adipocytes (**Ad**) occur mainly in the parotid, not often seen in the two other major salivary glands. 175×. *H&E.*

► **LM of a parotid at higher magnification.** Loose connective tissue (**CT**) of the stroma surrounds many secretory acini (**SA**) and two striated ducts (**SD**). Serous cells in each acinus have round basal nuclei and are arranged around a small central lumen. Simple columnar epithelium lines the larger lumina of striated ducts, so named because of striations in the basal cytoplasm of the lining cells. 340×. *H&E.*

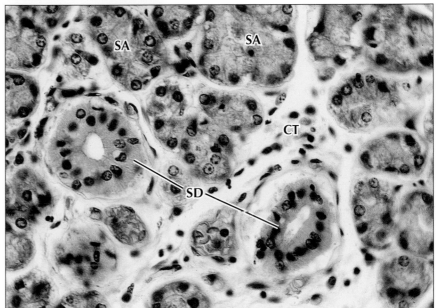

12.12 HISTOLOGY OF PAROTID GLANDS

A fibrous capsule encloses parenchyma of the parotid and sends in *septa* to divide it into *lobes* and *lobules*. The septa are a supportive framework for the gland and a conduit for blood vessels and autonomic nerves. The parotid, a **branched tubuloacinar gland,** is composed of clusters of elongated, branched **serous acini.** Pyramidal **serous cells** that surround a central lumen form each acinus. These cells have round basal nuclei and granular cytoplasm that is basophilic at the base and a bit more eosinophilic toward the apex. A basement membrane surrounds each acinus and encloses a few flat myoepithelial cells that are hard to see in conventional preparations. *Intercalated ducts,* the initial part of the duct system, are slender conduits formed of one layer of squamous or cuboidal epithelial cells. They drain into **striated ducts,** which are lined by columnar cells with basal striations. Both intercalated and striated ducts are intralobular and are **secretory ducts** because of their metabolic activities. A delicate, richly vascularized stroma surrounds secretory acini and **intralobular ducts.** These ducts connect with larger **interlobular ducts** between lobules. Initial segments of interlobular ducts are lined by stratified cuboidal **epithelium,** which gradually becomes stratified **columnar** and then **pseudostratified** as duct diameters increase. Near the main outlet of the major (Stensen's) duct, the epithelium becomes stratified squamous as it opens into the oral cavity vestibule.

CLINICAL POINT

Mumps, or **epidemic parotiditis,** is an *acute viral infection* caused by *paramyxovirus* and transmitted mainly via infected saliva. Before the vaccine, it was a common childhood communicable disease affecting both sexes equally. It causes swollen and painful parotid glands (both glands or one), plus headache, malaise, and fever. The parenchyma of the gland is diffusely infiltrated by plasma cells and macrophages, followed by degeneration of acini and vacuolation of ductal epithelium. Inflammation of the testes (**orchitis**) occurs in 25%-30% of infected males, but *infertility* is rare. Serious complications, such as *pancreatitis, encephalitis,* and *meningitis,* may develop.

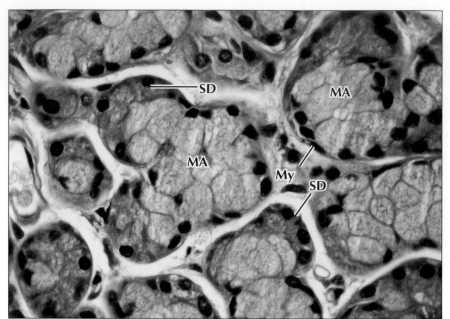

◀ **LM of part of a submandibular gland.** Mucous acini (**MA**) are made of pyramidal, pale-staining mucous cells with flattened basal nuclei. These cells surround small central lumina. Darker staining serous demilunes (**SD**) cap some acini. A few myoepithelial cells (**My**) are associated with acini and share a basement membrane with the mucous cells. 320×. *H&E.*

▼ **LM of part of a sublingual gland showing details of intralobular ducts.** An intercalated duct (**InD**) lined by simple squamous epithelium drains (**arrows**) two secretory acini (**SA**). The intercalated duct empties into a larger striated duct lined by tall columnar cells with basal striations. Surrounding stroma is loose, delicate connective tissue (**CT**). 800×. *H&E.*

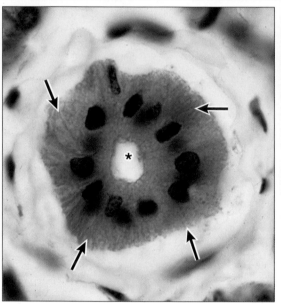

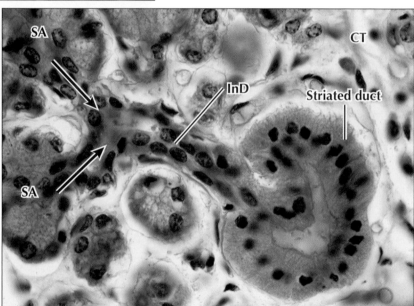

▲ **LM of a striated duct at high magnification.** Lightly eosinophilic columnar cells with basal striations (**arrows**) line a central lumen (✶). 1000×. *H&E.*

12.13 HISTOLOGY OF MIXED SALIVARY (SUBMANDIBULAR AND SUBLINGUAL) GLANDS

As in the parotid, an outer fibrous capsule surrounds the **submandibular gland** and sends in delicate septa to divide the gland into lobes and lobules. Unlike the parotid, however, the submandibular has both **serous** and **mucous acini,** the majority being serous. The gland also has mixed **seromucous acini,** in which lighter staining, larger **mucous cells** around a central **lumen** are capped by crescent-shaped **serous demilunes** of flattened **serous cells.** The basal nuclei of mucous cells are usually flattened, not rounded, and apical cytoplasm appears washed out because of large mucin droplets. Serous cells look similar to those in the parotid. Unlike

the parotid and submandibular glands, the **sublingual gland** lacks a clear fibrous capsule. The secretory part of the gland is made mostly of mixed seromucous acini. Both submandibular and sublingual glands have **intralobular** and **interlobular ducts** like those in the parotid, as well as a conspicuous feature unique to salivary glands—**striated ducts.** **Basal striations** in the simple **columnar epithelial cells** in these ducts set them apart from other parts of the duct system. Striations are basal infoldings of the plasma membrane. Hematoxylin and eosin (H&E) staining shows cells as intensely eosinophilic, indicating many mitochondria. Unlike the parotid, with variable amounts of adipose tissue in its stroma, and the sublingual gland, which has adipocytes, the submandibular gland usually lacks adipocytes.

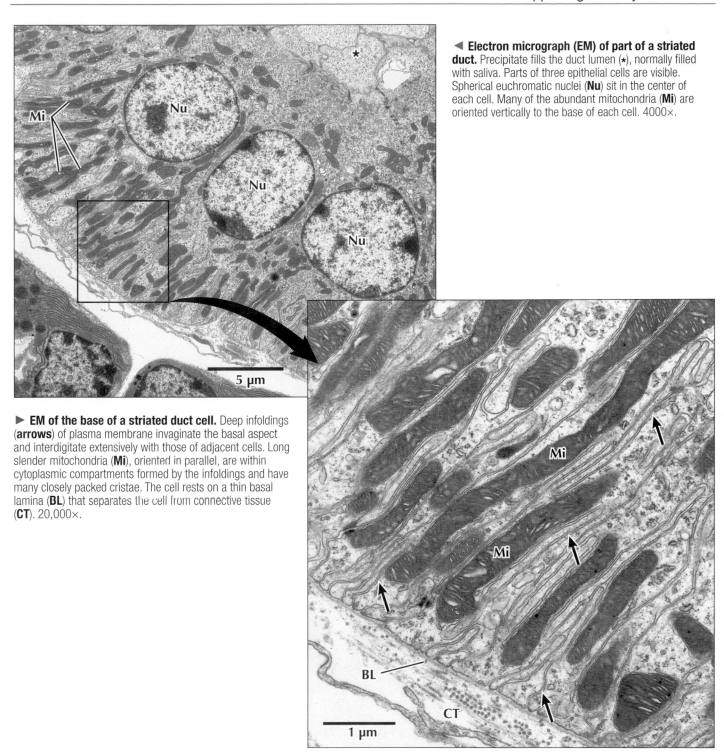

◄ **Electron micrograph (EM) of part of a striated duct.** Precipitate fills the duct lumen (⋆), normally filled with saliva. Parts of three epithelial cells are visible. Spherical euchromatic nuclei (**Nu**) sit in the center of each cell. Many of the abundant mitochondria (**Mi**) are oriented vertically to the base of each cell. 4000×.

► **EM of the base of a striated duct cell.** Deep infoldings (**arrows**) of plasma membrane invaginate the basal aspect and interdigitate extensively with those of adjacent cells. Long slender mitochondria (**Mi**), oriented in parallel, are within cytoplasmic compartments formed by the infoldings and have many closely packed cristae. The cell rests on a thin basal lamina (**BL**) that separates the cell from connective tissue (**CT**). 20,000×.

12.14 ULTRASTRUCTURE AND FUNCTION OF STRIATED DUCTS

The ultrastructure of striated ducts, unique to salivary glands, is consistent with an active role in electrolyte transport. The ducts modify the composition of *saliva* via resorption of Na^+, which makes saliva hypotonic. Cl^- moves across the cells passively in the same direction. In contrast, K^+ and HCO_3^-, formed by carbonic anhydrase in the cytosol, are excreted in a reverse direction into the duct lumen. The ultrastructure of these ducts resembles that of proximal renal tubules, although the tubules have brush border microvilli, and the striated duct does not. **Nuclei** are round and centrally placed, and cells rest on a **basal lamina. Basal striations**, which are perpendicular to the base of the cells, are the characteristic feature. Surface area is increased by many **infoldings** of the **basal plasma membrane**, which contains the ion pump Na^+,K^+-ATPase. The arrangement of elongated **mitochondria** in parallel rows between the infoldings facilitates active transport by providing energy, as ATP, where Na^+ is actively resorbed. Also, interdigitations between lateral borders of adjacent cells are intricate. Apical surfaces, which are in contact with the duct lumen, bear short stubby microvilli. These areas also contain *small secretory granules* that store *kallikrein*, a vasoactive substance, and secretory immunoglobulins.

▼ **Gross anatomy of the esophagus.**   ▼ **Histology of the esophagus at different levels.**

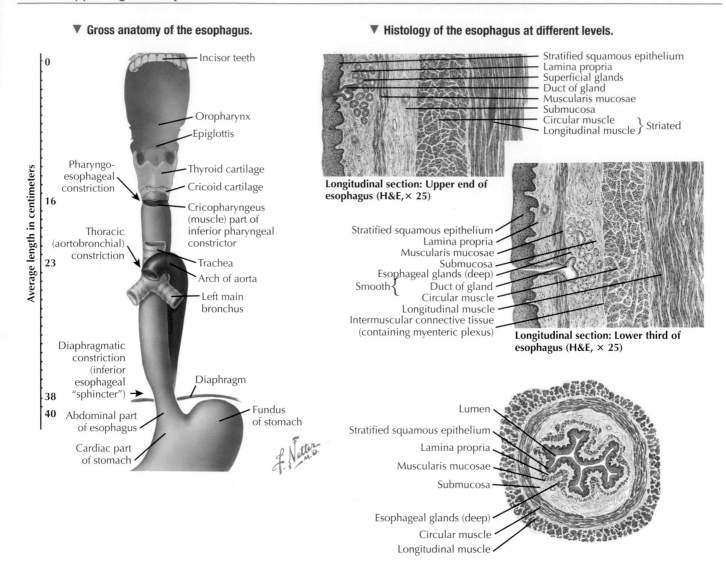

Longitudinal section: Upper end of esophagus (H&E, × 25)

Longitudinal section: Lower third of esophagus (H&E, × 25)

12.15 STRUCTURE AND FUNCTION OF THE ESOPHAGUS

The esophagus is a hollow tube, about 25 cm long in adults, that passes vertically through the mediastinum and connects the **pharynx** and **stomach.** It propels partly digested food by *peristalsis* from the laryngopharynx to the stomach. Like other parts of the digestive tract, it has four primary layers: **mucosa, submucosa, muscularis externa,** and **adventitia.** But unlike the other parts, its muscularis externa consists of two types of muscle tissue. The upper third of the esophagus has **skeletal muscle fibers;** the middle third, a mixture of smooth and skeletal muscle; and the lower third, only **smooth muscle.** The esophagus has sphincters at its two ends. The upper sphincter is an anatomically distinct structure of skeletal muscle fibers of the **cricopharyngeus muscle.** At the lower end (distal 5 cm), in contrast, is a physiologic sphincter, less well defined histologically, that usually prevents reflux of gastric contents. It is a zone of increased intraluminal pressure. At rest, the esophageal lumen is collapsed and plicated by temporary longitudinal folds. During passage of a food bolus, the distensible esophageal wall allows the folds to flatten out because of its high content of elastic tissue.

CLINICAL POINT

Esophageal varices—abnormally dilated submucosal veins—occur in the lower third of the esophagus. When portal blood flow is obstructed, these veins serve as collateral vessels between portal and systemic circulations. Varices often occur in patients with *cirrhosis* and *portal hypertension. Alcoholic liver disease* and *viral hepatitis* are leading causes. The varices are prone to rupture and hemorrhage, which may be life-threatening. The mortality rate is 40%-70%. Increased endothelin-1 (a vasoconstrictor) and decreased nitric oxide (a vasodilator) have been implicated in pathogenesis of portal hypertension and esophageal varices. Endoscopy is used for diagnosis and treatment.

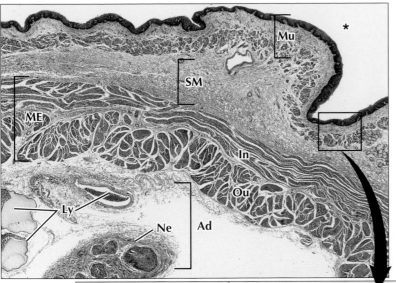

◄ **LM of the wall of the esophagus.** As in most other parts of the digestive tract, four tunics are seen: mucosa (**Mu**), next to the lumen (∗); submucosa (**SM**); muscularis externa (**ME**); and adventitia (**Ad**). The muscularis externa has inner (**In**) and outer (**Ou**) smooth muscle layers; the adventitia, nerves (**Ne**) and lymphatic channels (**Ly**). 6.5×. *H&E.*

▼ **Higher magnification LM of esophageal mucosa.** The superficial layers of the nonkeratinized stratified squamous epithelium (**SSE**) have a basket-weave appearance. Highly vascularized lamina propria (**LP**) sends connective tissue papillae (**arrows**), which carry capillaries (**Cap**), close to the epithelium. The muscularis mucosae (**MM**) is thicker in the esophagus than in other parts of the digestive tract. 135×. *H&E.*

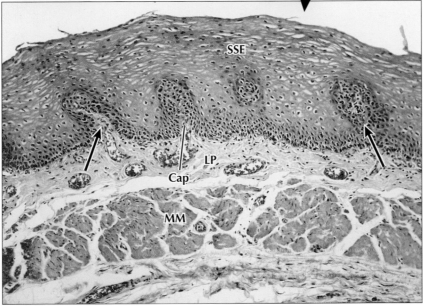

12.16 HISTOLOGY OF THE ESOPHAGUS: MUCOSA

The esophageal mucosa consists of **nonkeratinized stratified squamous epithelium** (continuous with that of the pharynx), underlying **lamina propria,** and prominent **muscularis mucosae.** The multilayer epithelium is 300-500 μm thick; is well suited to protect against friction, abrasion, and injury; and has basal, intermediate, and superficial layers. Basophilic cuboidal cells form the basal layer, which, as in other stratified epithelia, is mainly a mitotic and regenerative zone. Continuous renewal of epithelial cells normally takes 14-21 days as cells slowly migrate to the surface and desquamate. Above the basal layer, maturing cells become flatter and accumulate *glycogen,* which is seen as washed-out areas in conventional preparations. Cell nuclei slowly undergo *pyknosis* as cells approach the surface. The basal layer also contains scattered melanocytes and Merkel cells; the intermediate layer, Langerhans cells and T lymphocytes. The surface cells retain their nuclei, and their cytoplasm may have a few *keratohyalin granules.* These cells are usually nonkeratinized in humans but may become keratinized if subjected to an unusual degree of trauma. The lamina propria is loose fibroelastic connective tissue richly endowed with capillaries, nerves, and small lymphatic channels. Its conical **papillae** project into the epithelium at irregular intervals and usually penetrate up to two-thirds of the epithelial thickness. The muscularis mucosae has two ill-defined layers of smooth muscle cells, arranged helically and longitudinally, that contract to allow localized movements and folding of the mucosa.

CLINICAL POINT

In **Barrett esophagus**—*metaplasia* of the esophageal epithelium—columnar epithelium, similar to that of the stomach, replaces the usual stratified squamous epithelium. A response to esophagitis or injury, it can occur anywhere above the gastroesophageal junction. Diagnosis is by endoscopy, with biopsy for confirmation. A burning pain, known as *heartburn,* is a major symptom. It may rarely lead to the more serious **adenocarcinoma.** Patients with persistent *gastroesophageal reflux disease,* in which acid reflux disrupts the esophageal mucosal barrier, are predisposed to metaplastic change in the esophageal epithelium.

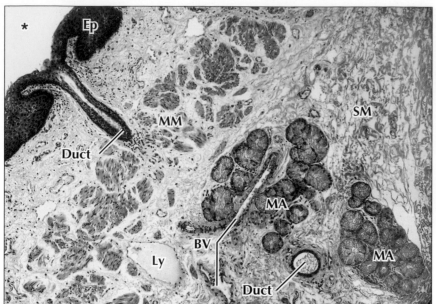

◀ **LM of a submucosal gland in the esophagus.** The secretory part of the gland contains groups of tightly packed mucous acini (**MA**) located in the submucosa (**SM**) and draining into ducts that penetrate the muscularis mucosae (**MM**). The duct at the left crosses the lamina propria and opens onto the surface (∗). Epithelium lining the duct merges with stratified epithelium (**Ep**) on the mucosal surface. The submucosa is richly vascularized connective tissue with many lymphatic channels (**Ly**) and blood vessels (**BV**). A predominance of elastic fibers in this layer provides the esophageal wall with considerable distensibility. 160×. *H&E.*

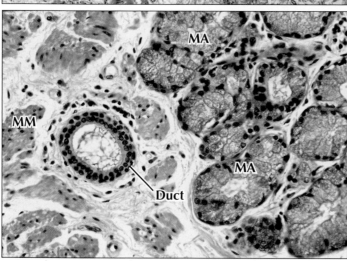

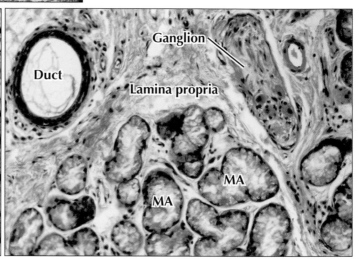

▲ **Higher magnification LM of a submucosal gland in the esophagus.** Mucous acini (**MA**) contain pale-stained secretory cells around a central lumen. Flattened nuclei of these cells are basally located. A duct, lined by stratified cuboidal epithelium, drains the acini and pierces the muscularis mucosae (**MM**) on its way to the mucosal surface. 270×. *H&E.*

▲ **LM of a cardiac gland in the esophageal mucosa.** Coiled mucous acini (**MA**) and a short duct (lined by low cuboidal epithelium) are in the lamina propria. A small autonomic ganglion is close to this tortuous gland. These glands are distinctive features of upper and lower ends of the esophagus. 270×. *H&E.*

12.17 HISTOLOGY OF MUCOUS GLANDS OF THE ESOPHAGUS

Epithelium lining the esophageal lumen is mainly protective, with mucous glands providing a thin, highly viscous film of *mucus* to lubricate the luminal surface. These glands derive embryonically from surface epithelium. During development, they migrate into underlying **connective tissue,** but they retain connections to the surface via ducts. Two types of mucous glands occur in the esophageal wall—named **superficial** or **submucosal glands** on the basis of location. Superficial glands are simple tubular glands that occur in the **lamina propria** only at proximal and distal ends of the esophagus, close to the cricopharyngeus muscle and gastroesoph-

ageal junction, respectively. They pursue a tortuous course in the mucosa and drain secretory product—a *neutral mucin*—by short **ducts** to the surface. They resemble small cardiac glands of the stomach, so they are also called *cardiac glands.* Deeper glands—whose secretory acini lie in the **submucosa**—are diffusely scattered along the entire esophagus. These small-compound tubular glands produce an *acidic mucin* and are drained by ducts that are initially composed of simple cuboidal epithelium, which then becomes **stratified cuboidal epithelium** with a double layer of cells. These ducts pierce the **muscularis mucosae** to merge with mucosal epithelium and open into the esophageal lumen.

▼ **Musculature of the esophagus.**

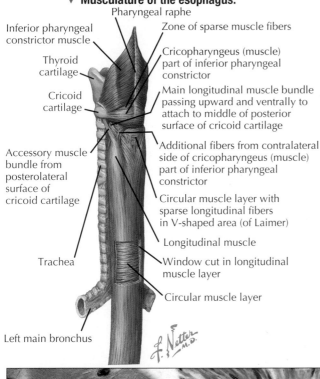

Pharyngeal raphe

Inferior pharyngeal constrictor muscle

Zone of sparse muscle fibers

Thyroid cartilage

Cricopharyngeus (muscle) part of inferior pharyngeal constrictor

Cricoid cartilage

Main longitudinal muscle bundle passing upward and ventrally to attach to middle of posterior surface of cricoid cartilage

Accessory muscle bundle from posterolateral surface of cricoid cartilage

Additional fibers from contralateral side of cricopharyngeus (muscle) part of inferior pharyngeal constrictor

Circular muscle layer with sparse longitudinal fibers in V-shaped area (of Laimer)

Longitudinal muscle

Trachea

Window cut in longitudinal muscle layer

Circular muscle layer

Left main bronchus

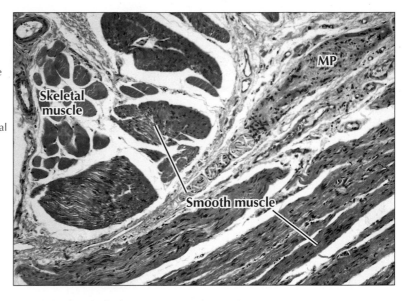

▲ **LM of the muscularis externa.** The middle third of the esophagus has a mixture of skeletal muscle fibers and smooth muscle cells. Part of a myenteric plexus (**MP**) is between the inner and outer muscle layers. 180×. *H&E.*

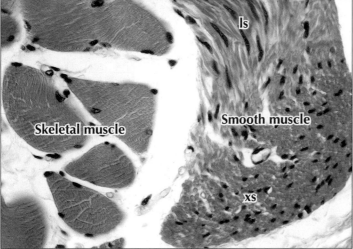

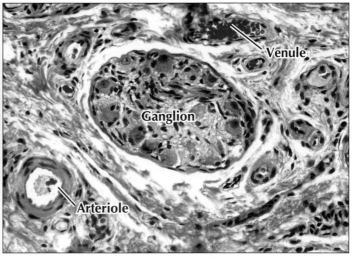

▲ **Higher magnification LM of two types of muscle tissue in the esophagus.** The larger skeletal muscle fibers are pleomorphic and have peripheral nuclei. The much smaller smooth muscle cells are sectioned transversely (**xs**) and longitudinally (**ls**). 280×. *H&E.*

▲ **LM of part of the adventitia of the esophagus.** This dense irregular connective tissue layer contains many blood vessels, nerves, and lymphatics that often travel together. An arteriole and venule are near a peripheral autonomic ganglion. 250×. *H&E.*

12.18 HISTOLOGY AND FUNCTION OF THE ESOPHAGUS: MUSCULARIS EXTERNA AND ADVENTITIA

The muscularis externa of the esophagus, 0.5-2 mm thick, is made of inner circular and outer longitudinal layers of muscle. Unlike most other parts of the digestive tract, in which the inner circular layer is usually thicker, the outer layer here is slightly thicker. In the upper third of the esophagus, both layers contain only **skeletal muscle fibers,** on which nerve fibers of cranial nerves IX and X end as motor endplates. These muscle fibers are unique, however, because their contraction is involuntary. In the middle third of the esophagus, **smooth muscle cells** are internal to skeletal muscle, and their number gradually increases distally. In the lower third

of the esophagus, inner and outer layers are purely smooth muscle, innervated by both parasympathetic and sympathetic nerves. Ganglia of the **myenteric (Auerbach) plexus** are found between outer and inner muscle layers along the whole esophagus. A plexus of lymphatic channels, as well as blood vessels, is especially prominent in the submucosa, muscularis, and adventitia. The **adventitia**—loose connective tissue that supports and protects—anchors the esophagus to nearby structures in the mediastinum. A short segment of esophagus is below the diaphragm, in the peritoneal cavity, where serosa surrounds it. The lack of serosa along most of the esophageal length may account for rapid spread of metastatic tumor cells outside esophageal boundaries.

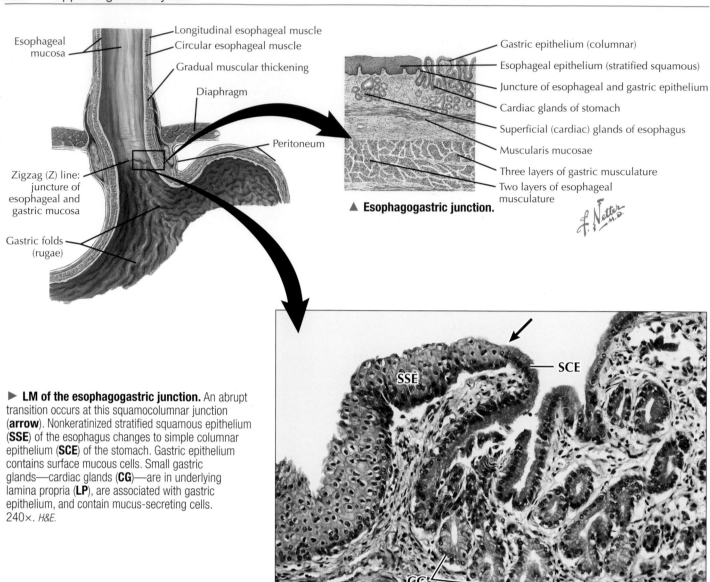

Esophageal mucosa
Longitudinal esophageal muscle
Circular esophageal muscle
Gradual muscular thickening
Diaphragm
Peritoneum
Zigzag (Z) line: juncture of esophageal and gastric mucosa
Gastric folds (rugae)

Gastric epithelium (columnar)
Esophageal epithelium (stratified squamous)
Juncture of esophageal and gastric epithelium
Cardiac glands of stomach
Superficial (cardiac) glands of esophagus
Muscularis mucosae
Three layers of gastric musculature
Two layers of esophageal musculature

▲ **Esophagogastric junction.**

▶ **LM of the esophagogastric junction.** An abrupt transition occurs at this squamocolumnar junction (**arrow**). Nonkeratinized stratified squamous epithelium (**SSE**) of the esophagus changes to simple columnar epithelium (**SCE**) of the stomach. Gastric epithelium contains surface mucous cells. Small gastric glands—cardiac glands (**CG**)—are in underlying lamina propria (**LP**), are associated with gastric epithelium, and contain mucus-secreting cells. 240×. *H&E.*

12.19 HISTOLOGY AND FUNCTION OF THE ESOPHAGOGASTRIC JUNCTION

An abrupt transition occurs in the epithelial lining at the esophagogastric junction. This serrated border, called the **Z line,** is clinically important, as it is the most common site of esophageal carcinoma. At the Z line, **nonkeratinized stratified squamous epithelium** of the esophagus changes to **simple columnar epithelium** of the stomach, and only basal cells of the esophageal epithelium continue into simple epithelium of the stomach. Endoscopy easily identifies the typical change in color from pale above to deep red below. A change in texture of the **mucosa** also occurs, from smooth proximally to plicated distally. The existence of a true anatomic sphincter at this junction is controversial. A slight thickening of inner circular and outer longitudinal smooth muscle layers may occur, but the *lower esophageal sphincter* is most

likely physiologic, not anatomic. Lymphoid tissue aggregates also occur in the **lamina propria** near the junction.

▼ **Intrinsic nerve supply of the digestive tract.**

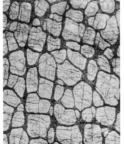

Myenteric (Auerbach) plexus lying on longitudinal muscle. (duodenum of guinea pig, Champy-Coujard, osmic stain, ×20)

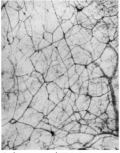

Submucosal (Meissner) plexus (ascending colon of guinea pig. Stained by gold impregnation, ×20)

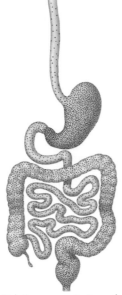

Relative concentration of ganglion cells in myenteric (Auerbach) plexus and in submucosal (Meissner) plexus in various parts of alimentary tract (myenteric plexus cells represented by maroon, submucosal by blue dots)

▼ **Innervation of the esophagus.**

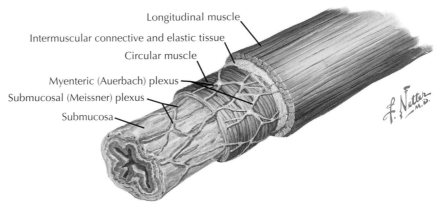

Longitudinal muscle
Intermuscular connective and elastic tissue
Circular muscle
Myenteric (Auerbach) plexus
Submucosal (Meissner) plexus
Submucosa

▶ **LM of a myenteric plexus (MP) in the muscularis externa of the esophagus.** This encapsulated collection of ganglion cells, with associated nerve fibers and supportive cells, lies between the two muscle layers of the muscularis externa. Smaller supportive cells and fibroblasts, which have more condensed nuclei, surround several large ganglion cells (**arrows**) with spherical, euchromatic nuclei. Nerve fibers (**NF**), which form an intricate network, have a wavy, washed-out appearance. Postganglionic sympathetic nerves and synapses between pre- and postganglionic parasympathetic nerves occur in the plexus. Smooth muscle cells (**Sm**) in the muscularis externa are sectioned longitudinally in the bottom and transversely in the top. The myenteric plexus is also seen in the stomach and intestines. 320×. *H&E.*

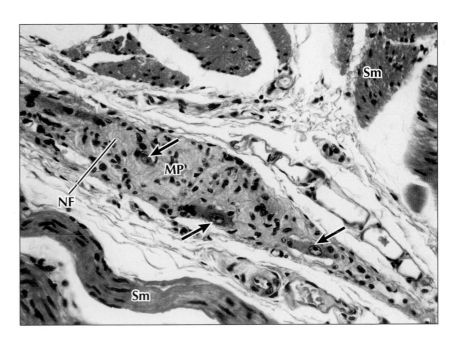

12.20 STRUCTURE AND FUNCTION OF THE ENTERIC NERVOUS SYSTEM

The digestive tract, from the esophagus to the anus, has its own intrinsic nerve supply—the enteric nervous system (ENS)—consisting of an extensive network of **nerve fibers,** clusters of **nerve cell bodies (ganglion cells),** and supportive (**glial**) cells. Neural components of this system (peripheral ganglia and nerve fibers) are found in all four layers of the digestive tract, but they are especially prominent in **muscularis externa** and **submucosa.** Derived embryonically from neural crest, the ENS comprises two distinct yet connected parts in the digestive tract wall. The larger **myenteric (Auerbach) plexus,** between inner and outer layers of smooth muscle in the muscularis externa, mainly regulates smooth muscle contraction, peristalsis, and gastrointestinal motility. The smaller **submucosal (Meissner) plexus** mostly regulates glandular secre-

tion and local blood flow. It also alters electrolyte and water transport. Areas of the digestive tract where these functions are minimal have a sparse submucosal plexus. At least 30 *neurotransmitters* and three functional types of *intrinsic neurons* occur in the ENS. *Motor neurons* modulate activity of targets such as smooth muscle, enteroendocrine, and glandular epithelial cells. *Sensory neurons* transmit impulses activated by mechanical or chemical stimuli in the mucosa. Interneurons, or *interstitial cells of Cajal,* are pacemaker cells that relay and integrate information between other neurons. More neurons are estimated to be in the ENS than in the spinal cord, perhaps as many as 10^8. ENS neurons act independently but are regulated by **parasympathetic** and **sympathetic** parts of the **autonomic nervous system,** which also link the ENS and central nervous system. Parasympathetic nerve fibers usually activate physiologic digestive processes; sympathetic nerves are mainly inhibitory.

13

LOWER DIGESTIVE SYSTEM

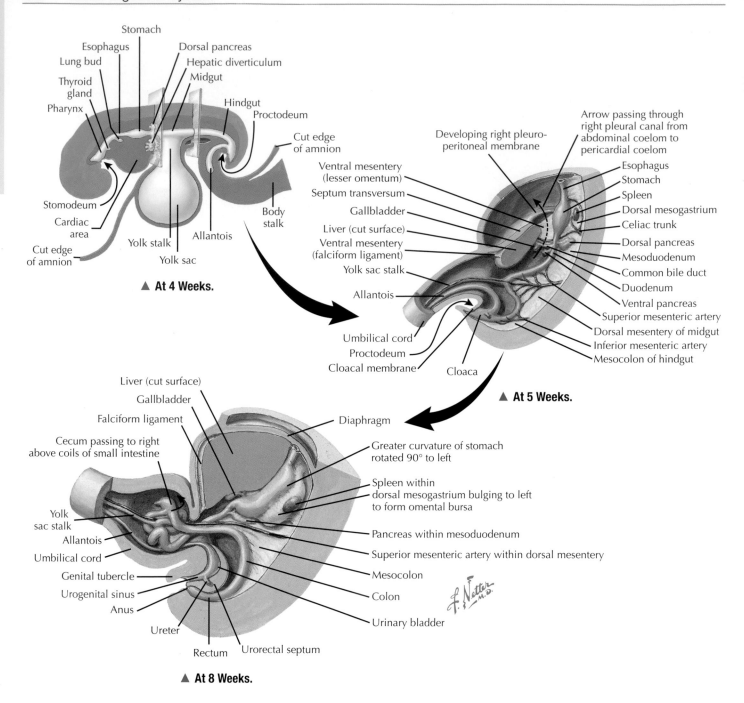

▲ At 4 Weeks.

▲ At 5 Weeks.

▲ At 8 Weeks.

13.1 DEVELOPMENT OF THE FOREGUT, MIDGUT, AND HINDGUT

The early **embryo** starts as a flattened, trilaminar disc with three primary germ layers: **ectoderm, mesoderm,** and **endoderm.** Its ventral surface, covered by endoderm, communicates with the **yolk sac.** Later, lateral and cephalocaudal folding forms a long, cylindrical endodermal tube extending the length of the embryo; this becomes the primitive gut tube and then the digestive tract. Splanchnic mesoderm externally surrounds an endodermal lining. In the head area, the proximal part of the tube gives rise to the foregut. The caudal part, which extends into the tail, becomes the hindgut. A midgut in the center at first communicates with the yolk sac but then loses the connection. The endoderm becomes mucosal epithelium of the digestive tract and gives rise to the

parenchyma and ducts of all intramural and accessory digestive glands. The overlying mesoderm becomes connective tissue, muscle, lymphatics, and blood vessels in the tube's wall. Neural crest ectoderm migrates to the gut wall to give rise to **myenteric** and **submucosal neural plexuses.** The foregut gives rise to the *pharynx,* **esophagus, stomach, proximal duodenum, liver, gallbladder,** and **pancreas.** The midgut becomes the rest of the duodenum, small bowel, cecum, ascending colon, and proximal transverse *colon.* The hindgut forms the rest of the transverse colon, descending colon, sigmoid colon, and *rectum.* The foregut rotates 90 degrees clockwise; the midgut, 270 degrees around its blood supply. Sheet-like **mesenteries,** derived from splanchnic mesoderm, suspend and attach parts of the tube to the body wall and serve as conduits for blood vessels, nerves, and lymphatics.

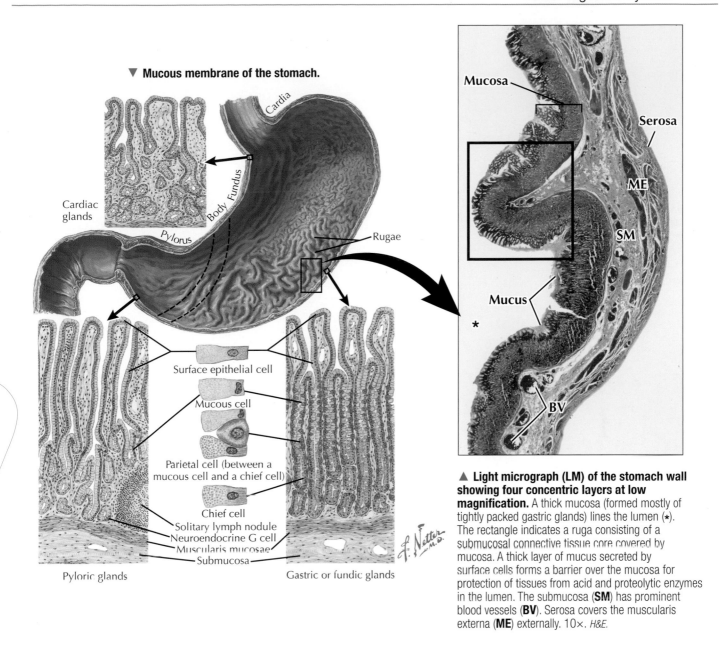

▼ **Mucous membrane of the stomach.**

Cardiac glands

Pyloric glands

Surface epithelial cell

Mucous cell

Parietal cell (between a mucous cell and a chief cell)

Chief cell

Solitary lymph nodule

Neuroendocrine G cell

Muscularis mucosae

Submucosa

Gastric or fundic glands

▲ **Light micrograph (LM) of the stomach wall showing four concentric layers at low magnification.** A thick mucosa (formed mostly of tightly packed gastric glands) lines the lumen (★). The rectangle indicates a ruga consisting of a submucosal connective tissue core covered by mucosa. A thick layer of mucus secreted by surface cells forms a barrier over the mucosa for protection of tissues from acid and proteolytic enzymes in the lumen. The submucosa (**SM**) has prominent blood vessels (**BV**). Serosa covers the muscularis externa (**ME**) externally. 10×. *H&E.*

13.2 STRUCTURE AND FUNCTION OF THE STOMACH

The stomach, the most dilated part of the digestive tube, is an expandable fibromuscular sac that connects the esophagus to the small intestine. In adults, it can hold about 1.5 L, or up to 3 L when distended. It stores and mixes food and reduces it to a semisolid mass, known as *chyme,* which it delivers to the duodenum. The stomach has four anatomic regions: **cardia, fundus, body,** and **pylorus.** As in other parts of the digestive tract, the wall has four concentric layers: **mucosa, submucosa, muscularis externa,** and **serosa.** The mucosa is 0.3-1.5 mm thick. The inner lining shows irregular longitudinal folds, known as **rugae,** which can be seen by the naked eye in a contracted stomach. They flatten as the stomach expands. Simple columnar epithelium of surface

mucous cells lines the lumen. This epithelium regularly dips to form small **gastric pits,** or **foveolae,** which lead to long tubular **gastric glands.** The total number of glands is about 15×10^6. Gastric pits and glands provide up to 800 m² of total surface area for secretion of *mucus, acid,* and *digestive enzymes.* The three types of glands have the same general structural plan but with regional histologic variations. **Cardiac glands,** in a small area around the esophageal (cardiac) orifice, are shortest, least numerous, and occupy less than 10% of the mucosa. In the body and fundus, main **gastric glands,** the largest and most numerous, make up about 75% of the mucosa. The pyloric area close to the duodenum contains small **pyloric glands** that constitute about 15% of the mucosa and resemble cardiac glands.

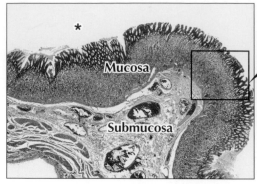

▲ **LM of a gastric ruga at low magnification.**
The mucosa is prominent; underlying submucosa
is richly vascularized connective tissue. The gastric
lumen (⋆) is above. 10×. *H&E.*

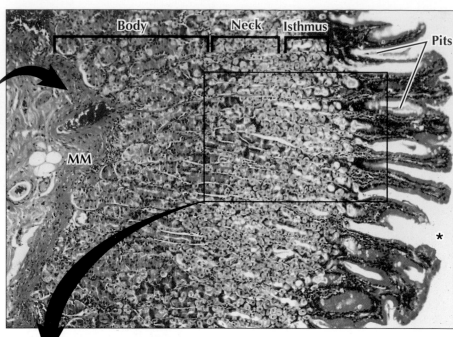

▲ **LM of the gastric mucosa.** Short gastric pits on
the surface lead into long tubular gastric glands that
extend through the isthmus, neck, and base to the
muscularis mucosae (**MM**). The gastric lumen (⋆) and
isthmus, neck, and body regions of a gland are
indicated. 120×. *H&E.*

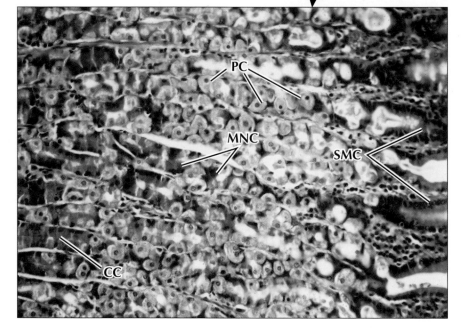

◀ **LM of part of the gastric mucosa.** The isthmus,
neck, and upper base of gastric glands are visible.
Columnar surface mucous cells (**SMC**) line the gastric
pits on the right. Large parietal cells (**PC**) with relatively
clear cytoplasm are interspersed with small, dark-
stained mucous neck cells (**MNC**) in the isthmus.
The upper base of the glands contain many
dark-stained, columnar chief cells (**CC**). 280×. *H&E.*

13.3 HISTOLOGY OF THE STOMACH: GASTRIC GLANDS AND PITS

Gastric mucosa consists of a **simple columnar epithelium,** underlying **lamina propria,** and deeper **muscularis mucosae.** Surface mucous cells line the luminal surface and gastric pits. Several gastric glands discharge contents into the bottom of each pit. The glands occupy the entire thickness of the mucosa and extend through the lamina propria to the muscularis mucosae. The loose, richly cellular lamina propria under the surface epithelium and between the glands contains various connective tissue cells and an extensive capillary network. Mucosal glands are so tightly packed that the lamina propria is hard to see and usually appears scanty. The main gastric glands, the most specialized glands, are long, straight, and often bifurcated. In longitudinal section, glands (especially those in the fundus) have three parts. The upper part—the **isthmus**—opens into the gastric pit. The midregion—the **neck**—contains a mixture of **mucous neck cells** and **parietal cells.** Both isthmus and neck contain proliferating stem cells, which give rise to cells in the glands, plus those on the surface. The bottom part is the **body** (or main part): the upper area contains parietal cells plus gastric **chief cells;** the lower, the **base,** contains mostly chief cells. Cardiac and fundic glands (compound tubular glands) contain mostly mucus-secreting cells.

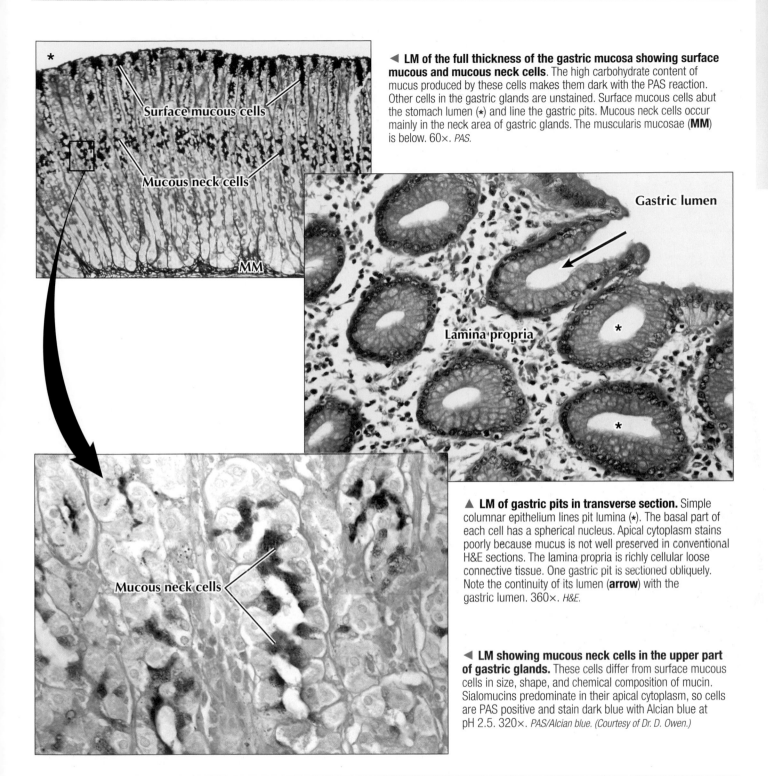

◀ **LM of the full thickness of the gastric mucosa showing surface mucous and mucous neck cells**. The high carbohydrate content of mucus produced by these cells makes them dark with the PAS reaction. Other cells in the gastric glands are unstained. Surface mucous cells abut the stomach lumen (∗) and line the gastric pits. Mucous neck cells occur mainly in the neck area of gastric glands. The muscularis mucosae (**MM**) is below. 60×. *PAS.*

▲ **LM of gastric pits in transverse section.** Simple columnar epithelium lines pit lumina (∗). The basal part of each cell has a spherical nucleus. Apical cytoplasm stains poorly because mucus is not well preserved in conventional H&E sections. The lamina propria is richly cellular loose connective tissue. One gastric pit is sectioned obliquely. Note the continuity of its lumen (**arrow**) with the gastric lumen. 360×. *H&E.*

◀ **LM showing mucous neck cells in the upper part of gastric glands.** These cells differ from surface mucous cells in size, shape, and chemical composition of mucin. Sialomucins predominate in their apical cytoplasm, so cells are PAS positive and stain dark blue with Alcian blue at pH 2.5. 320×. *PAS/Alcian blue. (Courtesy of Dr. D. Owen.)*

13.4 HISTOLOGY AND FUNCTION OF SURFACE MUCOUS AND MUCOUS NECK CELLS

A thin film of **mucus** secreted by surface mucous and mucous neck cells forms a highly viscous barrier that protects the stomach surface. The mucus consists mostly of glycoproteins rich in carbohydrates and bicarbonate (HCO_3^-) ions. It counteracts effects of HCl and proteolytic enzymes in the **gastric lumen.** Surface mucous cells—tall **columnar epithelial cells** with **basal nuclei**—form a continuous layer that lines the whole gastric lumen. The cells rest on a basement membrane (not easily seen by light microscopy). Junctional complexes link lateral cell borders. Apical parts of the cells are filled with **mucin granules**, which account

for pale-staining, washed-out cytoplasm. Surface mucous cells also contain many mitochondria (best seen by electron microscopy), which provide energy for HCO_3^- secretion into the lumen. Surface mucous cells extend into **gastric pits,** which lead into densely packed, branched tubular glands. Mucous neck cells in the upper (neck) parts of the glands are smaller and more cuboidal than are surface mucous cells in gastric pits and on the luminal surface. Hard to see in hematoxylin and eosin (H&E) sections, they are better visualized with PAS. Cells have a flattened basal nucleus and apical mucin granules. Unlike surface cells, whose mucus is alkaline, mucous neck cells elaborate a more acidic or neutral mucus such as sialomucin.

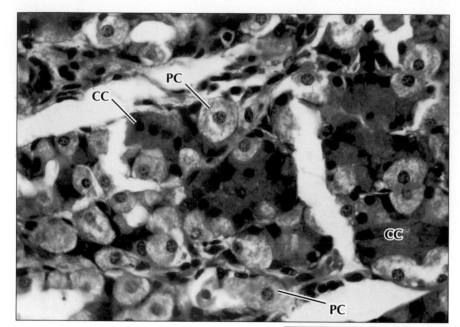

◀ **LM of the lower part of a gastric gland in the fundus of the stomach.** Large, round parietal cells (**PC**)—organized singly or in groups—are interspersed with smaller basophilic chief cells (**CC**). Each parietal cell is lightly eosinophilic and has a central spherical nucleus. At the base of some glands, most cells lining the glandular lumen are chief cells; parietal cells are more numerous in more superficial areas of the mucosa. 500×. *H&E.*

▶ **LM of gastric glands in transverse section.** Two cell types line the lumen (⋆) of each gland: parietal cells (**PC**) and chief cells (**CC**). Enteroendocrine cells (**EE**) with small granules and pale-stained nuclei are smaller, fewer, and harder to see than parietal and chief cells. Enteroendocrine cells do not face the glandular lumen but are polarized toward the lamina propria (**LP**). The lamina propria contains capillaries (**Cap**), venules, and connective tissue cells. 1000×. *Toluidine blue, plastic section.*

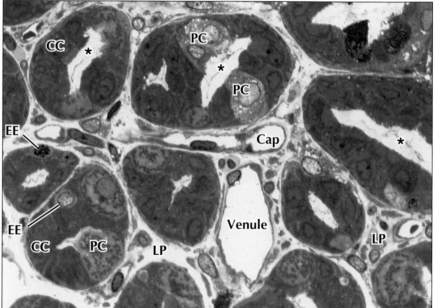

13.5   HISTOLOGY OF GASTRIC CHIEF CELLS AND PARIETAL CELLS

Main gastric glands in the mucosa of the **fundus** and body of the stomach are long, straight and branched tubular glands, which are perpendicular to the mucosal surface. Several glands usually open into the base of a **gastric pit.** Proliferating stem cells are in the isthmus and neck of the gastric glands. They migrate either up to renew cells on the surface or down to give rise to other cells deeper in gastric glands. **Parietal cells** are most numerous in the body of the glands but are also mixed with mucous neck cells in neck areas or with chief cells in basal areas of glands. They are large

(20-35 μm in diameter), rounded or polygonal cells with one central nucleus. Their deeply *eosinophilic* cytoplasm is due to abundant mitochondria and relative paucity of rough endoplasmic reticulum. Cuboidal to columnar **chief cells,** mostly in basal parts of glands, have a round basal nucleus. Their basal cytoplasm is *basophilic; secretory (zymogenic) granules* make their apical cytoplasm look more granular. Gastric glands also contain less numerous **enteroendocrine cells,** scattered with the other cells, that produce gut hormones and are hard to see in routine sections. Special immunocytochemical or electron microscopic methods are needed to identify them with certainty.

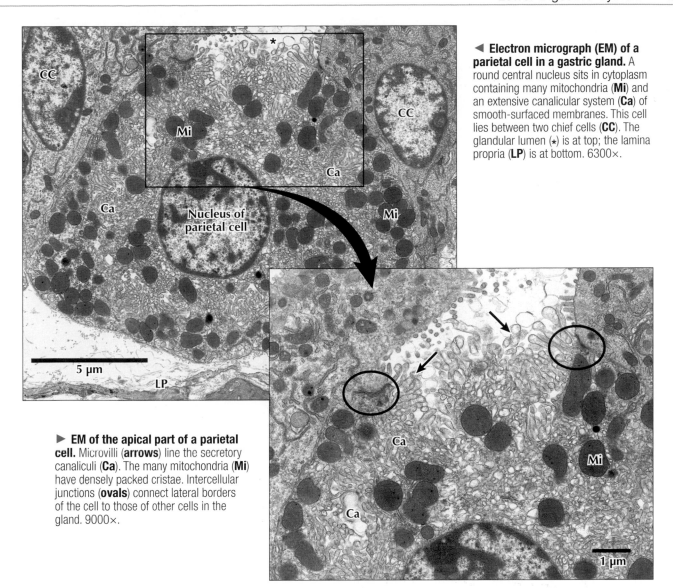

◀ **Electron micrograph (EM) of a parietal cell in a gastric gland.** A round central nucleus sits in cytoplasm containing many mitochondria (**Mi**) and an extensive canalicular system (**Ca**) of smooth-surfaced membranes. This cell lies between two chief cells (**CC**). The glandular lumen (★) is at top; the lamina propria (**LP**) is at bottom. 6300×.

▶ **EM of the apical part of a parietal cell.** Microvilli (**arrows**) line the secretory canaliculi (**Ca**). The many mitochondria (**Mi**) have densely packed cristae. Intercellular junctions (**ovals**) connect lateral borders of the cell to those of other cells in the gland. 9000×.

13.6 ULTRASTRUCTURE AND FUNCTION OF PARIETAL CELLS

Parietal cells secrete high concentrations of HCl, pH 0.8-2, into **gastric gland** lumina. Trench-like infoldings of apical cell membranes form a ramifying network of narrow channels (1-2 μm wide)—the **secretory canaliculi.** They occur throughout the cytoplasm and near the nucleus and open into glandular lumina. Canaliculi are lined by many densely packed **microvilli** for increased surface area. Membranes of canaliculi and microvilli contain the *proton pump H^+,K^+-ATPase* for acid secretion. Many **mitochondria** in the cytoplasm constitute up to 40% of cell volume, have densely packed **cristae** with many **matrix granules,** and provide energy for ion transport. *Lysosomes* are common and engage in turnover of organelles by *autophagocytosis.* An elaborate *tubulovesicular system,* which has Cl^- and K^+ conductance channels, also occurs near cell surfaces and canaliculi. Resting cells not producing HCl have many tubulovesicles, which during active secretion fuse with canaliculi membranes. The resulting decrease in tubulovesicle number occurs together with a large increase in microvilli and canaliculi. H^+ ions are actively transported across apical cell membranes and unite with luminal Cl^- ions to form HCl. Infoldings of basal plasma membrane also increase surface area to facilitate HCO_3^- transport in exchange for Cl^-. Basal membranes bear receptors for acetylcholine, gastrin, and histamine, which stimulate acid secretion. Parietal cells also synthesize *intrinsic factor,* a glycoprotein that facilitates vitamin B_{12} absorption in the proximal small intestine. For this function, the base of the cells contains a small Golgi complex, a few free ribosomes, and rough endoplasmic reticulum.

CLINICAL POINT

The gram-negative bacterium **Helicobacter pylori** inhabits gastric mucosa. Its mode of transmission is unclear, but infection rates are high in populations in developed (40%) and underdeveloped (85%) countries. It may cause inflammation of the stomach (**gastritis**) and **gastric ulcers** via urease, which damages the mucosa. Chronic infection may lead to gastric **adenocarcinoma.** Diagnosis is by endoscopic or histologic study of the mucosa and stool antigen and blood antibody tests. Treatment with antibiotics is usually very effective.

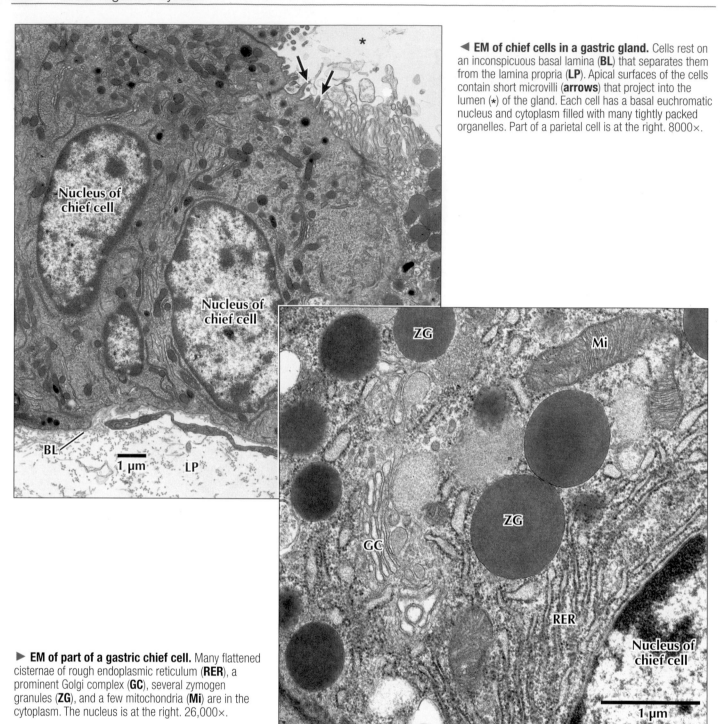

◄ **EM of chief cells in a gastric gland.** Cells rest on an inconspicuous basal lamina (**BL**) that separates them from the lamina propria (**LP**). Apical surfaces of the cells contain short microvilli (**arrows**) that project into the lumen (⋆) of the gland. Each cell has a basal euchromatic nucleus and cytoplasm filled with many tightly packed organelles. Part of a parietal cell is at the right. 8000×.

▶ **EM of part of a gastric chief cell.** Many flattened cisternae of rough endoplasmic reticulum (**RER**), a prominent Golgi complex (**GC**), several zymogen granules (**ZG**), and a few mitochondria (**Mi**) are in the cytoplasm. The nucleus is at the right. 26,000×.

13.7 ULTRASTRUCTURE AND FUNCTION OF GASTRIC CHIEF CELLS

Chief cells produce two distinct groups of *proteolytic enzymes,* called *pepsinogen I* and *II,* as inactive proenzymes. These classic protein-synthesizing cells have a basal nucleus and organelles for synthesis and secretion of protein. Their ultrastructure closely resembles that of pancreatic acinar cells. The basal aspect of each pyramidal cell rests on a **basal lamina;** its apical border contacts the **gastric gland** lumen. The basal cytoplasm contains extensive **rough endoplasmic reticulum** and many **free ribosomes,** which account for intense basophilia in H&E sections. The supranuclear cytoplasmic region has a prominent **Golgi complex. Mitochon-**dria are scattered in the cytoplasm and are especially large and numerous during cell secretion. Large, electron-dense membrane-bound *secretory vesicles,* the **zymogen granules,** are a salient feature of apical cytoplasm and emanate from the concave side of the Golgi. They discharge their contents by *exocytosis*—fusion of their limiting membranes with apical plasma membranes. Luminal plasma membranes contain short stubby **microvilli** that amplify surface area for secretion. Released pepsinogen is converted to pepsin, the active form of the enzyme, because of the low intraluminal pH in gastric glands. Chief cells also produce *lipase,* another digestive enzyme.

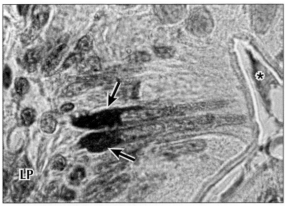

▲ **LM of enteroendocrine cells in the small intestine.** This stain detects vasoactive intestinal polypeptide hormone. The golden brown reaction product is concentrated at bases of the cells (**arrows**), toward the lamina propria (**LP**) and away from the lumen (٭). 1000×. *Diaminobenzidine and immunoperoxidase.*

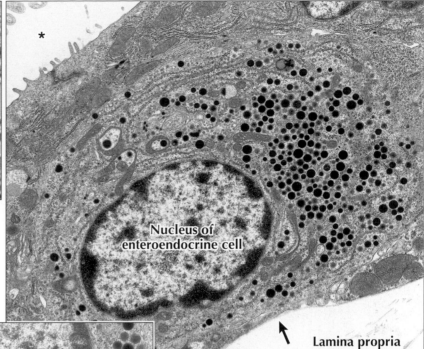

▲ **EM of an enteroendocrine cell in a gastric gland.** This granulated cell lies between other cells of the gland. It has an elliptical, euchromatic nucleus and many small electron-dense secretory vesicles. The basal surface (**arrows**) touches the lamina propria. The cell does not reach the glandular lumen (٭). Rather, other epithelial cells abut it. 9000×.

◄ **EM of part of an enteroendocrine cell in the stomach.** Many membrane-bound, electron-dense secretory vesicles (**arrows**) lie in the basal part of the cytoplasm. Rough endoplasmic reticulum (**RER**) and mitochondria (**Mi**) are sparse. Hormones in the vesicles are released by exocytosis into the lamina propria (**LP**). 15,000×.

13.8   ULTRASTRUCTURE AND FUNCTION OF ENTEROENDOCRINE CELLS

Enteroendocrine cells—hormone-producing cells of the gastrointestinal tract—are small pyramidal cells that are diffusely scattered in the epithelium, from the esophagus to the colon. Probably derived embryonically from endoderm, they are widespread in the mucosal lining, gastric glands, intestinal glands, and villi. They are called *argentaffin, argyrophil,* or *APUD* (amine precursor uptake and decarboxylation) cells on the basis of metabolic and staining properties. Cells are hard to see in routine sections, but immunocytochemistry and electron microscopy can reveal them. They make up a family of cells that belong to the *diffuse neuroendocrine system;* grouped together, these cells would form the largest endocrine organ in the body. The cell types are classed according to specific secretory product, but all conform to the same ultrastructural plan. Some may reach the lumen; most do not extend to the surface and are on the basal lamina, where they face the **lamina propria.** All have small, membrane-bound, electron-dense **secretory vesicles** concentrated in basal cell areas. One elliptical **nucleus** is usually euchromatic. The cytoplasm has a small Golgi complex, a few **mitochondria,** and scattered elements of **rough endoplasmic reticulum.** Cells produce various peptides and amines, which enter the bloodstream or act locally, with powerful effects on target cells. More than 30 gastrointestinal hormones, such as *gastrin, motilin, cholecystokinin, somatostatin, secretin,* and *vasoactive intestinal polypeptide,* are produced.

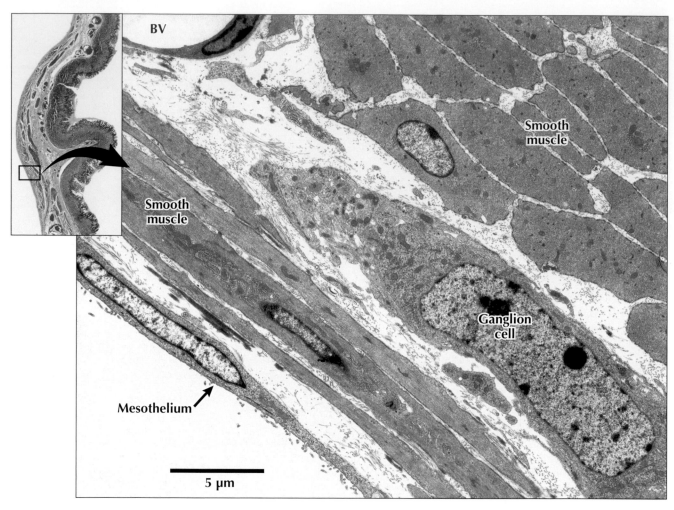

▲ **Top left. LM of the stomach wall.** 5×. *H&E.* **Center. EM of the outer wall of the stomach.** The serosa consists of one outer layer of flattened mesothelial cells and associated connective tissue. Smooth muscle cells in the muscularis externa sectioned longitudinally and transversely are seen. A blood vessel (**BV**) and part of a myenteric plexus with a ganglion cell are between the smooth muscle layers. 5000×.

13.9 ULTRASTRUCTURE OF THE SEROSA AND MUSCULARIS EXTERNA

A moist, slippery **serous membrane** (or *serosa*) that lines the *peritoneal cavity*, the **peritoneum**, is made of two layers. The *parietal peritoneum* lines abdominal and pelvic walls and the undersurface of the diaphragm. The *visceral peritoneum* covers the intraperitoneal parts of the digestive system and the suspensory folds, such as mesenteries and omentum. A serosa, which constitutes the visceral peritoneum, covers the stomach and intestines; suspensory folds also support these parts of the digestive tract. In contrast, parts of the duodenum and colon are retroperitoneal and are covered only anteriorly by parietal peritoneum. The serosa consists of one layer of **mesothelial cells,** which face the peritoneal cavity, an underlying basal lamina, and a deeper layer of loose **connective tissue.** Like mesothelial cells lining pleural and pericardial cavities, these simple squamous epithelial cells derive embryonically from mesoderm. Cells are linked by intercellular junctions and have microvilli on their surfaces. Cells produce a thin film of serous fluid, thus providing a slippery surface over which abdominal viscera can glide freely. The **muscularis externa** of the stomach is made of three layers of smooth muscle: outer longitudinal, middle circular, and inner oblique. Of these, the circular layer is the most continuous and well defined. Between muscularis externa layers is the **myenteric plexus** of **Auerbach**—a network of autonomic ganglia and nerves.

CLINICAL POINT

Peritonitis—localized or diffuse inflammation of the peritoneum—is usually due to entry of bacteria into the peritoneal cavity via an internal perforation of the digestive tract or an external penetrating wound. Infecting bacteria are most commonly *Escherichia coli* and *Enterococcus faecalis*. Clinical features are severe abdominal pain and distention, nausea, vomiting, and diarrhea. Major causes are *gastric (peptic) ulcer, appendicitis, diverticulitis, cholecystitis,* and *gangrenous obstruction* of the small intestine. Peritonitis may also be a complication of abdominal surgery. A medical emergency, it can be life-threatening if untreated.

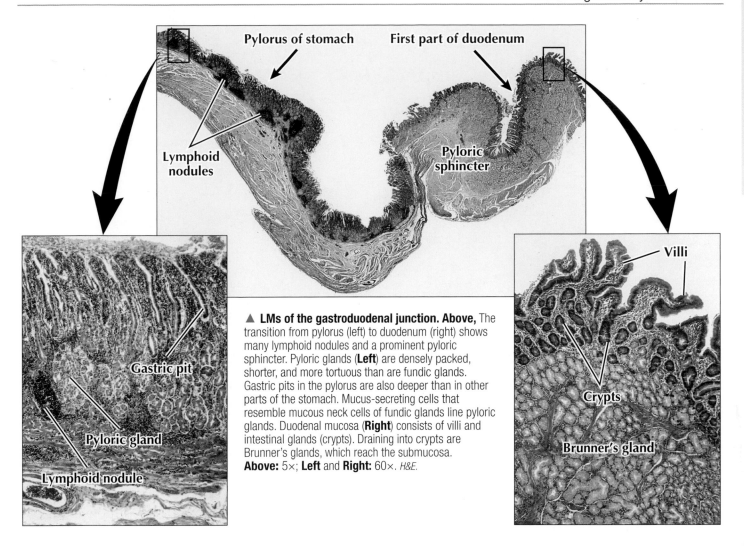

▲ **LMs of the gastroduodenal junction. Above,** The transition from pylorus (left) to duodenum (right) shows many lymphoid nodules and a prominent pyloric sphincter. Pyloric glands (**Left**) are densely packed, shorter, and more tortuous than are fundic glands. Gastric pits in the pylorus are also deeper than in other parts of the stomach. Mucus-secreting cells that resemble mucous neck cells of fundic glands line pyloric glands. Duodenal mucosa (**Right**) consists of villi and intestinal glands (crypts). Draining into crypts are Brunner's glands, which reach the submucosa. **Above:** 5×; **Left** and **Right:** 60×. *H&E.*

13.10 HISTOLOGY OF THE GASTRODUODENAL JUNCTION

The **pylorus** of the **stomach** is continuous with the first part of the **duodenum** in a broad transitional zone—the gastroduodenal junction. Its gross anatomy is well delineated, but its histology is not. In contrast to the esophagogastric junction—a discrete squamocolumnar junction—the gastroduodenal junction shows a gradual transition from **gastric mucosa** of the pylorus to **villous epithelium** of the **duodenal mucosa.** The junction is crenated with finger-like processes of gastric epithelium often extending up to 6 mm into the duodenum, which leads to islands of gastric mucosa on the duodenal side and small areas of duodenal mucosa on the gastric side. Branched tubuloalveolar, mucus-secreting **pyloric glands** are in gastric mucosa; multilobular, mucus-secreting **submucosal (Brunner's) glands** are on the duodenal side. Only *surface mucous cells* line gastric epithelium, but duodenal epithelium has two types of cells (*enterocytes* and *goblet cells*). The middle smooth muscle layer in the **muscularis externa** of the pylorus is thickened to form the **pyloric sphincter:** mucosa and submucosa are raised to form a circular thickening of the gastric wall. Peristaltic contractions of the muscle control the

amount of partly digested food moving from stomach to duodenum. Mucosa of the first part of the duodenum is smooth and flattened; more distal parts have circular folds (of Kerkring). The folds are made of mucosa and submucosa and are typical of the remaining small intestine. The lamina propria and submucosa of the pylorus and first part of the duodenum contain lymphoid tissue with variable numbers of **lymphoid nodules** with or without *germinal centers.*

CLINICAL POINT

Gastric and duodenal mucosae usually resist damage from gastric acid and proteolytic enzymes. **Peptic ulcers,** however, may develop in areas affected by acid and pepsin. These mucosal defects penetrate muscularis mucosae and cause pain and hemorrhage. Most peptic ulcers are caused by *Helicobacter pylori* infection, but they may also result from use of nonsteroidal antiinflammatory drugs (NSAIDs) and alcohol. Antibiotic treatment often promotes healing. A rare cause is *Zollinger-Ellison syndrome* (or *gastrinoma*)—a tumor of enteroendocrine (G) cells in the pylorus. It leads to overproduction of the hormone gastrin and increased HCl production by parietal cells.

▼ Topography and relations of transverse colon and greater omentum elevated exposing small intestine.

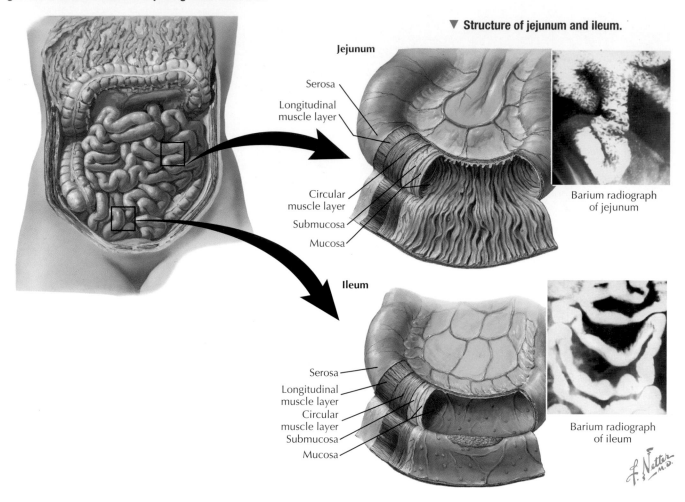

▼ Structure of jejunum and ileum.

Jejunum

Serosa
Longitudinal muscle layer
Circular muscle layer
Submucosa
Mucosa

Barium radiograph of jejunum

Ileum

Serosa
Longitudinal muscle layer
Circular muscle layer
Submucosa
Mucosa

Barium radiograph of ileum

13.11 STRUCTURE AND FUNCTION OF THE SMALL INTESTINE

The small intestine, 6-8 m long and the most convoluted part of the digestive tract, extends from the pylorus of the stomach to the ileocecal valve at the junction with the large intestine. It lies in the **abdominal cavity,** suspended by **mesenteries** that attach it to the body wall. It consists of three main segments. The horseshoe-shaped **duodenum** is the shortest, 25-30 cm long; its name (from Greek *dodekadaktulon*) denotes its length—about 12 finger-breadths. The **jejunum,** in the middle, is 2.5-3 m long and leads into the **ileum,** which is 4-4.5 m long. The transition between segments is gradual, but they all show the same histologic plan with minor variations. As in other parts of the digestive tract, from within outward, its wall consists of **mucosa, submucosa, muscularis externa,** and **serosa.** The small intestine conveys chyme from the stomach to the large intestine. It engages in processing and breakdown of ingested nutrients via action of enzymes produced by intramural cells and cells in extramural accessory glands (liver and pancreas). It absorbs end products of digestion, which move across the epithelium into capillaries and blind-ending lymphatic vessels (lacteals). The mucosa of the small intestine, with an area of 20-40 m², has specializations that markedly augment its surface area. Visible to the naked eye are circular folds called plicae: 3- to 10-mm-high permanent folds of mucosa with a central core of submucosa. Unique to this organ, villi—finger-like projections of mucosa facing the lumen—are 0.2-1.0 mm long. Microvilli, forming a striated border, greatly increase apical surfaces of enterocytes (or columnar absorptive cells) that line the intestinal lumen.

CLINICAL POINT
Ulcerative colitis (UC) and **Crohn's disease** (CD) are the most common forms of **inflammatory bowel disease.** CD may affect the small intestine and colon; UC is limited to the colon. Their causes are unknown, but genetic factors with multiple contributing genes may lead to their development. Bleeding, diarrhea, and abdominal pain occur and may result in life-threatening complications. UC produces distorted mucosal architecture, leukocyte infiltration of lamina propria, goblet cell depletion, and distal Paneth cell metaplasia. Abnormalities in CD, however, are transmural and penetrate all four layers of affected wall. Histologic changes include deep ulcerations, granulomas, prominent lymphoid aggregates, and dilated submucosal lymphatics.

▼ **Duodenal bulb and mucosal surface of duodenum.**

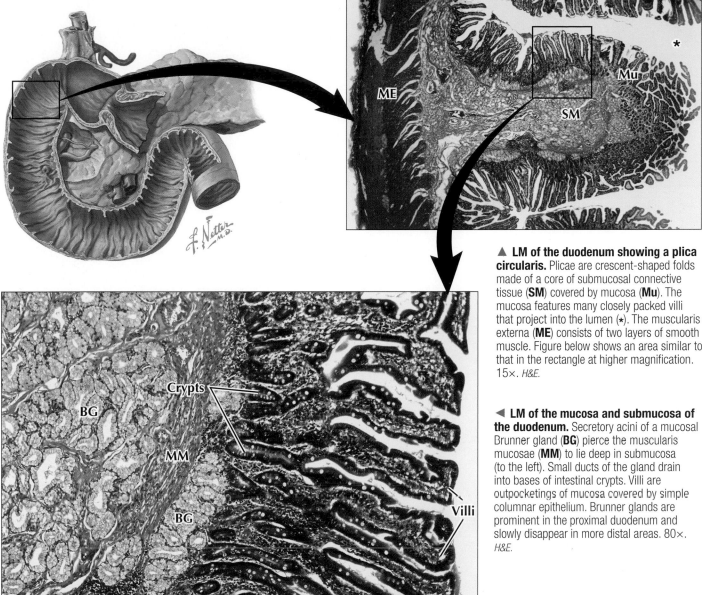

▲ **LM of the duodenum showing a plica circularis.** Plicae are crescent-shaped folds made of a core of submucosal connective tissue (**SM**) covered by mucosa (**Mu**). The mucosa features many closely packed villi that project into the lumen (✶). The muscularis externa (**ME**) consists of two layers of smooth muscle. Figure below shows an area similar to that in the rectangle at higher magnification. 15×. *H&E.*

◀ **LM of the mucosa and submucosa of the duodenum.** Secretory acini of a mucosal Brunner gland (**BG**) pierce the muscularis mucosae (**MM**) to lie deep in submucosa (to the left). Small ducts of the gland drain into bases of intestinal crypts. Villi are outpocketings of mucosa covered by simple columnar epithelium. Brunner glands are prominent in the proximal duodenum and slowly disappear in more distal areas. 80×. *H&E.*

13.12 HISTOLOGY AND FUNCTION OF THE DUODENUM

Villi and **intestinal crypts** characterize the **mucosa** of the entire small intestine. Villi—projections of epithelium and lamina propria—make the mucosal surface appear velvety. Duodenal villi are usually broad and leaf-shaped. The jejunum, however, has taller finger-shaped villi; the ileum, stubby club-shaped villi. **Simple columnar epithelium,** made of *enterocytes* and *goblet cells,* covers the villi. The relative number of goblet cells gradually increases toward the more distal small intestine. Between the villi, the epithelium dips down to form simple, tube-like invaginations called **intestinal glands,** or **crypts of Lieberkühn,** which extend to the **muscularis mucosae.** Because it is near the stomach, the proximal duodenum has distinctive **mucus-secreting glands of**

Brunner in its wall. These compound tubular glands appear similar to mucous glands in the pylorus of the stomach. Their **secretory acini** consist of tall cuboidal cells with flattened basal nuclei and pale vacuolated cytoplasm. Acini penetrate muscularis mucosae to reach the **submucosa,** where they form small lobules. Their short **ducts** drain into bases of crypts in the mucosa. The mucus, an alkaline glycoprotein (pH 8.1-9.3), has a high concentration of HCO_3^- ions that serves as a buffer to protect the mucosa from damage or erosion caused by gastric acid or by digestive enzymes draining into the duodenum from the pancreas. Brunner glands also produce urogastrone, a peptide hormone that inhibits HCl secretion. Enteroendocrine cells scattered among epithelial cells of secretory acini produce urogastrone.

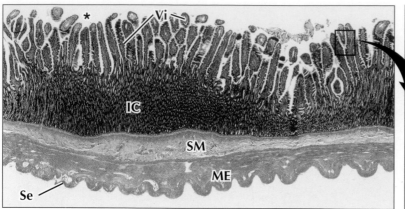

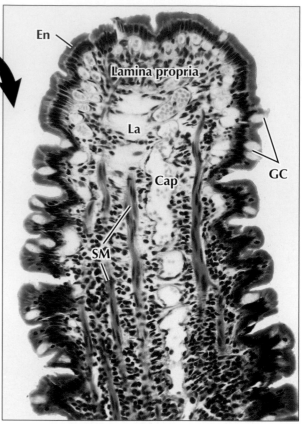

▲ **LM of the jejunum at low magnification.** Tall, slender villi (**Vi**) and intestinal crypts (**IC**) occupy the mucosa. The lumen (⋆), submucosa (**SM**), muscularis externa (**ME**), and serosa (**Se**) are indicated. 15×. *H&E.*

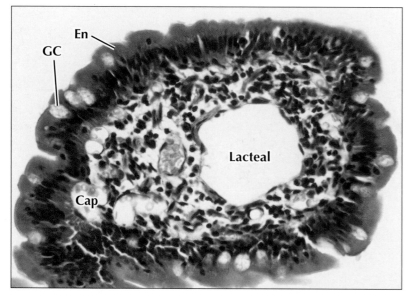

▲ **LM of a jejunal villus in transverse section.** Enterocytes (**En**) and goblet cells (**GC**) make up the layer of epithelial cells covering the villus. A lacteal and smaller systemic capillaries (**Cap**) are in the lamina propria. 380×. *H&E.*

▲ **LM of the tip of a jejunal villus in longitudinal section.** Simple columnar epithelium composed of enterocytes (**En**) and goblet cells (**GC**) covers the surface. The lamina propria, a highly cellular connective tissue, contains a central lacteal (**La**), blood capillary (**Cap**), and tufts of smooth muscle cells (**SM**). 300×. *H&E.*

13.13   HISTOLOGY OF THE JEJUNUM

Unlike the duodenum, which is almost all retroperitoneal, the jejunum and ileum are suspended by mesenteries. Compared with other parts of the small intestine, the jejunum has the largest surface area for luminal secretion and absorption. Its name is from the Latin, meaning empty, because at autopsy it usually looks empty. The division between jejunum and ileum is arbitrary, but the jejunum has a thicker wall and wider lumen than the ileum. The jejunal mesentery is more richly vascularized and contains less adipose tissue than that of the ileum. Barium x-ray studies show plicae circulares to be thicker, taller, and more numerous in the jejunum than in the ileum. The total thickness of the jejunal **mucosa,** which consists mostly of **villi** and **crypts,** is 0.5-1.5 mm. These tall, slender, finger-shaped villi in the

jejunum are 0.2-1.0 mm tall and lined by **simple columnar epithelium** composed mainly of two cell types. Most are **enterocytes**—tall columnar absorptive cells—that contain basal oval nuclei and have an apical striated border. Mucus-secreting **goblet cells** are mixed with enterocytes and have a washed-out cytoplasm because of **mucin granule** content. The core of each villus contains a richly vascularized, highly cellular **lamina propria.** Each villus also has small systemic **capillaries** and one larger **lymphatic lacteal. Smooth muscle cells** originating from the **muscularis mucosae** extend into each villus. A few solitary **lymphoid nodules** are found in the mucosa and sometimes penetrate the **submucosa.** Inner circular and outer longitudinal layers of smooth muscle constitute the **muscularis externa.** A **serosa** covers the jejunum externally.

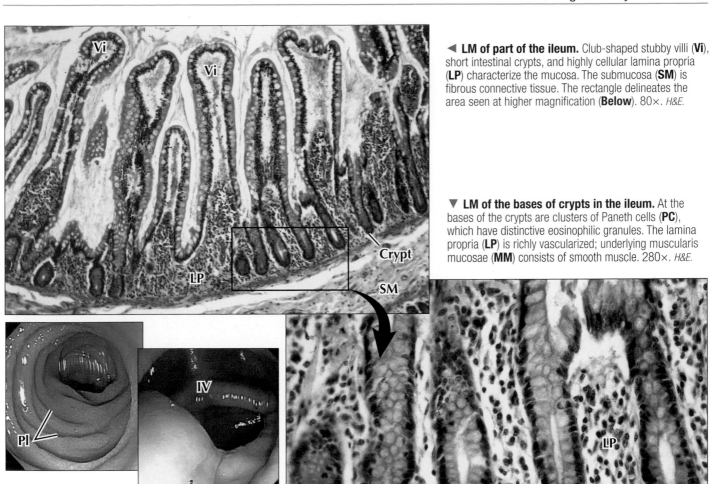

◀ **LM of part of the ileum.** Club-shaped stubby villi (**Vi**), short intestinal crypts, and highly cellular lamina propria (**LP**) characterize the mucosa. The submucosa (**SM**) is fibrous connective tissue. The rectangle delineates the area seen at higher magnification (**Below**). 80×. *H&E.*

▼ **LM of the bases of crypts in the ileum.** At the bases of the crypts are clusters of Paneth cells (**PC**), which have distinctive eosinophilic granules. The lamina propria (**LP**) is richly vascularized; underlying muscularis mucosae (**MM**) consists of smooth muscle. 280×. *H&E.*

▲ **Colonoscopic views of the ileum (Left) and ileocecal valve (Right).** Plicae circulares (**PI**) are a main feature of the ileum. The ileocecal valve (**IV**) between ileum and cecum is a sphincter formed by semilunar folds of mucosa supported internally by thickened smooth muscle.

13.14 HISTOLOGY OF THE ILEUM

The ileum shares many features with other parts of the small intestine, such as a wall with the usual four layers; a **mucosa** with **villi** and **crypts;** and villi containing a core of **loose connective tissue** covered by epithelium. Capillaries and isolated **smooth muscle cells** surround a central blind-ending lacteal. The ratio of goblet cells to enterocytes is greatest in the ileum, and a distinctive feature of the ileum is the presence of large amounts of *gut-associated lymphoid tissue (GALT),* a type of mucosa-associated lymphoid tissue. Besides many lymphocytes in the **lamina propria,** aggregated *lymphoid nodules,* called *Peyer's patches,* are most numerous in the distal ileum. At 8-20 cm in diameter, they are visible to the naked eye. They contain 10-250 lymphoid nodules, which lie in the submucosa, opposite the mesentery attachment. The 300 lymphoid nodules present at puberty diminish in size and number with age. They function in the immune response and serve as a source of plasma cells. Secretory **Paneth cells** occur in

all parts of the small intestine but are especially numerous in the ileum at bases of crypts. Crypts also harbor stem cells that replenish epithelial cells, which die and are extruded from villi. Protection of stem cells is thus essential for maintenance of the epithelium. The location of Paneth cells next to stem cells suggests a role in aiding epithelial cell renewal by secreting antimicrobial agents (e.g., *lysozyme*) into the crypts.

CLINICAL POINT

Colonoscopy enables the entire colon and terminal ileum to be evaluated at one examination. Gastroenterologists use it to screen for **colon cancer.** If needed, biopsy samples can be obtained during the procedure. Therapeutic colonoscopy is used for removal of **polyps,** which are abnormal elevations of colonic mucosa that can develop anywhere. They may progress from *adenomas* to *carcinomas.* Hereditary and dietary factors may play a role in formation of polyps and *colorectal neoplasms.*

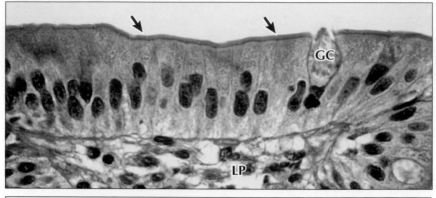

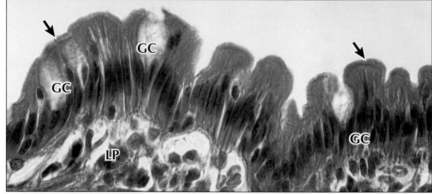

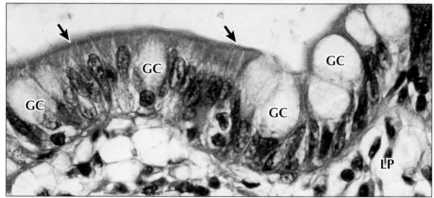

▲ **Contrasting LMs of the epithelium of the duodenum (Above), jejunum (Middle) and ileum (Below).** Enterocytes have a distinctive striated (or brush) border (**arrows**). They are interspersed with goblet cells (**GC**), which are most numerous in the ileum. Richly cellular lamina propria (**LP**) lies under the epithelium, which rests on a thin basement membrane. 800×. *H&E.*

13.15 HISTOLOGY AND CELL RENEWAL OF THE EPITHELIUM OF THE SMALL INTESTINE

Simple columnar epithelium lining the small intestine lumen consists of both **enterocytes** and **goblet cells.** They rest on a thin **basement membrane,** which separates them from the **lamina propria.** Enterocytes, about 25 μm high and 8-10 μm wide, have a basal oval nucleus. Their free surfaces show a prominent, distinctly **striated border.** Flask-shaped goblet cells, however, have pale cytoplasm and a cup-shaped, basally located nucleus. The three parts of the small intestine can be distinguished by the ratio of enterocytes to goblet cells. Enterocytes are most numerous in upper parts, their number slowly decreasing toward the lower end of the tract. In contrast, the number of goblet cells increases from duodenum to ileum. The number and height of **villi** also show regional variations. Duodenal villi are 0.2-0.5 mm high, relatively short, and often branched. Jejunal villi are more rounded, finger-like, and the tallest villi in the small intestine—0.2-1.0 mm high. Ileal villi are less numerous and slightly smaller than jejunal villi. The lifespan of enterocytes is about 5-6 days; goblet cells are replaced every 2-4 days. Both types are continuously extruded and lost at villi tips. Progenitor cells from deeper parts of the epithelium replenish them. For their replacement, mitotic *stem cells,* called *crypt base columnar cells,* reside in the lower half of the *crypts.* As they differentiate, they migrate up to the villi, ultimately to mature. Other cells of the intestinal epithelium (**Paneth cells, enteroendocrine cells**) also derive from this dynamic stem cell population.

▼ **Three-dimensional scheme of striated border of intestinal epithelial cells.**

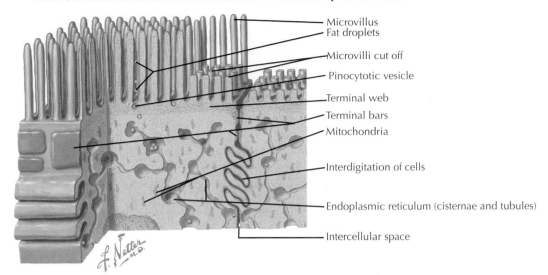

- Microvillus
- Fat droplets
- Microvilli cut off
- Pinocytotic vesicle
- Terminal web
- Terminal bars
- Mitochondria
- Interdigitation of cells
- Endoplasmic reticulum (cisternae and tubules)
- Intercellular space

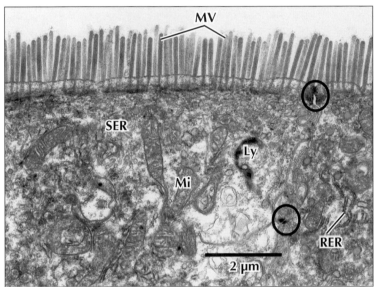
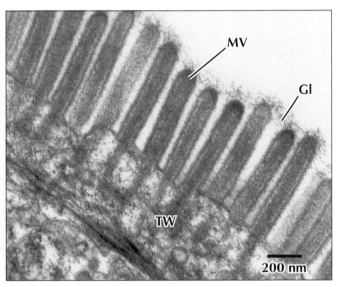

▲ **EMs of enterocytes at low (Left) and high (Right) magnification.** Apical microvilli (**MV**) make up a striated border and extend from free surfaces of the cells. A fuzzy glycocalyx (**Gl**) covers them. A terminal web (**TW**) of actin filaments in the apical cytoplasm reaches into microvilli. Intercellular junctions (**circles**) are between adjacent cells. The cytoplasm contains mitochondria (**Mi**), lysosomes (**Ly**), and smooth (**SER**) and rough (**RER**) endoplasmic reticulum. **Left:** 10,000×; **Right:** 50,000×.

13.16 ULTRASTRUCTURE AND FUNCTION OF ENTEROCYTES

Cells lining the lumen of the small and large intestine are mainly enterocytes, with ultrastructural features linked to a role in final breakdown of ingested nutrients. They also engage in end stages of absorption and intracellular processing via active transcellular transport to capillaries and lymphatics. The apical plasma membrane is studded with a prominent **striated border** of up to 3000 closely packed, parallel **microvilli** that greatly enhance surface area. Each microvillus is uniformly 1 μm long and 0.1 μm in diameter, with a surface covered by a glycoprotein-rich fuzzy coat (or **glycocalyx**), about 0.5 μm thick. Enterocytes synthesize *enzymes* such as disaccharidases, peptidases, enterokinase, and lipases, which are integral membrane proteins of the glycocalyx. Apical cytoplasm under the microvilli contains the **terminal web**—an elaborate network of **actin filaments** that are associated with myosin and other contractile and cytoskeletal proteins in the cell. A bundle of 20-40 parallel actin filaments extends into the core of each microvillus to provide stability. A cytoskeleton of *microtubules* and *intermediate filaments* courses through the remaining cytoplasm. Intercellular junctions that anchor adjacent cells link their lateral borders and provide a permeability barrier to macromolecules. Lateral cell membranes are highly infolded and contain ion pumps, such as H^+,K^+-ATPase, for ion transport and nutrient absorption. **Mitochondria, lysosomes,** elements of **rough** and **smooth endoplasmic reticulum,** and a supranuclear Golgi complex are also in the cytoplasm. The Golgi and smooth endoplasmic reticulum play a critical role in terminal lipid processing during fat absorption.

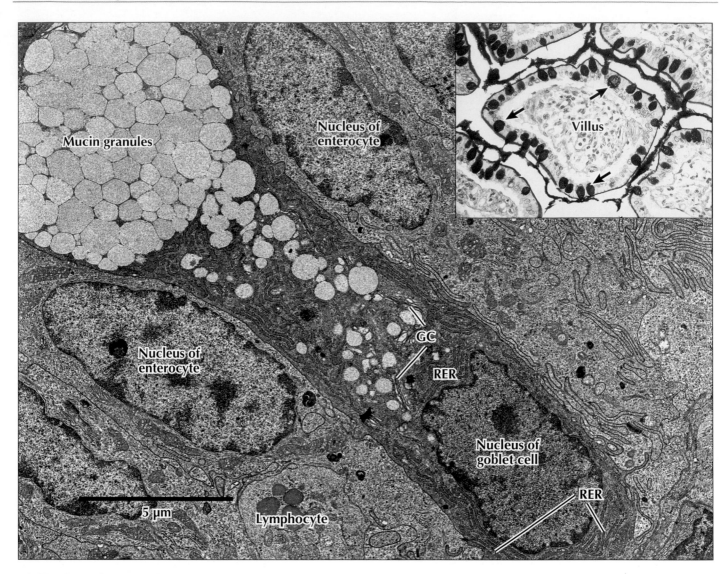

▲ **EM of part of the epithelium of the small intestine.** A goblet cell is insinuated between enterocytes. The narrow basal part of the goblet cell contains a nucleus that is surrounded by multiple flattened cisternae of rough endoplasmic reticulum (**RER**). A conspicuous supranuclear Golgi complex (**GC**) contains many dilated sacs. Mucin granules emanate from the Golgi and crowd into the apical cytoplasm. A lymphocyte crosses the epithelium, probably on its way to the lumen. 8000×. *(Courtesy of Dr. B. J. Crawford.)*

▼ **LM of a villus in the jejunum in transverse section (top right).** A high carbohydrate content of mucin makes the PAS-positive goblet cells (**arrows**) stain magenta. 200×. *PAS.*

13.17 ULTRASTRUCTURE AND FUNCTION OF GOBLET CELLS

Goblet cells produce copious amounts of protective **mucus** that covers the mucosa of the small and large intestine. Mucus, a high-molecular-weight *glycoprotein* with protein and carbohydrate moieties, is a highly viscous surface lubricant that also blocks bacteria from binding with epithelium. Each cell has a flask or wine goblet shape because its apical cytoplasm is distended with tightly packed, large (1-3 μm) **secretory vesicles** (or **mucin granules**). Moderately electron-dense, they originate from a prominent supranuclear **Golgi complex.** Elaborate **rough endoplasmic reticulum** consists of parallel, flattened **cisternae** in the basal cytoplasm. The indented or cup-shaped **nucleus** is displaced toward the attenuated basal part of the cell. Goblet cells have one or two secretory cycles in a lifespan of 2-4 days. They synthesize, store, and discharge mucus by *compound exocytosis,* whereby random fusion of separate vesicles occurs before release. In humans, newly synthesized mucin granules move from the Golgi to the apical surface in 12-24 hours. Goblet cells mingle with enterocytes in the epithelium, and *intercellular junctions* link their lateral borders. Apical cell membranes have short **microvilli** that project into the lumen. Precursors of goblet cells are undifferentiated stem cells, capable of cell division, that reside deep in crypts and migrate to the surface. Goblet cells secrete various types of mucus. Sialomucins predominate in the small intestine; sulfomucins, in the large intestine. Cholinergic stimulation, as well as bacterial and endotoxin exposure, causes massive mucin release by goblet cells.

▲ **LM of the base of an intestinal crypt showing Paneth cells (Left).** Large secretory granules in the apical cytoplasm, which are ultimately discharged into the lumen (∗) of the crypt, are a notable feature. 1000×. *Toluidine blue, plastic section.*

▲ **EM of Paneth cells.** Several cells line the lumen (∗) of a crypt, with a few short microvilli projecting into it. The basal part of each cell rests on a thin basal lamina (**arrows**), which abuts the lamina propria. Parallel arrays of rough endoplasmic reticulum (**RER**) surround the nucleus. A prominent Golgi complex (**GC**), many large secretory granules (**SG**), and a few mitochondria (**Mi**) are in the apical cytoplasm. 7600×.

13.18 ULTRASTRUCTURE AND FUNCTION OF PANETH CELLS

Paneth cells sit in the bases of **crypts** in the small intestine. Most numerous in the ileum, they are also in the normal appendix. They originate from undifferentiated stem cells in intestinal crypts and live for 20-30 days, which is longer than most other intestinal epithelial cells. Paneth cells exposed to bacteria or bacterial antigens produce *lysozyme,* which regulates the bacterial microenvironment of the crypts. They also contain zinc, an activator and stabilizer of lysozyme. Paneth cells phagocytose bacteria and immunoglobulins. They may also serve in host defense as antigen-presenting cells to T lymphocytes. Paneth cells resemble other protein-secreting cells—pyramidal cells with a basal nucleus and apical cytoplasm filled with large, conspicuous, electron-dense **secretory vesicles** (or **granules**). These spherical vesicles, with diameters of 5-20 nm, increase in density as they approach the apical cell surface. Vesicle contents are discharged by *exocytosis* into crypt lumina by fusion of the vesicle's limiting membrane with the cell's apical plasma membrane. Each cell contains a **Golgi complex,** abundant **rough endoplasmic reticulum** arranged as multiple flattened cisternae, and many **lysosomes.** Short stubby **microvilli** project from apical cell membranes into crypt lumina. Paneth cells secrete constantly, but feeding enhances the rate of secretion. *Hyperplasia* is associated with *adenocarcinoma* of the small intestine, and Paneth cell *metaplasia* occurs in *chronic ulcerative colitis.*

▼ **Structure of the colon (large intestine).**

Greater omentum (*cut away*)
Transverse mesocolon
Transverse colon
Omental taenia
Omental (epiploic) appendices
Omental taenia (*exposed by hook*)
Ascending colon
Free taenia (taenia libera)
Semilunar folds
Rectosigmoid junction
Cecum
Vermiform appendix
Rectum

Descending colon
Mesocolic taenia (*exposed by hook*)
Free taenia (taenia libera)
Sigmoid mesocolon
Sigmoid colon

▼ **Cross-section of large intestine.**

Lumen
Mucosa
Muscularis mucosae
Submucosa
Circular muscle
Longitudinal muscle
Visceral peritoneum

▲ **Colonoscopy of normal transverse colon.** The typical triangular lumen is due to the configuration of taenia coli and haustra.

▶ **LM of the mucosa of the colon.** The colon lacks villi. Invaginations of surface epithelium (**EP**) form intestinal crypts, which contain many washed-out goblet cells. A lymphoid nodule (**LN**) in the lamina propria (**LP**) extends into submucosa (**SM**). Epithelium over the nodule consists of M cells (**MC**), which are specialized columnar epithelial cells with microplicae—rather than microvilli—on the luminal surface. 120×. *H&E.*

13.19 STRUCTURE AND FUNCTION OF THE LARGE INTESTINE

The large intestine, or **colon**—a sacculated tube that is 1.5 m long and about 6.5 cm in diameter—begins at the **ileocecal junction** and ends at the **rectoanal junction.** It stores intestinal contents before discharge and absorbs water, electrolytes, bile acids, and some vitamins. It also secretes mucus for protection and lubrication and engages in nonenzymatic, bacterial digestion of foods. It consists of the **cecum; appendix** (a worm-like appendage of the cecum); **ascending, transverse,** and **descending** segments; **sigmoid colon;** and **rectum.** The colon has the four concentric layers of other parts of the digestive tract, with some changes. The *muscularis externa* consists of a complete inner circular layer of smooth muscle; the outer layer, of nonuniform thickness, has three equidistant longitudinal bands called **taenia coli.** Their state of partial contraction creates **haustra,** or saccules, between the

coli. These outward bulges are important surgical landmarks. Between them, the colon wall has crescent-shaped projections into the lumen called **plicae semilunares. Appendices epiploicae,** another unique feature of the colon, are subserosal pockets of adipose tissue that form pendulous bulges shaped like grapes.

CLINICAL POINT

Diverticulosis is the presence of diverticula, or herniations of mucosa and submucosa through the muscularis externa of the colon. Of unknown cause, it is most prevalent in developed countries where low-fiber diets are common. Inflammation of diverticula, or **diverticulitis,** can lead to perforations, tears, bleeding, and infection. Early symptoms are cramps, bloating, and constipation, often followed by blood in the stool. Antibiotic treatment is usually successful, but severe cases may need surgery. A high-fiber (25-30 g/day) diet may prevent the disorders.

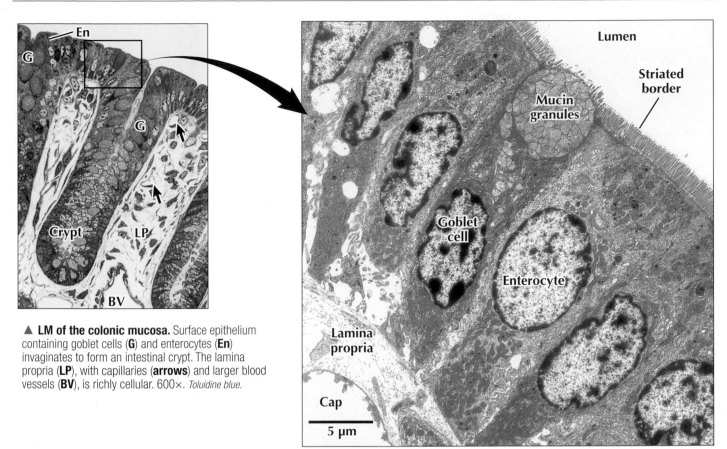

▲ **LM of the colonic mucosa.** Surface epithelium containing goblet cells (**G**) and enterocytes (**En**) invaginates to form an intestinal crypt. The lamina propria (**LP**), with capillaries (**arrows**) and larger blood vessels (**BV**), is richly cellular. 600×. *Toluidine blue.*

▲ **EM of the colonic mucosa.** Enterocytes have an apical striated border of microvilli that project into the lumen. These cells occur with goblet cells, which have apical mucin granules. The lamina propria contains a capillary (**Cap**). 3400×.

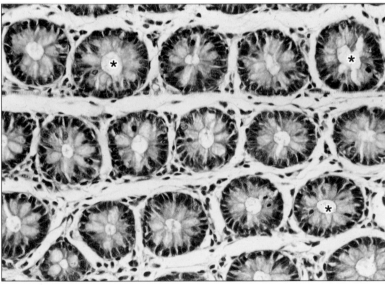

◀ **LM of intestinal crypts in the colonic mucosa.** The crypts, sectioned transversely, appear as regularly oriented, circular profiles surrounded by lamina propria. Simple columnar epithelium lines crypt lumina (✱). 600×. *H&E.*

13.20 HISTOLOGY OF THE LARGE INTESTINE

Unlike the small intestine mucosa, which has villi, the relatively flat colonic **mucosa** lacks them. The deep straight **intestinal glands** (or **crypts**) indenting its surface, at about 0.5 mm long, are two to three times longer than those in the small intestine. The layer of cells lining the surface and crypts forms a **simple columnar epithelium** similar to that seen elsewhere in the small intestine. The ratio of **goblet cells** to **enterocytes,** however, is greater in the colon than in the small intestine, and this ratio slowly increases from the cecum to the rectum. The highly cellular **lamina propria** contains many lymphoid nodules that may pierce the muscularis mucosae to reach the submucosa. Paneth cells are seen in the cecum and appendix but are normally missing from crypts of the rest of the colon. Crypts contain **stem cells** for epithelial renewal, as well as **enteroendocrine cells;** these are scattered among enterocytes and goblet cells. Epithelial cell replacement in the colon normally takes 5-6 days. The submucosa has the usual tissue components including large amounts of adipose tissue. The ascending and descending segments of the colon are retroperitoneal, so they are covered posteriorly by adventitia. Other parts of the colon, however, are invested by an incomplete serosa and suspended by mesentery.

▼ **Ileocecal region.**

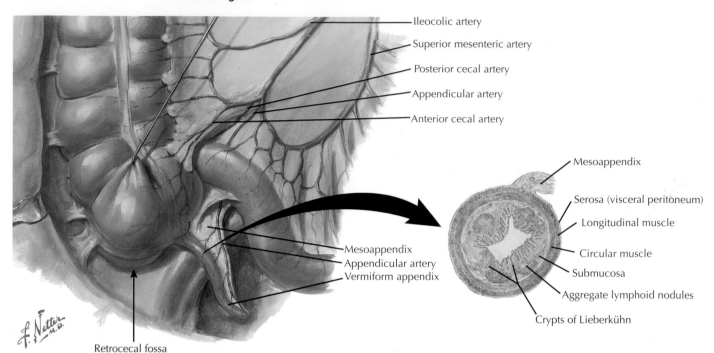

Ileocolic artery

Superior mesenteric artery

Posterior cecal artery

Appendicular artery

Anterior cecal artery

Mesoappendix

Appendicular artery

Vermiform appendix

Retrocecal fossa

Mesoappendix

Serosa (visceral peritoneum)

Longitudinal muscle

Circular muscle

Submucosa

Aggregate lymphoid nodules

Crypts of Lieberkühn

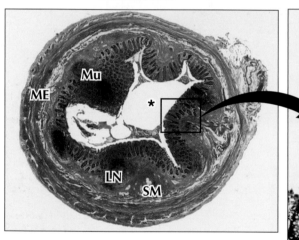

▲ **LM of the appendix in transverse section.**
Prominent mucosa (**Mu**) shows multiple lymphoid nodules (**LN**) bulging into a narrow stellate lumen (✶). Connective tissue makes up a submucosa (**SM**); the muscularis externa (**ME**) contains two layers of smooth muscle. 8×. *H&E.*

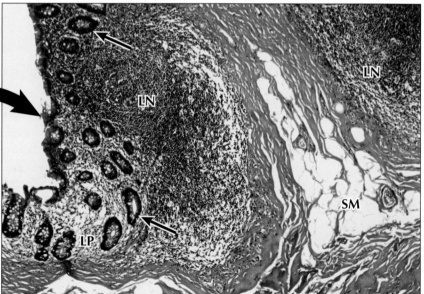

▲ **LM of part of the appendix.** Mucosa contains richly cellular lamina propria (**LP**) infiltrated with lymphoid nodules (**LN**) that extend into submucosa (**SM**). Shallow invaginations of the surface—intestinal crypts (**arrows**)—vary in length. The submucosa has some adipose tissue. 85×. *H&E.*

13.21 STRUCTURE AND FUNCTION OF THE APPENDIX

The appendix is a slender, worm-shaped tube, 7-10 cm long and 5-8 mm wide. It projects from the blind end of the cecum about 2 cm beyond the ileocecal junction. A short mesentery, the **mesoappendix,** attaches to the mesentery of the terminal ileum. It serves as a conduit for blood vessels, autonomic nerves, and lymphatics that supply the appendicular wall. The histology resembles that of other parts of the colon with some changes, such as the distinctive multiple, confluent **lymphoid nodules** that are part of

gut-associated lymphoid tissue (GALT). The nodules, in the lamina propria, protrude into the lumen, thereby narrowing it so it has a slit-like, stellate appearance. The lumen is wide and patent in early childhood but with age may become partly or completely obliterated. Lymphoid nodules in the mucosa pierce the muscularis mucosae to occupy the submucosa. The appendix has been assumed to be vestigial, but abundant lymphoid tissue in its wall and production of B-lymphocytes in germinal centers of nodules imply an immunologic defense function.

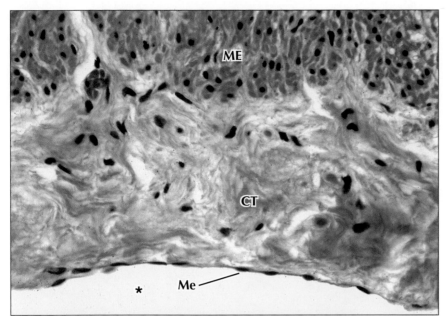

◀ **LM of the serosa of the appendix.** As in other parts of the digestive tract, the serosa is made of simple squamous epithelium—a mesothelium (**Me**). Its flattened cells face the peritoneal cavity (*). A dense irregular connective tissue (**CT**) layer is under the mesothelium, next to the outer layer of the muscularis externa (**ME**). Smooth muscle cells in this layer are parallel to the long axis of the appendix. 420×. *H&E.*

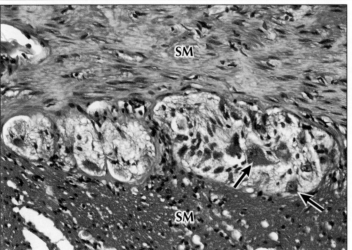

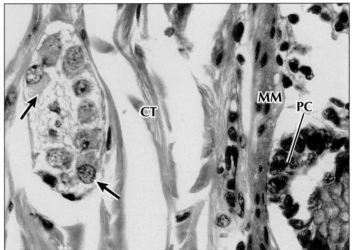

▲ **LMs of the myenteric (Left) and submucosal (Right) plexuses in the appendix.** These nerve cell bodies (**arrows**) and associated pale-stained nerve fibers are parts of the enteric nervous system. Smooth muscle (**SM**), connective tissue (**CT**), muscularis mucosae (**MM**), Paneth cells (**PC**). **Left:** 260×; **Right:** 720×. *H&E.*

13.22 HISTOLOGY OF THE APPENDIX

The appendix lacks villi, and invaginations of surface **epithelium** lead into straight tubular intestinal crypts. They are less abundant and shallower than those elsewhere in the colon. The simple columnar epithelium consists mostly of mixed enterocytes and goblet cells. M (or membranous) cells are also in the epithelium overlying many lymphoid nodules in the lamina propria. These cuboidal to columnar antigen-processing epithelial cells, best seen by electron microscopy, have short microvilli, or *microfolds,* on their apical surface. Crypts have many enteroendocrine cells and mitotically active stem cells. The **muscularis externa** lacks taenia coli and consists of complete outer longitudinal and inner circular layers of **smooth muscle.** As in other parts of the digestive tract,

elements of the **enteric nervous system** are seen: the **myenteric plexus** between the two smooth muscle layers, and the **submucosal plexus** in the **submucosa.**

CLINICAL POINT

Appendicitis—inflammation of the appendix—is caused by obstruction of the narrow lumen, which increases susceptibility to *bacterial infection.* Pain in the lower right quadrant, nausea, and vomiting result. Accurate diagnosis is by CT scan and white blood cell count. Acute appendicitis first affects the mucosa, where edema and leukocyte infiltration occur. Penetration of other layers may lead to abscess, necrosis, perforation into the peritoneal cavity, and a complication—*peritonitis* (inflammation of the peritoneum). Treatment is surgical removal of the inflamed appendix, or *appendectomy.*

▼ Rectum and anal canal.

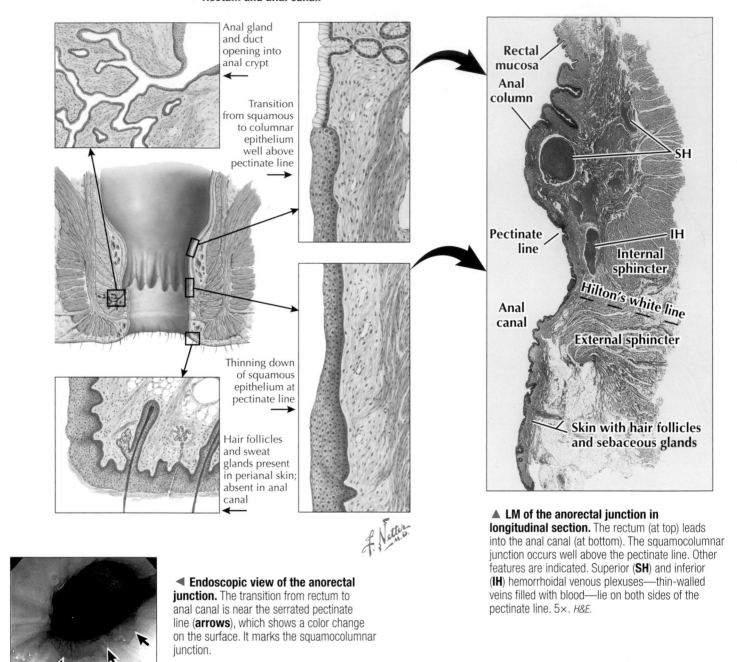

Anal gland and duct opening into anal crypt

Transition from squamous to columnar epithelium well above pectinate line →

Thinning down of squamous epithelium at pectinate line →

Hair follicles and sweat glands present in perianal skin; absent in anal canal →

Rectal mucosa
Anal column
SH
Pectinate line
IH
Internal sphincter
Hilton's white line
Anal canal
External sphincter
Skin with hair follicles and sebaceous glands

f. Netter

◄ **Endoscopic view of the anorectal junction.** The transition from rectum to anal canal is near the serrated pectinate line (**arrows**), which shows a color change on the surface. It marks the squamocolumnar junction.

▲ **LM of the anorectal junction in longitudinal section.** The rectum (at top) leads into the anal canal (at bottom). The squamocolumnar junction occurs well above the pectinate line. Other features are indicated. Superior (**SH**) and inferior (**IH**) hemorrhoidal venous plexuses—thin-walled veins filled with blood—lie on both sides of the pectinate line. 5×. *H&E.*

13.23 STRUCTURE AND FUNCTION OF THE ANORECTAL JUNCTION

The **rectum,** the distal part of the colon, is about 12 cm long; it extends from the S3 vertebral level to the pelvic diaphragm and continues to the **anal canal.** It lacks a mesentery, so an adventitia replaces a serosa. The **rectal mucosa** resembles that of the colon: it is lined by **simple columnar epithelium,** lacks villi, and has a smooth surface with periodic invaginations equivalent to intestinal crypts. These are longer—at 0.5-0.7 mm—than those elsewhere in the colon. They consist almost solely of *goblet cells.* Three transverse semilunar mucosal folds project into the rectal lumen and aid support of feces before defecation. Solitary lymphoid

nodules are in the lamina propria. The 2- to 3-cm-long anal canal ends at the anus, where its epithelial lining becomes continuous with epidermis of **skin.** The mucous membrane of the anal canal has 5-10 permanent longitudinal folds called *anal columns of Morgagni.* They are joined at their bases by cup-shaped folds, the *anal valves.* This area of the mucosa appears serrated and is called the **pectinate line** because it resembles a comb. In the submucosa at the base of each anal column are terminal branches of the *superior hemorrhoidal artery* and *vein.* The veins form an extensive **hemorrhoidal venous plexus,** which may develop varicosities and lead to *internal hemorrhoids.*

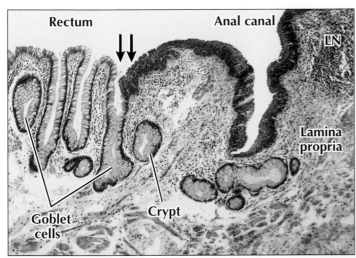

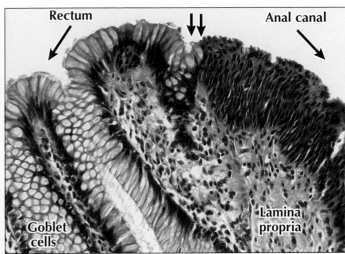

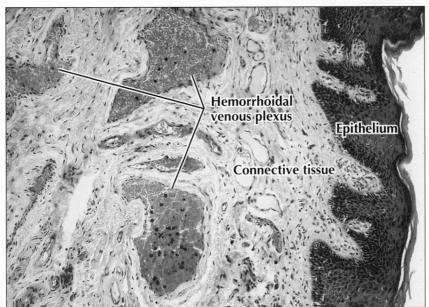

▲ **LMs of the anorectal junction at low (Left) and high (Right) magnifications.** An abrupt transition (**double arrows**) from simple columnar (left) to stratified columnar (right) epithelium occurs in this part of the pectinate line. Mucus-secreting goblet cells predominate on the mucosal surface and in rectal crypts. Highly cellular lamina propria under the epithelium contains lymphoid nodules (**LN**). **Right:** 80×; **Left:** 320×. *H&E.*

◄ **LM of the mucosa of the anal canal.** Further along the canal, epithelium becomes stratified squamous. Just below the pectinate line, it is nonkeratinized, but it becomes keratinized. In connective tissue under the epithelium is a plexus of thin-walled hemorrhoidal veins. 260×. *H&E.*

13.24 HISTOLOGY OF THE ANORECTAL JUNCTION

The **pectinate line** marks the boundary between **rectum** and **anal canal**. In this area, **simple columnar epithelium** changes abruptly to an intervening transitional zone of **stratified columnar epithelium,** which becomes **nonkeratinized stratified squamous.** As a common site of neoplastic change, the junction is clinically important. The arterial supply, venous return, lymphatic drainage, and innervation have different sources on the two sides of the line. The pectinate line corresponds to the fetal anal membrane, which marks the boundary between hindgut endoderm and the ectodermal part of the anal canal. Submucosa below the pectinate line has a plexus of **inferior hemorrhoidal veins.** The inner circular smooth muscle layer in the muscularis externa is thickened—the involuntary **internal sphincter.** Beyond this sphincter, skeletal muscle fibers of the levator ani form the voluntary **external sphincter.** Between the two sphincters lies a groove called

Hilton's white line, palpable at physical examination. At the lower end of the anal canal, the epithelium becomes keratinized and is continuous externally with **epidermis** of **skin.** Large apocrine sweat glands, the *circumanal glands,* are in the **dermis.**

CLINICAL POINT

Hemorrhoids—varicose submucosal veins of the hemorrhoidal plexus that protrude into the rectum or anal canal—are a common clinical condition. **Internal hemorrhoids** are above the pectinate line and originate from superior hemorrhoidal veins; **external hemorrhoids,** below the line, are from the inferior hemorrhoidal plexus. Causes may include genetic predisposition and increased pressure in the veins resulting from repeated straining from constipation or during pregnancy. Chronic congestion of the veins, which lack valves, leads to thrombosis and bleeding.

14

LIVER, GALLBLADDER, AND EXOCRINE PANCREAS

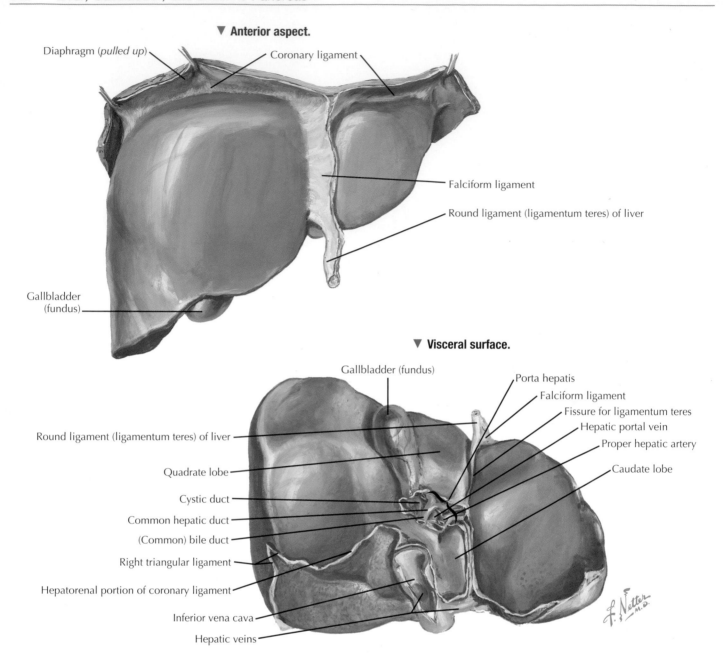

▼ **Anterior aspect.**

Diaphragm (*pulled up*)

Coronary ligament

Falciform ligament

Round ligament (ligamentum teres) of liver

Gallbladder (fundus)

▼ **Visceral surface.**

Gallbladder (fundus)

Porta hepatis

Falciform ligament

Fissure for ligamentum teres

Hepatic portal vein

Proper hepatic artery

Caudate lobe

Round ligament (ligamentum teres) of liver

Quadrate lobe

Cystic duct

Common hepatic duct

(Common) bile duct

Right triangular ligament

Hepatorenal portion of coronary ligament

Inferior vena cava

Hepatic veins

14.1 OVERVIEW OF THE LIVER

The wedge-shaped liver, the largest and heaviest internal organ (weighs about 1.5 kg in an adult), is essential to life and is the most versatile and vascular organ. It sits just below the diaphragm in the upper right quadrant of the abdominal cavity and is protected completely by the rib cage. It comprises **two main lobes** of almost equal size—**right** and **left**—separated by a falciform ligament and a round ligament (ligamentum teres). **Two smaller lobes—caudate** and **quadrate**—are seen on the inferior (visceral) surface but are poorly demarcated. Under a peritoneal serous covering, a thin connective tissue (**Glisson**) capsule surrounds the lobes. On the visceral surface is the **porta hepatis,** the gateway for the *hepatic*

ducts, portal vein, hepatic artery, lymphatics, and *nerves.* The liver arises in the embryo as a diverticulum of foregut endoderm. Parenchymal cells proliferating from this diverticulum pass into mesenchyme of the septum transversum and occupy meshes of a network of capillaries related to vitelline and umbilical vessels. The liver is an accessory gland—both **exocrine** and **endocrine**—of the digestive tract and plays a central role in three broad functional categories: metabolism of carbohydrates, proteins, and fats; modification of exogenous substances such as drugs and alcohol; and formation and exocrine secretion of **bile,** which is critical for fat digestion.

▼ **Blood and bile supply.**

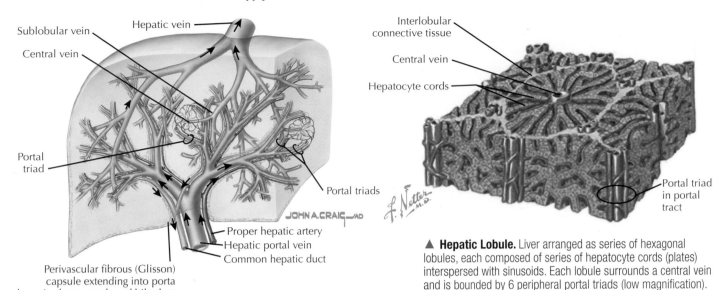

Sublobular vein
Hepatic vein
Central vein
Portal triad
Perivascular fibrous (Glisson) capsule extending into porta hepatis along vessels and bile duct
Proper hepatic artery
Hepatic portal vein
Common hepatic duct
Portal triads

JOHN A. CRAIG—AD

Interlobular connective tissue
Central vein
Hepatocyte cords
Portal triad in portal tract

▲ **Hepatic Lobule.** Liver arranged as series of hexagonal lobules, each composed of series of hepatocyte cords (plates) interspersed with sinusoids. Each lobule surrounds a central vein and is bounded by 6 peripheral portal triads (low magnification).

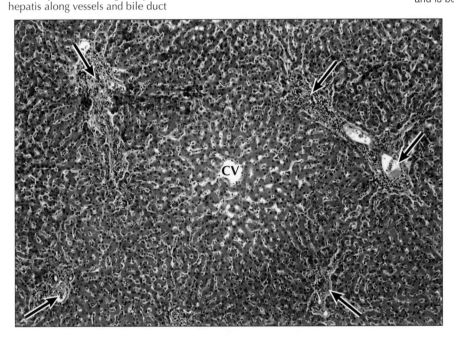

CV

◄ **Light micrograph (LM) of a hepatic lobule.** It is polyhedral and has a central vein (**CV**) as its morphologic axis, with plates of hepatocytes radiating from the vein. Its boundaries are marked by portal areas (**arrows**) at its corners, various amounts of connective tissue, and portal triads. The lobule shows an interlocking mosaic pattern with other lobules. 75×. *H&E.*

14.2 CLASSIC HEPATIC LOBULES

About 80% of liver tissue in the adult is **parenchyma** consisting of **hepatocytes** arranged as a labyrinth of cellular plates. The remaining 20% is **stroma,** a delicate supportive framework of **connective tissue** that forms the outer Glisson capsule. At the porta hepatis, this capsule is continuous with the arborization of connective tissue that accompanies the branching pattern of the entering hepatic artery and portal vein and the emerging bile duct. Branches of these three structures are the **portal triads.** They travel together throughout the liver's interior and divide repeatedly through 17-20 orders of branches. Their size progressively decreases to the terminal ramifications. Connective tissue in the liver indistinctly divides hepatic parenchyma into **classic hepatic lobules,** which are the liver's structural units. In humans, the lobules are poorly defined, the amount of connective tissue between lobules being scanty. In each lobule, a delicate stroma of *reticular fibers* forms a supportive network for hepatocytes and surrounding sinusoids.

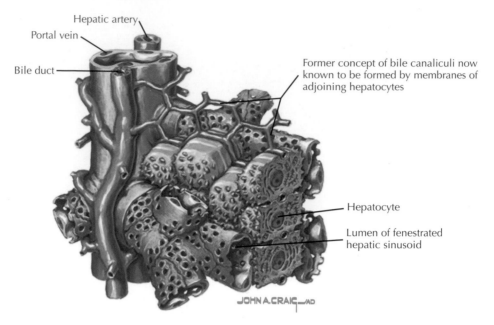

Hepatic artery
Portal vein
Bile duct
Former concept of bile canaliculi now known to be formed by membranes of adjoining hepatocytes
Hepatocyte
Lumen of fenestrated hepatic sinusoid

JOHN A. CRAIG—AD

▲ **Parts of hepatic lobule at portal triad (high magnification).**

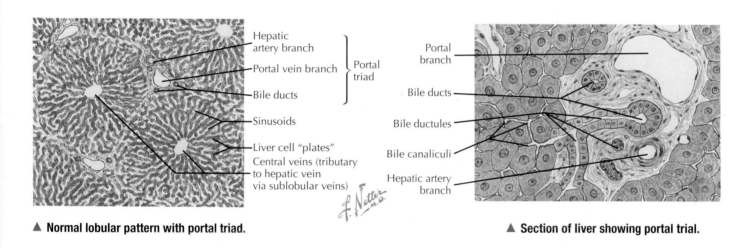

Hepatic artery branch
Portal vein branch } Portal triad
Bile ducts
Sinusoids
Liver cell "plates"
Central veins (tributary to hepatic vein via sublobular veins)

▲ **Normal lobular pattern with portal triad.**

Portal branch
Bile ducts
Bile ductules
Bile canaliculi
Hepatic artery branch

▲ **Section of liver showing portal trial.**

14.3 PORTAL TRIADS WITH BLOOD AND BILE SUPPLY

Each classic hepatic lobule has a prism form of about six sides, about 1 mm in diameter and 2 mm long. **Portal triads** surrounded by small amounts of interlobular connective tissue sit at corners of each lobule in areas called **portal tracts,** around which are limiting plates of hepatocytes. Triads also mark peripheral meeting places of adjacent **lobules,** which look like a mosaic of interlocking tiles. In transverse section, each lobule consists of plates of hepatocytes, one or two cells thick, which are separated by **hepatic sinusoids** and appear to radiate out from a small central vein. Hepatocyte arrangement resembles that of a sponge, with sinusoids represented by the spaces. Each triad consists of a branch of the bile duct, portal vein, and hepatic artery, which divide into smaller branches. Small lymphatic vessels often accompany them. A unique, unusual feature of the liver is a *dual blood supply.* The portal vein brings nutrient-rich blood from the gastrointestinal tract—75% of the total blood to the liver; hepatic arteries provide

25% of oxygenated blood. The liver receives about 1.5 L of blood each minute, and at least 20% of its volume is occupied by blood. Terminal branches of **portal veins,** about 300 μm in diameter, regularly give off inlet venules, which empty into thin-walled, fenestrated **hepatic sinusoids** that are in intimate contact with hepatocytes. Terminal branches of hepatic arteries, which ramify with portal vein branches, end as arterioles that drain into sinusoids, which thus receive a mixture of arterial and venous blood. Sinusoids converge toward a **central vein,** also called a terminal hepatic venule, and empty into it in the center of each lobule. A central vein is about 50 μm in diameter. Central veins unite to form **sublobular veins,** which lead into larger **hepatic veins** that travel alone and branch repeatedly. Hepatic veins coalesce to join the **inferior vena cava,** the main drainage route of blood from the liver. Important for understanding lobule organization and hepatocyte function, blood and bile flow through lobules in opposite directions.

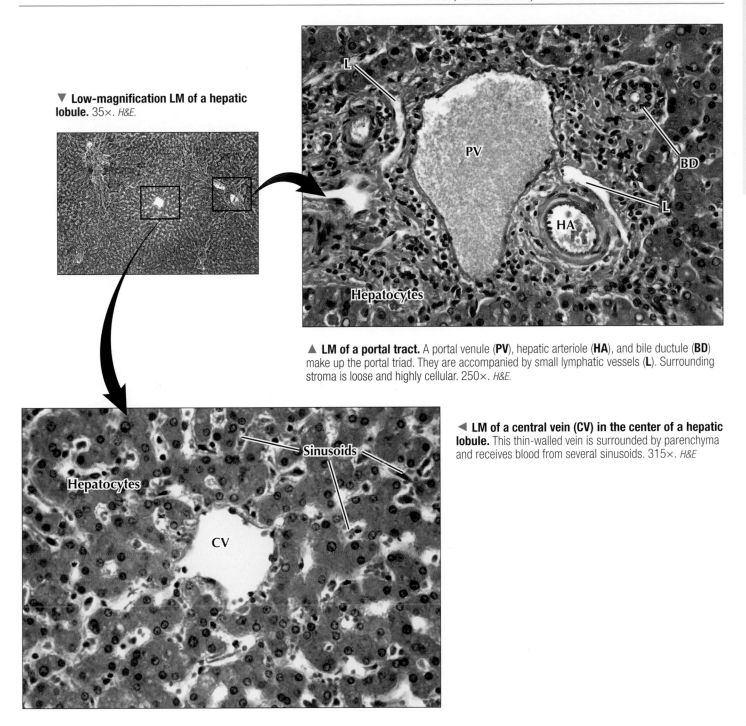

▼ **Low-magnification LM of a hepatic lobule.** 35×. *H&E.*

▲ **LM of a portal tract.** A portal venule (**PV**), hepatic arteriole (**HA**), and bile ductule (**BD**) make up the portal triad. They are accompanied by small lymphatic vessels (**L**). Surrounding stroma is loose and highly cellular. 250×. *H&E.*

◄ **LM of a central vein (CV) in the center of a hepatic lobule.** This thin-walled vein is surrounded by parenchyma and receives blood from several sinusoids. 315×. *H&E*

14.4   HISTOLOGY OF THE PORTAL TRACT AND CENTRAL VEIN

At their smallest branches, the three components of the portal triad are accompanied by small lymphatic vessels. **Connective tissue stroma** known as the **portal tract** encloses them all. In transverse section, the **hepatic arteriole** consists of one to three layers of smooth muscle cells and a relatively small lumen. The **portal venule** has a larger, often collapsed lumen with a more attenuated wall. The **bile ductule** is lined by simple cuboidal to columnar epithelium and drains exocrine secretions of hepatocytes from the liver. Biliary passages start with tiny **bile canaliculi**

between hepatocytes. Best seen by electron microscopy, they are small intercellular channels formed by groove-like invaginations of adjacent hepatocytes. As canaliculi approach the periphery of each lobule, they are drained by small ducts, known as **canals of Hering,** lined by a low simple cuboidal epithelium. These canals drain to larger **bile ducts** in portal tracts. As the ducts widen, their simple columnar epithelium becomes taller. Typical **central veins** are thin-walled venules with an attenuated endothelium. They normally lack significant investment of connective tissue stroma. The lumen of each central vein has numerous openings, which allows several hepatic sinusoids to drain freely into them.

▼ **Stereogram of liver cell plates.**

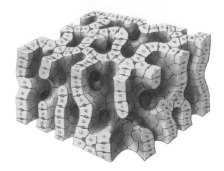

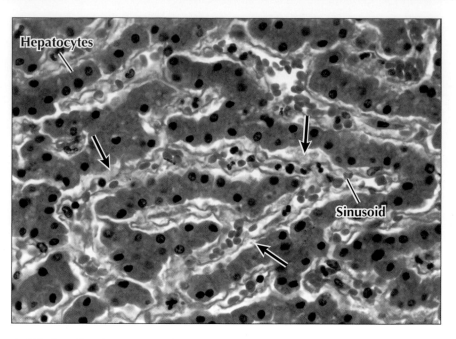

▲ **LM of the liver.** The parenchyma is made of hepatocytes arranged in regular, branching, interconnecting plates that are interposed with a network of thin-walled hepatic sinusoids. Shrinkage artifact helps highlight the narrow spaces of Dissé (**arrows**). 450×. *H&E.*

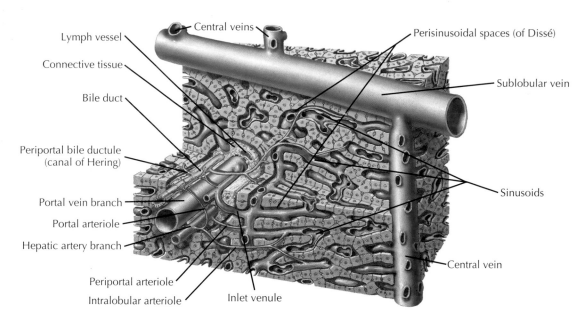

▲ **Three-dimensional schematic of liver structure.**

14.5 HISTOLOGIC ARRANGEMENT OF HEPATIC PARENCHYMA

Three-dimensional reconstructions of liver from serial sections provide insights into the arrangement of hepatic parenchyma and its relationship to vascular and biliary duct systems. The parenchyma consists of an anastomosing network of interconnecting plates, one or two cells thick, which resemble walls of a building with spaces in between. The hepatocytes in each plate can be likened to the building's bricks, and the hepatic sinusoids appear suspended within the spaces. In humans, one-cell-thick plates are most common in the normal adult liver; two-cell-thick plates

occur in the embryo and in adults during regeneration in certain diseases. Via electron microscopy or special light microscopic techniques, narrow fluid-filled perivascular spaces—spaces of Dissé (or perisinusoidal spaces)—can be seen separating the endothelial lining of sinusoids from the hepatocyte surfaces. These spaces allow plasma to flow between sinusoidal lumina and hepatocyte surfaces, which permits rapid exchange of soluble, noncellular substances between blood and parenchyma. In the fetus and in chronic anemias, these spaces are sites of extramedullary hematopoiesis. Hepatic lymph originates in these spaces and eventually drains to small lymphatic vessels in portal tracts.

▼ **Schematic view of a liver acinus.**

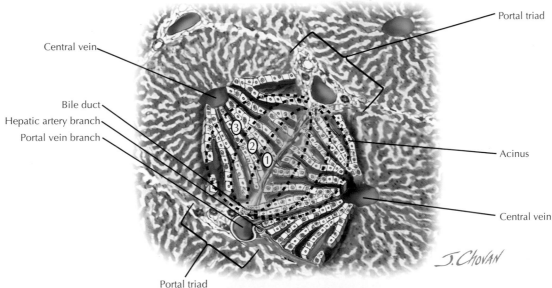

Central vein

Bile duct
Hepatic artery branch
Portal vein branch

Portal triad

Portal triad

Acinus

Central vein

J. CHOVAN

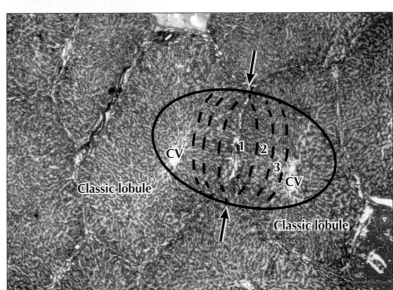

▶ **LM of the liver at low magnification showing approximate boundaries of a liver acinus.** Oval to ellipsoidal, the acinus comprises parts of two adjacent classic hepatic lobules. The border between the two lobules forms the central equatorial axis of the acinus, around which are three concentric zones (**1, 2, 3**). Peripheral landmarks of the acinus are two nearby central veins (**CV**) at the acinus poles, and two portal areas (**arrows**) at the ends of the equator. 23×. *H&E.*

CV
Classic lobule
1 2 3
CV
Classic lobule

14.6 STRUCTURE AND FUNCTION OF THE LIVER ACINUS

Another concept of liver lobulation is the **liver acinus**—an oval to diamond-shaped area of hepatic parenchyma defined in relation to blood supply from **terminal branches** of the **portal vein** and **hepatic artery**. It is smaller and harder to see than the classic hepatic lobule, but it is useful functionally and clinically because it is best for describing metabolic and pathologic changes in relation to many diseases. Its short axis runs along the border of two classic hepatic lobules; its long axis is an imaginary line between two central veins closest to the short axis. Hepatocytes in the acinus are arranged in *three concentric, elliptical zones* around the short axis. **Zone 1,** most central, is closest to the terminal distributing branches of the portal venule and hepatic arteriole. This zone first receives oxygen, hormones, and nutrients from the bloodstream, and most glycogen and plasma protein synthesis by hepatocytes occurs here. **Zone 3** is furthest from the distributing vessels; between zones 1 and 3 is the intermediate **zone 2.** A gradient of metabolic activity exists for many hepatic enzymes in the three zones. *Zone 3* is poorly oxygenated, is the first to show ischemic necrosis and fat accumulation if metabolism is altered, and is the site of most *drug and alcohol detoxification.* The classic hepatic lobule and liver acinus are not contradictory concepts of lobulation but rather complement each other.

CLINICAL POINT

Caused by hepatotropic viruses (A to E), **viral hepatitis** encompasses a broad array of acute or chronic inflammatory liver disorders. **Epstein-Barr virus, herpes simplex virus,** and **cytomegalovirus** may also cause acute hepatitis. Modes of transmission are fecal-oral, food/waterborne, sexual, parenteral, and perinatal. Acute hepatocellular injury, elevated serum aminotransferase and bilirubin levels, and presence of serum IgM and anti-HAV antibody characterize **hepatitis A.** The histologic hallmark of **hepatitis B** is the presence of ground-glass hepatocytes, caused by accumulation of hepatitis B surface antigen in endoplasmic reticulum. **Hepatitis C,** often transmitted via blood or blood products, may become chronic, which may lead to cirrhosis and hepatocellular carcinoma.

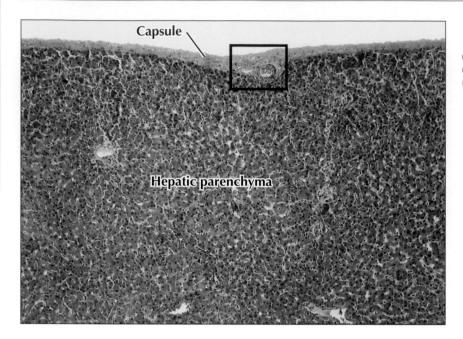

◄ **LM of the external aspect of the liver.** The Glisson capsule adheres tightly to underlying parenchyma. Area delineated in rectangle is seen at higher magnification (below left). 65×. *H&E.*

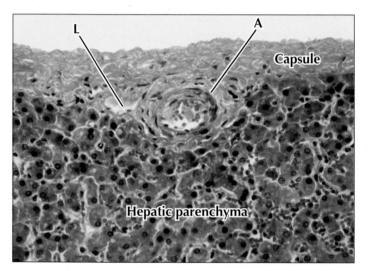

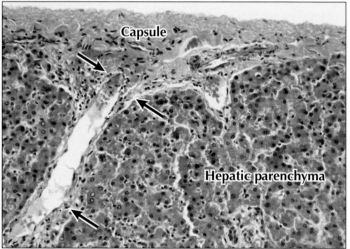

▲ **High-magnification LM of Glisson capsule.** Fibroblasts and small vessels, including an arteriole (**A**) and lymphatic channel (**L**), are interspersed with densely packed connective tissue fibers. Hepatocytes comprise parenchyma. 270×. *H&E.*

▲ **LM of the surface of the liver.** A thin extension of Glisson capsule (**arrows**) entering the hepatic parenchyma consists of connective tissue, which contains small blood vessels. 165×. *H&E.*

14.7   HISTOLOGY OF GLISSON CAPSULE

Except where the liver attaches to the diaphragm, it is surrounded by a dense fibrous **connective tissue capsule**, 70-100 μm thick. **Serous mesothelium** covers this capsule where it faces the peritoneal cavity. The mesothelium acts as a shield, especially against entry of pathogenic bacteria and other potentially harmful substances. The capsule comprises regularly arranged **collagen** and **elastic fibers** and provides external support and shape to the liver. It also contains a few small blood vessels and sends anchoring extensions into hepatic parenchyma, which contributes to its supportive stroma. Continuations of the capsule penetrate through the porta hepatis for support of blood and lymph vessels, ducts, and nerves. In part because of the thinness of the capsule, the liver, which has the consistency of table jelly, damages easily. Being richly vascularized, it bleeds profusely after injury. The capsule increases in thickness with aging and may undergo excessive proliferation in response to certain diseases. The stroma also proliferates after hepatocellular injury.

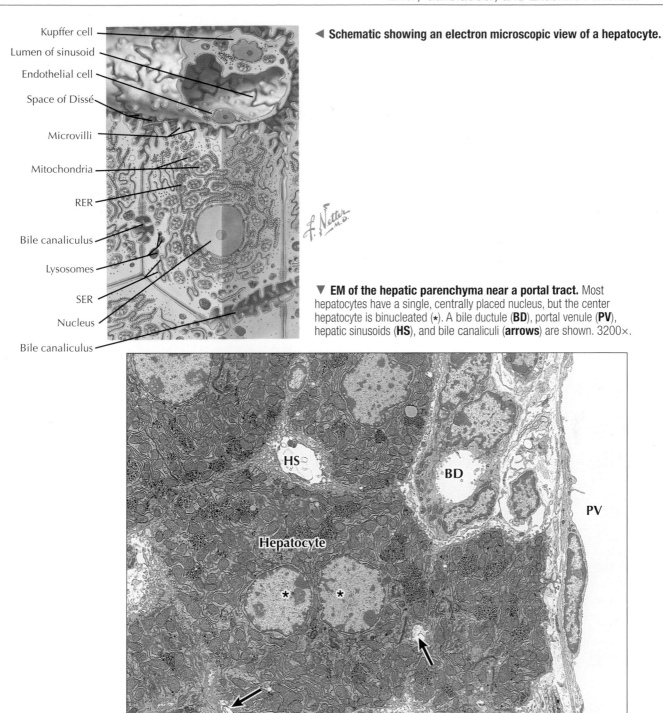

Kupffer cell
Lumen of sinusoid
Endothelial cell
Space of Dissé
Microvilli
Mitochondria
RER
Bile canaliculus
Lysosomes
SER
Nucleus
Bile canaliculus

◀ **Schematic showing an electron microscopic view of a hepatocyte.**

▼ **EM of the hepatic parenchyma near a portal tract.** Most hepatocytes have a single, centrally placed nucleus, but the center hepatocyte is binucleated (★). A bile ductule (**BD**), portal venule (**PV**), hepatic sinusoids (**HS**), and bile canaliculi (**arrows**) are shown. 3200×.

14.8   ULTRASTRUCTURE OF HEPATOCYTES

Hepatocytes are **polyhedral parenchymal cells,** about 20 µm by 30 µm in size, that are arranged in irregular plates between hepatic sinusoids. They usually have one centrally placed spherical nucleus, but binucleated cells and polyploid nuclei are common, with up to 20% of cells being binucleated. One or more prominent nucleoli, which function in ribosomal RNA production, are often present. Hepatocyte cytoplasm is densely packed with organelles and inclusions. The hepatocyte has **three functional surfaces: a canalicular** (secretory) surface, where a cylindrical space—a bile canaliculus—is formed by grooves of two adjoining membranes of neighboring hepatocytes, a **sinusoidal** (absorptive) surface studded with microvilli that faces the space of Dissé, and a surface between two closely apposed cells without special surface features other than junctional complexes.

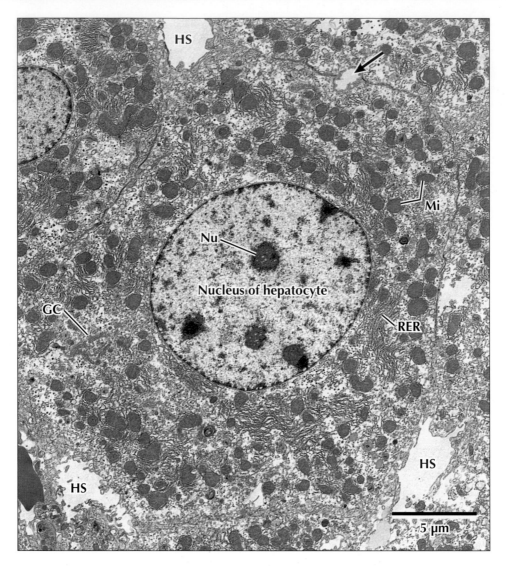

▲ **EM of a hepatocyte and its relationship to surrounding structures.** A polyhedral shape, one euchromatic nucleus with multiple nucleoli (**Nu**), and tightly packed cytoplasm are characteristic features. Mitochondria (**Mi**), a Golgi complex (**GC**), and rough endoplasmic reticulum (**RER**) are indicated. Hepatic sinusoids (**HS**) and a bile canaliculus (**arrow**) border the cell. 4600×.

14.9   ULTRASTRUCTURE AND FUNCTION OF HEPATOCYTES

Hepatocyte **cytoplasm** differs markedly in ultrastructure and content of organelles and inclusions depending on its functional state. Many round to elongated **mitochondria** with flattened or tubular cristae in the cytoplasm provide energy as ATP for various cell functions. Free **ribosomes** and multiple stacks of **rough endoplasmic reticulum** studded with ribosomes throughout the cytoplasm function in protein synthesis for internal use and export. Numerous **Golgi complexes** typically cluster close to a bile canaliculus or adjacent to the nucleus. The prominent **smooth endoplasmic reticulum** (SER)—a branching network of tubules and cisternae—often contains globules of low-density lipoprotein, which are eventually released into the bloodstream. SER also contains enzymes for *detoxifying drugs, converting glycogen to glucose,* and *cholesterol synthesis.* Variable amounts of glycogen are stored in cytoplasm, often close to the SER. **Lipid droplets** of variable size and **lysosomes** filled with digestive enzymes are abundant, and **peroxisomes** are close to the Golgi complex.

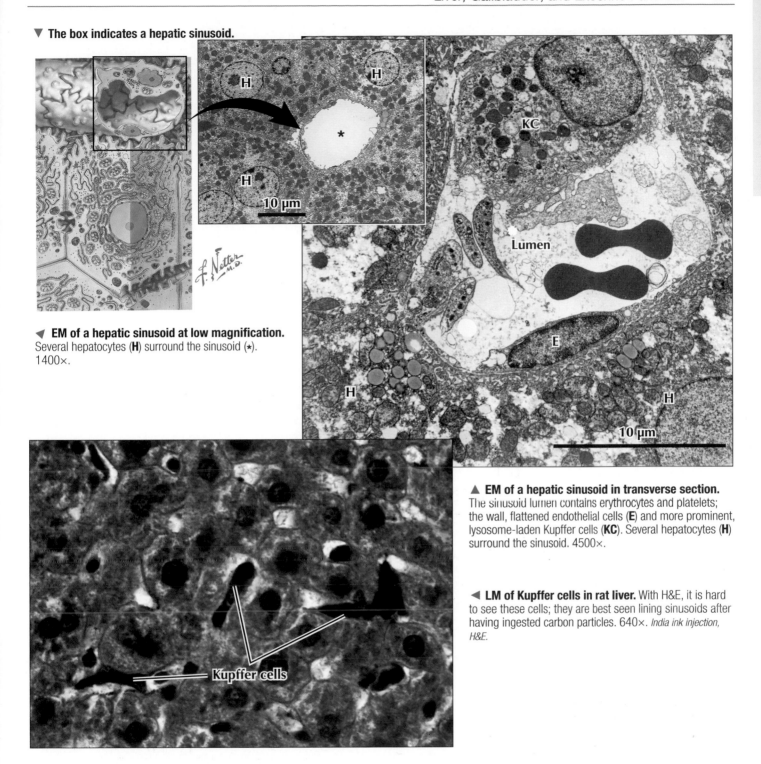

▼ The box indicates a hepatic sinusoid.

◀ **EM of a hepatic sinusoid at low magnification.**
Several hepatocytes (**H**) surround the sinusoid (∗).
1400×.

▲ **EM of a hepatic sinusoid in transverse section.**
The sinusoid lumen contains erythrocytes and platelets;
the wall, flattened endothelial cells (**E**) and more prominent,
lysosome-laden Kupffer cells (**KC**). Several hepatocytes (**H**)
surround the sinusoid. 4500×.

◀ **LM of Kupffer cells in rat liver.** With H&E, it is hard
to see these cells; they are best seen lining sinusoids after
having ingested carbon particles. 640×. *India ink injection,
H&E.*

14.10 ULTRASTRUCTURE OF HEPATIC SINUSOIDS

With a diameter of 9-15 μm, hepatic sinusoids are larger and less regular in shape than capillaries. Their extremely attenuated walls consist of **flattened endothelial** cells interspersed with plumper, irregularly shaped **Kupffer cells.** Intercellular spaces up to 2 μm wide are between the lining cells. Endothelial cells have **fenestrae** that lack diaphragms, are 100 nm wide, and enhance permeability. These cells, with no continuous basement membrane on their outer aspect, occur singly or in clusters and represent 6%-8% of the surface area of the sinusoidal endothelium. Endothelial cells have dark ovoid nuclei projecting into a lumen; Kupffer cells have pale-staining rounded nuclei. By electron microscopy, Kupffer cells are rich in **lysosomes,** with many filopodia and endocytotic vesicles. As macrophages, these phagocytic cells, derived from blood monocytes, remove bacteria, viruses, tumor cells, and parasites. Their cytoplasm contains abundant lysosomes, erythrocyte fragments, and phagocytosed particulate matter. Sinusoids are highly permeable for rapid exchange. Gaps between lining cells and endothelial fenestrae allow plasma proteins to pass but exclude blood cells or platelets. Narrow **spaces of Dissé** separate sinusoids from surrounding hepatocytes.

▼ **The box indicates a space of Dissé.**

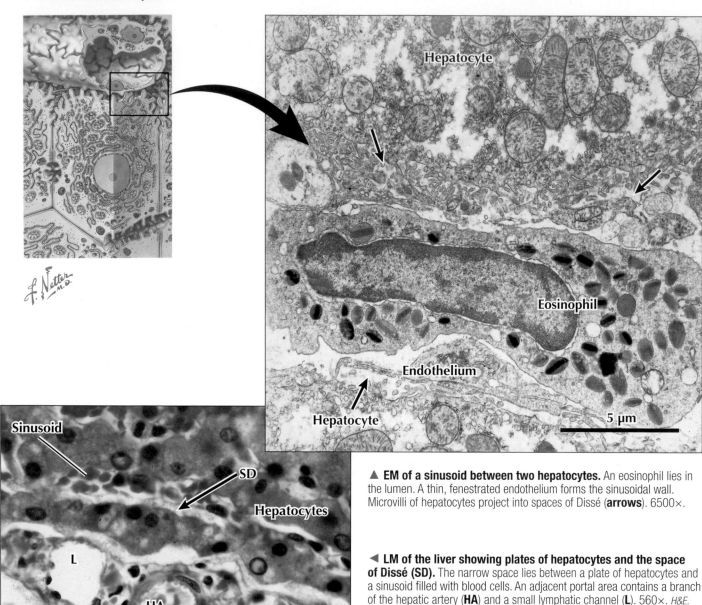

Hepatocyte

Eosinophil

Endothelium

Hepatocyte

5 µm

Sinusoid

SD

Hepatocytes

L

HA

▲ **EM of a sinusoid between two hepatocytes.** An eosinophil lies in the lumen. A thin, fenestrated endothelium forms the sinusoidal wall. Microvilli of hepatocytes project into spaces of Dissé (**arrows**). 6500×.

◄ **LM of the liver showing plates of hepatocytes and the space of Dissé (SD).** The narrow space lies between a plate of hepatocytes and a sinusoid filled with blood cells. An adjacent portal area contains a branch of the hepatic artery (**HA**) and a small lymphatic channel (**L**). 560×. *H&E.*

14.11   ULTRASTRUCTURE OF THE SPACE OF DISSÉ

Plasma in the sinusoidal lumen communicates with the space of Dissé via **fenestrations** in endothelial cells and the gaps between them. Hepatocytes thereby come in direct contact with plasma. Long, abundant **hepatocyte microvilli** project into the space of Dissé, which increases surface area and enhances the rate of exchange of metabolites between hepatocytes and bloodstream. Hepatocyte cytoplasm has many vesicles and vacuoles, with a large surface area for secretion and absorption. Fat-containing *cells of Ito* (also called stellate cells), which store exogenous vitamin A, are also found in spaces of Dissé. These cells usually secrete growth factors, cytokines, and extracellular matrix proteins. In some pathologic conditions, such as alcoholic liver disease, they may also aid development of fibrosis. Excess fluid and solutes in these spaces contribute to hepatic lymph formation.

CLINICAL POINT

Cirrhosis of the liver is the end stage of chronic liver disease caused usually by *alcohol abuse, biliary obstruction,* or *viral hepatitis.* Excessive deposition of connective tissue stroma produces abnormal fibrous septa made of collagen fiber bundles, which link portal tracts to each other and to hepatic veins. Resulting, persistent **liver cell necrosis** leads to nodules of regenerating hepatocytes encircled by fibrosis. This morphologic pattern advances to marked disruption in microscopic architecture of the entire liver. Disease progression causes distortion of the vascular supply, portal hypertension, reduced hepatocyte function, and liver failure.

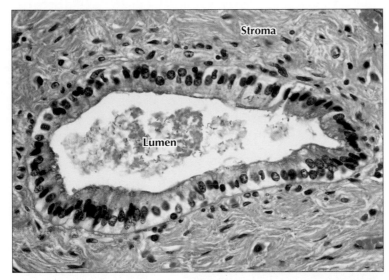

◄ **LM of an intrahepatic bile duct in transverse section.** The wall of this medium-sized duct consists of simple columnar epithelium. Flocculent material in the lumen is bile. Surrounding stroma is dense fibrous connective tissue. 240×. *H&E.*

► **Electron micrograph (EM) of a bile ductule in a portal tract in transverse section.** Several cuboidal cells line the central lumen. Short microvilli and a cilium (**arrow**) project into the lumen. The duct cells rest on a thin basement membrane (**BM**). 2600×.

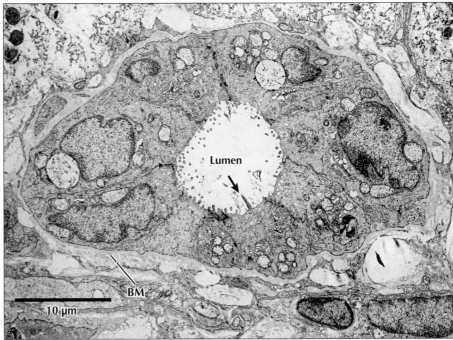

14.12 HISTOLOGY AND ULTRASTRUCTURE OF THE HEPATIC BILIARY DUCT SYSTEM

The smallest intrahepatic bile ducts have one layer of small **cuboidal cells,** each about 10 µm in diameter, surrounding a small lumen. Junctional complexes, composed of **tight junctions** and **desmosomes,** are close to the luminal surface and join cells together. Cells have the usual organelles and a round, centrally placed nucleus. Many **tonofilaments** occupy the cytoplasm, some attached to desmosomes and others found at the luminal terminal web. They may be contractile and aid peristalsis in the ductule. The luminal surface has short, fairly regular **microvilli** with occasional cilia that project into the lumen. The basal surface of the epithelium rests on a basement membrane, which is 20-30 nm thick. Ductal cells become more columnar as ducts get larger, and their nuclei become more basal. In larger ducts, adnexal mucous glands are associated with luminal epithelium. Connective tissue composed of **dense collagen fiber bundles** surrounds the ducts. Ducts are always found in portal tracts and travel with branches of the portal vein and hepatic artery.

CLINICAL POINT

Intrahepatic cholestasis is a pathologic state of reduced bile formation or flow. It leads to **jaundice,** a yellowing of the skin and sclera of the eyes, because of excess circulating *bilirubin*. Plug-like deposits of this bile pigment in dilated canaliculi, hepatocytes, and intrahepatic bile ducts are a histologic hallmark. By electron microscopy, microvilli of canaliculi are fewer or look blunted. Cholestasis may be due to an ion pump or permeability defect in the canalicular membrane or in contractile properties of canaliculi and bile ducts. Elevated levels of *serum alkaline phosphatase,* an enzyme in canaliculi and ductal epithelium, are diagnostic.

▼ **The box indicates a bile canaliculus.**

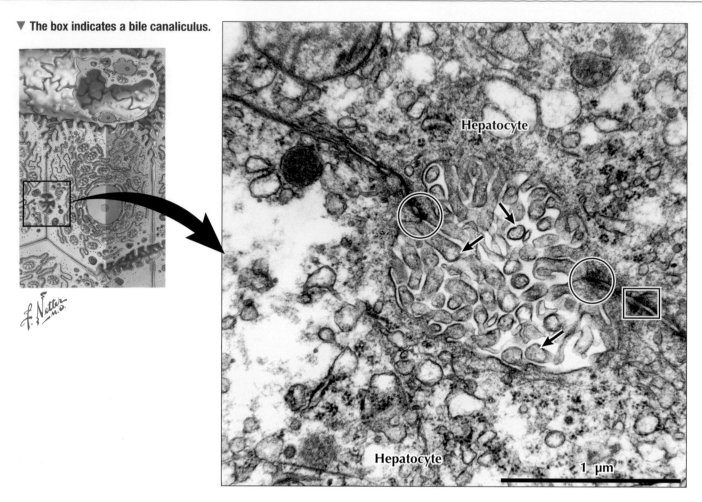

▲ **EM of a bile canaliculus in transverse section.** The lumen shows short stubby microvilli (**arrows**) of two hepatocytes. Desmosomes (**rectangle**) and tight junctions (**circles**) link cell membranes, which seals the canaliculus and prevents bile leakage to surrounding tissues. 47,000×.

14.13 ULTRASTRUCTURE AND FUNCTION OF BILE CANALICULI

The bile canaliculus is the first and smallest **biliary passage,** about 1 μm in diameter. It is an **intercellular space,** or channel, formed by opposing membranes of two adjoining hepatocytes. These cells secrete bile into canalicular lumina. Canaliculi, best demonstrated via special stains for light microscopy, enzyme histochemistry to detect ATPase activity, or electron microscopy, form a chicken wire-like network when viewed in a section that extends throughout the entire liver. About 0.5 mL of bile is produced by hepatocytes each minute. Bile contains **detoxified waste** for elimination via the alimentary canal. No communication usually exists between bile in the canaliculi and the bloodstream. The short, irregular **microvilli** of adjacent hepatocytes protrude into the canalicular lumen. Hepatocyte lateral borders are reinforced with **desmosomes,** and **tight junctions** sequester contents of canalicular lumina and prevent bile leakage.

CLINICAL POINT

The most common genetic liver disease in infancy and childhood is the **autosomal recessive α1-antitrypsin deficiency.** It is marked by abnormally low levels of this serum protease inhibitor, a glycoprotein usually produced by hepatocytes. A defect in migration of secretory protein from the rough endoplasmic reticulum (RER) to the Golgi complex results in accumulation of mutant protein in dilated RER cisternae. A distinctive feature—faintly eosinophilic, periodic acid Schiff-positive cytoplasmic inclusions, 1-10 μm in diameter—leads to severe damage to hepatocytes. This disorder causes *hepatitis* in newborns and often causes *cirrhosis,* for which liver transplantation may be indicated.

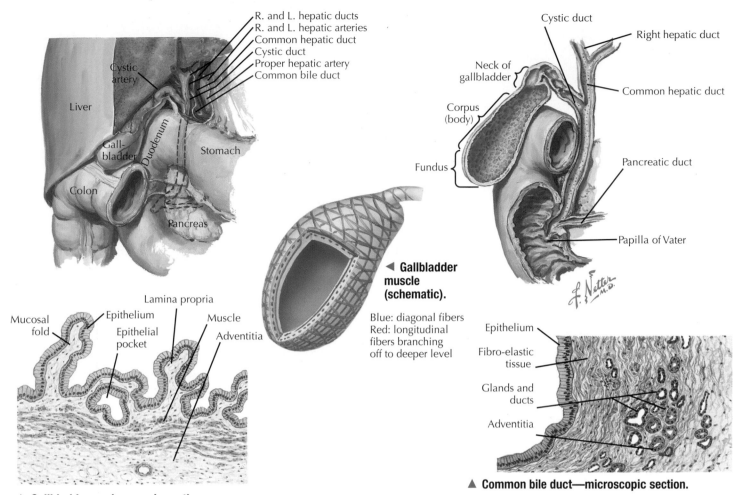

▼ **Anatomy and histology of the gallbladder and bile ducts.**

R. and L. hepatic ducts
R. and L. hepatic arteries
Common hepatic duct
Cystic duct
Proper hepatic artery
Common bile duct

Cystic artery

Liver

Gall-bladder

Duodenum

Stomach

Colon

Pancreas

Cystic duct

Right hepatic duct

Neck of gallbladder

Common hepatic duct

Corpus (body)

Fundus

Pancreatic duct

Papilla of Vater

◄ **Gallbladder muscle (schematic).**

Blue: diagonal fibers
Red: longitudinal fibers branching off to deeper level

Mucosal fold

Epithelium

Lamina propria

Muscle

Epithelial pocket

Adventitia

▲ **Gallbladder—microscopic section.**

Epithelium

Fibro-elastic tissue

Glands and ducts

Adventitia

▲ **Common bile duct—microscopic section.**

14.14 OVERVIEW OF THE GALLBLADDER

The gallbladder is a hollow, **pear-shaped organ** lying in a shallow fossa on the inferior surface of the liver. It is 3-5 cm in diameter and about 10 cm long. It has a blind end, known as the **fundus;** a main part, or **body;** and a **neck,** which joins the **cystic duct.** It distends easily and has a capacity of about 50 mL. The gallbladder stores **bile** and concentrates it by absorbing water and electrolytes. Connected to both liver and duodenum by the **biliary duct system,** the organ drains through the cystic duct, which joins the **common hepatic duct** to form the **common bile duct.** The gallbladder wall consists of three layers: a *mucosa,* a *muscularis propria,* and an adventitia, or *serosa.*

CLINICAL POINT

The presence of stones in the gallbladder or extrahepatic biliary ducts is known as **cholelithiasis.** Gallstones are made of various components of bile. They are often solid deposits of cholesterol or calcium salts. Most patients have no symptoms, but gallstones lodged in bile ducts between the liver and intestine can block bile flow and cause *jaundice* (or icterus) and severe abdominal pain known as *biliary colic.* Gallstones may also cause gallbladder inflammation or infection known as **cholecystitis,** marked by mucosal inflammation with abnormal thickening of the muscularis layer. The most common gallstone treatment method is laparoscopic surgery.

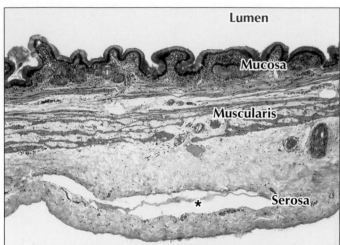

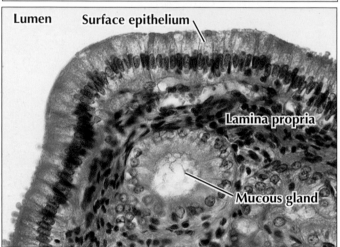

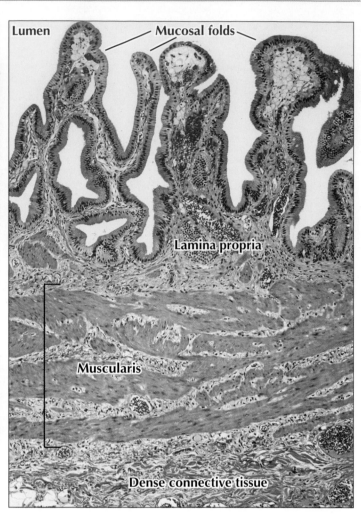

▲ **LM of the entire thin wall of the gallbladder in transverse section (above).** The wall has three layers. In an empty or contracted gallbladder, the mucosa shows many folds, which flatten out when the organ fills with bile. This slightly distended gallbladder has just a few small folds. Bundles of smooth muscle fibers form the middle muscularis. The serosa contains a rich network of lymphatic channels (⋆) and is covered externally by simple squamous mesothelium of the peritoneum. 57×. *H&E.*

▲ **LM of part of a nondistended gallbladder.** The mucosa shows many folds, which are lined by simple columnar epithelium. The epithelium rests on loose, richly vascularized connective tissue—the lamina propria. Mucosal folds extend to the upper part of the muscularis and bear a resemblance to villi, but unlike villi, they disappear in a distended organ. Smooth muscle cells in the muscularis are oriented in different directions: longitudinally, circularly, and obliquely. An outermost layer of dense irregular connective tissue constitutes the serosa (or adventitia). 85×. *H&E.*

▲ **LM of the gallbladder mucosa in the neck region (below).** Simple columnar epithelium lines the lumen. The highly cellular lamina propria contains parts of a mucous gland. Mucous glands occur in the neck area but are usually absent in other parts of the organ. 380×. *H&E.*

14.15 HISTOLOGY OF THE GALLBLADDER WALL

The **mucosa,** the thinnest layer, folds into ridges, the number depending on the degree of distention caused by bile in the lumen; the organ lacks a submucosa. **Simple columnar epithelial cells** with many **microvilli** on their **apical surface** line the organ. Underlying **lamina propria** is a highly cellular connective tissue with scattered **smooth muscle cells** from the **muscularis.** Interlacing bundles of smooth muscle with intervening connective tissue and blood vessels make up the muscularis. Smooth muscle bundles are circular, longitudinal, and oriented obliquely. The outer layer is an unusually thick fibrous connective tissue contain-

ing nerves, blood vessels, and a rich lymphatic plexus. This connective tissue is covered externally by **peritoneal mesothelium,** so it is more correctly called **a serosa.** The neck area has scattered mucous glands in the lamina propria whose number may increase in response to chronic infection. Sinuses of *Rokitansky-Aschoff*—epithelial invaginations that may extend deep into the muscle layer—are lined by the same epithelium as that on the surface and are thought to be initial pathologic changes in the wall. Aberrant vestigial bile *ducts of Luschka* may occur in the serosa next to the liver and may be a route of infection from liver to gallbladder. **Extrahepatic bile ducts** contain all layers of the gallbladder wall and are lined by an epithelium similar to that of the gallbladder.

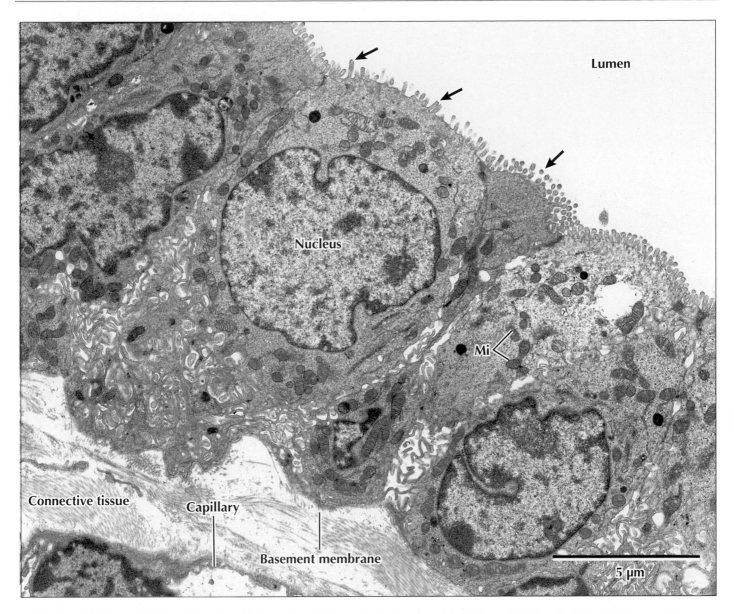

▲ **EM of gallbladder epithelium.** Short microvilli (**arrows**) project from apical cell surfaces into the lumen. Mitochondria (**Mi**) and other organelles are randomly dispersed in cytoplasm. Lateral cell borders are markedly interdigitated. A thin basement membrane separates epithelium from underlying connective tissue, which contains a capillary. Epithelial cells usually appear columnar, but anatomic and functional variations can cause them to look cuboidal, as here. 7800×.

14.16   ULTRASTRUCTURE AND FUNCTION OF THE GALLBLADDER MUCOSA

Lining the gallbladder mucosa is a layer of **simple columnar cells,** each with one oval to spherical nucleus usually, at the base or closer to the middle of the cell. Apical cytoplasm is lightly eosinophilic; an **apical brush border** contains many **short microvilli.** The epithelium rests on a delicate basement membrane that separates it from underlying **lamina propria.** By electron microscopy, junctional complexes, including **tight junctions,** link lateral cell membranes close to the lumen. Basal infoldings of plasma membrane and **interdigitations** of adjacent cell membranes reflect the role of these cells in ion transport. Water from the lumen is absorbed into lateral intercellular spaces between epithelial cells and then to the underlying, richly vascularized lamina propria. The gallbladder stores bile, which is released by reflex contraction of smooth muscle in its wall in response to the hormone *cholecystokinin.* Concomitantly, sphincters associated with the common bile duct and the ampulla relax to permit bile to enter the duodenum.

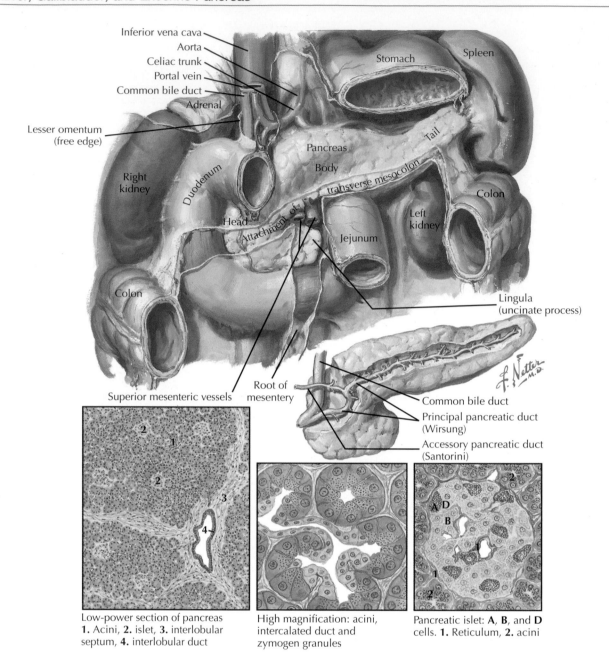

Low-power section of pancreas
1. Acini, **2.** islet, **3.** interlobular septum, **4.** interlobular duct

High magnification: acini, intercalated duct and zymogen granules

Pancreatic islet: **A**, **B**, and **D** cells. **1.** Reticulum, **2.** acini

14.17 OVERVIEW OF THE PANCREAS

The pinkish-yellow pancreas is an **accessory digestive gland,** 18-20 cm long and weighing about 100 g. Situated on the posterior wall of the abdominal cavity, the gland has a *retroperitoneal position* at the level of the first and second lumbar vertebrae. Its head lies in the concavity of the duodenum; its neck, body, and tail extend transversely to the spleen. Its serosa-covered anterior surface is separated by the *omental bursa* from the posterior stomach wall. Like other parenchymal glands, the pancreas is covered by a thin, indistinct **connective tissue capsule,** which sends inward projections, or **septa,** of loose connective tissue that partially subdivide the gland into indistinct **lobules.** The pancreas has both *exocrine* and *endocrine* parts. The exocrine part comprises 99% of the gland by weight and is made of secretory acini and their associated ducts. **Acinar cells** produce pancreatic juice, about 1.5 L/day, which contains digestive enzymes that empty through the excretory duct system into the duodenum. The endocrine part of the pancreas consists of *islets of Langerhans,* which produce several hormones that affect carbohydrate metabolism.

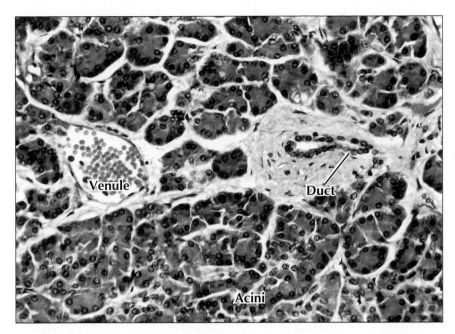

◄ **LM of the exocrine pancreas at low magnification.** Many round to oval acini make up the parenchyma of the gland. A small interlobular duct and a venule are in the stroma. The duct, lined by simple cuboidal epithelium, is invested by dense fibrous connective tissue. 300×. *H&E.*

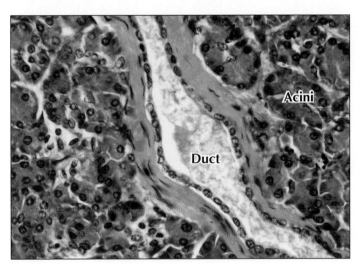

▲ **LM of the exocrine pancreas at high magnification.** A large interlobular duct is cut longitudinally and crosses the field of view. Dense fibrous connective tissue envelops its simple cuboidal epithelial lining. Surrounding areas of parenchyma contain tightly packed acini. 400×. *H&E.*

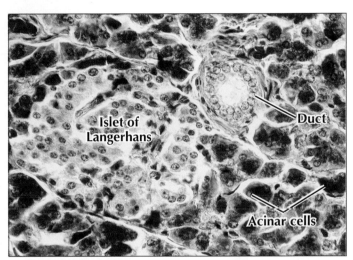

▲ **LM of the pancreas showing an intralobular duct with an islet of Langerhans.** The duct is lined by simple cuboidal epithelium surrounded by a small amount of connective tissue. Pale cells in the richly vascularized islet constitute the endocrine part of the gland. Clusters of acinar cells of the exocrine gland contain prominent eosinophilic zymogen granules. 295×. *Masson trichrome.*

14.18 HISTOLOGY OF THE EXOCRINE PANCREAS: DUCTS

The first part of the duct system consists of small, pale **centroacinar cells** that extend into the center of each **acinus**. They lead into small **intralobular intercalated ducts** that are lined by one layer of low cuboidal epithelial cells. **Intercalated ducts** lead into larger interlobular ducts outside the lobules and lined by simple cuboidal to low columnar epithelium. **Interlobular ducts** branch extensively, get larger, and empty into two main excretory ducts. The large **main pancreatic duct** traverses the entire gland, tail to head.

It opens into the duodenum, usually together with the bile duct. The smaller accessory pancreatic duct receives branches from the pancreatic head; it communicates with the main duct and opens about 2 cm above it. Both ducts are lined by simple columnar epithelium, surrounded by a layer of connective tissue. Small mucous glands open into the larger ducts and lubricate and protect the lining epithelium. The endocrine part of the pancreas—*islets of Langerhans*—secretes primarily insulin and glucagon.

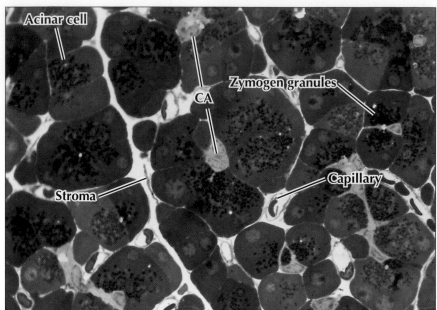

◀ **LM of the exocrine pancreas.** Several pancreatic acini in this part of the gland contain both acinar and centroacinar (**CA**) cells. The dark acinar cells surround a small central lumen and have apical zymogen granules. Lighter centroacinar cells project into the lumen of each acinus. 700×. *Toluidine blue, plastic section.*

▶ **LM showing pancreatic acini at high magnification.** Flask-shaped acini contain clusters of pyramidal acinar cells. Their apical cytoplasm appears granular and intensely eosinophilic; their bases stain darker. Centroacinar cells (**CA**) have rounded euchromatic nuclei and form the initial intra-acinar part of the duct system. 825×. *H&E.*

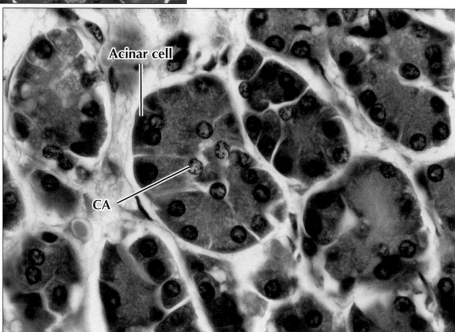

14.19 HISTOLOGY OF THE EXOCRINE PANCREAS: ACINI

The exocrine pancreas is a **compound tubuloacinar gland.** Each oval- to flask-shaped **acinus** consists of one layer of cuboidal to pyramidal cells around a central lumen. Each single, spheroid nucleus sits toward the basal part of the cell in the area with the most intense cytoplasmic basophilia. By electron microscopy, this area contains an extensive network of **rough endoplasmic reticulum,** consistent with intense protein synthesis in acinar cells. Apical parts of cells are filled with prominent **secretory** (zymogen) **granules** that stain intensely with eosin or acid dyes. Acinar cells synthesize and secrete a host of digestive enzymes or their inactive precursors, including *trypsin, chymotrypsin, amylase, lipase, and carboxypeptidase.* A unique feature of acini is the presence of initial parts of the excretory duct system, composed of **centroacinar** cells,

which partially protrude into the acinar lumen. These pale cells secrete a *bicarbonate-rich fluid*, as do intercalated duct cells. Centroacinar cells lead into intercalated ducts lined by simple cuboidal epithelium.

CLINICAL POINT

Acute pancreatitis is an inflammatory disorder of the exocrine pancreas often associated with alcoholism or excessive alcohol intake. Its clinical manifestations range from mild to life-threatening. Pancreatic acinar cells are normally protected from harmful effects of digestive enzymes that they secrete. However, acinar cell injury or pancreatic duct obstruction may lead to inappropriate extracellular leakage of activated digestive enzymes and *autodigestion* of pancreatic acini. Edema and progressive fibrosis of the stroma may ensue and cause hemorrhage and ultimately *pancreatic insufficiency*. Elevated serum amylase and lipase levels are diagnostic for this disorder.

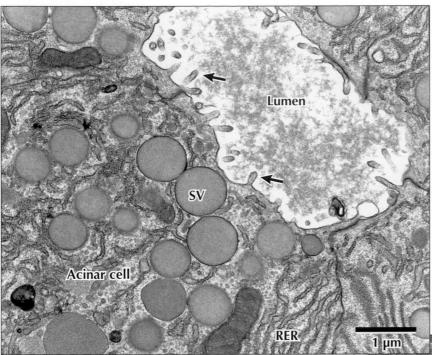

◄ **EM of the lumen of a pancreatic acinus.** Parts of several acinar cells border the lumen. Their apical cytoplasm contains many large, rounded secretory vesicles (**SV**). Abundant in the cytoplasm are also multiple cisternae of RER (**RER**). Luminal surfaces of the cells bear a few short microvilli (**arrows**). 15,000×.

► **EM of the lumen of a pancreatic acinus.** Several profiles of centroacinar cells show lateral interdigitations (**arrows**). These cells have a Golgi complex and scattered mitochondria (**Mi**) but relatively few other organelles. The apical part of an acinar cell (at bottom) with its prominent secretory vesicles (**SV**) also lines the lumen. Centroacinar cells lack these vesicles. 15,000×.

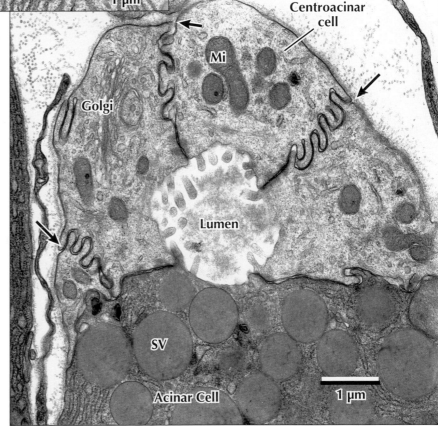

14.20 ULTRASTRUCTURE OF THE EXOCRINE PANCREAS

By electron microscopy, **acinar** and **centroacinar** cells of the exocrine pancreas are readily distinguished by ultrastructural features that reflect function. Acinar cells are **polarized secretory cells** with all the organelles involved in protein synthesis for export. An abundant rough endoplasmic reticulum (RER) and an extensive supranuclear Golgi complex are associated with large membrane-bound and moderately electron-dense **secretory vesicles.** Diges-tive enzymes or their inactive precursors are found in the vesicles, which collect at the cell apex. Stimulated vesicles migrate apically, fuse with plasma membrane, and release their contents via *exocytosis* into the lumen. **Centroacinar cells,** in contrast, are small flattened cells incompletely bordering the lumen of a pancreatic acinus. They have scattered mitochondria, a small Golgi complex, occasional RER, and extensive lateral interdigitations of cell borders.

Embryonic origin and development of the pancreas

Liver

Foregut

Dorsal pancreas

Hepatic diverticulum
- Hepatic duct
- Common bile duct
- Gallbladder
- Hepatico-pancreatic duct
- Ventral pancreas

Yolk sac (cutaway)

Hindgut

1. Bud formation

Stomach

Common hepatic duct

Portal vein

Gallbladder

Common bile duct

Ventral pancreas

Dorsal pancreas

Superior mesenteric vein

2. Beginning rotation of common duct and of ventral pancreas

Dorsal pancreas

Ventral pancreas

3. Rotation completed but fusion has not yet taken place

Accessory pancreatic duct (Santorini's)

Pancreatic duct (Wirsung's)

4. Fusion of ventral and dorsal pancreas and union of ducts

Formation of acini and islets from ducts. A–acini; I–islets in various stages of development

Relationship of intercalated duct and centroacinar cells to acini

14.21   DEVELOPMENT OF THE PANCREAS

In the 6-week embryo, the pancreas develops from two endodermal diverticula—**dorsal** and **ventral pancreatic buds**—that emanate from the part of the **foregut** destined to be the duodenum. The dorsal bud is the larger of the two; the ventral bud is close to the gallbladder part of the hepatic diverticulum. With rotation of the gut tube, the buds come to lie close to each other and fuse. Ducts develop in both buds and anastomose. The body and tail areas of the fused buds are drained by the duct of the ventral bud, which becomes the main pancreatic *duct of Wirsung*. The original duct of the dorsal pancreas becomes the *accessory duct of Santorini*. At this stage, the pancreas consists of a duct system of tubules lined by endodermally derived epithelium. Their blind ends are initially solid and become the **secretory acini** by forming a central cavity. The more proximal tubule areas become the excretory duct system that drains acini and delivers their secretions to duct openings in the duodenal wall. Along certain parts of the duct system, some cells lose their connections and form isolated clusters of endocrine cells that become *islets of Langerhans* scattered in the gland. Surrounding mesenchyme eventually gives rise to the gland's **capsule** and **stroma**.

15

RESPIRATORY SYSTEM

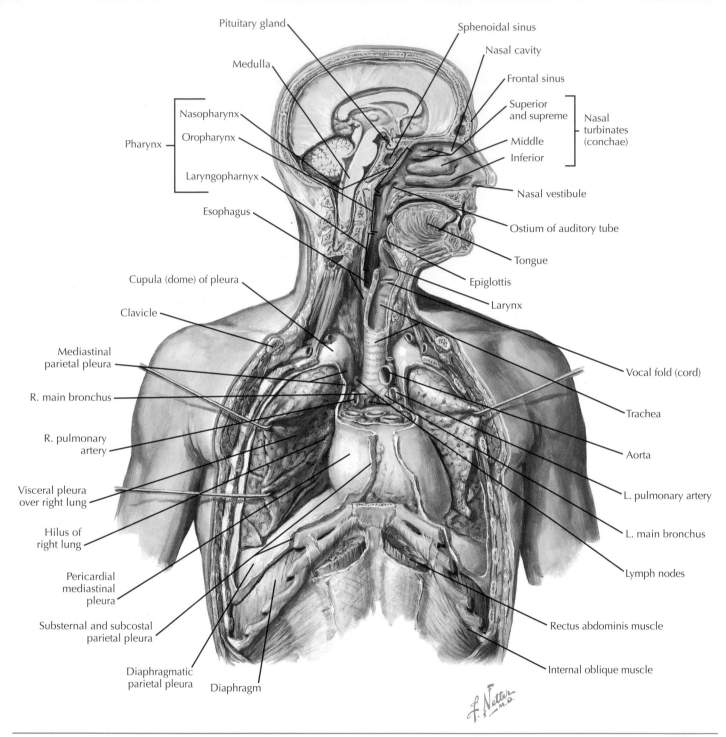

Pituitary gland

Medulla

Pharynx
- Nasopharynx
- Oropharynx
- Laryngopharynx

Esophagus

Cupula (dome) of pleura

Clavicle

Mediastinal parietal pleura

R. main bronchus

R. pulmonary artery

Visceral pleura over right lung

Hilus of right lung

Pericardial mediastinal pleura

Substernal and subcostal parietal pleura

Diaphragmatic parietal pleura

Diaphragm

Sphenoidal sinus

Nasal cavity

Frontal sinus

Superior and supreme

Middle

Inferior

Nasal turbinates (conchae)

Nasal vestibule

Ostium of auditory tube

Tongue

Epiglottis

Larynx

Vocal fold (cord)

Trachea

Aorta

L. pulmonary artery

L. main bronchus

Lymph nodes

Rectus abdominis muscle

Internal oblique muscle

15.1   OVERVIEW

The respiratory system is divided functionally into a *conducting* portion that conveys air from outside the body to the lungs and a *respiratory* portion where exchange of gases between the air and blood occurs. The conducting airways moisten, warm, and cleanse the air, whereas the respiratory portion provides O_2 obtained from the air and removes excess CO_2 from the bloodstream. The conducting passageways (the cavities and tubes) consist anatomically of the **nose** and **paranasal sinuses; pharynx,** which is the passageway for both air and food; **larynx,** which produces the voice; **trachea,** which divides into **bronchi** and **bronchioles** of decreasing size; and terminal bronchioles. The respiratory portion comprises respiratory bronchioles, which branch into alveolar ducts and pulmonary alveoli, where exchange of gases with adjacent

capillaries takes place. Pseudostratified ciliated columnar epithelium plus numerous mucus-secreting goblet cells line the mucous membrane of the upper airways of the conducting portion. This ciliated epithelium, commonly known as respiratory epithelium, is well suited for airway protection and cleansing and removal of particulate matter. The cilia beat in a rhythmic fashion toward the oral cavity and move debris and pathogen-laden *mucus* so it can be expectorated or swallowed. Subepithelial mucous and serous glands liberate their secretions onto the mucosal surface to also aid in entrapment of particulate matter, lubrication, and moistening. Accessory structures needed for proper functioning of the respiratory system include the pleurae, diaphragm, thoracic wall, and muscles that raise and lower ribs during *inspiration* and *expiration*.

▼ Frontal section of the nasal cavity and sinuses.

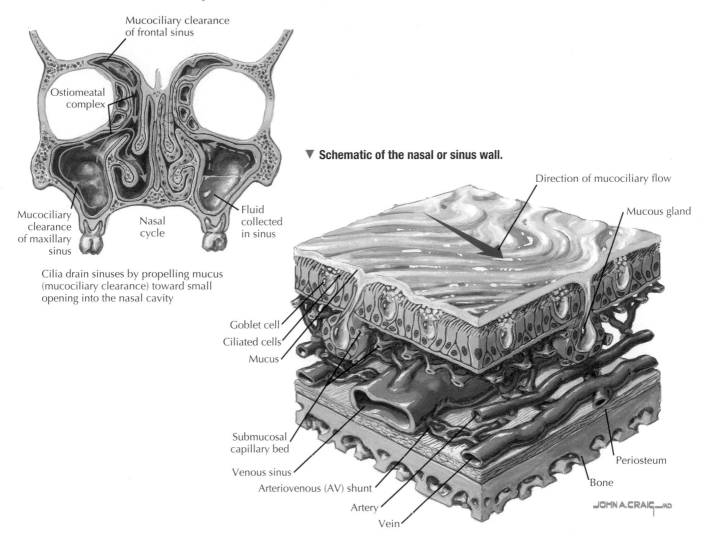

Mucociliary clearance of frontal sinus

Ostiomeatal complex

Mucociliary clearance of maxillary sinus

Nasal cycle

Fluid collected in sinus

Cilia drain sinuses by propelling mucus (mucociliary clearance) toward small opening into the nasal cavity

▼ Schematic of the nasal or sinus wall.

Direction of mucociliary flow

Mucous gland

Goblet cell

Ciliated cells

Mucus

Submucosal capillary bed

Venous sinus

Arteriovenous (AV) shunt

Artery

Vein

Periosteum

Bone

JOHN A. CRAIG—AD

15.2 STRUCTURE OF THE NASAL CAVITIES AND PARANASAL SINUSES

The nasal cavities—paired passages separated by a nasal septum—are the first structures of the conducting part of the respiratory system. Each cavity consists of an anterior vestibule and nasal cavity proper. The vestibule, which is lined by epidermis containing many sebaceous glands, sweat glands, and hair follicles, leads into the nasal cavity proper, which is lined by mucosa consisting of pseudostratified ciliated columnar epithelium interspersed with goblet cells and resting on a prominent basement membrane. The underlying lamina propria, a thick, vascular connective tissue rich in collagen and elastic fibers, attaches firmly to the **periosteum** and **perichondrium** of the bony and cartilaginous walls of the nasal cavity, which provide rigidity during inspiration. **Seromucous glands** are also found in the lamina propria and drain onto the epithelial surface via small ducts. **Cilia** on the epithelial surface beat to move surface secretions toward the nasopharynx. In the lamina propria are large **venous plexuses** whose major role is to warm inspired air via heat exchange. The plexuses may become engorged during an allergic reaction or nasal infection, which leads to mucous membrane swelling and restricted air passage.

Paranasal sinuses—**frontal, ethmoidal, sphenoidal,** and **maxillary**—are air-filled cavities that communicate with nasal cavities. Their mucosa, consisting of respiratory epithelium with numerous goblet cells, is continuous with that of the nasal cavities, a feature that favors the spread of infection. The lamina propria is very thin and blends with the periosteum of surrounding bony tissue. A few small seromucous glands are found in the mucosa of paranasal sinuses.

CLINICAL POINT

Sinusitis is a common clinical condition referring to *inflammation* of the mucous membrane of the sinuses. Often associated with the common cold or allergies, it may be caused by bacterial, viral, or fungal infection. Acute and chronic forms affect 30-40 million people in North America annually. The mucosal lining of the nasal and paranasal sinuses produces about 750 mL of mucus daily. Inflamed sinuses become blocked with mucus and can become infected. In cases of chronic sinusitis, the drainage pathways of the sinuses are obstructed and do not function properly. The mucous glands produce thick secretions that stay in the cavities, which increases bacterial overgrowth and thickens the lining.

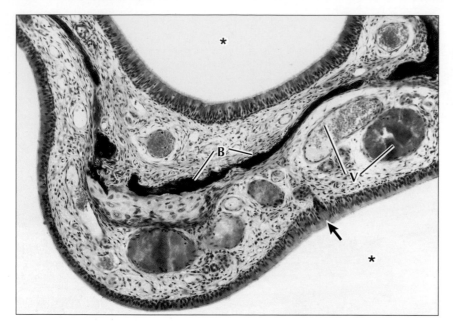

◄ **Low-magnification light micrograph (LM) of a nasal concha.** Respiratory epithelium covers the concha externally and is in direct contact with the nasal cavity lumen (∗). Its central core of loose connective tissue contains several thin-walled venous sinuses (**V**) and bony trabeculae (**B**). A small gland in the lamina propria is drained by a duct that opens onto the surface (**arrow**). 100×. *H&E.*

▶ **LM of respiratory mucosa lining the nasal cavity.** The tall pseudostratified epithelium consists of basal cells (**B**), goblet cells (**G**), and columnar cells bearing apical cilia (**short arrow**). Note the particulate matter (**long arrow**) on the ciliated surface. A thin, imperceptible basement membrane (**BM**) separates the epithelium from underlying lamina propria, which is highly cellular and richly vascularized. This lamina contains a network of capillaries (**C**). 300×. *H&E.*

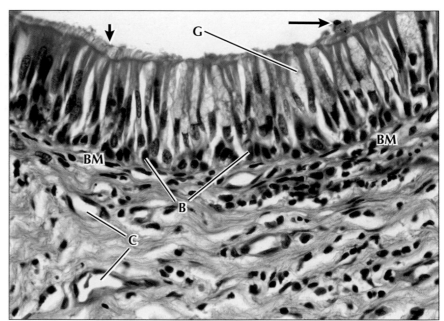

15.3 HISTOLOGY OF THE NASAL CAVITIES AND PARANASAL SINUSES

Each nasal cavity is a narrow passage that communicates posteriorly via a small orifice, the choana, with the nasopharynx. The cavity's surface area is dramatically increased by **nasal conchae** consisting of **bony trabeculae** covered by **mucous membrane**. The **pseudostratified ciliated columnar epithelium** of the mucous membrane has abundant, unevenly distributed mucus-secreting goblet cells. Many branched **seromucous glands** extend into the underlying **lamina propria** and are connected to the surface via small **ducts**. An extensive, tortuous network of **venous sinuses,** arteriovenous anastomoses, and capillaries characterizes the lamina propria. In certain areas of the nasal mucosa, thin-walled venous sinuses that are superficially located resemble erectile tissue and warm inspired air via heat exchange. A surface layer of

mucus produced by goblet cells and seromucous glands entraps foreign particles and is constantly moved by cilia. This process, known as *mucociliary clearance*, sweeps particulate matter toward the nasopharynx, where it is swallowed or expectorated. The lining epithelium in the paranasal sinuses is lower than that of the nasal cavities, with fewer goblet cells than in the nasal cavities. Three types of cells characterize the respiratory epithelium: **basal, ciliated,** and **goblet cells.** Basal cells serve as reserve cells, which continuously replace other epithelial cells that are shed. They are small rounded cells in a monolayer resting on the **basement membrane.** Goblet cells sit on the basement membrane and extend to the surface, where they have a relatively wide apical region that appears pale or washed out because of a varying content of mucus.

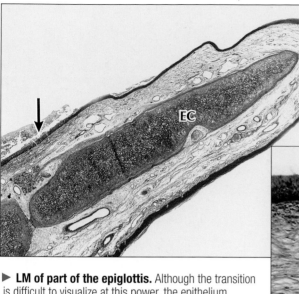

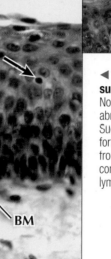

◀ **LM of the tip of the epiglottis at low magnification.** The epiglottis has a core of elastic cartilage (**EC**). Its lingual surface (at bottom) and free margin (upper right) are covered by nonkeratinized stratified squamous epithelium. Halfway along the laryngeal surface (**arrow**), the epithelium undergoes a transition; it eventually becomes respiratory epithelium. 15×. *H&E.*

▶ **LM of part of the epiglottis.** Although the transition is difficult to visualize at this power, the epithelium (at top) undergoes an abrupt change from stratified squamous (**SSE**) to stratified columnar (**SCE**). The lamina propria (**LP**) is highly cellular and contains many blood vessels and nerves. Elastic cartilage (**EC**) covered by perichondrium (**PC**) is below. 70×. *H&E.*

◀ **Details of the epithelial transition at the laryngeal surface of the epiglottis at high magnification.** Nonkeratinized stratified squamous epithelium (to the right) abruptly changes to stratified columnar epithelium (to the left). Such areas of epithelial transition may be sites of tumor formation. A thin basement membrane (**BM**) separates the epithelium from underlying lamina propria, which consists of loose connective tissue (**CT**). **Arrows** point to several intraepithelial lymphocytes. 500×. *H&E.*

15.4   HISTOLOGY OF THE EPIGLOTTIS

The epiglottis is an unpaired leaf-shaped structure below the root of the tongue that covers the entrance to the **larynx.** It has a core of **elastic cartilage,** which is highly flexible and attaches to the hyoid bone. Its **lingual surface** is covered by a protective mucosa with a **nonkeratinized stratified squamous epithelium** that is directly continuous with the epithelium covering the dorsal surface of the tongue. This epithelium continues onto the laryngeal undersurface of the epiglottis. Deep along this surface, the epithelium becomes a transitional zone of **stratified columnar epithelium** and then **pseudostratified ciliated columnar epithelium** with goblet cells, commonly known as **respiratory epithelium.** Scattered **seromucous glands** are found between the plates

of elastic cartilage or close to the mucosa lining the undersurface. **Lamina propria** of **loose connective tissue** underneath the epithelium contains numerous blood and lymphatic vessels, nerves, and scattered mononuclear connective tissue cells. The **perichondrium** surrounding the elastic cartilage attaches firmly to the lamina propria. At rest, the epiglottis is usually upright and allows air to pass into the larynx and the rest of the lower respiratory airways. During swallowing, it folds back like a flap to cover the entrance to the larynx, to prevent food and liquid from entering the trachea. A sore throat—*infection* or *inflammation* of the tonsils, pharynx, or larynx—can obstruct the trachea and make breathing more labored, which may be fatal unless promptly treated.

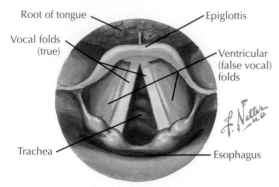

▲ **Laryngoscopic view of the larynx: inspiration.**

▶ **Frontal section of the larynx.** The vocal cord (**VC**) contains elastic fibers; the false vocal fold (**FF**) contains seromucous glands. Nonkeratinized stratified squamous epithelium covers both folds (**arrows**). An intervening laryngeal ventricle (**LV**) and the vocalis muscle (**VM**) are shown. 15×. *H&E.*

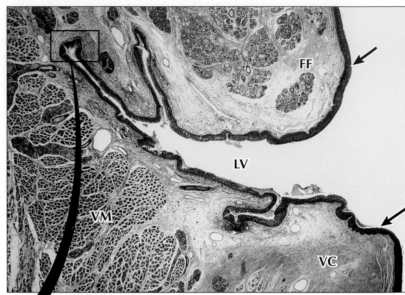

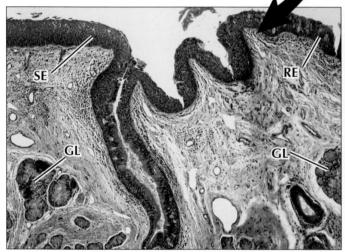

▲ **LM of a ventricular recess in the larynx.** Nonkeratinized stratified squamous epithelium (**SE**) and respiratory epithelium (**RE**) line the mucosal surface. Seromucous glands (**GL**) occupy the lamina propria. 60×. *H&E.*

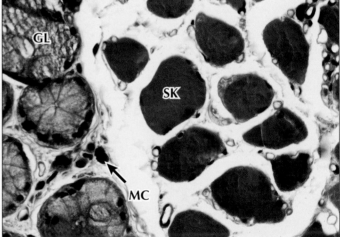

▲ **LM of part of the vocalis muscle of the larynx.** Skeletal muscle fibers (**SK**) in transverse section are close to mucous acini of a gland (**GL**). A mast cell (**MC**) can be seen in the connective tissue. 300×. *H&E.*

15.5 HISTOLOGY OF THE LARYNX AND VOCAL CORDS

The larynx lies between the **pharynx** and **trachea** and is 4-5 cm long. Part of the respiratory conducting system, it plays a critical role in *phonation* and closes during *swallowing*, thereby preventing food from entering the lower airways. Its wall is made of a framework of hyaline and elastic cartilage united by **connective tissue** and associated with **skeletal muscles.** The laryngeal **mucous membrane** has two sets of prominent folds that project inward: **false** (or **ventricular**) **folds** and **true vocal folds** (or **cords**). Between the folds lies a space, the **laryngeal ventricle,** with narrow pouch-like invaginations known as ventricular recesses. The vocal folds contain vocal ligaments of **elastic fibers** to which skeletal muscle fibers of the vocalis part of the **thyroarytenoid muscles** attach. Contraction of the **vocalis muscle** relaxes elastic fibers of the vocal ligaments, thereby changing the shape of the laryngeal ventricles and allowing production of different sounds. The mucous membrane of the larynx consists mainly of **respiratory epithelium,** but over the vocal folds it becomes **nonkeratinized stratified squamous epithelium;** this change is a function of active movement of the folds and wear and tear induced by friction. The epithelium at the junction of the two types of folds is ciliated stratified columnar. Beneath the epithelium is the lamina propria of loose, highly cellular connective tissue, with lymphoid nodules near the laryngeal recesses. Mixed **seromucous glands,** which are invaginations of the epithelium, occur in the ventricular folds but not in the vocal cords. The larynx is unusually replete with **mast cells** that release histamine during allergic responses, which results in *edema* that may become life threatening (can occlude the airway).

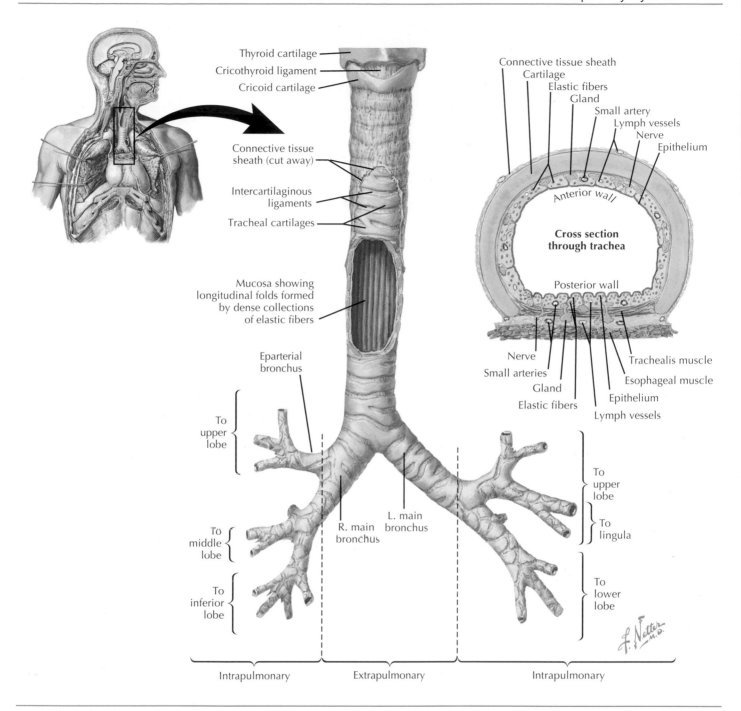

Thyroid cartilage
Cricothyroid ligament
Cricoid cartilage

Connective tissue
sheath (cut away)

Intercartilaginous
ligaments

Tracheal cartilages

Mucosa showing
longitudinal folds formed
by dense collections
of elastic fibers

Eparterial
bronchus

To
upper
lobe

To
middle
lobe

To
inferior
lobe

R. main
bronchus

L. main
bronchus

Connective tissue sheath
Cartilage
Elastic fibers
Gland
Small artery
Lymph vessels
Nerve
Epithelium

Anterior wall

**Cross section
through trachea**

Posterior wall

Nerve
Small arteries
Gland
Elastic fibers

Trachealis muscle
Esophageal muscle
Epithelium
Lymph vessels

To
upper
lobe

To
lingula

To
lower
lobe

Intrapulmonary   Extrapulmonary   Intrapulmonary

15.6 STRUCTURE OF THE TRACHEA AND MAJOR BRONCHI

The **tracheobronchial tree,** a conduit for air traveling to and from alveoli in the lungs, comprises the trachea and the right and left bronchi and their subdivisions. The outer anterolateral aspect of the trachea contains 16-20 crescent-shaped rings of **hyaline cartilage** that provide rigidity, maintain shape, and ensure patency of the tracheal lumen. With aging, the cartilage often shows degenerative changes and may calcify. Posteriorly, the ends of the cartilage rings are spanned by a fibrous membrane containing smooth muscle fibers that constitute the **trachealis muscle.** Contraction of this muscle, which is mainly circular in orientation, causes the tracheal lumen to narrow. Pseudostratified ciliated columnar epithelium lines the lumen and rests on a prominent basement membrane, one of the thickest in the body. *Metaplasia* of the epithelium occurs in response to local friction and chronic coughing. Goblet cells interspersed in the epithelium secrete *mucus,* which lubricates the tracheal surface and traps foreign particulate matter such as dust and bacteria. Small seromucous glands characterize the underlying submucosa. A layer of longitudinally oriented **elastic fibers,** rather than muscularis mucosae, separates **mucosa** from underlying submucosa. Cilia in the tracheal epithelium sweep particles trapped by mucus upward in a synchronized wave-like fashion. Mononuclear cells—lymphocytes, plasma cells, and macrophages—heavily infiltrate the richly vascularized lamina propria. The bronchi resemble the trachea histologically but have a smaller diameter and thinner walls, as well as irregular cartilage plates that are discontinuous and circumferential in orientation. Smooth muscle completely encircles the lumen of each bronchus.

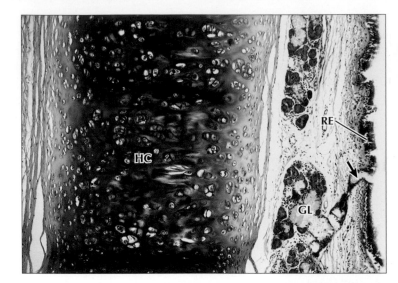

◀ **LM of the wall of the trachea in transverse section.** The tracheal lumen (to the right) is lined by respiratory epithelium (**RE**). A mixed seromucous gland (**GL**) in the submucosa drains to the epithelial surface via a small duct (**arrow**). Hyaline cartilage (**HC**) surrounded by perichondrium is situated on the outer aspect of the airway. 60×. *H&E.*

▶ **LM of a tracheal seromucous gland at higher magnification.** A mix of mucous acini (**MA**), serous acini, and serous cells, many of which are organized as demilunes (**SD**), constitutes the secretory part of this gland. Mucous cells are relatively large, pale cells with flattened nuclei at the base. Serous cells are smaller, more darkly stained cells with rounded nuclei. Surrounding stroma is highly cellular. 265×. *H&E.*

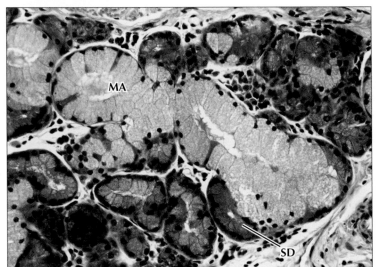

15.7 HISTOLOGY OF THE TRACHEA

The trachea is a semirigid tube, 15-20 cm long and 2-3 cm in diameter, between the larynx and the carina, which is the site of its bifurcation into two main bronchi. The tracheal **wall** consists of four concentric tunics surrounding a central **lumen.** The first tunic, the innermost **mucosa,** consists of pseudostratified ciliated columnar epithelium with goblet cells (the **respiratory epithelium**). It rests directly on an unusually thick basement membrane, which separates the epithelium from an underlying lamina propria of loose connective tissue rich in elastic fibers. The lamina propria also contains diffuse lymphoid tissue and scattered lymphatic nodules. The next tunic, the **submucosa,** contains mixed **seromucous glands.** Mucous and serous **acini** produce secretions that pass via ducts to the mucosa for discharge at the luminal surface. Small stellate myoepithelial cells are scattered along the bases of the acini and, by contraction, assist in expelling secretions into the ducts. The third tunic is a fibromuscular layer of **hyaline cartilage** rings bound together by dense fibroelastic connective tissue, which merges with the **perichondrium** surrounding the cartilage. The cartilage rings ensure that the trachea will not collapse and obstruct free flow of air into the lungs. Posteriorly, trachealis muscle fibers, stretched between the free ends of the cartilage rings, run in a transverse and oblique longitudinal orientation. These fibers play a role in regulating the caliber of the tracheal lumen. The outermost tunic, the adventitia, is loose connective tissue containing small blood vessels and nerves that supply the trachea. The adventitia blends imperceptibly with the surrounding connective tissue.

CLINICAL POINT

Cystic fibrosis is an autosomal recessive disorder caused by defective transport of chloride ions in mucous cells of seromucous glands in the respiratory tract as well as in cells producing sweat, saliva, and pancreatic secretions elsewhere in the body. A defective gene alters a membrane-associated protein with an active transport function. Known as *CF transmembrane conductance regulator,* this protein is a channel that controls movement of chloride in and out of cells. Defective chloride ion transport results in thick and sticky mucus, which predisposes patients to chronic lung infections, among other symptoms. Respiratory failure is the most dangerous consequence and can be life-threatening. Patients with cystic fibrosis are good candidates for *gene therapy.*

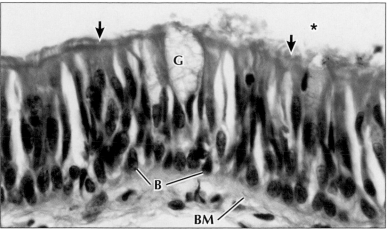

◄ **LM of respiratory epithelium in the trachea.** Small, rounded basal cells (**B**) rest on the basement membrane (**BM**). Goblet cells (**G**) have a distinctive shape and washed-out appearance. Both of these cell types intermingle with tall, columnar cells bearing apical cilia (**arrows**) that are in contact with the lumen (⋆). 420×. *H&E.*

▼ **Ultrastructural schematic: trachea and large bronchi.**

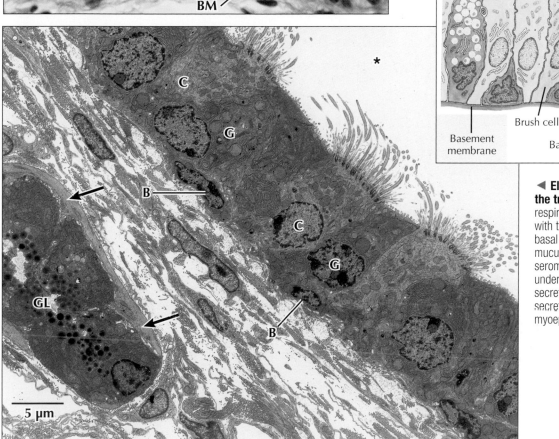

◄ **Electron micrograph (EM) of the tracheal mucosa.** The respiratory epithelium is in contact with the lumen (⋆) and comprises basal cells (**B**), ciliated cells (**C**), and mucus-secreting goblet cells (**G**). A seromucous gland (**GL**) in the underlying submucosa contains secretory cells, with prominent secretory vesicles, and underlying myoepithelial cells (**arrows**). 2500×.

15.8 ULTRASTRUCTURE OF TRACHEAL AND BRONCHIAL EPITHELIUM

The surface epithelium of both the trachea and the bronchi consists mainly of tall, **ciliated columnar cells** intermixed with goblet-shaped mucous cells (**goblet cells**) and small, rounded to triangular **basal cells.** Because not all cells reach the lumen and their nuclei are found at various levels, the epithelium is known as **pseudostratified.** This appearance is gradually lost in distal bronchi as cells become simple columnar and then cuboidal. The ciliated cell is the most prominent cell type and extends from the luminal surface to the basement membrane. Cells attach firmly to one another via apical *tight junctions*. Arising from the surface of ciliated cells are 200-250 *cilia* and numerous shorter *microvilli*. Goblet cells constitute about 20%-30% of cells in the more proximal airways and decrease in number distally. Many membrane-bound **mucus droplets** expand the apical part of these cells, whereas the basal portion is attenuated and has fewer organelles, thus producing the goblet shape. Basal cells sit in a single row close to the basement membrane, and their apices do not reach the lumen. They show little specialization in the cytoplasm and serve as stem cells for continuous replacement of other epithelial cells. As in other parts of the respiratory tract, several other cell types, which are better seen by electron microscopy, occur in the epithelium. **Brush cells** with small apical microvilli and **intermediate cells** with no special features are also found, although their functions remain uncertain. Occasional **serous cells,** resembling those seen in underlying submucosal glands, and neuroendocrine (*Kulchitsky, or K*) cells, with small membrane-bound secretory granules and analogous to enteroendocrine (*diffuse neuroendocrine*) cells of the gastrointestinal tract, are also present.

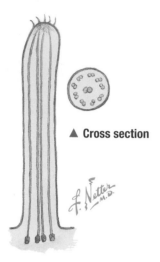

▲ **Cross section**

▲ **Magnified detail of cilium.**

▶ **EM of a ciliated cell of the trachea.**
Many cilia project from the cell surface and
protrude into the tracheal lumen. They
originate from basal bodies (**BB**) in the cell
apex immediately under the plasma
membrane and contain a complex array of
microtubules in their core. Smaller microvilli
(**arrows**) with a relatively simple cytoplasmic
structure are interposed between the cilia.
Mitochondria (**Mi**) are abundant in ciliated
cells and provide energy for ciliary motility.
Part of an adjacent goblet cell (**GC**) is seen.
20,000×.

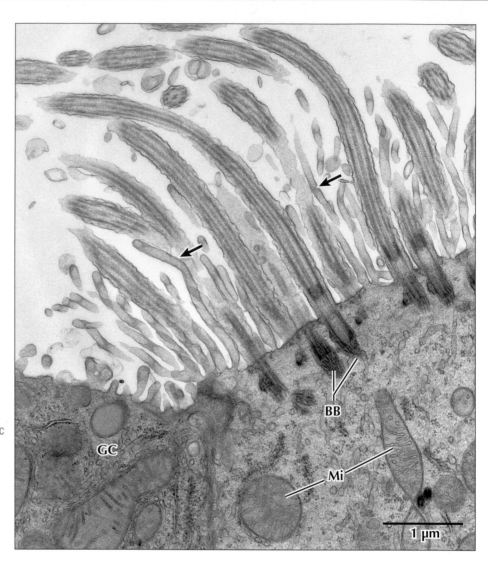

15.9 ULTRASTRUCTURE AND FUNCTION OF RESPIRATORY CILIA

Ciliated epithelial cells are found along the respiratory tract from the nasal cavity to the respiratory bronchioles. **Cilia** are luminal surface projections of the cells; one cell may contain several hundred. Their primary role is to move mucus and entrapped particulate matter, including dust and dead cells, over the surface of the cells toward the oral cavity, where they are eliminated or swallowed. They measure 0.25 µm in diameter and vary in length from 5 to 10 µm. The base of a cilium is fixed by cytoplasmic microtubules and a basal body consisting of a basal foot and rootlet. The beating of cilia resembles the breast stroke in swimming: a forward, rapid power stroke is followed by a recovery stroke that is slower and more flexible. Movement of a cilium depends on its central shaft, or **axoneme,** which consists of two central pairs of **microtubules** surrounded by nine peripheral microtubular doublets and their associated proteins. *Tubulin* is the main structural protein of microtubules; *nexin* links them mechanically. Each doublet consists of an A tubule and a B tubule. Projections or side arms from the A tubules occur regularly along the tubule length and are arranged in two rows. They contain *ciliary dynein*, which hydrolyzes ATP to generate the sliding force that causes bending. During movement, the outer doublets slide past each other with no shortening of microtubules. Because they are linked to each other by nexin, bending occurs. Cilia beat, at 10-25 beats per second, in a coordinated, unidirectional pattern characterized by successive waves of whip-like movements. Genetics determines the direction of the beat.

CLINICAL POINT
Kartagener syndrome (or **primary ciliary dyskinesia,** an **immotile cilia syndrome**) is a rare genetic disorder characterized by situs inversus (reversal of body organ positioning during prenatal development), sinusitis, and bronchiectasis (chronic enlargement of bronchial airways). This syndrome is inherited via an autosomal recessive pattern; its etiology is unknown. Electron microscopy reveals a deficiency of dynein arms in the cilia, which leads to their motility defect. This syndrome may become evident in neonatal life, with clinical manifestations including chronic upper and lower respiratory tract disease resulting in defective mucociliary clearance. Males demonstrate infertility secondary to immotile spermatozoa.

▼ **Schematic section of a large bronchus.**

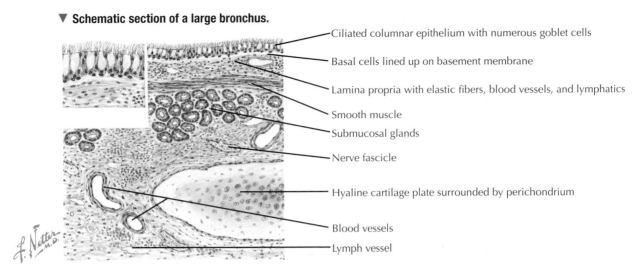

Ciliated columnar epithelium with numerous goblet cells

Basal cells lined up on basement membrane

Lamina propria with elastic fibers, blood vessels, and lymphatics

Smooth muscle

Submucosal glands

Nerve fascicle

Hyaline cartilage plate surrounded by perichondrium

Blood vessels

Lymph vessel

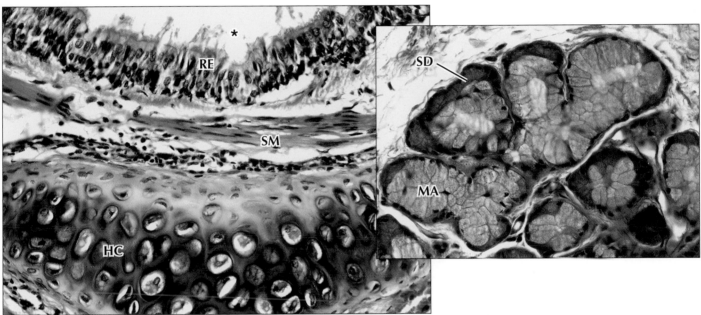

▲ **LM section of the wall of a bronchus.** Ciliated respiratory epithelium (**RE**) lines the lumen (⋆). Smooth muscle (**SM**) is in the underlying lamina propria. A plate of hyaline cartilage (**HC**) is situated on the outer aspect of the airway. A seromucous gland appears to the right. 300×. *H&E.*

◀ **LM of a bronchial seromucous gland.** It contains pale-stained mucous acini (**MA**), darkly stained serous demilunes (**SD**), and flattened myoepithelial cells that surround the demilunes on the outside. 300×. *H&E.*

15.10 HISTOLOGY OF THE BRONCHI

Although extrapulmonary bronchi have a smaller diameter compared with the trachea, they closely resemble the trachea histologically. The **hyaline cartilage** and **smooth muscle** have the same configuration in these larger bronchi as in the trachea. At the hilum, primary bronchi branch dichotomously as they enter the substance of the lung. Hyaline cartilage in bronchial walls prevents wall collapse and, as bronchi subdivide into smaller bronchi, the cartilage takes the form of irregular plates. In the area interior to the cartilage is a network of collagen and longitudinally oriented **elastic fibers** in which are embedded smooth muscle cells arranged in criss crossing bands that completely encircle the lumen of intrapulmonary bronchi. *Parasympathetic* vagal stimulation causes contraction of bronchial smooth muscle, whereas *sympathetic*

stimulation leads to relaxation. Bronchial **seromucous glands** in the submucosa immediately above the cartilage consist of **mucous** and **serous cells** arranged in **demilunes.** Their small ducts lead to the mucosal surface, where their contents are liberated to provide a moist, highly viscous, protective surface coating of mucus. Serous cells produce a watery, proteinaceous low-viscosity secretion that most likely flushes out the secretion of the mucous cells. Small accumulations of lymphatic tissue, often as lymphoid nodules, are common in the **lamina propria.** They provide immunologic defense against pathogens and may represent sites of B lymphocyte differentiation (germinal centers) for production of antibody-secreting plasma cells. As bronchi get smaller, they continue to branch, with a reduction in height of the epithelium and a gradual decrease in numbers of goblet and ciliated cells.

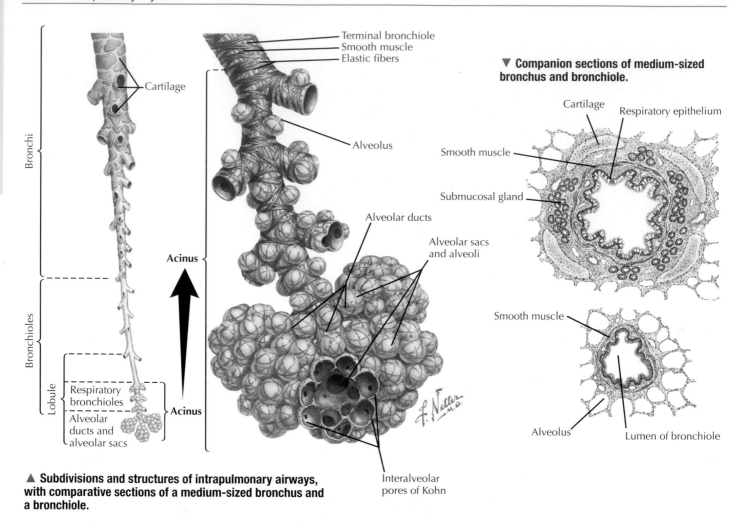

▲ **Subdivisions and structures of intrapulmonary airways, with comparative sections of a medium-sized bronchus and a bronchiole.**

15.11 STRUCTURE OF INTRAPULMONARY AIRWAYS

Intrapulmonary airways are characterized by successive, dichotomous branching, with about 20 generations extending from the **bronchi** to the **respiratory bronchioles. Cartilage** plates in the bronchi become sparser toward the periphery and, in the last generations, occur only at branching points. Terminal bronchioles are distal to the bronchi, past the last cartilage plate, and lead into respiratory bronchioles, which have small, spherical alveolar outpocketings in their walls. Beyond the respiratory bronchioles are **alveolar ducts** and rotunda-shaped **alveolar sacs,** which lead into **alveoli** proper. The smallest anatomic unit in relation to the branching pattern of airways is the **pulmonary acinus,** defined as the portion of the lung supplied by the terminal bronchiole and all its branches. At 6-10 mm in diameter in humans, the acinus can be visualized radiologically; pathologists utilize the acinus to help delineate the spread of lung disease. A larger respiratory unit, the **pulmonary lobule,** measures about 2.5 cm in diameter and is demarcated by fibrous connective tissue septa. Each lobule is a pyramidal area of lung tissue, with its tip toward the hilum and its base facing the visceral pleura. A bronchus enters at the tip of the lobule and immediately loses its cartilage to become a bronchiole, which branches and ends as clusters of pulmonary alveoli. Five to eight acini make up a lobule. Collateral air passage occurs between acini via small round to oval holes in the alveolar walls, which are known as **interalveolar pores of Kohn.** These openings also allow air to pass from one alveolus to another and may permit the spread of infection.

CLINICAL POINT

Lung cancer is a leading cause of cancer mortality worldwide, with more than 85% of deaths due to effects of cigarette smoking. Most tumors are **carcinomas** arising from respiratory epithelium of the tracheobronchial tree or pneumocytes of pulmonary alveoli. Histologic study confirms diagnosis and helps with clinical staging and prognosis. *Non-small-cell carcinomas*—the most common—grow rapidly, usually metastasize, and respond poorly to chemotherapy or radiation. *Small-cell* (formerly *oat-cell*) *carcinomas* make up about 20% of tumors, usually arise from bronchial epithelium, and are highly malignant. *Carcinoid tumors*—slow-growing neuroendocrine neoplasms from pluripotential basal cells of respiratory epithelium—account for about 5% of lung cancers.

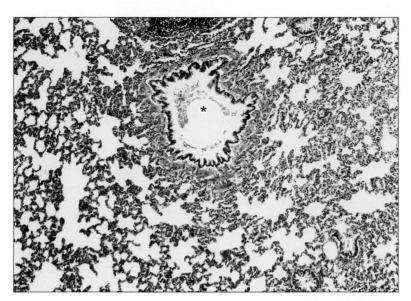

◀ **LM of the lung in transverse section that shows a terminal bronchiole at low magnification.** A thin wall and relatively simple histologic structure characterize this airway. Partial contraction of its smooth muscle causes the stellate lumen (∗). Many closely packed alveoli constituting the lung parenchyma surround the bronchiole. 150×. *H&E.*

▶ **Higher magnification view of a respiratory bronchiole.** Simple columnar epithelium lines the lumen and consists of dome-shaped Clara cells (**arrows**) plus ciliated cells. Pulmonary alveoli form outpocketings (∗) in the wall of the respiratory bronchiole and are also seen (**A**) in surrounding areas of the lung. 270×. *H&E.*

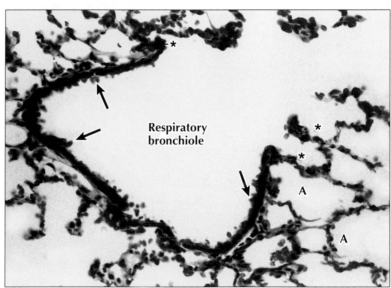

Respiratory bronchiole

15.12 HISTOLOGY OF TERMINAL AND RESPIRATORY BRONCHIOLES

When airways reach a diameter of 1 mm or less and their walls lack cartilage, they are called bronchioles. These small conducting tubes branch repeatedly and have thin walls with a simple histologic structure. They are lined by a **simple columnar epithelium.** Many **ciliated cells** are present, but dome-shaped nonciliated secretory cells called **Clara cells** replace the goblet cells of the upper airways. The cilia beat synchronously and sweep dust particles upward toward the bronchi. In contrast to the upper airways, no glands underlie the bronchiolar epithelium. A relatively large amount of helically arranged **smooth muscle** occupies the airway walls that, by contraction, can constrict the lumen and shorten the airway. The surrounding loose connective tissue stroma is continuous with that of surrounding **pulmonary alveoli** and contains abundant elastic fibers, which are mostly longitudinal in orientation. Terminal bronchioles give rise to respiratory bronchioles, which show at least two orders of successive branching, and each respiratory bronchiole branches into 2-10 alveolar ducts that, in turn, lead into clusters of pulmonary alveoli. Although

their histology resembles that of the conducting bronchioles, respiratory bronchioles have extremely thin walls and are lined by low simple cuboidal epithelium, which in smaller branches has no cilia. Respiratory bronchiole walls contain many small outpocketings of alveoli between the criss-crossing bundles of smooth muscle. These small sacculations have extremely attenuated walls lined by simple squamous epithelium.

CLINICAL POINT

Asthma, a disorder characterized by a heightened response of the tracheobronchial tree to numerous stimuli, affects millions of people annually. Symptoms of dyspnea, coughing, respiratory distress, and wheezing result from bronchospasm, bronchial wall edema, and hypersecretion of mucous glands. Pathologic features include mucosal and submucosal edema in bronchi and bronchioles, thickening of the basement membrane, hypertrophy of smooth muscle, and profuse infiltration of leukocytes, chiefly eosinophils. Intraluminal mucous plugs are highly viscous, adhere to the bronchial walls, and narrow the airway lumina. Hypercontraction of smooth muscle compounds these effects and increases resistance to airflow.

▼ Schematic of an electron microscopic view of bronchiolar epithelium.

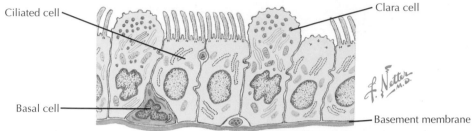

Ciliated cell

Clara cell

Basal cell

Basement membrane

▶ **EM showing salient features of bronchiolar epithelium.** A mixture of Clara cells (**Cl**) and ciliated cells (**Ci**) characterizes this epithelium. Adjacent cells are sealed by apical tight junctions (**circles**). Apical regions of Clara cells protrude into the lumen (∗) and contain abundant and tightly packed (**SER**) and numerous electron-dense secretory vesicles (**arrows**). A thin basement membrane separates the epithelium from underlying tissue, which contains smooth muscle cells (**SM**). 5000×.

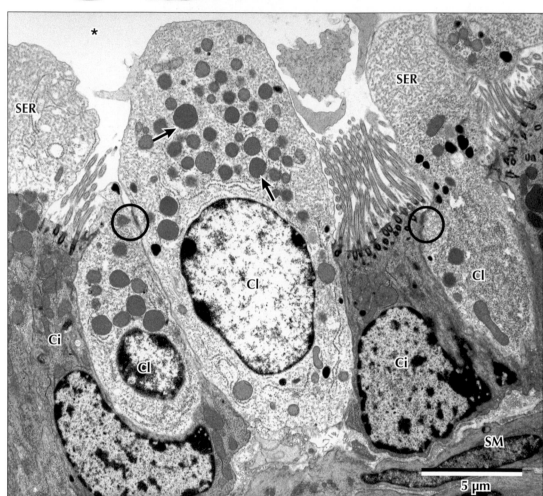

15.13 ULTRASTRUCTURE OF BRONCHIOLAR EPITHELIUM: CLARA CELLS

Clara cells are nonciliated columnar cells unique to **bronchioles.** They constitute 75%-80% of the epithelial cells lining the lumina of these airways. They are mainly secretory cells that discharge their products directly into these lumina. Electron microscopy reveals highly compartmentalized cells: they have protuberant apical cytoplasm with large, ovoid, electron-dense **secretory vesicles** containing unique proteins that are discharged in a *merocrine* fashion. Clara cells can segregate and pinch off the apical region from the supranuclear region and discharge material into the airway lumen. Their secretions are believed to play antiinflammatory roles. The apical cytoplasm also contains a prominent cap of closely packed **smooth endoplasmic reticulum** (SER) arranged as tubular aggregates. The SER is believed to play a role in *detoxifica-*

tion, because Clara cells can detoxify many inhaled noxious substances such as nitrogen dioxide. The cytoplasm also contains many mitochondria, which suggests a high oxidative capacity. Rough endoplasmic reticulum and variable amounts of glycogen are often seen in basal regions of the cells. Clara cells also secrete a surfactant-like protective material that coats the bronchiolar epithelial surface; proteolytic enzymes that break down mucus produced in the upper tracheobronchial tree; a leukocyte protease inhibitor that may be important in maintaining the integrity of the bronchiolar epithelium; and lysozymes. In addition, these cells are involved in transport of water and electrolytes, especially release of chloride ions. They act as progenitor (stem) cells for normal renewal of nonciliated and ciliated bronchiolar epithelial cells, particularly in response to injury.

► **Schematic of intrapulmonary blood circulation.**

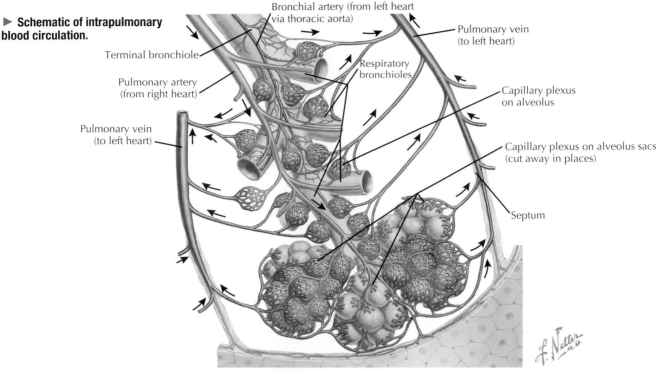

Bronchial artery (from left heart via thoracic aorta)

Terminal bronchiole

Pulmonary artery (from right heart)

Pulmonary vein (to left heart)

Respiratory bronchioles

Pulmonary vein (to left heart)

Capillary plexus on alveolus

Capillary plexus on alveolus sacs (cut away in places)

Septum

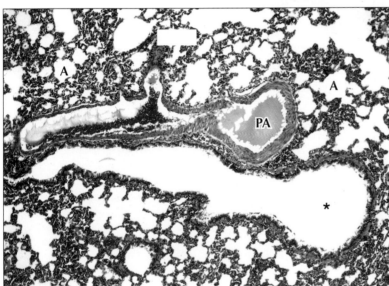

◄ **LM of the lung that shows the close relationship between a branch of the pulmonary artery (PA) and a terminal bronchiole (*).** The pulmonary artery is sectioned obliquely and has smooth muscle in its wall. It accompanies the bronchiole, which appears to get progressively smaller to the left. Pulmonary alveoli (**A**) occupy surrounding areas of the lung. 105×. *H&F*

15.14 INTRAPULMONARY BLOOD CIRCULATION

The lungs have a **dual blood supply**—one from each side of the heart—that enters at the hilum. **Pulmonary arteries** from the right ventricle deliver deoxygenated blood under low pressure to an extensive network of pulmonary capillaries in the alveolar walls, where CO_2 is exchanged for O_2. Details of intrapulmonary circulation are best understood in relation to the branching pattern of peripheral airways. Pulmonary arteries and their branches accompany the airways in a sheath of connective tissue. The more proximal arteries are the elastic type and extend to the junctions of bronchi and bronchioles. The more distal arteries are muscular arteries, which lead into arterioles ending around alveolar sacs and ultimately deliver blood to an extensive, intercommunicating network of pulmonary capillaries. **Bronchial arteries** from the thoracic aorta deliver oxygenated blood under high pres-

sure to the walls of the airways from the hilum to the respiratory bronchioles. These arteries function as nutrient vessels that drain into plexuses of capillaries extending into the mucosa of these airways. Bronchial arteries also supply blood to the visceral pleura covering the lungs. Venous blood from pulmonary and bronchial systems drains through pulmonary veins that carry blood to the left atrium of the heart. Pulmonary arteries and veins do not run together in the lobules: arteries travel with the airways, and veins run in the septa. The lungs also have a dual and extensive lymphatic drainage system. A superficial lymphatic plexus drains visceral pleura and transports lymph to the hilum of the lungs—the location of several lymph nodes. A deeper lymphatic plexus is associated with bronchioles and bronchi and also delivers lymph to hilar lymph nodes. Within lung lobules, lymphatics typically run in the septa, not with the airways or interalveolar walls.

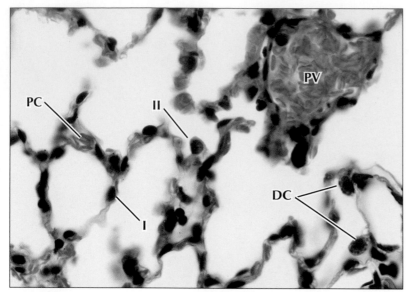

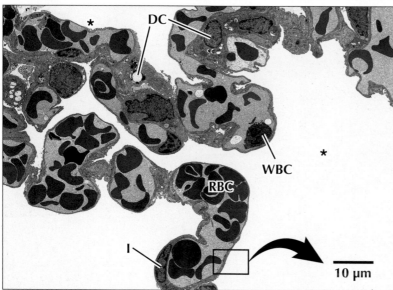

◀ **LM of the parenchyma of the lung.** Pulmonary alveoli are lined by flattened type I pneumocytes (**I**), with darkly stained nuclei, and cuboidal type II pneumocytes (**II**), with more euchromatic nuclei. Pulmonary capillaries (**PC**) filled with erythrocytes traverse the interalveolar septa. Alveolar macrophages (dust cells, **DC**) are clearly seen after they have ingested particulate matter. A small branch of the pulmonary vein (**PV**) has a thin wall and collects venous blood from the pulmonary capillaries. 675×. *H&E.*

▼ **Schematic of alveoli and interalveolar septum.**

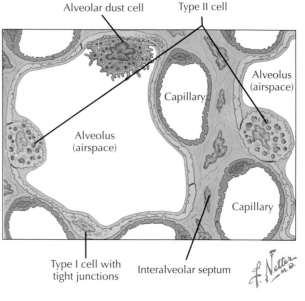

▲ **EM of the alveoli of the lung.** Red (**RBC**) and white (**WBC**) blood cells occupy lumina of pulmonary capillaries, which travel in interalveolar septa. Alveolar spaces (✱) are lined by type I pneumocytes (**I**), which are best seen in the region of their elongated nuclei. Alveolar macrophages (dust cells, **DC**) in the interstitium are recognizable by their content of lysosomes. The area delineated by the rectangle is seen at higher magnification in Fig. 15.16. 1000×. *(Courtesy of Dr. B. J. Crawford)*

15.15 HISTOLOGY AND ULTRASTRUCTURE OF PULMONARY ALVEOLI

Pulmonary alveoli are small, cup-shaped outpocketings of respiratory bronchioles, alveolar ducts, and sacs that can be likened to closely packed cells of a honeycomb. They measure 200-250 μm in diameter. Very slender partitions—the **interalveolar septa**—demarcate and separate adjacent alveoli. Features of these septa are difficult to distinguish by conventional light microscopy. Alveoli have a continuous lining of simple squamous epithelium less than 0.2 μm thick that is composed of contiguous cells, known as pneumocytes, which rest on a basal lamina that is better seen via electron microscopy. Two types of pneumocytes make up this epithelium: **type I cells** are flattened and possess a large surface area to facilitate gas exchange. Their attenuated cytoplasm, except for the part of the cell containing the single, elongated, darkly stained nucleus, is beyond the limit of resolution of the light microscope. Type I pneumocytes cover about 95% of the alveolar surface, even though they constitute only 40% of all the epithelial cells. **Type II pneumocytes** account for the remaining 60% of cells lining the alveoli. However, because of their shape—more cuboidal—they account for only 5% of the lining cells. Resting on a basement membrane, type II cells usually sit between type I cells near corners where two alveoli meet. **Alveolar macrophages (dust cells)** protect alveolar spaces by scavenging the surface. Interalveolar septa are supported by a delicate connective tissue stroma—pulmonary interstitium—that is rich in elastic fibers. The main component of the septa is an extensive network of anastomosing **pulmonary capillaries** that undertake a convoluted course. Most cells in the septa are endothelial cells of capillaries; scattered fibroblasts, macrophages, and occasional mast cells also occur.

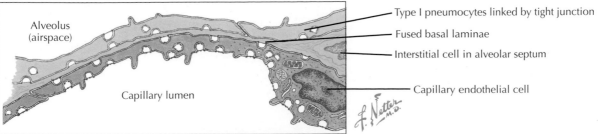

Schematic of fine structure of an alveolar capillary unit.

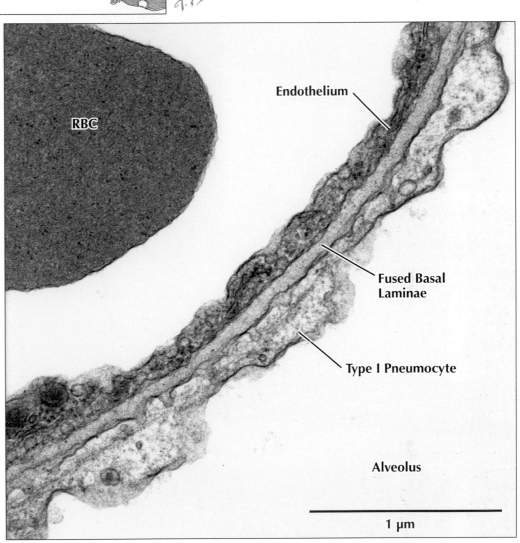

▶ **EM of the blood-air barrier at high magnification.** This interface between blood and air favors passive diffusion of gases. An erythrocyte (**RBC**) is in the lumen of a pulmonary capillary, and the lumen of a pulmonary alveolus is seen to the right. The attenuated endothelium of the capillary, the slender process of a type I pneumocyte, and their fused basal laminae constitute the main elements of this barrier. A few scattered organelles, including cytoplasmic vesicles, are in the cytoplasm of both the endothelial cell and pneumocyte. A layer of surfactant normally covers the epithelial lining of the alveolus but is not clearly seen in this micrograph and appears washed out (a fixation artifact). 47,000×.

15.16   ULTRASTRUCTURE OF THE BLOOD-AIR BARRIER

Gas exchange between blood and air occurs across a highly specialized region of the **pulmonary alveolus**—the blood-air barrier, or **alveolar-capillary membrane**—which is readily permeable to gases via diffusion. Less than 2 μm wide, it is best seen by electron microscopy. It comprises the attenuated **endothelium** of **pulmonary capillaries, type I pneumocytes** lining the alveolus, and their fused **basal laminae.** A thin layer of *surfactant* produced by type II pneumocytes also covers the alveolar surface. In the area of minimal thickness, type I pneumocytes have a thin rim of cytoplasm with few organelles except for many **cytoplasmic vesicles,** which suggests an active role in fluid and solute transport. Adjacent pneumocytes are sealed by **tight junctions,** which prevent leakage of fluid and solutes. The capillary endothelium, the continuous, non-

fenestrated type, also contains tight junctions. Ultrastructurally, endothelial cells are arranged as an interlocking, contiguous mosaic. Many small **microvilli** on the luminal surface greatly increase surface area. Immunocytochemistry has shown that microvilli react to antibodies to angiotensin-converting enzyme (ACE), whose inhibitors are used to treat congestive heart failure. Cytoplasm of endothelial cells contains (near the nucleus) mitochondria, Golgi complex, microtubules, microfilaments, Weibel-Palade bodies, and rough endoplasmic reticulum. Organelles are almost entirely absent in slender extensions of endothelial cells, which in some areas may be quite thin—only 0.1 μm. The most striking feature of these cells is the presence of numerous vesicles, which are free in the cytoplasm or closely associated with luminal and abluminal cell surfaces and whose main function is to transport fluid and proteins between blood and surrounding **interstitium.**

▼ **Ultrastructural schematic of type II pneumocyte and surfactant layer.**

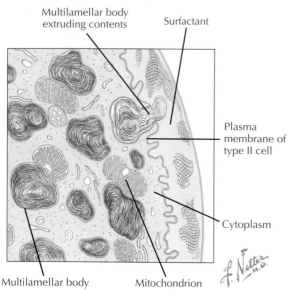

Multilamellar body extruding contents

Surfactant

Plasma membrane of type II cell

Cytoplasm

Multilamellar body

Mitochondrion

f. Netter M.D.

▶ **EM of a type II pneumocyte.** Its cytoplasm is replete with distinctive multilamellar bodies (**MB**), one of which is in the process of extrusion from the cell surface (**long arrow**). Short, stubby microvilli project from other parts of the cell surface (**small arrows**). The euchromatic nucleus suggests a high level of functional activity. Profiles of pulmonary capillaries (**Cap**) and portions of alveolar spaces (✱) are also visible. 9000×.

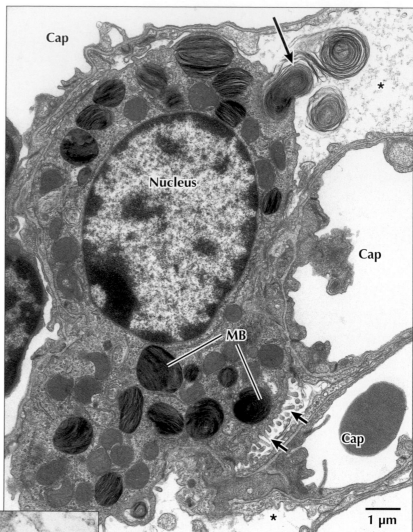

Cap

Nucleus

Cap

MB

Cap

✱

✱

1 μm

MB

OL

0.2 μm

◀ **EM of surfactant at high magnification.** In this optimally preserved specimen, the fingerprint structure typical of surfactant is clear. Surfactant appears as parallel sheets of osmiophilic lamellae (**OL**) that are rich in lipoprotein. The lamellae are continuous with a recently released multilamellar body (**MB**). 45,000×.

15.17   ULTRASTRUCTURE OF TYPE II PNEUMOCYTES

Type II pneumocytes are cuboidal cells that measure 10-12 μm in diameter and possess a distinctive ultrastructural appearance. They have a single, centrally placed, rounded **nucleus,** which is usually euchromatic, with one or two prominent nucleoli. Short stubby **microvilli** project from the cellular surface into the alveolar lumen. Their **cytoplasm** contains a well-developed Golgi complex, profiles of rough and smooth endoplasmic reticulum, scattered **mitochondria,** and peroxisomes. Large, pleomorphic membrane-bound **multilamellar bodies,** a unique feature of these cells, can be observed extruding their contents into alveolar spaces. The bodies are filled with electron-dense lamellar material

and represent **secretory vesicles.** They are derived from the Golgi complex and are ultimately discharged by *exocytosis* at the cell surface. Type II cells synthesize and secrete **pulmonary surfactant,** which contains complexes of phospholipids, protein, and carbohydrate that become part of the fluid coating the alveolar surfaces. Surfactant's detergent-like property prevents collapse of alveoli by reducing surface tension, thereby facilitating alveolar inflation during inspiration. Many type II cells are mitotically active and renew the alveolar surface via differentiation into type I pneumocytes. This replicative potential is important for healing after lung injury, because the large surface area of type I cells makes them especially susceptible to damage.

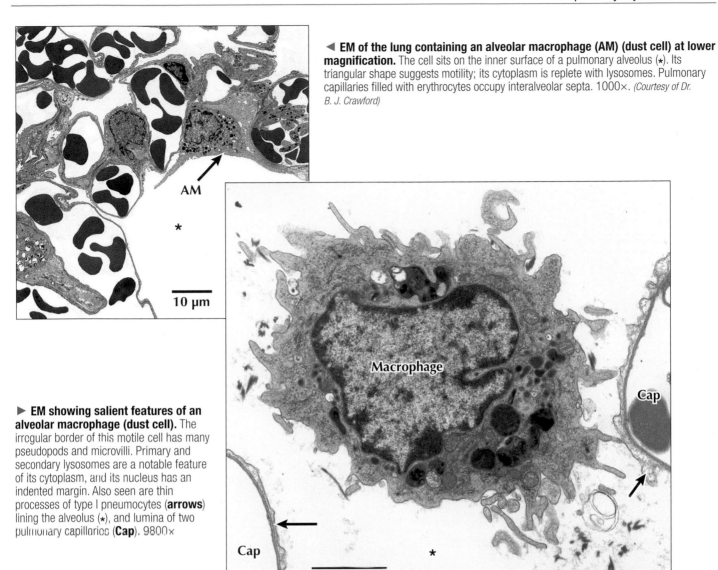

◄ **EM of the lung containing an alveolar macrophage (AM) (dust cell) at lower magnification.** The cell sits on the inner surface of a pulmonary alveolus (∗). Its triangular shape suggests motility; its cytoplasm is replete with lysosomes. Pulmonary capillaries filled with erythrocytes occupy interalveolar septa. 1000×. *(Courtesy of Dr. B. J. Crawford)*

AM

∗

10 μm

► **EM showing salient features of an alveolar macrophage (dust cell).** The irregular border of this motile cell has many pseudopods and microvilli. Primary and secondary lysosomes are a notable feature of its cytoplasm, and its nucleus has an indented margin. Also seen are thin processes of type I pneumocytes (**arrows**) lining the alveolus (∗), and lumina of two pulmonary capillaries (**Cap**). 9800×

Macrophage

Cap

Cap

∗

2 μm

15.18 ULTRASTRUCTURE OF ALVEOLAR MACROPHAGES

Alveolar macrophages are large rounded cells with a diameter of 15-50 μm. They are usually seen bulging into the alveolar space, often situated at junctions between adjacent interalveolar septa. They have a single, centrally placed **nucleus** that is often deeply indented. Their **cytoplasm** contains various organelles, including many **primary** and **secondary lysosomes**. Because of their dusty appearance after ingestion of carbon particles, they are also known as alveolar **dust cells.** Their main function is to ingest dust and other foreign particles that have entered alveolar spaces during inspiration. Electron microscopy has shown that the cells have an irregular shape and a surface studded with **pseudopodia** and short **microvilli**. These **motile cells** are derived from blood monocytes whose precursors arise in **bone marrow.** They migrate across the walls of **pulmonary capillaries** to the **interalveolar septa.** They undergo maturational division in the interstitium of the lung and then enter alveolar spaces to lie free in the lumina. After they remove debris from alveoli, they move up the bronchial tree, where they are carried by cilia and are eventually swallowed or expectorated with mucus. In certain types of heart disease, such as *congestive heart failure*, erythrocytes from the bloodstream may escape into pulmonary alveolar spaces, where alveolar macrophages may phagocytose them. These swollen macrophages with ingested hemosiderin may be seen in sputum and are known as *heart failure cells.*

CLINICAL POINT

Infant respiratory distress syndrome, formerly called **hyaline membrane disease,** is a common disorder affecting 10% of premature infants. Signs include labored breathing and cyanosis, which are caused by inability of pulmonary alveoli to expand or remain open after inspiration. It is due to an inadequate supply of surfactant at birth, which is related to deficient surfactant production or failure of development and maturation of type II pneumocytes. Treatment options depend on disease severity and prematurity of the infant and include supply of O_2 to assist respiration, mechanical ventilation, corticosteroid therapy, and delivery of artificial surfactant to the lungs.

▼ **Developing respiratory tract (top) at 4–5 weeks and bronchi and lungs (bottom) at 5–6 weeks.**

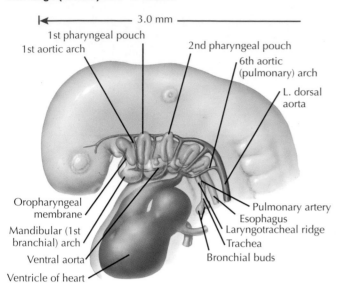

▼ **Ventral View of Pharynx.**

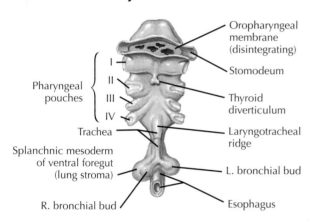

► **LM of fetal lung.** At this pseudoglandular developmental stage, the lung has a glandular appearance with many thin-walled tubes and sacs (∗) lined by simple squamous to cuboidal epithelium. A matrix of loose mesenchymal connective tissue separates the developing airways. Visceral pleura covering the lung (**arrows**) is derived from mesenchyme and is a simple cuboidal layer of mesothelial cells. 95×. *H&E.*

▼ **Developing airways in the fetal lung.**

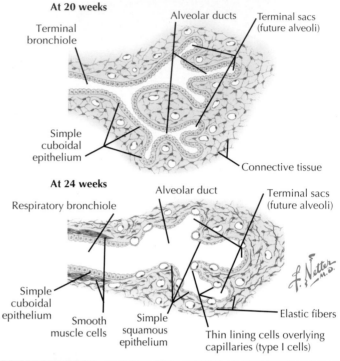

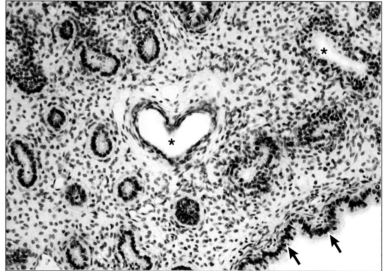

15.19 DEVELOPMENT OF THE LOWER RESPIRATORY SYSTEM

In the 4-week embryo, a midline endodermal bud, known as the **laryngotracheal ridge,** develops immediately caudal to the **pharyngeal pouches.** It forms a ridge in the floor of the pharynx and grows caudally to become a tube. The future larynx develops from the upper part of the tube; the **trachea,** from the caudal part. Two knob-like thickenings at its most distal end become the **bronchial buds,** which undergo about 20 successive divisions before birth, followed by continued postnatal growth. Growth of **endodermal epithelium** is accompanied by invasion and condensation of surrounding **splanchnic mesenchyme,** which envelops the tube. The mesenchyme gives rise to connective tissue, smooth muscle, and cartilage of the airways; endoderm is the source of the epithelium and its associated intramural glands. Bronchi and lungs develop like an exocrine gland: bronchi are equivalent to extralobular ducts, whereas bronchioles are counterparts of intralobular ducts. Five phases of lung development include the *embryonic period* from 26 days to 6 weeks, with initial development of lobar bronchi. In the *pseudoglandular phase* between 6 and 16 weeks, terminal bronchioles, which appear as blind tubules lined with cuboidal or columnar epithelium, develop further. The *canalicular period,* 16-28 weeks, includes development of acini accompanied by invasion of capillaries from surrounding mesenchyme. The *saccular period,* 28-36 weeks, is followed by the *alveolar period,* from 36 weeks to birth. At 28 weeks, type I and type II pneumocytes begin to develop, with initial production of surfactant. After birth and up to 8 years of age, development of alveoli continues.

16

URINARY SYSTEM

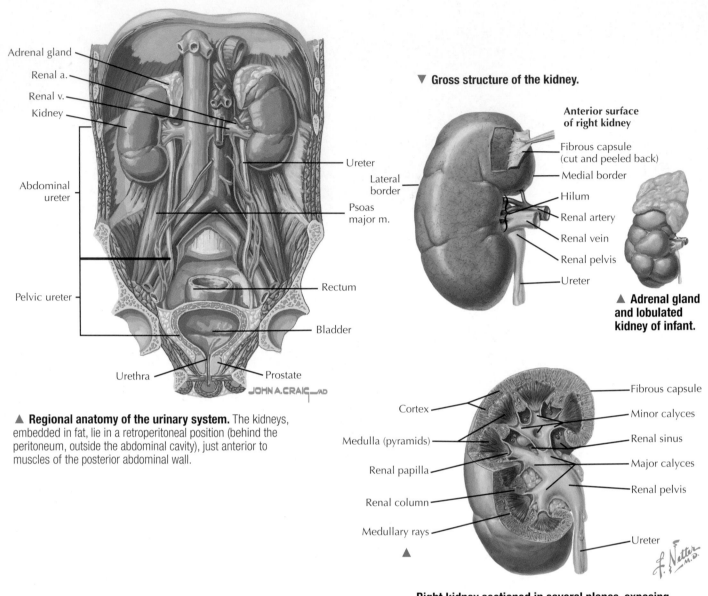

Adrenal gland

Renal a.

Renal v.

Kidney

Abdominal ureter

Pelvic ureter

Ureter

Psoas major m.

Rectum

Bladder

Urethra

Prostate

JOHN A. CRAIG _AD

▲ **Regional anatomy of the urinary system.** The kidneys, embedded in fat, lie in a retroperitoneal position (behind the peritoneum, outside the abdominal cavity), just anterior to muscles of the posterior abdominal wall.

▼ **Gross structure of the kidney.**

Anterior surface of right kidney

Lateral border

Fibrous capsule (cut and peeled back)

Medial border

Hilum

Renal artery

Renal vein

Renal pelvis

Ureter

▲ **Adrenal gland and lobulated kidney of infant.**

Cortex

Medulla (pyramids)

Renal papilla

Renal column

Medullary rays

Fibrous capsule

Minor calyces

Renal sinus

Major calyces

Renal pelvis

Ureter

f. Netter M.D.

Right kidney sectioned in several planes, exposing parenchyma and renal pelvis.

16.1   OVERVIEW

The urinary system comprises two **kidneys,** two **ureters,** a **urinary bladder,** and a **urethra.** Kidneys filter blood and produce *urine,* by which waste products and foreign substances leave the body. Urine formation involves *filtration, secretion,* and *reabsorption* of fluid by **renal corpuscles** and **tubules** in kidneys. About 180 L of fluid is filtered daily, but only 1-2 L of urine is produced, with the remaining fluid reabsorbed by renal tubules to reenter the vascular system. Kidneys control acid-base balance, maintain extracellular fluid volume, and regulate total body water. They also produce two hormones: *renin* aids regulation of systemic arterial blood pressure; *erythropoietin* stimulates production of erythrocytes in bone marrow. The flattened bean-shaped kidneys have an indented slit, or **hilum,** on the medial surface through which ureters, blood vessels, lymphatics, and nerves pass. Kidneys are *compound tubular glands* covered by a thin **capsule** of dense con-

nective tissue and embedded in a layer of fat. The parenchyma is divided into an outer dark-red **cortex,** a lighter striated **medulla,** and a funnel-shaped **pelvis** that lies in a shallow cavity—the **renal sinus.** The medulla consists of 12-15 cone-shaped **renal pyramids,** each with a broad base bordering on the cortex and an apex forming a nipple-like projection, or **papilla,** which extends into the sinus. Parts of the cortex dip down into spaces between the pyramids to form **renal columns.** The renal pelvis, a fan-shaped expansion of the ureter, forms two or three cup-like **major calyces** at its widest border. These divide into **minor calyces,** each being a drain for the papilla of a pyramid. Parenchyma served by one papilla is a **renal lobe;** each human kidney has 12-15 lobes. Urine flows from pyramids through calyces into the renal pelvis, then out of the kidneys and into ureters. Ureters deliver it to the bladder, where it is stored before urination via the urethra.

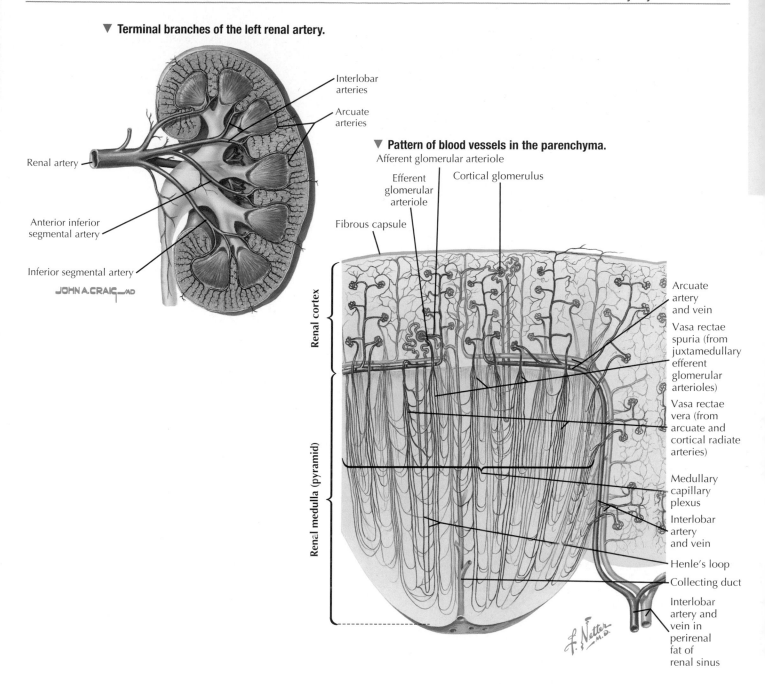

▼ Terminal branches of the left renal artery.

Interlobar arteries

Arcuate arteries

Renal artery

Anterior inferior segmental artery

Inferior segmental artery

JOHN A.CRAIG—MD

▼ Pattern of blood vessels in the parenchyma.

Afferent glomerular arteriole

Efferent glomerular arteriole

Cortical glomerulus

Fibrous capsule

Renal cortex

Renal medulla (pyramid)

Arcuate artery and vein

Vasa rectae spuria (from juxtamedullary efferent glomerular arterioles)

Vasa rectae vera (from arcuate and cortical radiate arteries)

Medullary capillary plexus

Interlobar artery and vein

Henle's loop

Collecting duct

Interlobar artery and vein in perirenal fat of renal sinus

16.2 ORGANIZATION OF THE RENAL VASCULATURE

The highly vascular **kidneys** receive nearly 25% of cardiac output, and their histologic organization and functions center on blood supply. Blood vessel arrangement provides arterial blood directly to **glomeruli** (site of *ultrafiltration*) of **renal corpuscles** and around all parts of renal **tubules** (site of *reabsorption* of substances). Arterial blood from the **renal artery**—a branch of the *aorta*—reaches a kidney at the hilum and passes into **interlobar arteries,** which distribute blood to glomeruli via **arcuate arteries** at the corticomedullary junction. Blood is then taken to **interlobular arteries,** which cross the cortical parenchyma radially, and in between medullary rays. Almost all blood goes first to **afferent arterioles,** which supply renal corpuscles. The capillary

network in the corpuscle is unique because it comprises an afferent and an **efferent arteriole.** The afferent arteriole branches into a tuft of 20-40 loops of **fenestrated capillaries**—the glomerulus. Filtered blood leaves a glomerulus via an efferent arteriole and travels through the extensive *peritubular capillary network* around cortical renal tubules to regain some water and solutes. Almost all blood to renal tubules comes from glomeruli. Also, efferent arterioles from juxtamedullary nephrons give off recurrent capillary loops, the **vasa recta,** which run in parallel into the medulla along medullary rays. Vasa recta drain into **arcuate veins** at the corticomedullary junction. Venous return from both cortex and medulla drains into **interlobular veins,** and venous blood follows the course of the arteries to the hilum, where it empties into the **renal vein,** which takes it to the *inferior vena cava* and the heart.

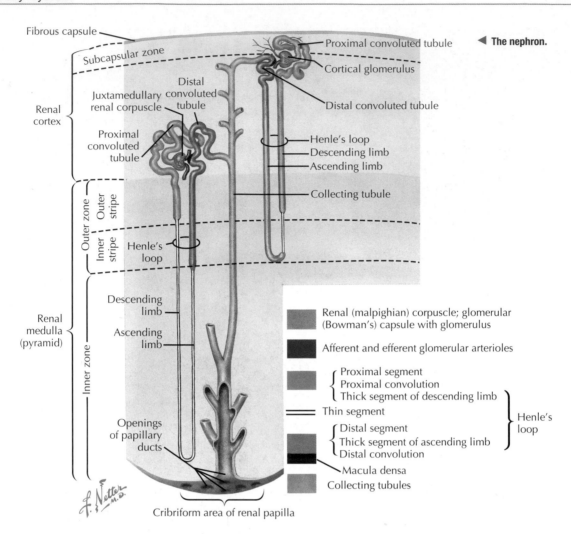

◀ **The nephron.**

Fibrous capsule
Subcapsular zone
Renal cortex
Juxtamedullary renal corpuscle
Distal convoluted tubule
Proximal convoluted tubule
Outer zone
Outer stripe
Inner stripe
Henle's loop
Renal medulla (pyramid)
Inner zone
Descending limb
Ascending limb
Openings of papillary ducts

Proximal convoluted tubule
Cortical glomerulus
Distal convoluted tubule
Henle's loop
Descending limb
Ascending limb
Collecting tubule

Renal (malpighian) corpuscle; glomerular (Bowman's) capsule with glomerulus
Afferent and efferent glomerular arterioles
Proximal segment
Proximal convolution
Thick segment of descending limb
Thin segment
Distal segment
Thick segment of ascending limb
Distal convolution
Macula densa
Collecting tubules

Henle's loop

Cribriform area of renal papilla

16.3 ANATOMY OF THE URINIFEROUS TUBULE (NEPHRON AND COLLECTING DUCT)

The functional unit of the kidney—the uriniferous tubule—consists of the secretory highly coiled **nephron,** which is 30-40 mm long and involved in production of urine; and the excretory **collecting ducts,** which are about 20 mm long and are conduits for urine. They derive embryonically from different sources, which fuse during development: nephrons originate from *metanephric diverticulum;* collecting ducts, from *ureteric buds.* Both originate from *mesoderm.* A nephron is a blind-ended tubule composed of several parts, each with structure reflecting functional differences. The initial blind-ended part of the nephron is the **renal corpuscle,** which consists of a tuft of **glomerular capillaries** in the double-walled sac-like **Bowman capsule,** which is made of epithelium. It receives filtrate of blood from glomerular capillaries. The nephron also consists of a **proximal tubule,** a segment that makes a hairpin turn and is called the **loop of Henle,** and a **distal tubule.** The proximal tubule has convoluted, straight, and thin segments; the distal tubule, straight, macula densa, convoluted, and connecting parts. Henle's loop includes descending, thin ascending, medullary thick ascending, and cortical thick ascending limbs. Nephrons empty into collecting tubules, which coalesce to form larger collecting ducts in *medullary rays* and *pyramids* that reach the

papilla. Collecting ducts take urine to the *renal pelvis.* Usually, renal corpuscles and convoluted parts of proximal and distal tubules are in the **cortex,** but their straight parts are in medullary rays. About 80% of nephrons, the **cortical nephrons,** have short Henle's loops and are in the peripheral cortex; the other 20%, the **juxtamedullary nephrons,** are closer to the corticomedullary junction and have longer Henle's loops. Henle's loops and most collecting ducts are in the **medulla.** Each adult kidney has more than 1 million uriniferous tubules.

HISTORICAL POINT

Marcello Malpighi (1628-1694), an Italian histologist and pioneer in use of the microscope, discovered renal corpuscles and tubules, which were named for him (malpighian). He set the stage for later discoveries about the kidney. German anatomist and pathologist **Friedrich Gustav Henle** (1809-1885) published the first systematic treatise on histology and contributed to study of human epithelial tissues. The thin, looped part of the nephron bears his name. Sir **William Bowman** (1816-1892), an English histologist and ophthalmologist, used the microscope to describe many previously unknown body structures. He identified the capsule of the renal corpuscle—the Bowman capsule.

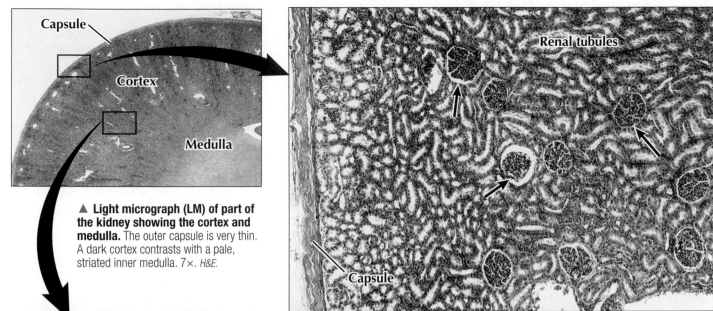

Capsule

Cortex

Medulla

▲ **Light micrograph (LM) of part of the kidney showing the cortex and medulla.** The outer capsule is very thin. A dark cortex contrasts with a pale, striated inner medulla. 7×. *H&E.*

Renal tubules

Capsule

▲ **LM of the outer part of the renal cortex.** The capsule is dense fibrous connective tissue. Spherical renal corpuscles (**arrows**) are interspersed with a tortuous network of closely packed, convoluted renal tubules, seen in transverse, oblique, and longitudinal views. Most in the cortical parenchyma are proximal and distal tubules. Very little intervening connective tissue is seen. 78×. *H&E.*

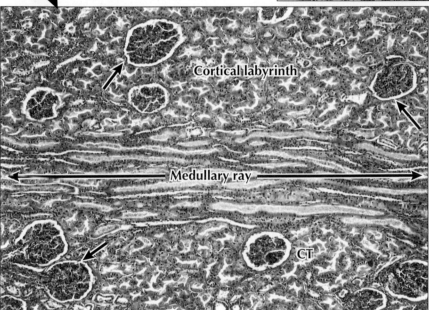

Cortical labyrinth

Medullary ray

CT

◀ **LM of a deeper part of the renal cortex.** Here, close to the corticomedullary junction, columns of straight tubules—medullary rays—radiate out from the medulla. They alternate with areas of cortical parenchyma, called cortical labyrinths, that contain renal corpuscles (**arrows**) and convoluted tubules. 78×. *H&E.*

16.4 HISTOLOGY AND FUNCTION OF THE RENAL CORTEX

A thin, tough outer **capsule** of **dense fibrous connective tissue** invests the kidney. It consists of regularly arranged *collagen fibers* interspersed with *fibroblasts.* The capsule is nearly nondistensible, loosely attached, and easily peeled off. The kidney and its capsule lie in a mass of *adipose tissue,* which cushions and protects the kidney. With routine stains, interstitial connective tissue in the kidney looks quite scanty and inconspicuous. It forms the *stroma,* which supports many blood vessels of various sizes that are closely associated with the renal **parenchyma.** The parenchyma consists of long, tortuous, tightly packed **renal tubules.** The cortex usually appears dark and granular because of its many spherical **renal corpuscles** and convoluted **uriniferous tubules.** Its uniform

granularity is mostly due to myriad **proximal** and **distal tubules** that are sectioned randomly in different planes. Corpuscles in the cortex are scattered between other parts of the uriniferous tubules. Each corpuscle, together with a renal tubule, constitutes a **nephron.** Corpuscles of **cortical nephrons** in the outer cortex are uniform in size; the slightly larger **juxtamedullary nephrons** are especially active in water reabsorption and urine concentration. Parallel groups of *loops of Henle* and *collecting ducts* form **medullary rays,** which extend into the cortex from the deeper medulla. Each medullary ray and its cortical parenchyma make up an ill-defined *renal lobule.* Blood filters through the glomerular capillary loops of each corpuscle into its renal tubule, and as filtrate passes down the segments of the renal tubule, it is modified by removal or addition of components, the ultimate product being urine.

▼ Histology of a renal corpuscle.

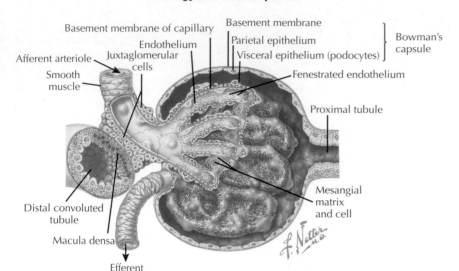

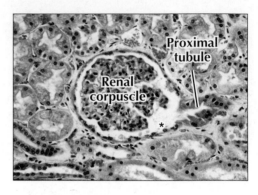

▲ **LM showing the urinary pole of a renal corpuscle.** Here, Bowman's space (∗) of the corpuscle is confluent with the lumen of a proximal tubule. 170×. *H&E.*

▶ **LM of a renal corpuscle and its juxtaglomerular complex (JG).** The parietal layer of Bowman's capsule (**arrows**), a simple squamous epithelium, surrounds Bowman's space (∗). The afferent arteriole forms a tuft of glomerular capillaries in the corpuscle. Erythrocytes (**RBC**) are in the lumina of these capillaries. Renal tubules in the area are sectioned transversely, obliquely, and longitudinally. Part of another corpuscle is seen (upper left). 470×. *H&E.*

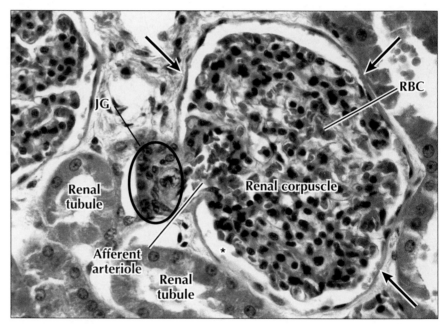

16.5 HISTOLOGY OF RENAL CORPUSCLES

At about 200 μm in diameter, the spherical renal corpuscles are just visible to the naked eye. They are found only in the **cortex** of the kidney and represent the initial, expanded part of the nephron. They have a *vascular pole* (where afferent and efferent arterioles enter and leave) and a *urinary pole* (where the proximal tubule begins). Each corpuscle consists of an epithelial part called **Bowman's capsule** and a vascular part consisting of a tuft of **glomerular capillaries** formed by a branching **afferent arteriole**. An **efferent arteriole** drains this lobulated tuft of 20-40 capillary loops. The double-layered epithelial Bowman's capsule forms the corpuscle's external covering. The outer layer of Bowman's capsule, the *parietal layer,* consists of **simple squamous epithelium** resting on an indistinct basement membrane. The inner *visceral layer* of the capsule consists of highly specialized cells called *podocytes.* Their name derives from the Greek and means foot-like cells. These highly branched podocytes are reflected over the capillary loops in direct contact with the **basement membrane**

of glomerular capillaries. The two layers of Bowman's capsule are continuous with each other at the vascular pole. **Bowman's (urinary) space** is between the two layers of the capsule and at the urinary pole becomes continuous with the proximal tubule lumen.

CLINICAL POINT

Immune, circulatory, and metabolic kidney diseases can affect renal corpuscles. These disorders can be evaluated via biopsy and light or electron microscopy. **Alport syndrome,** or **hereditary nephritis,** is an inherited progressive *nephropathy.* A genetic mutation results in abnormal type IV collagen in the glomerular basement membrane and leads to renal failure. Electron microscopy shows abnormal thickening of the basement membrane with irregular lamina densa splitting. Patients have blood (*hematuria*) and protein in urine, which is due to leakage of erythrocytes and plasma proteins across the defective membrane.

▼ **Fine structure of the renal corpuscle.**

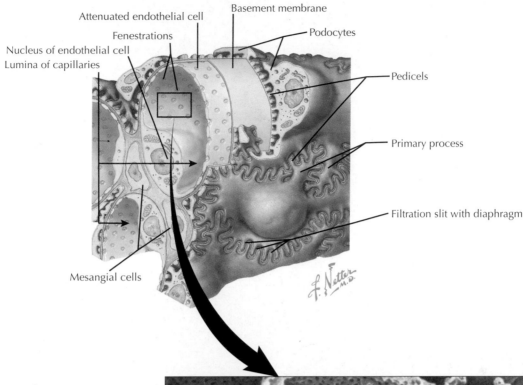

▶ **High-resolution scanning electron micrograph (HRSEM) of the luminal aspect of a glomerular capillary.** This three-dimensional perspective of fenestrated endothelium was taken from within the lumen, which is not easily done by conventional microscopy. Many round fenestrations of endothelial cells cause the sieve-like appearance. 10,000×.
(Courtesy of Dr. M. J. Hollenberg)

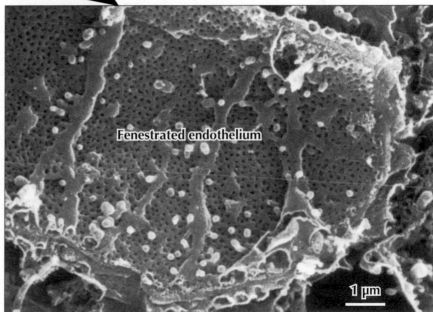

16.6 ULTRASTRUCTURE OF RENAL CORPUSCLES

The organization of renal corpuscles correlates with a role in *glomerular filtration, transport,* and *permeability.* The complex filter, through which fluid passes from blood in **glomerular capillaries** to **Bowman's (urinary) space,** comprises three distinct, closely apposed parts: **glomerular capillary endothelium,** intervening **basement membrane,** and **visceral layer** of *Bowman's capsule.* Lining glomerular capillaries is an attenuated endothelium with multiple **fenestrae,** each with an average diameter of 70 nm. Fenestrae lack **diaphragms,** are highly permeable, and are typically larger and more irregular in shape than those of fenestrated capillaries elsewhere in the body. Nuclei of endothelial cells sit close to the *mesangium* at the base of the capillary tuft where **mesangial cells** also reside. External to the endothelium is a continuous basement membrane formed by glomerular capillary endothelial cells and adjacent **podocytes.** Podocytes, highly specialized cells that form the visceral layer of Bowman's capsule, intimately embrace the outer endothelium. Each podocyte has several primary **processes (trabeculae),** which give rise to many secondary **processes** that end as **pedicels.** Pedicels of adjacent podocytes interdigitate and form a series of **filtration slits,** about 20-25 nm wide, between them. A thin, nonmembranous diaphragm—the **slit membrane**—spans each filtration slit.

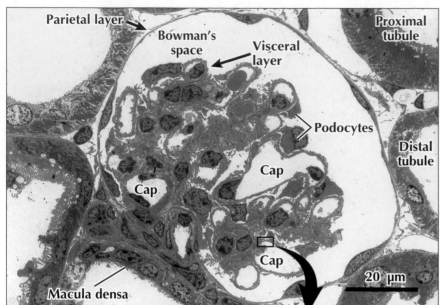

◄ **EM of a renal corpuscle at low magnification.** Between parietal and visceral layers of Bowman's capsule is Bowman's space, which in life contains glomerular filtrate. Loops of glomerular capillaries (**Cap**) are close to podocytes of the visceral layer. Proximal and distal tubules surround the corpuscle. The macula densa of the JG complex is also seen. 1000×.

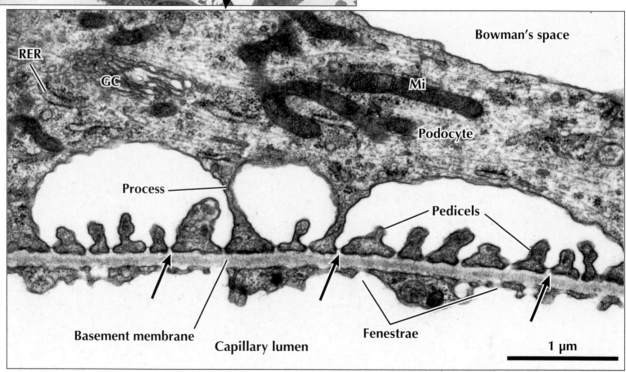

▲ **EM demonstrating the intricate renal filtration barrier in the renal corpuscle.** The endothelium of a glomerular capillary (**below**) is very attenuated and has many fenestrae. A Golgi complex (**GC**), scattered mitochondria (**Mi**), cisternae of rough endoplasmic reticulum (**RER**), and a criss-crossing network of cytoskeletal elements occupy the cytoplasm of the podocyte (at top). Its processes end as pedicels on the basement membrane. Membranes (**arrows**) span filtration slits between pedicels. 30,000×. *(Courtesy of Dr. W. A. Webber)*

16.7 ULTRASTRUCTURE AND FUNCTION OF RENAL CORPUSCLES

Transmission and scanning electron micrographs of renal corpuscles provide details of the **renal filtration barrier** related directly to function. Fluid from the **glomerular capillary** is filtered into **Bowman's space** by first passing through **fenestrae** of the **capillary endothelium.** High-resolution scanning electron microscopy is quite useful in providing surface views of fenestrated endothelium. Fenestrae are transcellular circular openings without diaphragms. Fluid passes through fenestrae and then the basement membrane, which is analogous to fine blotting or filter paper. It prevents passage of only large molecules. Fluid then passes through filtration slits between **pedicels** of **podocytes,** where a thin diaphragm, like a fine sieve, prevents passage of smaller molecules. The **basement membrane** between endothelium and podocyte is made of a central electron-dense layer, the *lamina densa,* and two external *laminae rara.* In humans, the glomerular basement membrane is 320-340 nm wide and consists of *laminin, fibronectin,* and several types of *collagen.* It also contains *proteoglycans* and *heparan sulfate*-rich anionic sites, which are arranged in a regular lattice-like network.

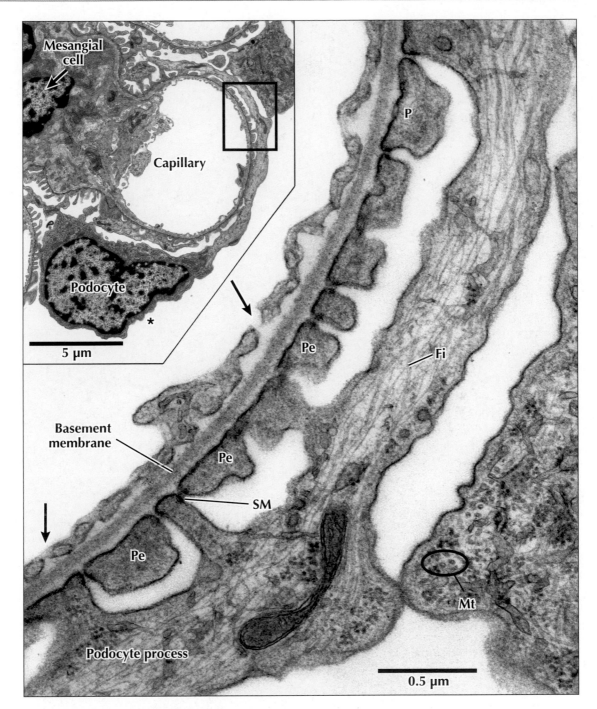

▲ **EMs of part of a renal corpuscle. Above left.** Relationship of mesangial cell, podocyte, and capillary to Bowman's space (✱). 5000×. **Below.** Details of the filtration barrier. Podocyte processes and pedicels (**Pe**) contain a network of cytoplasmic filaments (**Fi**) and microtubules (**Mt**). The basement membrane is between interlocking podocyte pedicels and fenestrated (**arrows**) endothelium of a glomerular capillary. The gaps forming the filtration slits between pedicels are spanned by slit membranes (**SM**). 53,000×.

16.8 ULTRASTRUCTURE AND FUNCTION OF THE RENAL FILTRATION BARRIER

The tripartite renal filtration barrier allows water and ions to pass from a capillary lumen to **Bowman's space** but retains large molecules and cells. **Pedicels** of **podocytes** interdigitate and envelop the abluminal aspect of the **glomerular capillary**. **Filtration slits** between pedicels are bridged by a ribbon-like filtration **slit mem-** brane that is 7-10 nm thick and has a unique filamentous mesh substructure. *Actin* **microfilaments** dominate podocyte cytoplasm, so these cells can contract and thereby widen the slits. **Mesangial cells** are between capillary loops, where they provide support and serve a phagocytic role in helping maintain **basement membrane** components. They can also contract, thus regulating blood flow in glomerular capillaries.

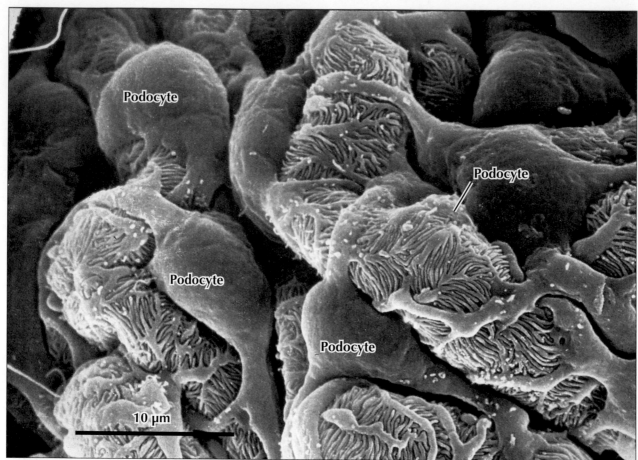

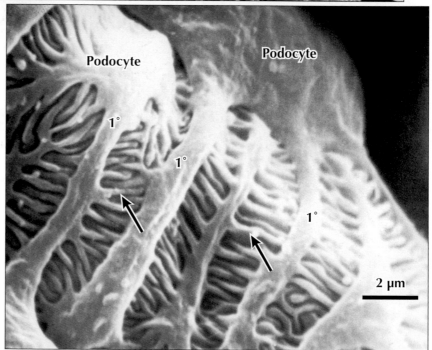

▲ **Low-magnification SEM of podocytes in a renal corpuscle.** Podocyte processes interdigitate on the outer surface of glomerular capillary walls. Bowman's space is external to the podocytes and in life contains glomerular filtrate. 4200×. *(Courtesy of Dr. T. Fujita)*

▶ **SEM of podocytes at higher magnification.** Primary (**1°**) and secondary (**arrows**) podocyte processes have regular shapes, sizes, and branching patterns with extensive interdigitation. 7800×. *(Courtesy of Dr. W. A. Webber)*

16.9 SCANNING ELECTRON MICROSCOPY OF RENAL PODOCYTES

Podocytes are highly modified epithelial cells with a remarkable ultrastructural appearance. Each cell body houses a nucleus and associated *cytoplasmic organelles*. Its three to six thick **primary processes** branch into multiple smaller **secondary processes.**

They may then divide into smaller branches or end directly as slender end-feet, named **pedicels,** which attach to the outer wall of **glomerular capillaries.** Each podocyte resembles an octopus perched on the outside of the capillary with its pedicels interdigitating with those of adjacent podocytes.

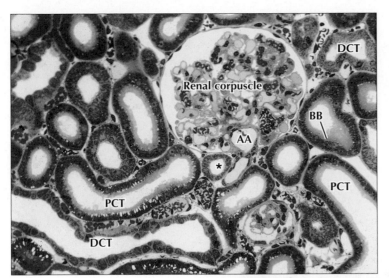

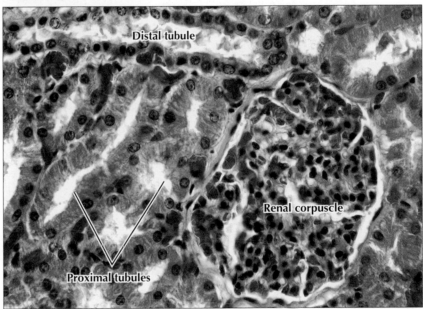

◄ ▼ Companion LMs of parts of the renal cortex.
The plastic section (**Left**) shows proximal (**PCT**) and distal
(**DCT**) convoluted tubules around a renal corpuscle.
Proximal tubules have prominent brush borders (**BB**)
and many clear vesicles in apical cytoplasm. Distal
tubules lack a brush border and have smaller, more
closely packed cells than do proximal tubules. An
afferent arteriole (**AA**) is at the vascular pole of the
corpuscle, close to the macula densa of a distal
tubule (✶). The paraffin LM (**Below**) shows several
proximal tubules and part of a distal tubule near a renal
corpuscle. Proximal tubules stain deeply and have
cells that are larger and more elongated than those
of distal tubules. Less numerous distal tubules have
pale cells. Plastic sections usually provide better
resolution than conventional paraffin sections.
Left: 270×. Toluidine blue, plastic section;
Below: 420×. *H&E.*

16.10 HISTOLOGY OF PROXIMAL AND DISTAL TUBULES

Proximal tubules are highly convoluted in the **cortex** and become straighter toward the **medulla.** The longest segment of the *nephron,* they constitute most of the cortical parenchyma. In transverse section, proximal tubules are round to oval. Usually four to six round nuclei are in the center or toward the base of each cell. Their walls, made of simple cuboidal or low columnar epithelium, surround a central, irregularly shaped lumen. Many *mitochondria* in the cytoplasm make the lining cells of proximal tubules appear granular and intensely eosinophilic. Proximal tubules have a shaggy inner border because apical cell margins bear many **microvilli** that make up a prominent **brush border.** Lateral cell borders are usually indistinct by light microscopy, partly because of extensive interdigitations. Distal tubules, however, are divided into a *thick ascending limb* and a **distal convoluted tubule.** Distal tubules are easily distinguished from proximal tubules: they are shorter than proximal tubules; their convolutions are less complex; smaller, less eosinophilic cuboidal cells line them; they

have smaller diameters; and the lumen is typically wider than that of proximal tubules. A brush border is absent in distal tubules, but cells may bear occasional stubby microvilli. The cells also show *basal striations,* which are due, just as in proximal tubule cells, to mitochondria in channels created by infolding of basal *plasma membrane.* These features are best seen by electron microscopy.

CLINICAL POINT

Acute tubular necrosis is a serious disorder with the histologic feature of destruction of epithelial cells of proximal and distal tubules, which leads to impaired renal function. Tubular cells are especially vulnerable to ischemia and toxins, in that they have a high rate of energy consumption and can absorb and concentrate toxins. They are thus susceptible to interference with oxidative and other metabolic pathways. Sloughing and necrosis of epithelial cells, plus a denuded brush border, lead to tubular obstruction and increased intraluminal pressure. This disorder is the most common cause of **acute renal failure.**

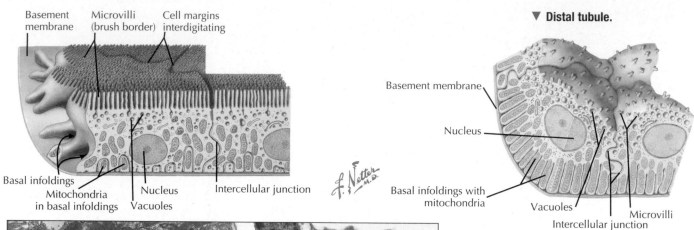

▼ **Proximal tubule.**

Basement membrane · Microvilli (brush border) · Cell margins interdigitating

Basal infoldings · Mitochondria in basal infoldings · Nucleus · Vacuoles · Intercellular junction

▼ **Distal tubule.**

Basement membrane · Nucleus · Basal infoldings with mitochondria · Vacuoles · Intercellular junction · Microvilli

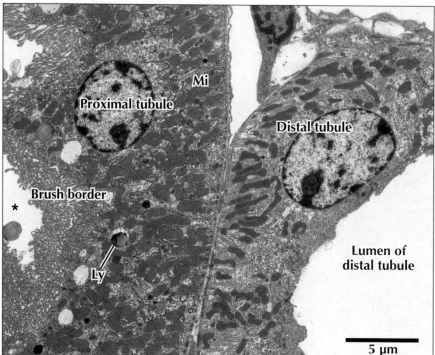

Mi

Proximal tubule

Distal tubule

Brush border

*

Ly

Lumen of distal tubule

5 µm

◄ **EM of parts of proximal and distal convoluted tubules.** Proximal tubule cells are usually more robust in size and in content of organelles and surface specializations than distal tubule cells. An elaborate apical brush border protrudes into the lumen (*) of the proximal tubule; distal tubule cells lack a brush border. Mitochondria (**Mi**) and lysosomes (**Ly**) are larger and more numerous in the proximal tubule, and lateral cell borders are indistinct in both. Cells of both tubules have round euchromatic nuclei. 4000×.

16.11 ULTRASTRUCTURE AND FUNCTION OF PROXIMAL AND DISTAL TUBULES

Despite subtle differences, the ultrastructure of both proximal and distal tubules reflects a role in *absorption* and *transport*. Most absorption occurs in the proximal tubule, so its cells usually have a greater variety of cytoplasmic **organelles** (e.g., **lysosomes**) and **inclusions** than distal tubule cells. Many tightly packed **microvilli** of the apical **brush border** in proximal tubules provide an enormous surface area for reabsorption of solutes and water from the lumen. For better diffusion, elaborate infoldings of basal **plasma membranes** increase surface area in both types of tubules. These folds also allow proximity of basal cell membranes and **mitochondria.** The arrangement of mitochondria, which are elongated and longitudinally oriented, creates a pattern of *basal striations*. These features are consistent with providing energy for active transport, both secretory and absorptive. Also, apical cytoplasm in proximal tubules has many *canaliculi* that open into the lumen between microvilli and engage in absorption. *Endocytotic vesicles* arise from

canaliculi and are close to apical cell membranes. Lateral cell membranes in both types of tubules interdigitate in a complex way, so that cell boundaries look irregular and separate cells are often hard to see. Cells of both tubule types also have one spherical **nucleus,** which is usually *euchromatic*.

CLINICAL POINT

Renal cell carcinoma, usually arising from proximal tubule epithelium, accounts for more than 90% of malignant kidney tumors. It is characterized by a lack of early warning signs, diverse clinical signs, and resistance to treatment by radiation or chemotherapy once *metastasis* has occurred. Both sporadic (nonhereditary) and hereditary forms are associated with structural alterations of the short arm of chromosome 3. Genetic studies of families at high risk for this carcinoma have led to cloning of genes (tumor suppressors or oncogenes) whose alteration causes tumor. Less common kidney tumors are *transitional cell carcinoma, Wilms' tumor,* and *renal sarcoma*.

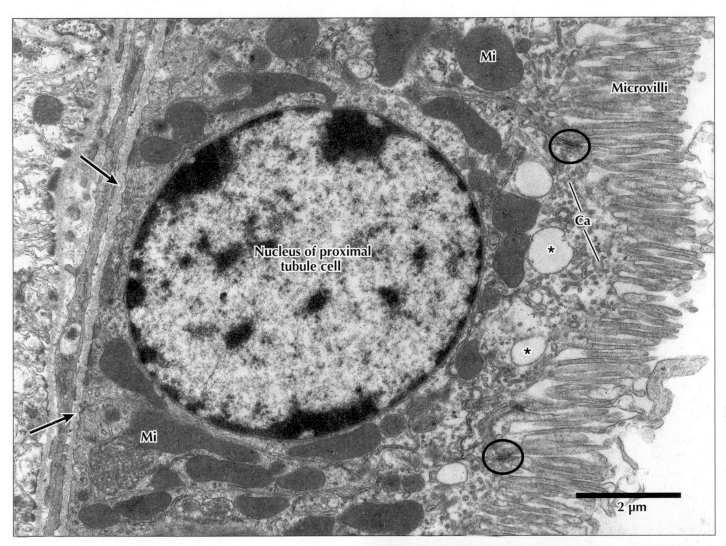

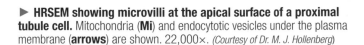

▲ **EM of the wall of a proximal tubule.** The wall consists of simple low columnar epithelium. Each cell has a spherical euchromatic nucleus surrounded by cytoplasm filled with organelles. An apical brush border of many closely packed microvilli lines the lumen. Apical canaliculi (**Ca**), numerous vesicles (∗), and many pleomorphic mitochondria (**Mi**) are seen. A thin basement membrane underlies the basal aspect of the cell (**arrows**). Intercellular junctions (**circles**) link apical membranes of adjacent cells. 14,000×.

▶ **HRSEM showing microvilli at the apical surface of a proximal tubule cell.** Mitochondria (**Mi**) and endocytotic vesicles under the plasma membrane (**arrows**) are shown. 22,000×. *(Courtesy of Dr. M. J. Hollenberg)*

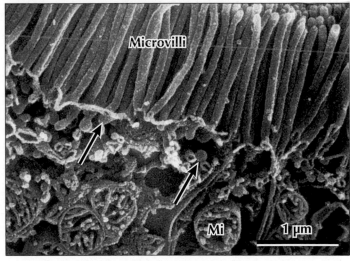

16.12 ULTRASTRUCTURE AND FUNCTION OF PROXIMAL TUBULES

Epithelial cells lining the lumen of proximal tubules are simple cuboidal to columnar with a distinctive, prominent **brush border.** Tightly packed **microvilli** are up to 1 μm long. Extensive interdigitations of **plasma membranes,** which are linked by **intercellular junctions,** make lateral cell boundaries indistinct. The large, abundant **mitochondria** have densely packed internal *cristae.* Apical parts of cells show tubular invaginations of the cell membrane and many **vesicles** and **canaliculi** in the cytoplasm. These morphologic features are consistent with epithelial cells involved in active transport. Proximal tubules resorb more than 60% of the glomerular filtrate, including most of the water, glucose, amino acids, bicarbonate, ascorbic acid, and all of the protein.

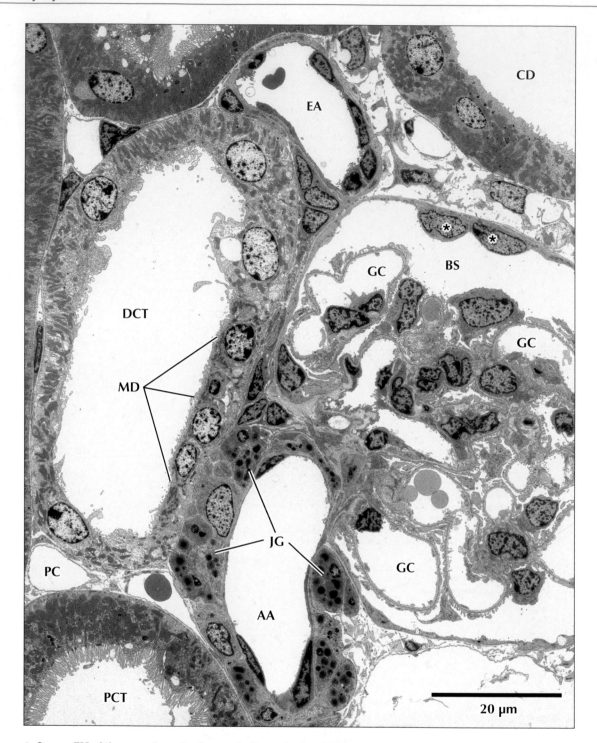

▲ **Survey EM of the vascular pole of a renal corpuscle showing features of the JG complex.** JG cells in the wall of an afferent arteriole (**AA**) are closely apposed to the macula densa (**MD**) of a distal convoluted tubule (**DCT**). A proximal convoluted tubule (**PCT**), peritubular capillary (**PC**), efferent arteriole (**EA**), and collecting duct (**CD**) are seen, as are glomerular capillaries (**GC**) and Bowman's space (**BS**). Nuclei of simple squamous cells of the parietal layer of Bowman's capsule are indicated (★). 1750×.

16.13   ULTRASTRUCTURE OF THE JUXTAGLOMERULAR COMPLEX

The juxtaglomerular (JG) complex near the **vascular pole** of the **renal corpuscle** has several components. The ascending thick limb of the **distal tubule** returns to the renal cortex and contacts the vascular pole of its own renal corpuscle between **afferent** and **efferent arterioles.** At this contact site, a cluster of dark-stained cuboidal cells with closely packed nuclei constitutes the **macula densa** of the distal tubule. These distinctive epithelial cells, plus JG cells of the afferent arteriole and pale *(lacis)* cells of the extraglomerular mesangium, make up the JG complex. JG cells are modified *smooth muscle cells* in the tunica media of the afferent arteriole and are closely related, functionally and structurally, to the macula densa, separated by only a thin *basement membrane.* JG cells have conspicuous Golgi-derived *secretory granules* and secrete the hormone *renin* into the circulation.

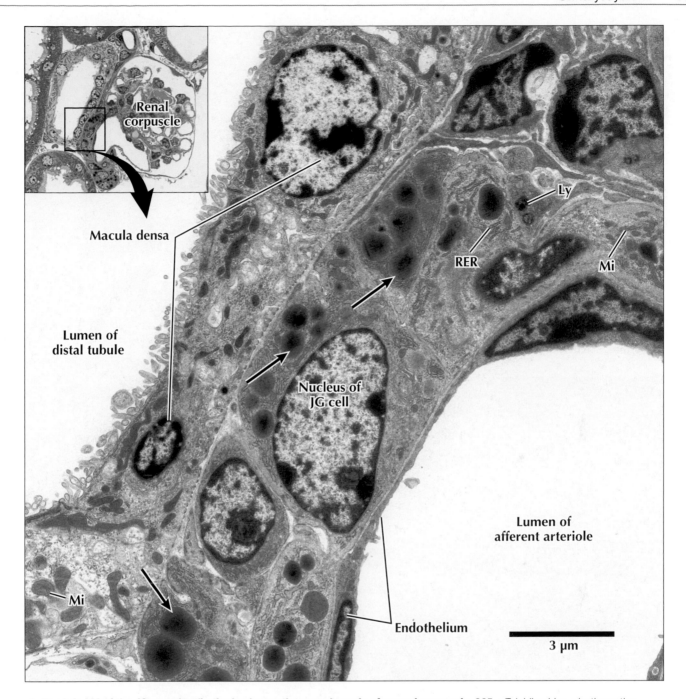

▲ **Top left. LM of the JG complex (in the box) near the vascular pole of a renal corpuscle.** 365×. Toluidine blue, plastic section.
Bottom. EM showing details of the macula densa of a distal tubule and JG cells in the tunica media of an afferent arteriole.
Electron-dense JG granules (**arrows**) dominate JG cell cytoplasm. Both distal tubule and JG cells contain many mitochondria (**Mi**). A lysosome (**Ly**) and several cisternae of rough endoplasmic reticulum (**RER**) are also in the JG cell. Flattened endothelial cells line the afferent arteriole lumen. 7500×.

16.14 ULTRASTRUCTURE AND FUNCTION OF CELLS OF THE JUXTAGLOMERULAR COMPLEX

Large oval to elongated JG cells have an eccentric **nucleus;** many small **mitochondria; rough endoplasmic reticulum;** a well-developed *Golgi complex;* and **secretory vesicles,** which are called **JG granules.** These membrane-bound vesicles (10-40 nm in diameter) have a moderately electron-dense core, often with a crystalline interior. They contain the hormone *renin* or its precursor and are polarized toward the cell membrane, adjacent to the afferent arteriole endothelium. Rather than contract, these modified smooth muscle cells secrete the hormone and release it into the lumen of the afferent arteriole. Renin regulates systemic arterial blood pressure and influences sodium ion (Na^+) concentration. Renin is also engaged in feedback control of glomerular filtration rate in individual nephrons via the *renin-angiotensin system.* Cells of the **macula densa** are narrow, closely packed epithelial cells of the **distal tubule.** They have many organelles, including a prominent Golgi complex, that are oriented toward the basal surface and face JG cells. The macula densa monitors Na^+ levels and ultrafiltrate volume in the distal tubule lumen.

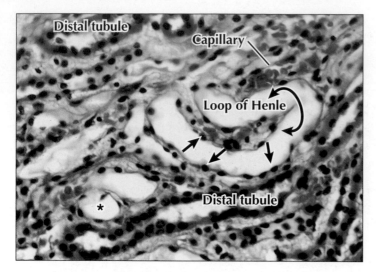

▲ **LM of loops of Henle in the renal medulla**. One—in the shape of a hairpin loop (**curved arrow**)—is sectioned longitudinally. It is lined by a thin layer of simple squamous epithelial cells, which have nuclei (**small arrows**) protruding into the lumen. Another loop (∗) is sectioned transversely. Other areas contain blood capillaries and ascending (straight) portions of distal tubules. 370×. *H&E.*

▼ **Thin segment.**

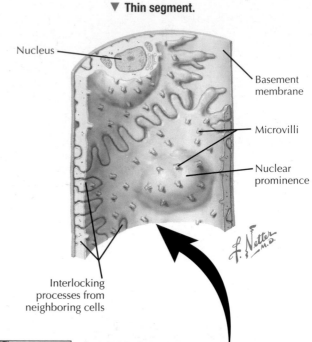

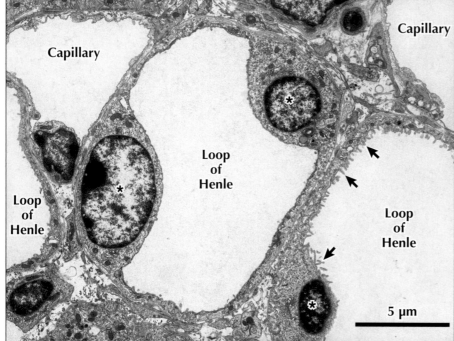

▲ **EM of loops of Henle in transverse section.** Loops consist of flattened epithelial cells with nuclei (∗) that bulge slightly into the lumen. Short, stubby microvilli (**arrows**) are on apical cell surfaces. Capillaries that form the vasa recta are close to the loops and have very thin walls. 5000×.

▲ **EM of a loop of Henle in transverse section.** Interlocking cell processes form its simple squamous epithelium. Sparse organelles, such as vesicles (**Ve**) and a few lysosomes (**Ly**), characterize the cytoplasm. Adjacent cells have intercellular junctions (**circles**). Except for a somewhat thicker wall and lack of blood cells, Henle's loops resemble systemic capillaries. 4000×. *(Courtesy of Dr. W. A. Webber)*

16.15 HISTOLOGY AND ULTRASTRUCTURE OF LOOPS OF HENLE (THIN SEGMENTS)

Loops of Henle—thin segments—are located in the *renal medulla* and are made of **simple squamous epithelium** that rests on a thin basement membrane. The segments, 12-15 μm in diameter, have a relatively large lumen. The flattened cells are 1-2 μm thick and have lenticular, closely spaced nuclei that protrude into the lumen. Henle's loops closely resemble blood capillaries, but their epithelium is thicker than the endothelium of surrounding capillaries.

Adjacent epithelial **cell processes** in Henle's loops usually interdigitate, so electron microscopy shows up to 12 or more processes in transverse section with relatively few nuclei. **Intercellular junctions,** including *tight junctions* and *desmosomes,* link cell processes laterally. There are few, if any, short, stubby *microvilli* on apical surfaces. Highly permeable to water, Henle's loops play a role in the *countercurrent multiplication* part of urinary concentration by setting up a concentration gradient in tissue fluid.

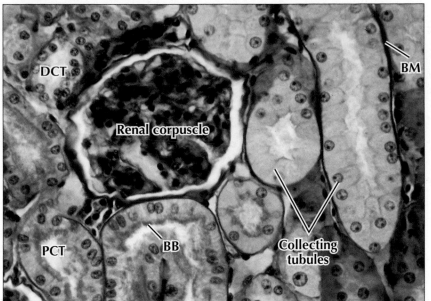

◄ **LM of collecting tubules in the renal cortex.** Lined by large, pale cells with round nuclei, the tubules normally cross medullary rays that penetrate the cortex. The brush border (**BB**) of proximal tubules (**PCT**), the basement membrane (**BM**) of renal tubules, and Bowman's capsule of the renal corpuscle show a positive (magenta) reaction to this stain. A distal convoluted tubule (**DCT**) is also seen. 440×. *PAS.*

▼ **LM of collecting tubules and loops of Henle in the renal medulla in transverse section.** Simple cuboidal to low columnar epithelium characterizes collecting tubules (★); the smaller loops of Henle are made of simple squamous epithelium. Vasa recta filled with erythrocytes are in the stroma. These vessels are intimately associated with loops of Henle and collecting ducts and function as countercurrent exchangers. 810×. *H&E.*

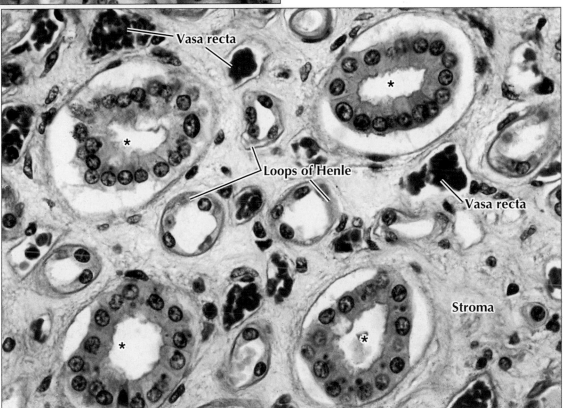

16.16 HISTOLOGY OF COLLECTING DUCTS

Collecting tubules, which join **distal convoluted tubules** to collecting ducts, vary in diameter from 40 μm in proximal parts to 200 μm as they approach collecting ducts in the *renal pelvis*. Conduits for urine, they begin in the **cortex** as *arched collecting tubules,* which extend toward the **medulla** in *medullary rays.* They then merge with other arched tubules to form *straight collecting tubules* that run in the medulla. In the medulla's inner zone, six or seven straight tubules join at acute angles to form the terminal *papillary duct of Bellini.* At tips of *medullary pyramids,* papillary ducts perforate the *renal papilla* to form the *area cribrosa.* In transverse section, most collecting tubules show a large lumen; proximal and distal tubules have relatively narrow lumina. Along their extent, the collecting tubule diameter gradually increases, as does the height of the epithelium. Lining cells bulging into the lumen form a **simple epithelium,** which ranges from cuboidal to low columnar. Their bases rest on a thin **basement membrane,** and their apical surfaces contact a large central lumen. A lack of intercellular projections or invaginations makes lateral cell borders more distinct than in other parts of the *uriniferous tubule.* Each cell has a round, central nucleus, pale cytoplasm, and relative paucity of *organelles* when compared with other parts of the uriniferous tubule. Around nuclei is often a halo pattern, which is due mostly to *glycogen* that by light microscopy usually looks washed out.

▼ Collecting tubule (duct).

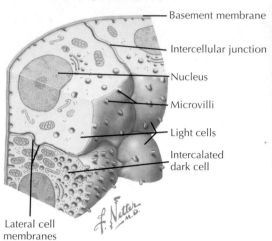

Basement membrane
Intercellular junction
Nucleus
Microvilli
Light cells
Intercalated dark cell

Lateral cell membranes

f. Netter M.D.

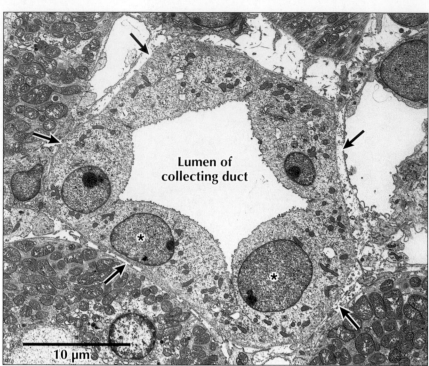

Lumen of collecting duct

10 μm

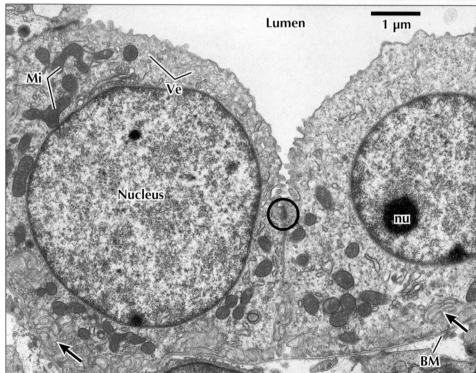

Lumen
1 μm

Mi
Ve
Nucleus
nu
BM

▲ **EM of a collecting duct in transverse section.** One continuous layer of cuboidal epithelial cells (**arrows**) lines the lumen. Convex apical borders of the cells contact the duct lumen. Each cell has a rounded nucleus (★) and cytoplasm packed with various organelles. 3000×.

◄ **EM showing parts of two epithelial cells of a collecting duct.** The rounded, euchromatic nucleus often has a nucleolus (**nu**). Randomly oriented mitochondria (**Mi**) are dispersed in the cytoplasm. Many small vesicles (**Ve**) are in apical cytoplasm. Short basal infoldings of plasma membrane (**arrows**) increase surface area and contain ion pumps. Tight junctions (**circle**) link apicolateral cell borders and seal the lumen from the extracellular space. Cells rest on a thin basement membrane (**BM**). 13,000×.

16.17 ULTRASTRUCTURE AND FUNCTION OF COLLECTING DUCTS

As a rule, collecting ducts have two types of epithelial cells with subtle ultrastructural differences—**light (principal) cells** and **dark (intercalated) cells**—that likely represent different functional stages. Dark cells, which may play a more active role in urine acidification, have more organelles, **apical vesicles,** and **basal infoldings** than do light cells. Apical surfaces of dark cells also have more numerous and stubby **microvilli;** light cells may bear a single cilium. **Tight junctions** connect both cell types; basal plasma membranes rest on a thin **basement membrane.** Collecting tubules take urine from *nephrons* to the renal pelvis, with some water absorption, which is controlled by *antidiuretic hormone* (ADH) from the posterior pituitary. ADH increases water permeability in collecting ducts; aldosterone from the zona glomerulosa of the adrenal cortex mainly regulates reabsorption of Na^+ and Cl^-. Collecting ducts also actively secrete H^+ and HCO_3 and reabsorb K^+. Thus, not only are collecting ducts conduits, but they also play a role in concentrating *urine* and regulating *acid-base balance.*

◄ **Section through the pronephros.**

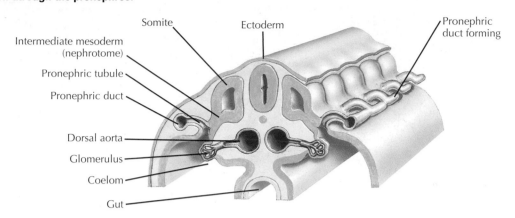

Somite — Ectoderm — Pronephric duct forming

Intermediate mesoderm (nephrotome) — Pronephric tubule — Pronephric duct — Dorsal aorta — Glomerulus — Coelom — Gut

▶ **Topography of the pronephros, mesonephros, and metanephric primordium.**

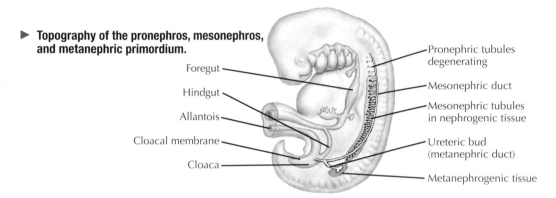

Foregut — Hindgut — Allantois — Cloacal membrane — Cloaca

Pronephric tubules degenerating — Mesonephric duct — Mesonephric tubules in nephrogenic tissue — Ureteric bud (metanephric duct) — Metanephrogenic tissue

◄ **Section through the mesonephros.**

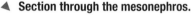

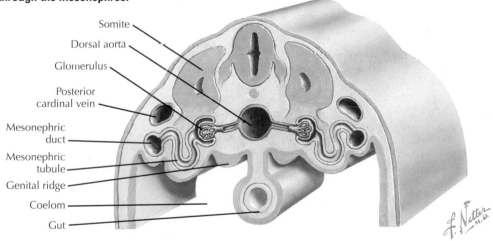

Somite — Dorsal aorta — Glomerulus — Posterior cardinal vein — Mesonephric duct — Mesonephric tubule — Genital ridge — Coelom — Gut

16.18 PRONEPHROS, MESONEPHROS, AND METANEPHROS

The **urinary** and **genital** (reproductive) **systems** develop in close association in the embryo, and kidney development recapitulates phylogeny. Both systems arise from **mesoderm:** At 4 weeks of gestation, **intermediate mesoderm** separates from successive somites to form segmentally arranged **nephrotomes,** which are just lateral to the genital ridge. They give rise, in a cranial to caudal direction, to three successive kidneys—pronephros, mesonephros, and metanephros. The pronephros forms seven pairs of pronephric tubules and a pronephric duct, which extends to the caudal part of the embryo to reach the cloaca. The vestigial and

nonfunctional human pronephros is quickly replaced caudally by the mesonephros, which serves briefly as an excretory organ in the fetus. The mesonephros consists of tubules that fuse with an extension of the pronephric duct, called the **mesonephric (wolffian) duct.** Successive formation of tubules in the caudal part of intermediate mesoderm continues for several weeks, with degeneration of tubules more cranially. Primitive renal glomeruli form in the mesonephros between blind ends of tubules and capillaries derived from branches of the dorsal aorta. The transitory mesonephros drains embryonic urine into the cloaca. After mesonephros regression, the metanephros (permanent kidney) appears in the fifth week of gestation.

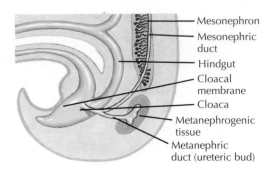

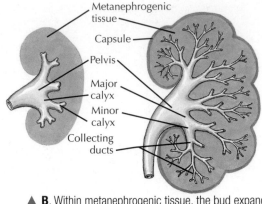

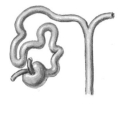

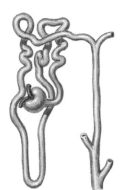

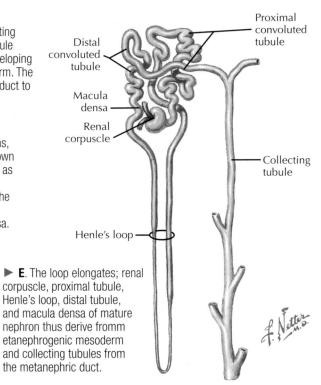

▲ **A**. The metanephric duct (ureteric bud) has grown out from the mesonephric duct, close to termination of latter in cloaca, and has invaded metanephrogenic mesoderm.

▲ **B**. Within metanephrogenic tissue, the bud expands to form a pelvis, which branches into calyces, which, in turn, bud into successive collecting ducts.

◄ **C**. Distal ends of collecting ducts connect with the tubule system of the nephron developing from metanephric mesoderm. The nephron extends from the duct to the renal corpuscle.

◄ **D**. The tubule lengthens, coils, and begins to dip down toward to the renal pelvis, as Henle's loop; one part of the tubule stays close to the glomerular mouth, as the future macula densa.

► **E**. The loop elongates; renal corpuscle, proximal tubule, Henle's loop, distal tubule, and macula densa of mature nephron thus derive fromm etanephrogenic mesoderm and collecting tubules from the metanephric duct.

16.19   DEVELOPMENT OF THE METANEPHROS

The metanephros consists of two mesodermally derived parts: the **ureteric bud** and **metanephrogenic tissue.** The bud—an outgrowth of the mesonephric duct—gives rise to **ureters, renal pelvis, renal calyces, collecting ducts,** and **collecting tubules.** These tubules undergo dichotomous branching, and by the 20th developmental week, about 10-12 generations of ducts have formed. Pelvis and calyces also enlarge. Metanephrogenic tissue from the caudal part of intermediate mesoderm gives rise to remaining parts of **nephrons: proximal** and **distal tubules, Henle's loop,** and **Bowman's capsule** of the **renal corpuscle.** Terminal branches of collecting tubules are first covered at distal ends by cellular aggregates of metanephrogenic tissue. These aggregates form hollow vesicles that become primitive tubules with a central lumen, which then become nephrons. The tubules, lined by *simple epithelium,* become covered externally by continuous *basement membrane,* elongate, and eventually reach their

convoluted adult form. Epithelium covering distal (free) ends of the tubules becomes flattened and is invaded by a tuft of *glomerular capillaries* to form a renal corpuscle. The primitive nephron lines up with the collecting tubule and the two fuse to form a passage for urine.

CLINICAL POINT

Wilms' tumor (or **nephroblastoma**) is a malignant tumor of the kidney in infants and children. It presents as an abdominal mass with *hematuria* (blood in urine). As the tumor progresses it invades, permeates, and replaces the whole kidney. Histologically, tumor cells form cords resembling fetal kidney. They consist of immature and mature mesenchymal tissues mingled with abortive glomeruli and renal tubules. Loss of the growth-regulating gene *WT-1* probably causes the tumor, which likely originates during differentiation of kidneys from metanephric mesodermal blastema. Surgery and chemotherapy result in fairly effective cures.

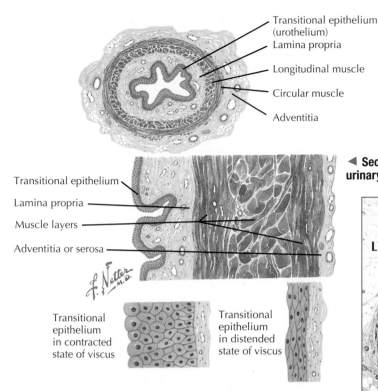

Transitional epithelium (urothelium)
Lamina propria

◄ **Section through the ureter.**

Longitudinal muscle

Circular muscle

Adventitia

Transitional epithelium

Lamina propria

Muscle layers

Adventitia or serosa

◄ **Section through the urinary bladder.**

Transitional epithelium in contracted state of viscus

Transitional epithelium in distended state of viscus

► **LM of the ureter in transverse section.** The irregular stellate contracted lumen is lined by urothelium, which rests on a lamina propria of loose connective tissue. Two layers of loosely arranged smooth muscle are easily seen in the upper part of the ureter; three layers occur in its lower part. An adventitia surrounds the ureter externally. 37×. *H&E.*

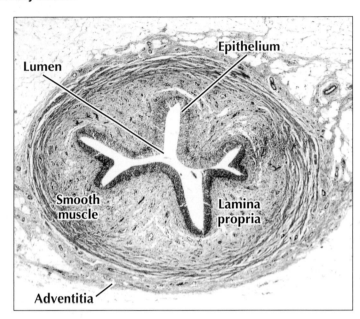

Epithelium

Lumen

Smooth muscle

Lamina propria

Adventitia

16.20 HISTOLOGY OF THE URETERS AND URINARY BLADDER

The ureters and urinary bladder follow a common histologic plan, with walls made of four concentric layers. First, a **urothelium (transitional epithelium)** lines the **lumen** and is expandable. Epithelium in the upper part of the ureter consists of two or three cell layers; it gradually changes to four or five layers in the lower third. The bladder has five to seven layers. Epithelium thickness depends on the degree of distention and varies markedly from thinner in the distended state to relatively thick in the collapsed (or empty) state. Plasma membranes of the most superficial epithelial cells, which are in direct contact with the lumen, have an accordion-like pleating capability. Also, the epithelium is almost impermeable to movement of water or ions, so the concentration of urine remains fairly constant as it passes down ureters into the bladder. Second, an underlying cellular and fibrous **lamina propria** supports the epithelium. Epithelium and lamina propria together constitute the *mucosa* (or *mucous membrane*) of both ureters and bladder. Third, a *muscularis externa* consists of **smooth muscle** arranged in layers that are opposite in orientation to those in the digestive tract wall. An outer oblique layer is found, especially in the bladder, but it is irregularly arranged, so it is not well defined. The fourth, outer layer is an **adventitia** (or **serosa**), which consists mostly of **loose connective tissue** with autonomic nerves and plexuses, blood vessels, and lymphatics.

CLINICAL POINT

Urinary incontinence—involuntary loss of bladder control and voiding of urine—is common in the elderly and is more prevalent in women than in men. Normal neurologic control of bladder and urethral function involves smooth muscle receptors for neurotransmitters of both sympathetic and parasympathetic nervous systems. Many neurologic disorders and systemic diseases may cause it, urinary tract infection being a common one; drugs may also disrupt normal function.

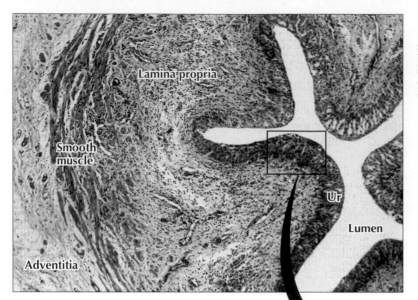

◀ **LM of the wall of the ureter in transverse section.** Urothelium (**Ur**) lines the star-shaped lumen. The lamina propria is highly vascular and cellular connective tissue. Interlacing smooth muscle bundles occupy the muscularis externa, which is invested by an outer adventitia. 75×. *H&E.*

▶ **Higher magnification LM of the mucosa of the ureter showing details of the multilayer urothelium.** Surface cells of the epithelium appear rounded when the ureter is contracted (empty) and flattened when it is distended with urine. The richly cellular lamina propria has many small blood vessels. 340×. *H&E.*

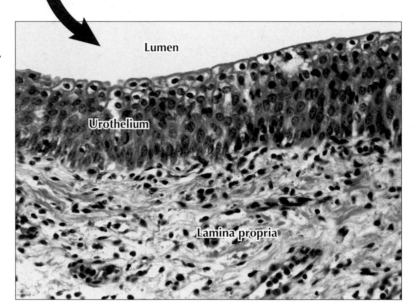

16.21 HISTOLOGY OF THE URETERS

The ureters are hollow fibromuscular tubes, each 4-5 mm in diameter and 14 cm long, that deliver urine, via waves of peristaltic **smooth muscle** contraction, from the *renal pelvis* to the *urinary bladder.* The wall is made of **mucosa,** which consists of **urothelium** that rests on a **lamina propria** of fairly dense collagenous and elastic **connective tissue.** The lamina propria is less dense and more cellular in deeper areas near the *muscularis externa.* This highly distensible layer allows marked changes in lumen caliber. The lamina propria also contains variable amounts of diffuse *lymphatic tissue* and occasionally small *lymphoid nodules.* Unlike the digestive tract with a distinct *submucosa,* no submucosa is found in either ureters or bladder. The muscularis externa of the upper two-thirds of the ureter has two layers of smooth muscle—an inner longitudinal and an outer circular. The lowest part of the ureter contains a third, discontinuous layer of longitudinal smooth muscle, outside the circular layer. This layer becomes more prominent in the bladder. All three smooth muscle layers are loosely arranged with variable amounts of areolar connective tissue with

the muscle cells. *Plexuses* of both *myelinated* and *unmyelinated nerve fibers* occur between the muscle layers. The ureters pierce the bladder wall obliquely as they enter it, so their walls are pressed together when the bladder fills with urine, which helps prevent backflow. The **adventitia** of loose connective tissue blends imperceptibly with that of surrounding structures.

CLINICAL POINT

The common condition **urolithiasis—kidney stones** or **renal calculi**—occurs mostly in males. Most stones form in the calyces or renal pelvis and either stay there or move to lower parts of the urinary tract. A pliable urothelium, which can stretch without rupturing, and longitudinal mucosal folds in the ureter usually allow unimpeded passage of stones. Severe cases, however, may involve urinary obstruction and erosion of urinary mucosa, causing blood in urine *(hematuria).* The many causes include *urinary infection, inborn errors of metabolism* (such as *hereditary cystinuria*), and *hyperparathyroidism,* which leads to increased excretion of calcium salts.

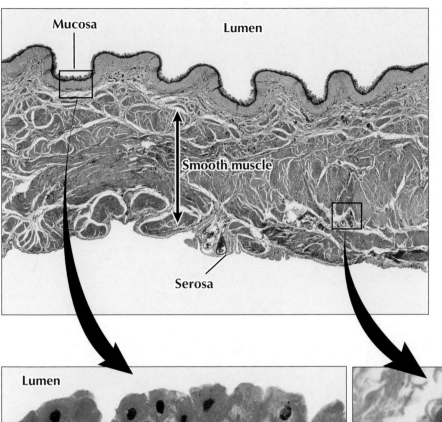

◄ **LM of the wall of the urinary bladder in transverse section.** The mucosa, according to the degree of distention, may look corrugated, with irregular longitudinal folds created by shape changes. Smooth muscle in the muscularis externa is thicker than that of the ureter. The superior bladder surface is covered externally by a serosa of peritoneum rather than by adventitia, the usual outer layer in the rest of the bladder. The serosa consists of connective tissue covered externally by thin, simple squamous epithelium made of a continuous layer of mesothelial cells (not seen at this magnification). 17×. *H&E.*

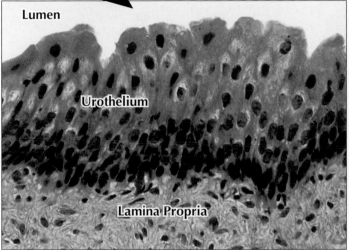

▲ **LM of the mucosa of the bladder at high magnification.** In the empty bladder the urothelium has an increased thickness—up to 8-10 cell layers. The lamina propria is highly fibrous with scattered connective tissue cells and a few capillaries. 420×. *H&E.*

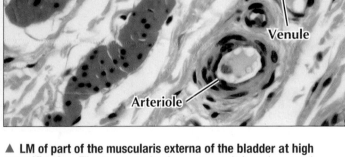

▲ **LM of part of the muscularis externa of the bladder at high magnification.** Fibrous connective tissue surrounds irregular smooth muscle cell bundles. An arteriole and venule are in the area. 420×. *H&E.*

16.22 HISTOLOGY OF THE URINARY BLADDER

Layers of the urinary bladder wall are basically the same as those of the lower part of the ureter: **urothelium, lamina propria,** three layers of **smooth muscle,** and **adventitia** or **serosa.** The epithelium thickness varies according to the degree of distention of the organ. In the contracted (empty) bladder, the urothelium is six to eight cell layers thick, and the most superficial cells are round to pear-shaped. Surface cells of this stratified epithelium can change shape and position by sliding over each other, so that when the bladder is distended, the cells are in only three or four layers and the cells become flattened. Electron microscopy shows apical plasma membranes of surface cells to possess unusually thick *plaques,* and apical cytoplasm to contain *fusiform vesicles.* Also, *desmosomes* and adluminal *tight junctions* link lateral borders of the cells. These features correlate with a tight permeability barrier; thus, the epithelium and underlying tissues are impermeable to urine. Lamina propria supports the epithelium and contains small blood vessels that provide oxygen and nutrients to the epithelium. The prominent muscularis externa is arranged in inner and outer longitudinal and middle circular layers. Smooth muscle bundles of the different layers are closely associated, so the three layers are often difficult to discern as discrete.

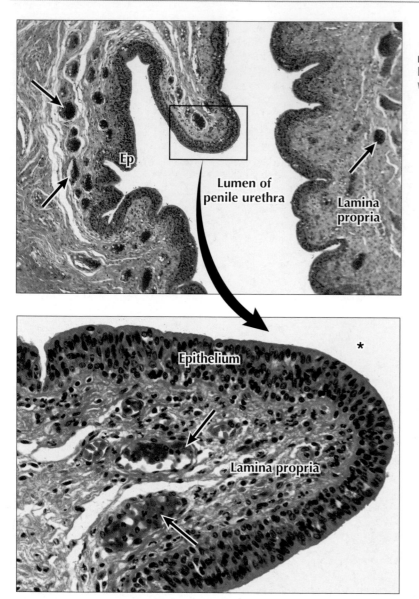

◀ **LM of the penile urethra showing key features at low magnification.** The mucosa has folds and pit-like invaginations. Deep to the epithelium (**Ep**) is an underlying lamina propria, which is richly vascularized (**arrows**). 65×. *H&E.*

▼ **Female Urethra.**

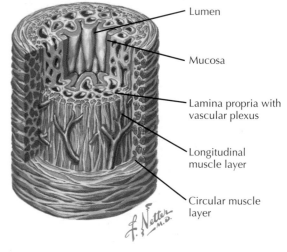

▲ **LM of the mucosa of the penile urethra at higher magnification.** Stratified columnar epithelium lines the lumen (∗). A rich vascular plexus (**arrows**) occupies the lamina propria. 260×. *H&E.*

16.23 HISTOLOGY OF THE MALE AND FEMALE URETHRA

The male urethra, 15-20 cm long, carries urine from the urinary bladder to the penile opening and is a conduit for semen during ejaculation. It is divided into three segments: *prostatic, membranous,* and *spongy.* The prostatic urethra, passing from the bladder to cross the *prostate gland,* is lined by **urothelium** with intervening patches of **stratified columnar epithelium.** The membranous urethra, the shortest part, is lined by stratified columnar epithelium. The terminal spongy urethra passes through the *corpus spongiosum* of the penis. Its stratified columnar epithelium is gradually replaced by *nonkeratinized stratified squamous epithelium.* A loose, richly vascularized, fibroelastic **lamina propria** underlies the epithelium. The small pits or invaginations of the irregular urethral

mucosa lead to branched, tubular, mucus-secreting *Littre glands* and *bulbourethral glands.* The female urethra is relatively short, about 4 cm long and 8 mm wide. Near the urinary bladder its crescent-shaped lumen is lined by mucosa of urothelium that is gradually replaced by stratified columnar epithelium in an intermediate zone, and then nonkeratinized stratified squamous epithelium at its opening into the *vestibule.* Invaginations of epithelium form mucus-secreting *urethral glands.* A lamina propria of *loose connective tissue* contains an extensive **venous plexus** that resembles cavernous tissues in the male corpus spongiosum. Like the membranous urethra in the male, the *muscularis externa* in the female urethra consists of inner longitudinal and outer circular layers. The tunica adventitia is a thin layer of loose connective tissue.

17

MALE REPRODUCTIVE SYSTEM

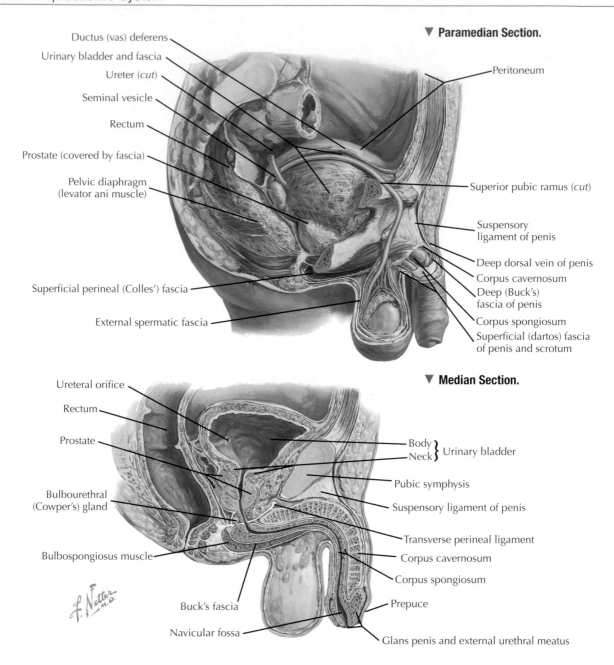

▼ **Paramedian Section.**

Ductus (vas) deferens
Urinary bladder and fascia
Ureter (*cut*)
Seminal vesicle
Rectum
Prostate (covered by fascia)
Pelvic diaphragm (levator ani muscle)
Superficial perineal (Colles') fascia
External spermatic fascia

Peritoneum
Superior pubic ramus (*cut*)
Suspensory ligament of penis
Deep dorsal vein of penis
Corpus cavernosum
Deep (Buck's) fascia of penis
Corpus spongiosum
Superficial (dartos) fascia of penis and scrotum

▼ **Median Section.**

Ureteral orifice
Rectum
Prostate
Bulbourethral (Cowper's) gland
Bulbospongiosus muscle
Buck's fascia
Navicular fossa

Body ⎫
Neck ⎭ Urinary bladder
Pubic symphysis
Suspensory ligament of penis
Transverse perineal ligament
Corpus cavernosum
Corpus spongiosum
Prepuce
Glans penis and external urethral meatus

17.1 OVERVIEW

The male **reproductive system** includes the paired primary sex organs, the **testes,** which have both *exocrine* and *endocrine* functions, and several secondary sex organs consisting of excretory ducts and accessory glands. The **scrotum** and **penis,** an erectile organ through which the distal **urethra** passes, are external genitalia. The testes reside outside the body cavity in the scrotum, where they are suspended and maintained in position. Testes and associated spermatic cords are invested by distinct layers of tissue acquired during descent of male gonads from their original retroperitoneal position in the abdominal cavity to the scrotum. Testes contain small convoluted **seminiferous tubules,** whose germinal epithelium produces male germ cells known as *spermatozoa*, and

interstitial connective tissue. **Leydig (interstitial) cells** produce *testosterone,* the hormone responsible for male secondary sex characteristics. After spermatozoa are produced in the testes, they travel a long, tortuous route: from seminiferous tubules to the paired **rete testis, efferent ductules (ductuli efferenti), epididymis, ductus (vas) deferens,** and **ejaculatory ducts,** and to the single urethra and penis. The accessory glands include two **seminal vesicles,** single **prostate gland,** and paired **bulbourethral glands** that secrete into ejaculatory ducts and urethra. Three key functions of this system are production of spermatozoa, delivery of these cells via *semen* into the female reproductive tract, and production of testosterone.

▼ **Schematic of tubules and ducts.**

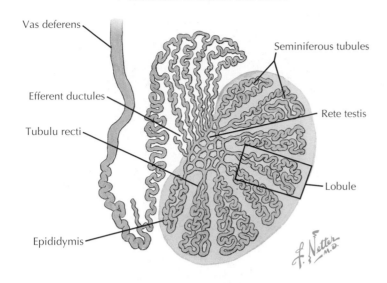

▼ **Seminiferous tubules and rete testis.**

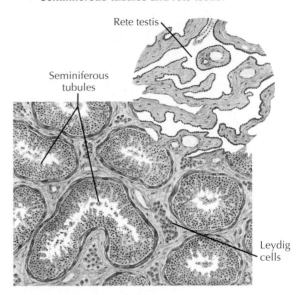

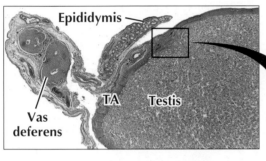

▲ **Light micrograph (LM) of part of the testis at low magnification.** A thick capsule—the tunica albuginea (**TA**)—covers it externally. Parts of the ductus deferens and epididymis are also seen. 3×. *H&E.*

▶ **LM of testis showing the tunica albuginea and mediastinum testis at low magnification.** Seminiferous tubules make up the glandular parenchyma. Rete testis forms a sponge-like network in the mediastinum. The thick tunica albuginea contains mostly regularly arranged collagen fibers, plus smooth muscle cells for contraction of the capsule. 30×. *H&E.*

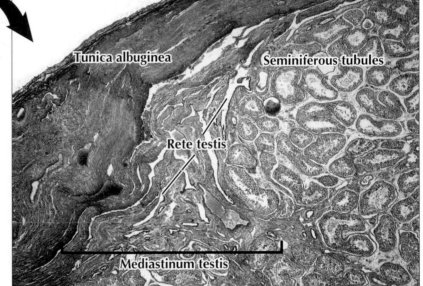

17.2 ANATOMY AND HISTOLOGY OF TESTES

The testis, an ovoid gland weighing about 15 g, is encased in a thick capsule of dense fibroelastic connective tissue known as the **tunica albuginea,** because it appears white in life. An outer visceral layer of the tunica vaginalis invests the capsule externally. Along the posterior border of the testis, the capsule projects inward as a thickened ridge, known as the **mediastinum testis.** This ridge corresponds to the hilum of other glands—the site where ducts, blood vessels, lymphatics, and nerves connect to the gland interior. Thin fibrous partitions, or septa, radiate from the mediastinum and form wedge-shaped lobules, about 250 in the human. The lobules contain **seminiferous tubules,** which are

sectioned in different planes because they have a convoluted course. Each testis has 600-1200 seminiferous tubules, with a total length of 280-400 m. In the mediastinum, seminiferous tubules empty into **tubuli recti** and **rete testis,** which coalesce to form six to eight **efferent ductules.** These ducts drain testicular fluid and spermatozoa to the proximal part of the **epididymis.** The rete testis is a labyrinthine network of collecting chambers of simple cuboidal epithelium. Interstitial connective tissue constitutes 20%-30% of the substance of the gland and consists of vascularized connective tissue with clusters of hormone-producing **Leydig cells.**

▼ **Spermatogenesis showing successive stages in development.**

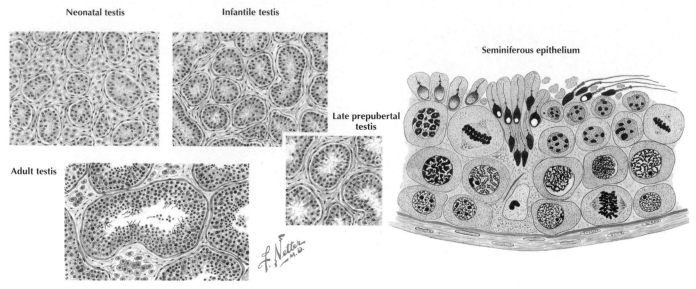

Neonatal testis

Infantile testis

Late prepubertal testis

Seminiferous epithelium

Adult testis

▼ **Mature spermatozoon.**

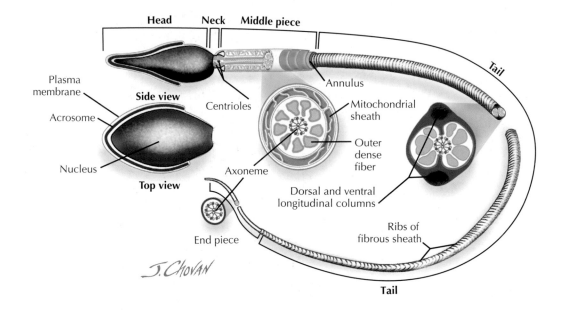

Head   Neck   Middle piece

Tail

Plasma membrane

Acrosome

Nucleus

Side view

Top view

Centrioles

Axoneme

End piece

Annulus

Mitochondrial sheath

Outer dense fiber

Dorsal and ventral longitudinal columns

Ribs of fibrous sheath

Tail

17.3 TESTICULAR DEVELOPMENT AND SPERMATOGENESIS

Testes derive from embryonic intermediate mesoderm that initially gives rise to primary epithelial sex cords, the precursors of **seminiferous tubules.** In the 4-week embryo, primordial germ cells migrate from yolk sac endoderm to the cords. Newborn testis consists of solid cords of germ cells arranged in layers and closely associated with epithelial cells that will be supporting **Sertoli cells.** The cords remain solid until puberty, when they lengthen, increase in diameter, and acquire a lumen. Leydig cells develop from mesenchyme between the seminiferous tubules. At puberty, primitive germ cells—**spermatogonia**—enlarge and become mitotically active. These cells undergo the process of *spermatogenesis,* in which diploid spermatogonia in seminiferous epithelium give rise to haploid **spermatozoa.** During differentiation, spermatozoa move toward the lumen of the tubules as they undergo mitosis, meiosis, and maturation. This process takes 64-74 days, is coordinated by Sertoli cells, and continues throughout life.

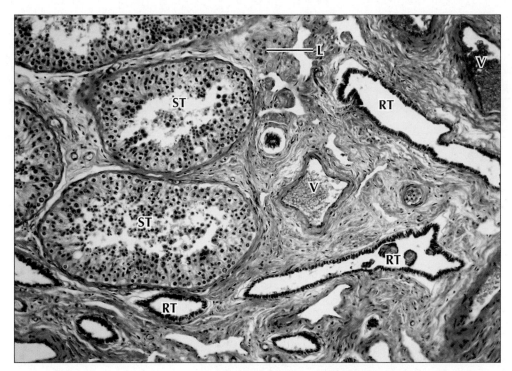

◀ **LM of the mediastinum testis.**
Seminiferous tubules (**ST**) are
embedded in a stroma rich with vessels
(**V**). A network of branching channels
constitutes the rete testis (**RT**). Clusters
of Leydig cells (**L**) occupy angular
spaces in the stroma. 115×. *H&E.*

▶ **LM of a seminiferous tubule
in transverse section.** A capsule
(**arrows**) surrounds seminiferous
epithelium. Spermatogonia (**Sg**)
are at the tubule base; large
spermatocytes (**Sp**) and smaller
spermatids (**S**) are closer to the
lumen. Pillar-shaped Sertoli
cells (**SC**) are interspersed with
germ cells. A clump of Leydig
cells is in adjacent stroma.
450×. *H&E.*

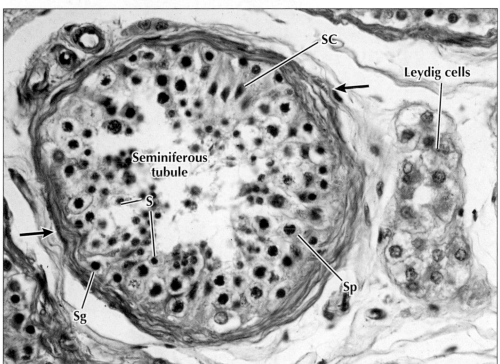

17.4 HISTOLOGY OF SEMINIFEROUS TUBULES

A distinct connective tissue **capsule,** a layer of flattened myoid cells, and a basement membrane surround seminiferous tubules. The **seminiferous epithelium** is an unusual, complex stratified epithelium with two cell populations: **spermatogenic** (or **germ**) **cells** and nonproliferating **Sertoli cells.** In a seminiferous tubule, germ cells are at various stages of *spermatogenesis.* The cells closest to the basement membrane with spherical nuclei are **spermatogonia.** Larger cells with spherical nuclei but with distinctive spaghetti-like chromatin are **primary spermatocytes.** The haploid **secondary spermatocytes** are seldom seen; almost as soon as they form they divide and produce **spermatids.** During a transformation period, spermatids attach to the relatively few Sertoli cells, which are tall and pillar-like. The bases of the Sertoli cells rest on the basement membrane; the free ends of the cells extend radially and reach the lumen. Spermatids, which are known as early and late, do not divide but mature into **spermatozoa,** which are released into the lumen and carried into efferent ducts.

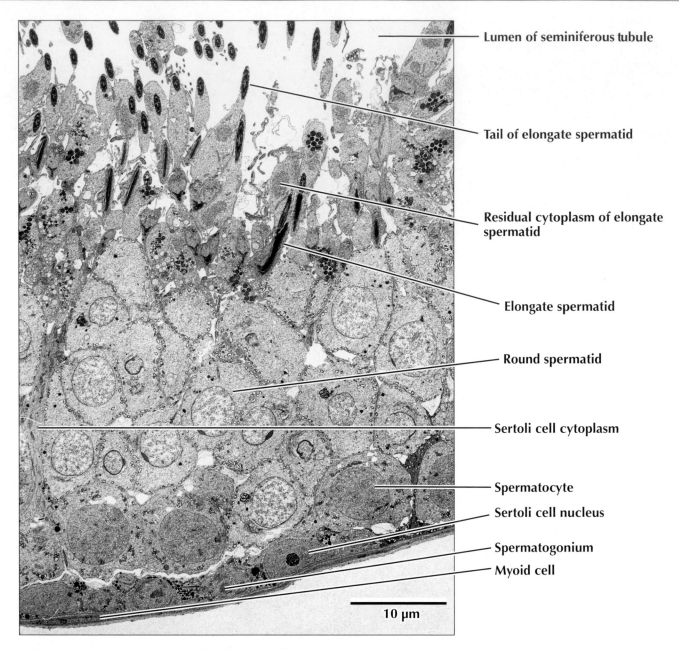

Lumen of seminiferous tubule

Tail of elongate spermatid

Residual cytoplasm of elongate spermatid

Elongate spermatid

Round spermatid

Sertoli cell cytoplasm

Spermatocyte

Sertoli cell nucleus

Spermatogonium

Myoid cell

10 μm

▲ **Panoramic electron micrograph (EM) of the seminiferous epithelium.** Ultrastructural features of germ cells at different stages of development and their relationship to Sertoli cells in the wall of the seminiferous tubule are clear. Myoid cells surround a thin outer capsule. 2500×. *(Courtesy of Dr. B. J. Crawford)*

17.5 ULTRASTRUCTURE OF SEMINIFEROUS TUBULES AND SPERMATOGENESIS

Spermatogonia are a continuously renewing stem cell population next to the **basement membrane** of the seminiferous tubule. They are diploid stem cells, with a diameter of about 12 μm and a relatively large spherical nucleus, and are the most immature group. On division, they give rise to **primary spermatocytes,** which have relatively large nuclei and are in the middle third of the seminiferous epithelium. After 10-22 days, these cells undergo meiotic division and give rise to smaller secondary spermatocytes, which

rapidly undergo a second meiotic division with no DNA replication. The resulting round **spermatids** have a diameter of about 9 μm and a haploid chromosome number and DNA content. Spermatids are embedded in invaginations of **Sertoli cells.** As spermatids move toward the tubule lumen, they elongate and undergo an elaborate process of maturation without mitosis, known as *spermiogenesis.* Resulting spermatozoa are highly specialized cells with a single flagellum and a small, condensed, conical nucleus. Spermatozoa, about 300 million being produced daily, are released into the lumen.

▶ **EM of an early spermatid in seminiferous epithelium.** In this plane of section, the spermatid appears close to the base of the seminiferous tubule. It has a round euchromatic nucleus and a large acrosome (⋆) at its anterior pole. A Sertoli cell is in contact with the spermatid. The tubule capsule (**arrow**) and an underlying capillary (**Cap**) are also seen. 5000×.
(Courtesy of Dr. A. W. Vogl)

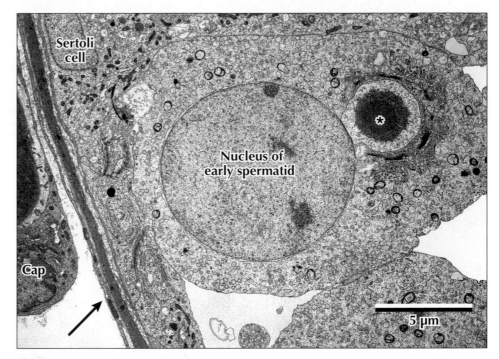

◀ **EM of the juxtanuclear region of an early spermatid.** Acrosomal vesicles (**arrows**) of various sizes and internal density are close to the Golgi complex. The largest vesicle shows an electron-dense acrosomal granule (⋆). The acrosome adheres to the outer aspect of the nuclear envelope. Many atypical mitochondria (**Mi**) are in cytoplasm. 20,000×. *(Courtesy of Dr. A. W. Vogl)*

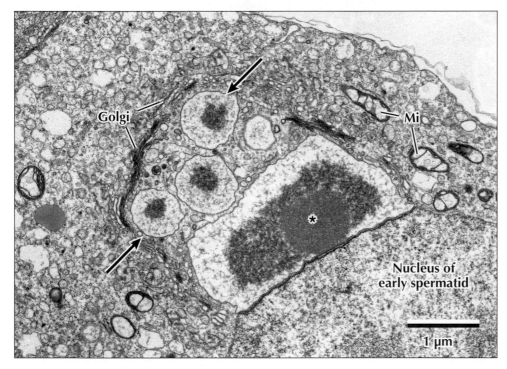

17.6   ULTRASTRUCTURE OF GERM CELLS AND EARLY SPERMIOGENESIS

Spermatids undergo an elaborate process of maturation known as *spermiogenesis*. Sequential changes take place whereby spherical, nonmotile spermatids become elongated, motile **spermatozoa.** Occurring in the upper layers of seminiferous epithelium, these changes include condensation of nuclear chromatin, elongation of the **nucleus,** formation of the **acrosome,** migration of cytoplasmic organelles to positions typical of mature cells, formation of a single flagellum, and loss of residual cytoplasm. At first, several small **acrosomal vesicles** form from the juxtanuclear **Golgi complex.** They coalesce into a single large membrane-bound **acrosome,** which adheres to the **nuclear envelope.** An electron-dense **acrosomal granule** forms within the vesicle, which gradually spreads to cap the anterior surface of the nucleus and ultimately becomes the front of the mature spermatozoon. The acrosome, a modified lysosome, contains hyaluronidase, lysosomal hydrolases, and protease enzymes that allow spermatozoa to penetrate the corona radiata and zona pellucida of the oocyte in the female at fertilization.

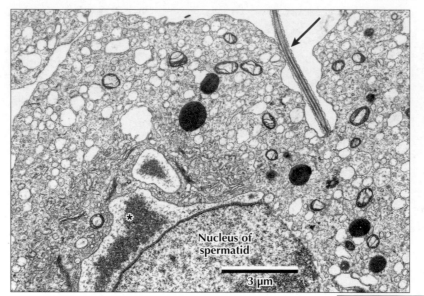

◀ **EM of a spermatid near the lumen of a seminiferous tubule.** Its developing acrosome (∗) is flattened and caps the anterior nuclear pole. A single flagellum (**arrow**) projects from its posterior pole into the lumen. 6000×. *(Courtesy of Dr. A. W. Vogl)*

▶ **EM of several elongated spermatids at the lumen of a seminiferous tubule.** The conical nuclei (∗) of the spermatids are electron dense. The spermatids are embedded in crypt-like recesses of the apical part of a Sertoli cell. Many organelles pack Sertoli cell cytoplasm. Residual cytoplasm of the spermatids, which will be shed, is at the top. 6000×. *(Courtesy of Drs. D. M. Pfeiffer and A. W. Vogl)*

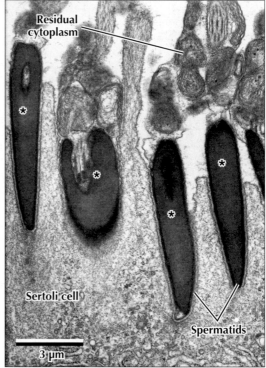

17.7 ULTRASTRUCTURE OF GERM CELLS AND LATER SPERMIOGENESIS

At a later stage of spermiogenesis, a pair of centrioles migrates to the opposite pole of the spermatid **nucleus,** and a single **flagellum** grows out from one. Its core has an axoneme with two central microtubules and nine peripheral microtubular doublets, which provides substrate for sperm tail motility. Mitochondria migrate toward the flagellum and form a sheath or collar around it. Residual cytoplasm and superfluous organelles are shed and are then phagocytosed by adjacent **Sertoli cells.** The highly specialized spermatozoa are about 60 μm long and are typically divided into five distinct regions. A small, condensed conical nucleus is in the head piece with the **acrosome;** a centriole pair occupies the neck piece. A middle piece contains helically arranged mitochondria that provide energy to propel the spermatozoon. The last two regions—principal and end pieces—contain the axoneme surrounded by coarse longitudinal fibers.

CLINICAL POINT

Seminomas are invasive germinal cell tumors accounting for 95% of solid tumors in men 15-35 years old. Their etiology and pathogenesis remain obscure, but they are thought to arise from germinal epithelium because seminoma cells are morphologically similar to spermatogonia. They tend to be localized or involve retroperitoneal lymph nodes. Although **testicular tumors** in children are rare, the developmental anomaly known as *cryptorchidism*, or undescended testis, predisposes boys to develop germ cell tumors. With advances in radiologic staging, serum tumor marker surveillance, and chemotherapy for advanced disease, the overall survival rate is >90%.

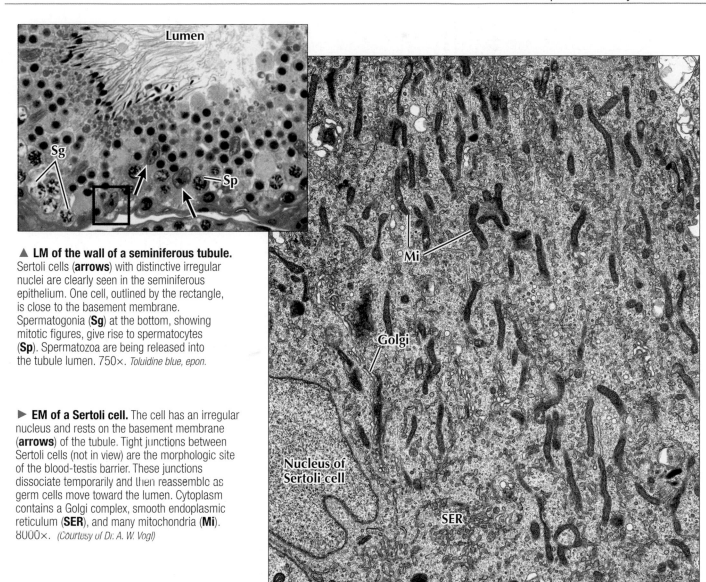

▲ LM of the wall of a seminiferous tubule.
Sertoli cells (**arrows**) with distinctive irregular
nuclei are clearly seen in the seminiferous
epithelium. One cell, outlined by the rectangle,
is close to the basement membrane.
Spermatogonia (**Sg**) at the bottom, showing
mitotic figures, give rise to spermatocytes
(**Sp**). Spermatozoa are being released into
the tubule lumen. 750×. *Toluidine blue, epon.*

▶ EM of a Sertoli cell. The cell has an irregular
nucleus and rests on the basement membrane
(**arrows**) of the tubule. Tight junctions between
Sertoli cells (not in view) are the morphologic site
of the blood-testis barrier. These junctions
dissociate temporarily and then reassemble as
germ cells move toward the lumen. Cytoplasm
contains a Golgi complex, smooth endoplasmic
reticulum (**SER**), and many mitochondria (**Mi**).
8000×. *(Courtesy of Dr. A. W. Vogl)*

17.8 ULTRASTRUCTURE AND FUNCTION OF SERTOLI CELLS

Sertoli cells play a critical role in support and maturation of **spermatozoa**. After puberty, they constitute about 10% of cells in the seminiferous epithelium. These columnar cells, with borders that are hard to distinguish, extend from the **basement membrane** to the lumen of the **seminiferous tubule.** Their apices bear crypt-like recesses that hold spermatids until release of newly formed spermatozoa into the lumen. Each cell has a jagged, euchromatic **nucleus** with a prominent nucleolus. The cytoplasm contains microtubules and intermediate filaments forming a prominent cytoskeleton, as well as long, slender mitochondria, a conspicuous smooth endoplasmic reticulum, large numbers of lipid droplets, and lipofuscin-laden lysosomes. Adjacent cells are linked by basolateral **tight junctions,** such that the epithelium is divided into basal and adluminal compartments. The resulting **blood-testis permeability barrier** separates spermatogonia and primary spermatocytes from more apical secondary spermatocytes and spermatids. Contents in the seminiferous tubule lumen are thus isolated from circulating antigens, thereby protecting spermatocytes and spermatids from autoimmune reactions and blood-borne substances. Sertoli cells *phagocytose* spermatid remnants and secrete fluid and many substances, including androgen-binding protein, essential for spermatozoa survival. Cell junctions are closely related to actin filaments and endoplasmic reticulum at sites called ectoplasmic specializations, which may adjust to changes in junctional architecture as spermatozoa move toward the lumen. The extensive cytoskeletal network of Sertoli cells helps provide for spermatozoa movement.

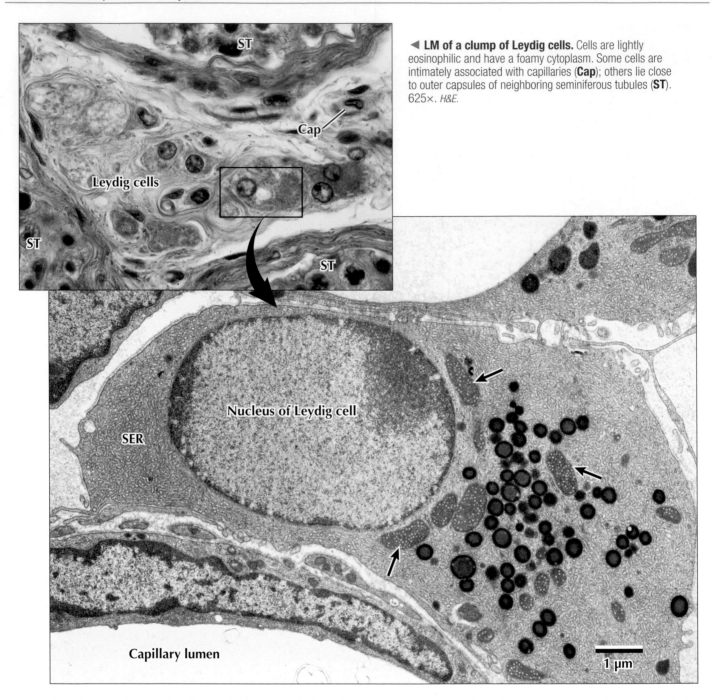

◀ **LM of a clump of Leydig cells.** Cells are lightly eosinophilic and have a foamy cytoplasm. Some cells are intimately associated with capillaries (**Cap**); others lie close to outer capsules of neighboring seminiferous tubules (**ST**). 625×. *H&E.*

▲ **EM of a Leydig cell close to a capillary.** The polyhedral cell has an eccentric, euchromatic nucleus and cytoplasm packed with abundant SER (**SER**). Spherical lipid droplets are electron dense, and tubulovesicular mitochondria (**arrows**) are scattered in cytoplasm. 12,000×. *(Courtesy of Dr. A. W. Vogl)*

17.9 HISTOLOGY AND ULTRASTRUCTURE OF LEYDIG CELLS

In loose connective tissue between seminiferous tubules are clusters of eosinophilic Leydig cells. Their foamy, washed-out cytoplasm is due to high lipid content, as they store cholesterol for synthesis of *testosterone*. These large polyhedral cells have an eccentric spherical **nucleus** with one or two prominent nucleoli, and cell surfaces have numerous small microvilli. They often lie close to **fenestrated capillaries** and small lymphatic vessels. Their cytoplasm contains abundant, tightly packed **smooth endoplasmic reticulum** (SER), a feature typical of steroid-secreting cells.

Relatively few ribosomes and rough endoplasmic reticulum, numerous scattered **mitochondria** with **tubulovesicular cristae,** a large juxtanuclear Golgi complex, and many spherical **lipid droplets** of various sizes also occupy the cytoplasm. Rectilinear crystalloid inclusions (crystals of Reinke) possessing a highly ordered pattern of internal structure also occur in human Leydig cells, but their function remains enigmatic. These inclusions are not present before puberty and are most common with advancing age. The amount of lipofuscin pigment associated with tertiary lysosomes also increases in old age.

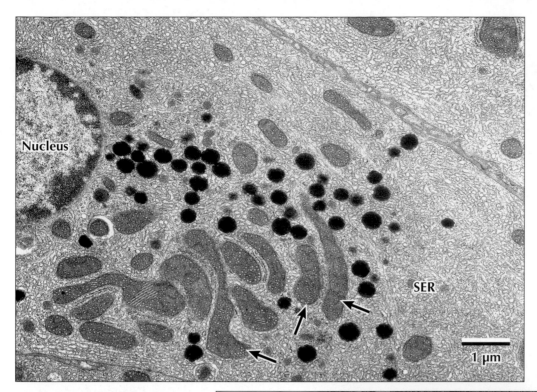

◀ **EM of part of a Leydig cell.** Elaborate, tightly packed SER is closely related to dark lipid droplets and pleomorphic mitochondria (**arrows**). 12,000×. *(Courtesy of Dr. A. W. Vogl)*

▶ **EM of part of a Leydig cell in contact with a capillary endothelial cell.** Many short microvilli project from the cell surface and abut the outer aspect of the capillary endothelium. The tubulovesicular cristae of mitochondria (**arrows**) appear similar to those in other steroid-secreting cells. Structural complexity of the inner mitochondrial membranes in this cell most likely enhances surface area for function. 18,200×. *(Courtesy of Dr. A. W. Vogl)*

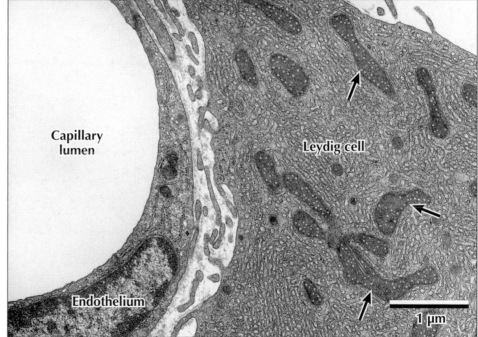

17.10 ULTRASTRUCTURE AND FUNCTION OF LEYDIG CELLS

Many organelles and inclusions in Leydig cells coordinate the synthesis and secretion of *testosterone,* the most abundant organelle being SER. Testosterone is derived from its precursor, cholesterol, which is either synthesized directly on SER membranes or derived from circulating low-density lipoprotein molecules taken up from the bloodstream. Non-membrane-bound **lipid droplets** store cholesterol until needed. After transport proteins move cholesterol to their inner **cristae, mitochondria** play a role in converting cholesterol to pregnenolone under the influence of luteinizing hormone. Once produced, pregnenolone is transferred from mitochondrial membranes to SER. Enzymes on the SER further modify pregnenolone and convert it to testosterone. Produced continuously by these cells, testosterone diffuses across the cell membrane, which is studded with **microvilli** that amplify its surface area. Testosterone released into the extracellular space associates rapidly with steroid-binding proteins in the circulation.

▼ **Testis, epididymis & vas deferens.**

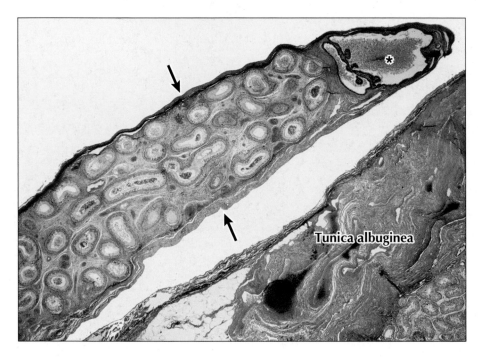

Ductus (vas) deferens

Appendix epididymis

Epididymis

Testis (covered by visceral layer of tunica vaginalis)

Epididymis

Efferent ductules

Tunica albuginea

Rete testis in mediastinum

Lobules

f. Netter m.d.

◀ **LM of the epididymis on the posterior pole of the testis.** The crescent-shaped epididymis consists mainly of a highly tortuous duct held together by loose connective tissue and covered by the visceral tunica vaginalis (**arrows**). Several profiles of spermatozoa are seen in the lumen. A dilated cyst-like structure (✶) in the head of the epididymis corresponds to the appendix epididymis, a mesonephric duct remnant. A thick tunica albuginea covers the surface of the testis. 20×. *H&E.*

Tunica albuginea

17.11 ANATOMY AND HISTOLOGY OF THE EPIDIDYMIS

The epididymis caps the posterior part of each **testis,** its main component being a tightly packed, tortuous duct about 6 m long and 400 µm in diameter. The epididymis, derived from the mesonephros in the embryo, is divided into three parts: an **initial (head) segment,** a **body** (the main part of the duct), and a **caudal (tail) region.** The head consists of tightly coiled parts of efferent ductules. Several cross and oblique views of the same duct are usually seen in histologic sections—evidence of the extremely convoluted nature of the duct. In 25% of males, the head contains a pedunculated cystic structure, the **appendix epididymis,** which is believed to be an embryologic remnant. The head receives efferent ductules that emerge from the rete testis and is engaged primarily in absorption of fluid and particulate matter. The efferent

ductules are lined by ciliated columnar epithelium; the cilia beat in the direction of the epididymis and may aid movement of spermatozoa.

CLINICAL POINT

Infections of the epididymis are common after puberty. Bacteria most often cause *inflammation* of the epididymis, known as **epididymitis.** Scrotal pain and edema are characteristic. In young males it usually arises as a complication of gonorrhea or as a sexually acquired infection with *Chlamydia.* Retrograde spread of infection from the urethra and lower urinary tract often occurs. In older men, this disorder is commonly associated with urinary tract infections caused by coliform bacteria such as *Escherichia coli.* Chronic epididymitis is characterized histologically by accumulation of plasma cells and macrophages followed by fibrosis and duct obstruction. In severe cases, bilateral epididymitis can lead to *male infertility.*

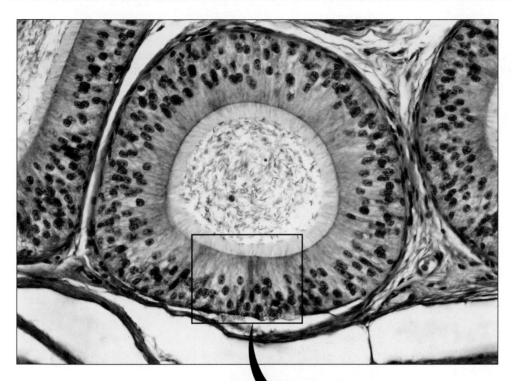

◀ **LM of the duct of the epididymis in transverse section.** The wall consists of tall pseudostratified epithelium of uniform thickness with apical nonmotile stereocilia. Spermatozoa are in the lumen. Surrounding lamina propria is loose, richly vascular connective tissue. The rectangle indicates an area similar to that seen **below**. 320×. *H&E.*

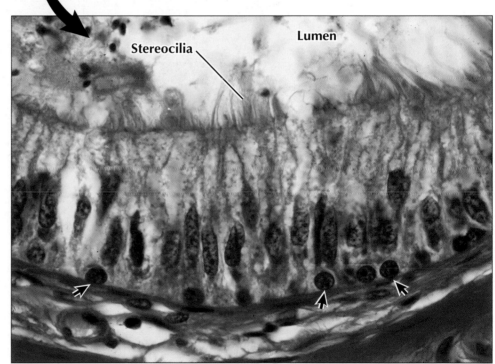

Stereocilia   Lumen

▶ **High-magnification LM of the epithelium of the epididymis.** The two major cell types of the epithelium rest on a basement membrane. Tall columnar cells have elongated, euchromatic nuclei and long, apical stereocilia. Small, round basal cells (**arrows**) on the basement membrane do not reach the luminal surface. They are most likely germinative stem cells for the epithelium. Underlying fibrous connective tissue contains smooth muscle. 525×. *H&E.*

17.12   HISTOLOGY AND FUNCTION OF THE EPIDIDYMIS

High magnification reveals the wall of the duct of the epididymis as consisting of a very high, **pseudostratified epithelium** containing **basal (stem) cells** and tall **columnar (principal) cells** with long, apical, nonmotile **stereocilia** projecting into the lumen. Stereocilia amplify the cell surface area and function in absorption of excess fluid that accompanies **spermatozoa** from the testis. The epididymis is also a long storage duct through which spermatozoa

pass slowly, their journey taking one to several weeks. In transit, spermatozoa mature and acquire motility and fertilizing capacity. Loose connective tissue and some circularly arranged **smooth muscle** are also found outside the ducts. The smooth muscle in the head of the epididymis undergoes spontaneous peristaltic contractions. In the epididymis tail, however, contraction is stimulated by adrenergic innervation during sexual stimulation, which promotes *ejaculation.*

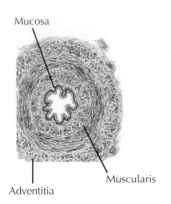

Mucosa

Adventitia

Muscularis

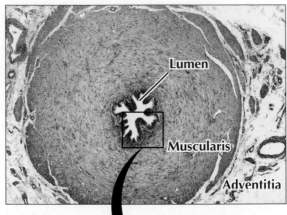

Lumen

Muscularis

Adventitia

◀ **LM of the ductus deferens in transverse section.** Folds of mucosa produce a stellate lumen. Around the mucosa is a prominent three-layer coat of tightly spiraled smooth muscle, the muscularis. Blood vessels, nerves, and lymphatics travel through an adventitia of loose connective tissue that covers the ductus externally. 35×. *H&E.*

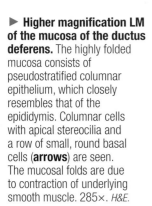

▶ **Higher magnification LM of the mucosa of the ductus deferens.** The highly folded mucosa consists of pseudostratified columnar epithelium, which closely resembles that of the epididymis. Columnar cells with apical stereocilia and a row of small, round basal cells (**arrows**) are seen. The mucosal folds are due to contraction of underlying smooth muscle. 285×. *H&E.*

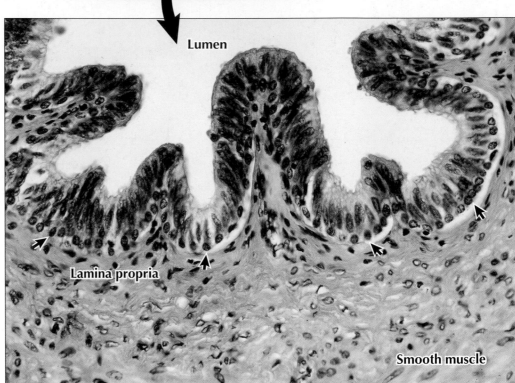

Lumen

Lamina propria

Smooth muscle

17.13 HISTOLOGY OF THE DUCTUS (VAS) DEFERENS

The ductus deferens, a continuation of the epididymis, is a hollow tube 35-40 cm long. It ends in the excretory duct of the **seminal vesicle** to form the ejaculatory duct, which passes through the prostate to drain into the prostatic part of the **urethra.** It derives embryologically from the mesonephric (wolffian) duct. **Pseudostratified columnar epithelium,** composed of columnar cells and basal cells, lines the tube; its lumen diameter is about 0.5 cm. Underlying **lamina propria** is rich in elastic fibers. The wall has a thick three-layer **smooth muscle** coat and an inner **mucosa** in longitudinal folds. The well-developed smooth muscle coat is 1-1.5 mm thick and consists of a prominent middle circular layer enclosed by thinner inner and outer longitudinal layers. The outermost **adventitia** is **loose connective tissue** containing blood vessels and nerves, which blend with surrounding tissues. Via sympathetic stimulation, smooth muscle contractions force spermatozoa along the duct during *ejaculation.* Functionally, the ductus is more than just a passive conduit for spermatozoa from epididymis to urethra; ultrastructural data suggest that it has both secretory and absorptive functions. The presence of apical **stereocilia** and lysosomes is consistent with absorptive and phagocytic functions. After *vasectomy,* spermatozoa are phagocytosed by epithelial cells of both ductus deferens and epididymis.

CLINICAL POINT

A **vasectomy** is a minor surgical procedure to produce permanent sterility by preventing transport of spermatozoa out of the testis. After the ductus deferens is exposed, it may be cut and then the two ends either tied or cauterized, or it may be blocked with surgical clips. Normal sexual intercourse with ejaculation is possible after vasectomy. Almost all vasectomies are 15- to 30-minute outpatient procedures done with local anesthesia. Microsurgery can reverse a vasectomy and restore fertility but is successful in only about 70% of cases. More than 500,000 vasectomies are done annually in North America.

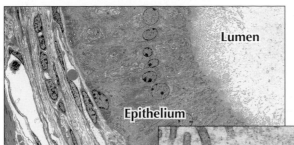

▶ **Higher magnification EM of apical surfaces of principal cells of the mouse ductus deferens.** Long, slender stereocilia greatly enhance apical cell surface area for absorption. They contain a supportive core of actin filaments. Apical blebs are also characteristic of these cells. Junctional complexes (**circles**) link lateral cell borders at the apex. Elongated mitochondria, vesicles, and vacuoles occupy apical cytoplasm. 12,500×.

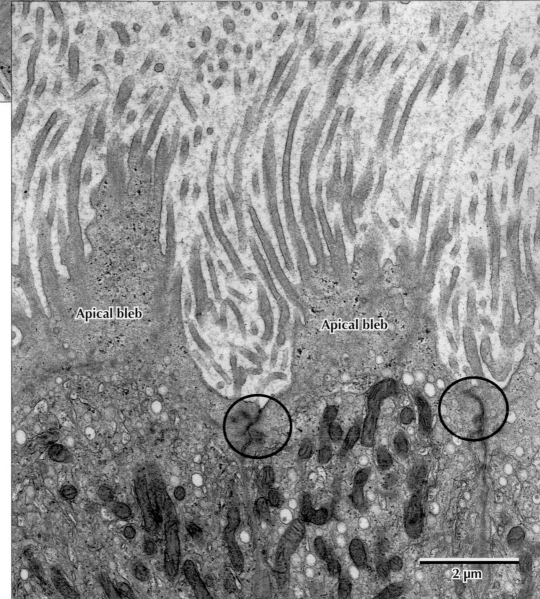

17.14 ULTRASTRUCTURE AND FUNCTION OF THE DUCTUS (VAS) DEFERENS

Columnar epithelial cells of the ductus deferens, called **principal cells,** share a common ultrastructural organization with similar cells in the epididymis that reflects their secretory and absorptive functions. Principal cells here synthesize and secrete various substances including glycoproteins. They have all organelles needed for two types of secretions—*merocrine* and *apocrine*. Also, the presence of **stereocilia,** a typical feature, is consistent with an absorptive function. Areas of **apical cell cytoplasm** that protrude out between stereocilia are called **apical blebs** and function in apocrine secretion. The secretory protein is thought to interact with spermatozoa and affect their mobility. Apical blebs form continuously and detach from the cell surface. Once released, they fragment and liberate their contents into the lumen. The presence of abundant **vesicles** and **vacuoles** in apical cytoplasm correlates with endocytosis, which occurs at the apical surface.

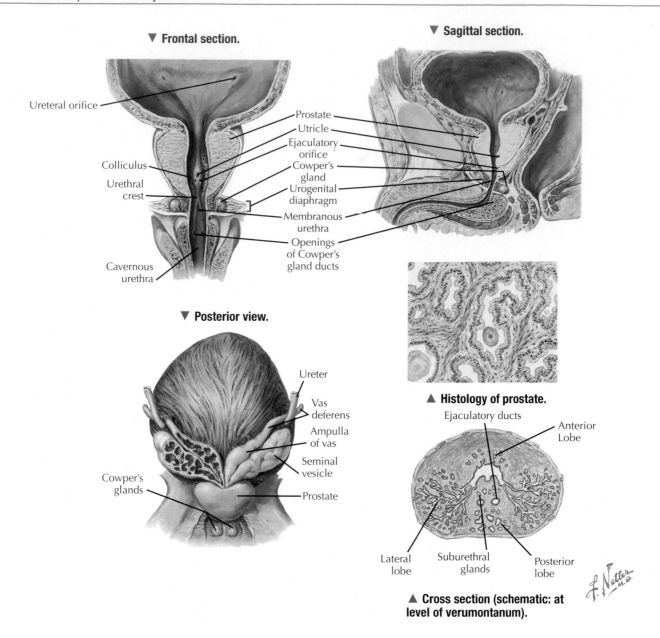

▼ **Frontal section.**

Ureteral orifice

Prostate
Utricle
Ejaculatory orifice
Cowper's gland
Colliculus
Urethral crest
Urogenital diaphragm
Membranous urethra
Openings of Cowper's gland ducts
Cavernous urethra

▼ **Sagittal section.**

▼ **Posterior view.**

Ureter
Vas deferens
Ampulla of vas
Seminal vesicle
Cowper's glands
Prostate

▲ **Histology of prostate.**

Ejaculatory ducts
Anterior Lobe
Lateral lobe
Suburethral glands
Posterior lobe

▲ **Cross section (schematic: at level of verumontanum).**

17.15 ANATOMY AND HISTOLOGY OF THE PROSTATE AND SEMINAL VESICLES

The normal adult prostate is the size of a chestnut and weighs about 20 g. This retroperitoneal organ encircles the neck of the urinary bladder and **urethra.** It is covered by a thin, indistinct fibroelastic connective tissue capsule mixed with smooth muscle and is traversed posteriorly by **ejaculatory ducts.** The prostate, a collection of up to 50 **compound tubuloalveolar glands,** has traditionally been divided anatomically into several lobes. Because the lobes are indistinct and some organs may be atrophic in normal adult humans, the prostate is better divided into three concentric zones, which are best seen in the sagittal plane. The peripheral zone constitutes 70% of the organ and contains the main glands. The central zone represents 25% of the prostate and consists of submucosal glands. A transitional zone of mucosal glands makes up 5% of the prostate. This pattern has clinical significance: in most cases *benign prostatic hyperplasia* arises in the transitional zone; the peripheral zone is the one most susceptible to inflammation and the site of most *prostatic adenocarcinomas.* The paired **seminal vesicles** lie behind the posterior wall of the urinary bladder. Their ducts fuse with the distal end of the paired **ductus deferens** to form ejaculatory ducts, which enter the prostate and end in the prostatic urethra.

CLINICAL POINT

Benign prostatic hypertrophy is a common clinical condition affecting 30% of men older than 50 years. Its frequency and severity increase with aging. It is caused by *hyperplasia* of glandular and stromal cells in the prostate and leads to nonmalignant enlargement of the gland. Other histopathologic features include squamous metaplasia, increased smooth muscle, reduced elastic tissue, and lymphocyte infiltration. Resulting periurethral nodules may compress the urethra so that urine flow is reduced and the bladder difficult to empty. The drugs used for treatment include α_1-*adrenergic receptor blockers,* which inhibit contraction of prostatic smooth muscle and may help alleviate symptoms.

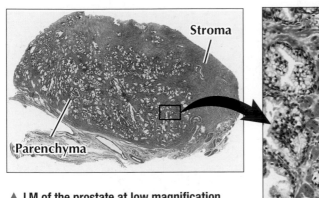

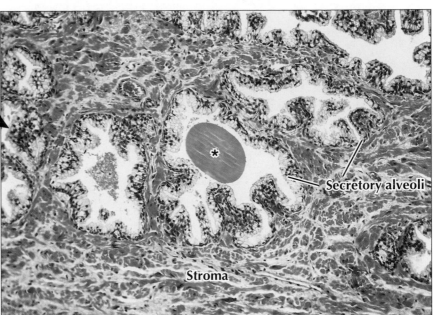

▲ **LM of the prostate at low magnification.**
Glandular parenchyma and fibromuscular stroma
make up the gland. Note the branching nature
of the tubuloalveolar glandular units. 5×. *H&E.*

▶ **LM of part of the prostate.** Glandular
epithelium lines irregularly shaped secretory alveoli.
A prostatic concretion (∗) is in an alveolus lumen.
Underlying stroma is a mixture of smooth muscle
and connective tissue.115×. *H&E.*

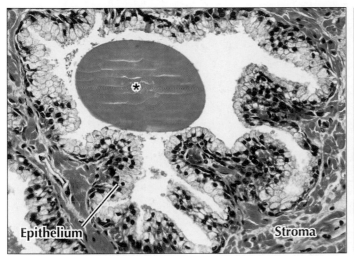

▲ **Higher magnification LM of the prostate.** Pseudostratified epithelium,
consisting of columnar cells and small basal cells, lines a secretory alveolus.
A prostatic concretion (∗) is in the alveolar lumen. A prominent fibromuscular
stroma is in adjacent areas. 220×. *H&E.*

▲ **Higher magnification LM of a secretory alveolus in the prostate.**
Columnar epithelial cells, which have lightly stained apical cytoplasm, line
the lumen. Smooth muscle cells in the stroma are red; connective tissue
(**CT**) is blue. 300×. *Masson's trichrome.*

17.16 HISTOLOGY AND FUNCTION OF THE PROSTATE

The prostate develops from mesenchyme around the urogenital
sinus during the 12th gestational week. The adult prostate is made
of numerous individual **tubuloalveolar** glandular units, irregularly shaped, that open by separate branching ducts into the prostatic urethra. They are embedded in fibromuscular **stroma**, dense
with collagen and irregularly arranged smooth muscle. The stroma
is continuous with the capsule and forms somewhat indistinct
lobules. The prostate contributes about 15% of fluid to the ejaculate. The secretory nature of the glandular epithelium is clear at
high magnification: the **pseudostratified epithelium** has both

basal and **secretory cells.** Secretory cells produce a white serous
fluid containing acid phosphatase, citric acid, zinc, **prostate-
specific antigen** (PSA), and other proteases and fibrolytic enzymes
involved in liquefaction of semen. PSA is a serine protease
that is used to diagnose some prostatic diseases. With aging, **prostatic concretions**—ovoid, eosinophilic, concentrically lamellated
bodies—may be found in **alveolar lumina.** These bodies increase
in number and calcify with age. They are thought to be a mixture
of prostatic secretions and debris from degenerated epithelial cells.
Testosterone may cause the glandular component of the prostate
to undergo *hyperplasia* and *hypertrophy.*

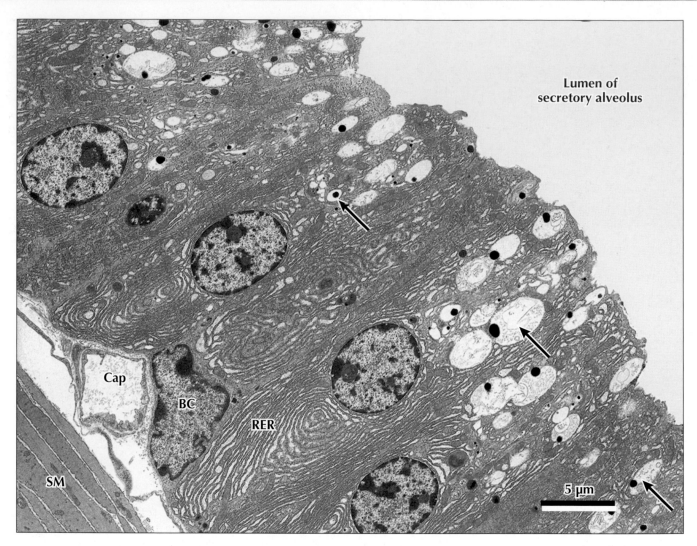

Lumen of
secretory alveolus

Cap

BC

RER

SM

5 µm

▲ **Survey EM of mouse prostatic epithelium.** The secretory nature of the columnar epithelial cells is clear, even if individual cell borders are difficult to distinguish. Multiple **RER** cisternae occupy basal cytoplasm; large secretory vesicles (**arrows**) are supranuclear. Small basal cells (**BC**) are next to the basement membrane. Underlying lamina propria contains a fenestrated capillary (**Cap**) and smooth muscle cells (**SM**). 4000×.

17.17   ULTRASTRUCTURE OF THE PROSTATE

The salient ultrastructural features of prostatic **epithelial cells** reflect their role in *synthesis* and *secretion*. Their organelles have a polarized arrangement. A well-developed **rough endoplasmic reticulum** (RER) in the basal cytoplasm either appears distended or is organized as parallel flattened **cisternae.** A prominent Golgi complex in the supranuclear region of each cell gives rise to membrane-bound **secretory vacuoles** and **vesicles,** which are pleomorphic, vary in size, and may appear empty or contain flocculent or electron-dense material. As in other protein-synthesizing cells, proteins from the RER are shuttled via small transport vesicles to the cis side of the Golgi complex. In the Golgi complex, secretory products are modified and then sorted into secretory vesicles destined for the cell surface. After fusion with the apical cell membrane, secretory vesicles and vacuoles release

their contents into the lumen. The function of **basal cells** is not completely understood. They most likely are reserve cells, as they proliferate during organ repair.

CLINICAL POINT

Adenocarcinoma of the prostate is one of the most common malignant tumors in males. It mostly affects the peripheral zone of the gland and causes elevated plasma levels of *prostate-specific antigen (PSA)*. This serine protease is a product of prostatic epithelium. Cytologic features include hyperchromatic enlarged nuclei in secretory epithelium and absence of the basal cell layer. Causes remain uncertain, but androgens are thought to influence the pathogenesis, and several risk factors including age, race, and family history may play a role in etiology. Treatments include surgery, radiation, and hormonal therapy

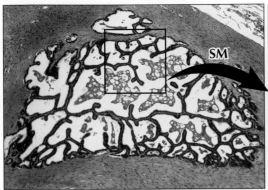

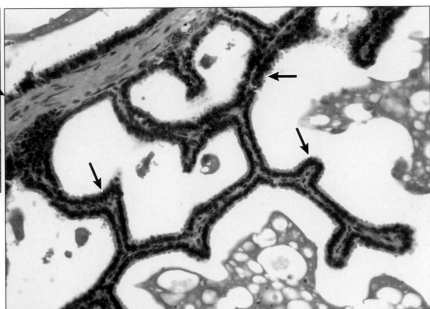

▲ **LM of the seminal vesicle.** The gland's mucosal folds are complex, and its wall has smooth muscle (**SM**) arranged tightly in inner circular and outer longitudinal layers. Flocculent eosinophilic material fills the lumen. 50×. *H&E.*

▲ **Higher magnification LM of the mucosa of the seminal vesicle.** The honeycombed mucosa has an epithelium (**arrows**) composed of columnar cells and basal cells. Semen consists of spermatozoa formed in germinal epithelium of the testis and seminal fluid, the components of which are secreted by the excretory duct sytem and accessory glands. Most of this fluid is produced in seminal vesicles. 280×. *H&E.*

◄ **High-magnification LM of the mucosa of the seminal vesicle.** The epithelium is usually pseudostratified, but it may be simple columnar in places. Its height varies with age, phase of secretion, and hormonal influence. Columnar cells with eosinophilic, dome-shaped apical cytoplasm (**arrows**) are normally interspersed with small rounded basal cells (**BC**). 500×. *H&E.*

17.18   HISTOLOGY OF SEMINAL VESICLES

Paired seminal vesicles are diverticula of the ductus deferens, about 2 cm wide and 4 cm long. These convoluted tubulosaccular glands have internal folds of connective tissue forming crests and ridges lined by **secretory epithelium** projecting into the lumen. The elaborately folded **mucosa** resembles a branching, anastomosing honeycomb. Underlying lamina propria is connective tissue with abundant elastic fibers. In histologic sections, the large lumen comprises separate cavities of various sizes, which communicate with each other throughout the gland. The lumen contains coagulated eosinophilic material thought to be stored secretion. Like the prostate, seminal vesicles depend on androgen and develop fully only after puberty. The epithelium, like that in

other areas of the male reproductive tract, is mostly pseudostratified with **basal cells** and **columnar cells.** By electron microscopy, polarized columnar cells show features typical of secretory epithelium—well-developed Golgi complex, abundant rough endoplasmic reticulum, numerous mitochondria, and apical secretory vesicles. Seminal vesicles contribute up to 70% of *seminal fluid.* The main secretory product is fructose used by spermatozoa as an energy source for motility, in addition to water, K$^+$ ions, prostaglandins, and other agents that modify spermatozoa activity in the ejaculate. As in other glands associated with the male reproductive tract, seminal vesicles have a thick wall of **smooth muscle,** which contracts during the emission phase of ejaculation.

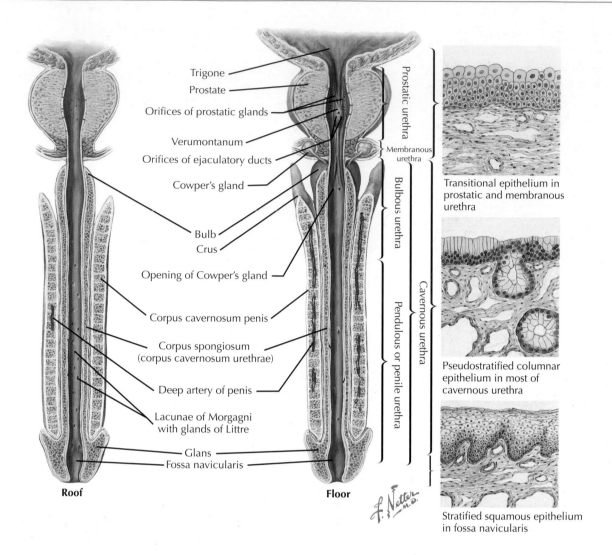

Trigone
Prostate
Orifices of prostatic glands
Verumontanum
Orifices of ejaculatory ducts
Cowper's gland
Bulb
Crus
Opening of Cowper's gland
Corpus cavernosum penis
Corpus spongiosum
(corpus cavernosum urethrae)
Deep artery of penis
Lacunae of Morgagni
with glands of Littre
Glans
Fossa navicularis

Prostatic urethra
Membranous urethra
Bulbous urethra
Pendulous or penile urethra
Cavernous urethra

Roof   **Floor**

Transitional epithelium in
prostatic and membranous
urethra

Pseudostratified columnar
epithelium in most of
cavernous urethra

Stratified squamous epithelium
in fossa navicularis

17.19 ANATOMY AND HISTOLOGY OF THE URETHRA AND PENIS

The male urethra conducts urine from the urinary bladder to the body's exterior, as well as *semen* during ejaculation. It comprises three anatomic parts, with mucosa and associated epithelium varying regionally. The **prostatic urethra,** next to the bladder, is about 2 cm long and is lined mostly by **transitional epithelium** associated with a richly cellular lamina propria with isolated smooth muscle cells. The prostatic urethra floor contains openings of ducts from the **prostate gland** and of paired **ejaculatory ducts.** The shorter **membranous urethra,** about 2 mm long, traverses the deep perineal pouch and perineal membrane; its mucosa is lined by **stratified columnar epithelium.** The **penile,** or **spongy, urethra** is the longest segment and extends through the center of the **corpus spongiosum.** Its mucous membrane changes from stratified columnar epithelium to **stratified squamous epithelium** at the **fossa navicularis,** the terminal enlargement of the urethra. Underlying lamina propria contains a rich plexus of venous sinuses. Ducts from pea-sized **bulbourethral (Cowper's) glands** open in the proximal penile urethra. Small, multiple, mucous-secreting **glands of Littre** drain, by small ducts along the penile urethra, directly into epithelium or into small recesses called **lacunae of Morgagni.**

CLINICAL POINT

Male circumcision is surgical removal of the foreskin, which covers the tip of the penis. It is usually performed on newborns under local anesthesia. A decision to circumcise may be based on religious ritual, family or cultural tradition, personal hygiene, or preventive health care. Possible medical benefits remain controversial, but circumcision may reduce the incidence of *urinary tract infections* and *penile carcinoma,* and perhaps sexually transmitted diseases such as infection with *human immunodeficiency virus* (HIV), the cause of AIDS, and *human papillomavirus* (HPV), which may cause *genital warts* or *cervical carcinoma.*

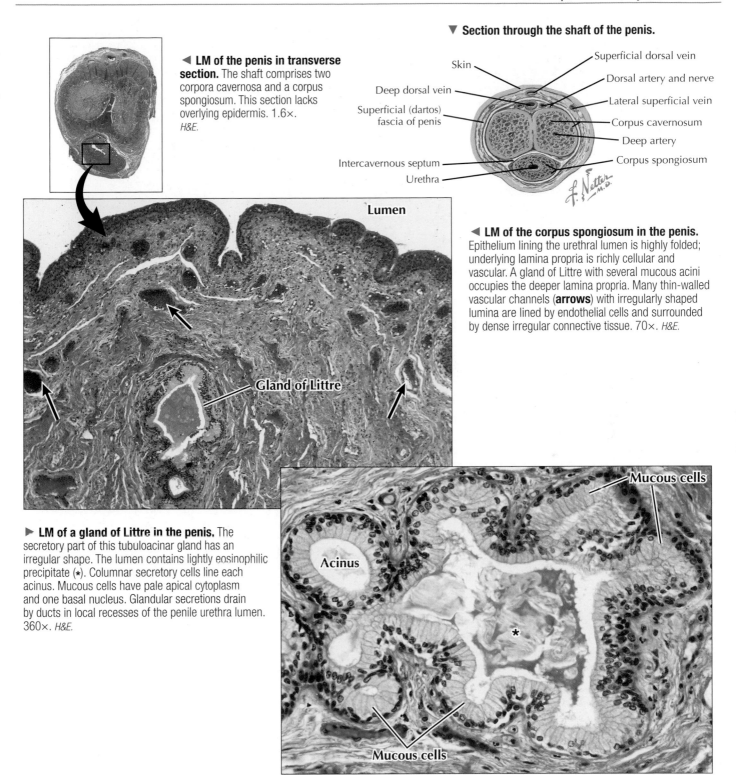

◄ **LM of the penis in transverse section.** The shaft comprises two corpora cavernosa and a corpus spongiosum. This section lacks overlying epidermis. 1.6×. *H&E.*

▼ **Section through the shaft of the penis.**

Skin
Superficial dorsal vein
Deep dorsal vein
Dorsal artery and nerve
Superficial (dartos) fascia of penis
Lateral superficial vein
Corpus cavernosum
Deep artery
Intercavernous septum
Corpus spongiosum
Urethra

Lumen

◄ **LM of the corpus spongiosum in the penis.** Epithelium lining the urethral lumen is highly folded; underlying lamina propria is richly cellular and vascular. A gland of Littre with several mucous acini occupies the deeper lamina propria. Many thin-walled vascular channels (**arrows**) with irregularly shaped lumina are lined by endothelial cells and surrounded by dense irregular connective tissue. 70×. *H&E.*

Gland of Littre

Mucous cells

Acinus

*

Mucous cells

► **LM of a gland of Littre in the penis.** The secretory part of this tubuloacinar gland has an irregular shape. The lumen contains lightly eosinophilic precipitate (✱). Columnar secretory cells line each acinus. Mucous cells have pale apical cytoplasm and one basal nucleus. Glandular secretions drain by ducts in local recesses of the penile urethra lumen. 360×. *H&E.*

17.20 HISTOLOGY OF THE PENIS

The penis consists of three cylindrical bodies: paired **corpora cavernosa,** separated by an incomplete midline septum, and a **corpus spongiosum,** located ventrally and containing the **penile urethra** at its center. A fibrous **tunica albuginea** surrounds each cavernous body; thin skin covers all three cylinders. These erectile tissues—corpora cavernosa and spongiosum—are masses of labyrinthine trabeculae of **fibroelastic connective tissue** and **smooth muscle** ramified by an extensive, cavernous network of **vascular sinuses,** which fill with blood during erection. Endothelium typically lines the sinuses. The penis is not only richly vascularized but also profusely innervated: many nerve fascicles and specialized sensory receptors, including Pacinian corpuscles, are abundant throughout. The penile urethra lies at the center of the corpus spongiosum and has a somewhat folded mucosa. The **epithelium** of the penile urethra is mostly stratified columnar and changes to stratified squamous near the end of the urethra. Invaginations form urethral **glands of Littre** in the lamina propria that secrete mucus as a preejaculatory emission, which is also thought to protect the epithelium against urine.

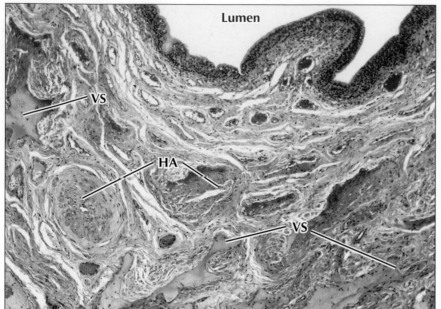

Lumen

VS

HA

VS

◀ **LM of the corpus spongiosum.** The mucosa lining the urethral lumen is corrugated. Erectile tissue in deeper layers contains helicine arteries (**HA**), veins, and venous sinuses (**VS**). 110×. *H&E.*

▲ **LM of the penile urethra at higher magnification.** The stratified columnar nature of the epithelium, with an underlying basement membrane (**arrowheads**) is clear. The lamina propria is loose connective tissue and contains several venules close to the surface. 400×. *H&E.*

▼ **LM of helicine arteries in the corpus spongiosum.** These highly coiled arterioles have a thick tunica media with an inner layer of longitudinally oriented smooth muscle that forms thickenings (**arrows**) of tunica intima. Contraction of this smooth muscle constricts the arteriolar lumen. These arteries drain directly into venous sinuses. 300×. *H&E.*

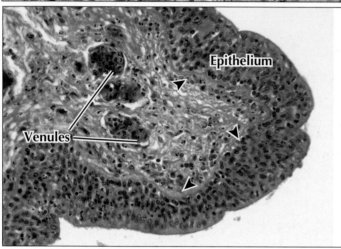

Epithelium

Venules

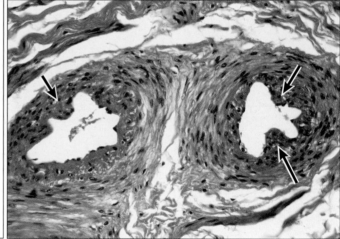

17.21 HISTOLOGY AND FUNCTION OF THE PENIS

Erectile tissue of the penis is made of dense, irregular connective tissue, which extends inward from the tunica albuginea and contains many elastic fibers, smooth muscle cells, and irregular cavernous spaces—the **venous sinuses.** These sinuses are lined by endothelium and are continuous with muscular arteries supplying them and with draining veins. The mechanism of *erection* is complex. Under parasympathetic stimulation, the primary blood supply of the penis is directed through convoluted **muscular (helicine) arteries,** which dilate and open into thin-walled venous sinuses. The tunica intima of these arteries has ridge-like thickenings, which partially occlude their lumina and act like valves. These vessels and sinuses become engorged with blood, which expands the **corpora cavernosa** and compresses the thin-walled veins beneath the tunica albuginea. The veins are effectively closed, so rigidity and enlargement of the organ increase. The **urethra** is not occluded during erection because the capsule of connective tissue around the **corpus spongiosum** is thinner and less rigid

than the more prominent tunica albuginea around the corpora cavernosa. After *ejaculation,* which is under sympathetic control, helicine arteries contract and their **intimal ridges** reduce the volume of incoming blood. Arteries regain normal tone, venous pressure falls, and normal blood flow to the region is restored.

CLINICAL POINT

Male erectile dysfunction (ED), or **impotence,** is the inability to achieve and maintain an erection for sexual intercourse. Although many physical and psychological causes exist, ED is a common problem causing progressive difficulty with aging. Use of a novel, potent class of drug, the *phosphodiesterase-5 (PDE5) inhibitors,* has become a safe, effective treatment. PDE5 inhibitors act selectively on endothelial cells in blood vessels of the corpus cavernosum, which increases nitric oxide production. Then, relaxation of penile vascular smooth muscle cells increases blood flow to the penis, thus enhancing penile engorgement and erection.

18

FEMALE REPRODUCTIVE SYSTEM

▼ **Topography of the female pelvic viscera: medial and paramedial sagittal views.**

Median (sagittal) section

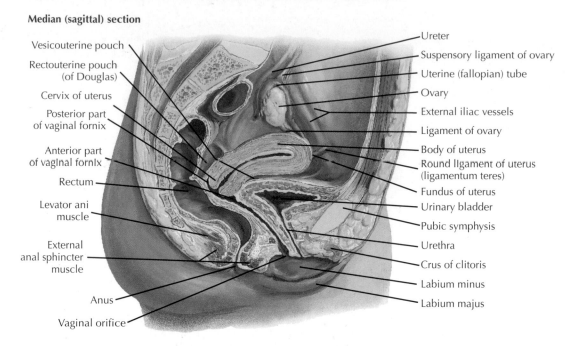

Vesicouterine pouch

Rectouterine pouch
(of Douglas)

Cervix of uterus

Posterior part
of vaginal fornix

Anterior part
of vaginal fornix

Rectum

Levator ani
muscle

External
anal sphincter
muscle

Anus

Vaginal orifice

Ureter

Suspensory ligament of ovary

Uterine (fallopian) tube

Ovary

External iliac vessels

Ligament of ovary

Body of uterus

Round ligament of uterus
(ligamentum teres)

Fundus of uterus

Urinary bladder

Pubic symphysis

Urethra

Crus of clitoris

Labium minus

Labium majus

Paramedian (sagittal) dissection

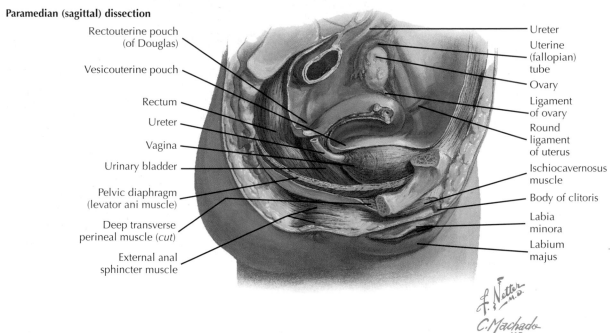

Rectouterine pouch
(of Douglas)

Vesicouterine pouch

Rectum

Ureter

Vagina

Urinary bladder

Pelvic diaphragm
(levator ani muscle)

Deep transverse
perineal muscle (cut)

External anal
sphincter muscle

Ureter

Uterine
(fallopian)
tube

Ovary

Ligament
of ovary

Round
ligament
of uterus

Ischiocavernosus
muscle

Body of clitoris

Labia
minora

Labium
majus

18.1   OVERVIEW

The female reproductive system consists of paired **ovaries** and the **genital tract,** including **fallopian tubes** (**oviducts,** or **uterine tubes**), **uterus,** and **vagina,** located in the pelvis—the **internal genitalia. External genitalia** consist of **labia majora, labia minora,** and **clitoris.** Mammary glands (see Chapter 2) and placenta are not classified as genital organs but are functionally associated with them. Ovaries, the center of cyclic changes in the female reproductive system, produce female germ cells (ova) and steroid hormones. Fallopian tubes are sites for fertilization of ova, and the uterus harbors fertilized ova during gestation. Like ovaries, the uterus undergoes a regular sequence of changes known as the *menstrual cycle.* The vagina connects the internal genitalia with the exterior. Embryonic development of the female reproductive

system, as in the male, closely parallels that of the urinary system. The system derives mainly from a urogenital ridge of intermediate mesoderm in the posterior abdominal wall. At 6 weeks of gestation, primordial germ cells migrate from their origin in the yolk sac endoderm to the urogenital ridge. Gonad development proceeds with interaction of germ cells with surrounding mesenchyme and coelomic surface epithelium. Germ cells in the primitive ovary develop into oogonia; surface epithelium differentiates into follicular cells. The female genital duct system and external genitalia then develop under the influence of circulating fetal hormones. The paramesonephric (Müllerian) duct system gives rise to most of the genital duct system, and the lower part of the vagina originates from the urogenital sinus.

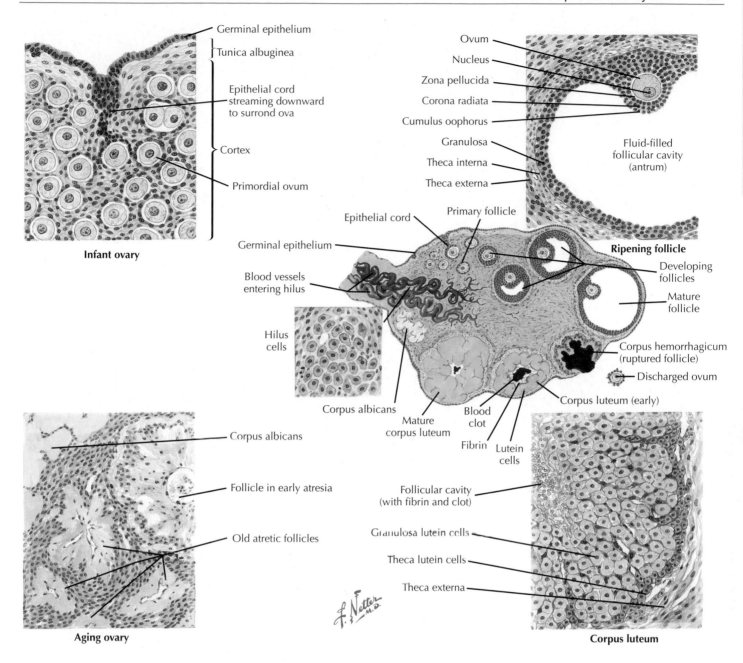

Germinal epithelium
Tunica albuginea
Epithelial cord streaming downward to surround ova
Cortex
Primordial ovum

Infant ovary

Ovum
Nucleus
Zona pellucida
Corona radiata
Cumulus oophorus
Granulosa
Theca interna
Theca externa

Fluid-filled follicular cavity (antrum)

Ripening follicle

Epithelial cord
Primary follicle
Germinal epithelium
Blood vessels entering hilus
Developing follicles
Mature follicle
Hilus cells
Corpus hemorrhagicum (ruptured follicle)
Discharged ovum
Corpus luteum (early)
Corpus albicans
Mature corpus luteum
Blood clot
Fibrin
Lutein cells

Corpus albicans
Follicle in early atresia
Old atretic follicles

Aging ovary

Follicular cavity (with fibrin and clot)
Granulosa lutein cells
Theca lutein cells
Theca externa

Corpus luteum

18.2 OVARIAN STRUCTURES AND DEVELOPMENT

The ovaries—solid, almond-shaped glands—are 3 cm long and 2 cm wide in adults, although their size and histologic appearance differ during menstrual cycles, pregnancy, and postmenopausal period. One side of the ovary has a mesentery—the mesovarium—which attaches the ovary at its **hilum** to the broad ligament. Ovaries are covered by a reflection of visceral peritoneum, originally known as **germinal epithelium** but better termed **ovarian surface epithelium.** Germinal epithelium is a misnomer, as its cells are not the source of ova but are modified mesothelial cells lining the peritoneal cavity. An ovary is divided into an outer **cortex** and an inner **medulla,** which are not clearly demarcated. Under the surface epithelium is a dense fibrous connective tissue, the **tunica albuginea,** which encapsulates the whole ovary. The

remaining cortex is richly cellular connective tissue arranged in a whorl-like pattern and harboring oocyte-containing **ovarian follicles** of various sizes and at different stages of maturation and degeneration. In childhood, the cortex contains numerous **primordial follicles;** in sexually mature women, **corpora lutea** form at sites of ruptured follicles. The ill-defined medulla consists of loose connective tissue with many convoluted **blood vessels,** nerves, and lymphatics. Ovaries at birth hold about 400,000 primary oocytes, which developed from oogonia; by puberty, about 40,000 oocytes remain after degeneration or **atresia.** In women, an ovum is liberated from an ovary via *ovulation* about every 28 days. Like testes, ovaries have both *exocrine* (cytogenic) and *endocrine* functions: they produce the hormones *estrogen* and *progesterone.*

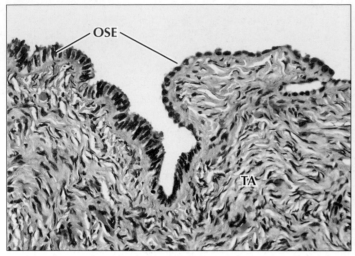

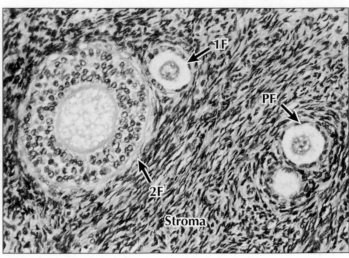

▲ **Light micrograph (LM) of the surface of the ovary.** The ovarian surface epithelium (**OSE**) consists of one layer of cuboidal to columnar cells. A basement membrane separates them from underlying tunica albuginea (**TA**). 390×. *H&E.*

▲ **LM of part of the ovarian cortex.** Markedly cellular connective tissue stroma surrounds primordial (**PF**), primary (**1F**), and secondary (**2F**) ovarian follicles. 295×. *H&E.*

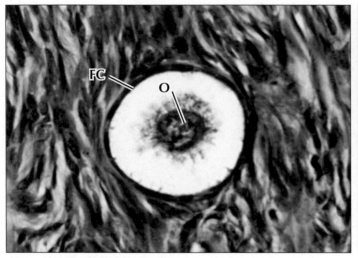

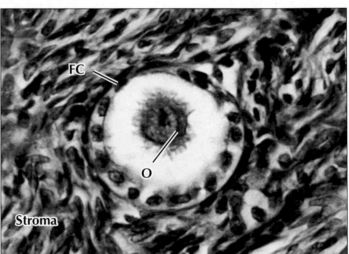

▲ **LM of a primordial follicle in the ovarian cortex.** One layer of squamous follicular cells (**FC**) surrounds a primary oocyte (**O**). The oocyte has a large vesicular nucleus. The clear space between oocyte and follicular cells is a cell shrinkage-related preparation artifact. 790×. *H&E.*

▲ **LM of a primary follicle.** One layer of cuboidal follicular cells (**FC**) envelops an oocyte (**O**). Surrounding stroma is highly cellular and contains elongated cells, some of which will become theca interna cells. The space between oocyte and follicular cells is a preparation artifact. 790×. *H&E.*

18.3 HISTOLOGY OF THE OVARIAN CORTEX

Development of **ovarian follicles,** which consist of an **oocyte** and surrounding epithelial layer of **follicular cells,** is complex. By birth, all oogonia have become **primary oocytes,** which have reached prophase of the first division of *meiosis.* Follicles in the cortex may be resting, or **primordial; maturing** (known as **primary** and **secondary follicles**); or **mature (Graafian).** Primordial follicles are just under the **tunica albuginea** and have not yet begun to develop. They contain a primary oocyte, measuring about 25 μm in diameter, that has an eccentric **nucleus** with a prominent nucleolus. One layer of **squamous epithelial cells,** the follicular cells, surrounds it. A thin basal lamina lies on the outer surface of these cells and separates them from surrounding **connective tissue stroma.** After puberty, about 20 primordial follicles become activated monthly during *menstrual cycles.* Usually, one follicle among them becomes dominant and moves to the next developmental stage by becoming a primary follicle. This follicle is slightly larger, with an oocyte, 40-45 μm in diameter, containing a large clear nucleus with distinct nucleolus. Surrounding follicular cells undergo cell division and become cuboidal. Their cytoplasm assumes a granular appearance, so the cells are now known as **granulosa cells,** which are surrounded by a basal lamina. Interstitial (stroma) cells adjacent to the follicle differentiate into a concentric sheath of **theca interna cells.**

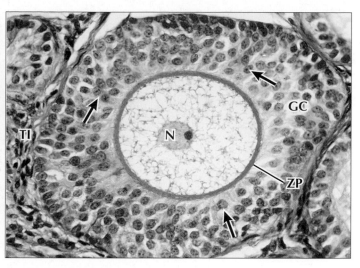

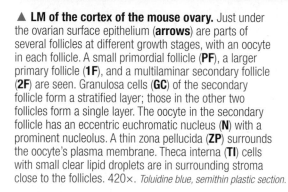

▲ **LM of the cortex of the mouse ovary.** Just under the ovarian surface epithelium (**arrows**) are parts of several follicles at different growth stages, with an oocyte in each follicle. A small primordial follicle (**PF**), a larger primary follicle (**1F**), and a multilaminar secondary follicle (**2F**) are seen. Granulosa cells (**GC**) of the secondary follicle form a stratified layer; those in the other two follicles form a single layer. The oocyte in the secondary follicle has an eccentric euchromatic nucleus (**N**) with a prominent nucleolus. A thin zona pellucida (**ZP**) surrounds the oocyte's plasma membrane. Theca interna (**TI**) cells with small clear lipid droplets are in surrounding stroma close to the follicles. 420×. *Toluidine blue, semithin plastic section.*

▲ **LM of a preantral secondary follicle.** The euchromatic nucleus (**N**) of the oocyte has a small, prominent eccentric nucleolus. A densely stained, eosinophilic zona pellucida (**ZP**) surrounds pale vesicular cytoplasm. Several layers of granulosa cells (**GC**), some undergoing mitosis (**arrows**), lie concentrically around the oocyte. Surrounding stroma shows early organization into a theca interna (**TI**). 375×. *H&E.*

▶ **LM of a late-term secondary follicle.** Granulosa cells surround the oocyte and its zona pellucida (**ZP**). Next to the outer layer of granulosa cells is a sheath of stromal cells: the theca interna. Several irregular intercellular spaces, or antral lakes (**arrows**), are among the granulosa cells. As the spaces accumulate fluid, they enlarge, become confluent, and give rise to a cavity—the follicular antrum. 270×. *H&E.*

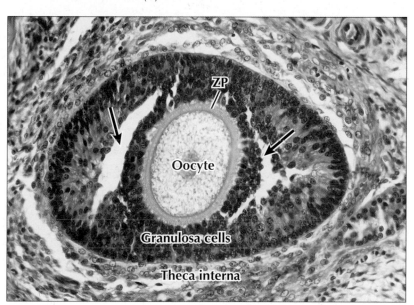

18.4 HISTOLOGY OF DEVELOPING OVARIAN FOLLICLES

The **follicular epithelium** and surrounding **stroma** are involved in the maturation process of follicles and undergo both *hyperplasia* and *hypertrophy*. They form a solid multilaminar **secondary follicle** in which mitotically active **granulosa cells** become stratified and form several layers of concentrically arranged, closely packed cells. The **primary oocyte** diameter increases, and a homogeneous, eosinophilic extracellular layer, the **zona pellucida,** surrounds the cell's **plasma membrane.** Both oocyte and granulosa cells synthesize the zona pellucida, which is rich in proteoglycans. As the follicle enlarges and consists of 8-12 layers of granulosa

cells, small, irregular fluid-filled spaces develop among the cells, and the follicle is called a **secondary** (vesicular, or antral) **follicle.** When the growing follicle has a diameter of about 200 μm, spaces coalesce (and accumulate more fluid) to form a single cavity known as the follicular antrum. The clear, viscous fluid within the antrum—the *liquor folliculi*—is rich in hyaluronic acid, growth factors, and steroid hormones produced by granulosa cells. **Theca interna** cells become vascularized and secrete the steroid androstenedione, from which granulosa cells produce estrogens. An outer layer of theca externa cells also forms and is continuous with connective tissue cells of the stroma.

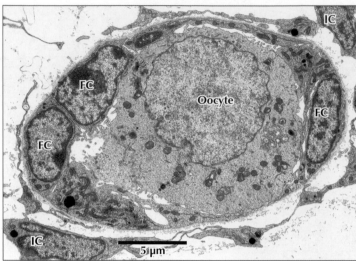

◀ **Electron micrograph (EM) of a primordial follicle in a mouse ovary.** Flattened follicular cells (**FC**) around an oocyte rest on a thin basal lamina; two interstitial cells (**IC**) are outside the follicle. The oocyte has a smooth surface with occasional small microvilli. Its large euchromatic nucleus has finely dispersed chromatin. A few mitochondria and vesicular structures are seen throughout the relatively pale cytoplasm. 3400×.

▶ **EM of part of a primary follicle.** The zona pellucida between the oocyte and granulosa cells consists of amorphous material rich in glycoproteins and proteoglycans. It contains profiles of small, irregularly shaped microvilli that emanate from granulosa cells and oocyte. Granulosa cells at this stage contain abundant ribosomes and RER. 6300×.

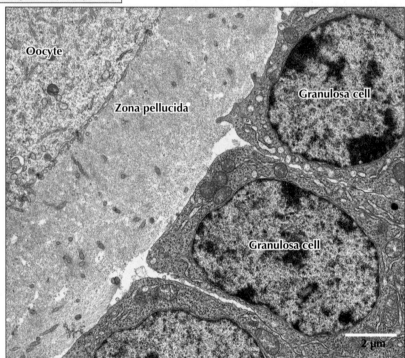

18.5 ULTRASTRUCTURE OF DEVELOPING OVARIAN FOLLICLES

Follicular and **granulosa cells** display a high mitotic activity during development of **ovarian follicles.** These cells are involved in synthesis and maintenance of the **zona pellucida.** Their **cytoplasm** is rich in **rough endoplasmic reticulum** (RER) and free **ribosomes;** mitochondria, lipid droplets, and lysosomes, although present, are not abundant. Junctional complexes occur between granulosa cells. Desmosomes probably reinforce the structural integrity of the follicle, zona pellucida, and corona radiata during ovulation. Gap junctions are sites of electrical and ionic communication between cells. The large round **oocyte** has a spherical, eccentrically placed **nucleus** with dispersed **chromatin** and an irregular nuclear envelope. The surrounding oocyte cytoplasm contains an array of organelles including closely packed cytoplasmic filaments, spherical mitochondria, free ribosomes, assorted

vesicles, and profiles of endoplasmic reticulum. The zona pellucida is a thick extracellular layer between the oocyte and the granulosa cells of the follicle. Slender **microvilli** of the oocyte and granulosa cells extend into the zona pellucida.

CLINICAL POINT

In developed countries, about 40 in 1000 births result from **multiple pregnancies,** most of which produce twins. **Identical (monozygotic) twins** come from a single oocyte that splits into two zygotes during early development. Identical twins share the same placenta but usually have separate amnions. **Fraternal (dizygotic) twins** develop when two oocytes are fertilized by separate spermatozoa. Fraternal fetuses have separate placentas and amnions. The number of fraternal twin births has greatly increased since 1980 as *infertility treatment* has become more common: multiple fetuses conceived with *assisted reproductive technology* are almost always fraternal.

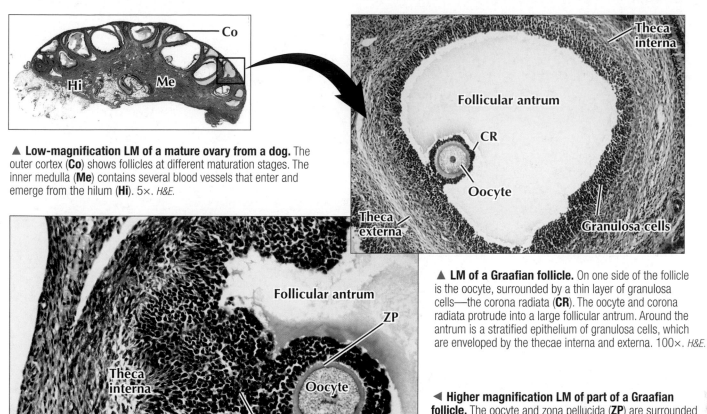

▲ **Low-magnification LM of a mature ovary from a dog.** The outer cortex (**Co**) shows follicles at different maturation stages. The inner medulla (**Me**) contains several blood vessels that enter and emerge from the hilum (**Hi**). 5×. *H&E.*

▲ **LM of a Graafian follicle.** On one side of the follicle is the oocyte, surrounded by a thin layer of granulosa cells—the corona radiata (**CR**). The oocyte and corona radiata protrude into a large follicular antrum. Around the antrum is a stratified epithelium of granulosa cells, which are enveloped by the thecae interna and externa. 100×. *H&E.*

◀ **Higher magnification LM of part of a Graafian follicle.** The oocyte and zona pellucida (**ZP**) are surrounded by a corona radiata (**CR**) that protrudes into a large follicular antrum. The cumulus oophorus (**CO**) is a mass of granulosa cells. The surrounding theca has differentiated into two layers—interna and externa. The antrum contains some flocculent eosinophilic precipitate. 176×. *H&E.*

18.6 HISTOLOGY OF MATURE GRAAFIAN FOLLICLES

After 12-14 days, the mature Graafian (tertiary) follicle is the final stage in development. With a diameter of 1.5-2.5 cm, it contains an **oocyte** that has reached a maximum size of about 150 µm. The primary oocyte sits in a local eccentric thickening of the granulosa cell layer, the **cumulus oophorus,** which projects into the **antrum.** One or more layers of **granulosa cells** are attached to the oocyte as the **corona radiata** and accompany it after *ovulation.* The antrum, the largest part of the follicle, is surrounded by multiple granulosa cell layers, which are, in turn, surrounded by **thecae interna** and **externa.** The **zona pellucida** is now 5-10 µm thick and anchors the oocyte to the corona radiata. The dominant follicle occupies the full breadth of the **cortex** and usually bulges above the ovarian surface. At their point of contact—the **stigma**—the tunica albuginea and the thecae become attenuated on the surface. The oocyte and corona radiata detach from the follicular wall and float freely in the fluid-filled antrum. Shortly before ovulation, the oocyte resumes meiosis to form a large secondary oocyte and a smaller polar body that disintegrates. The secondary oocyte, with a *haploid* number of chromosomes, is arrested in metaphase of the second meiotic division until fertilization. Increased luteinizing hormone on about day 14 of the *menstrual cycle* is thought to stimulate this meiotic division just before ovulation and may cause a follicle to rupture. Ovaries of young women usually have several Graafian follicles that may stay at this stage for several months. At ovulation, a follicle ruptures and releases the oocyte and corona radiata, which enter the fallopian tube infundibulum.

CLINICAL POINT

Nearly 90% of **ovarian malignancies** are *epithelial ovarian carcinomas* arising from the ovarian surface (germinal) epithelium. Ovarian cancer is one of the most common gynecologic cancers and the fifth most frequent cause of death in women. The risk of ovarian cancer increases with age, so this cancer occurs mostly in postmenopausal women. About 10% of ovarian cancers are familial, three distinct hereditary patterns having been identified. In most families affected by the *breast and ovarian cancer syndrome,* a genetic linkage on the *BRCA1* locus of chromosome 17q21 has been found. Ovarian cancer usually spreads by local shedding into the peritoneal cavity followed by implantation in the peritoneal surface.

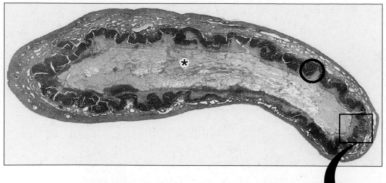

◀ **Low-power LM of the ovary.** The section passes through a corpus luteum. Its outer aspect is highly folded (**circle**) and contains tightly packed granulosa and theca lutein cells, which surround a central cavity (✱) filled with coagulated blood and fibrous scar tissue. 6.5×. *H&E.*

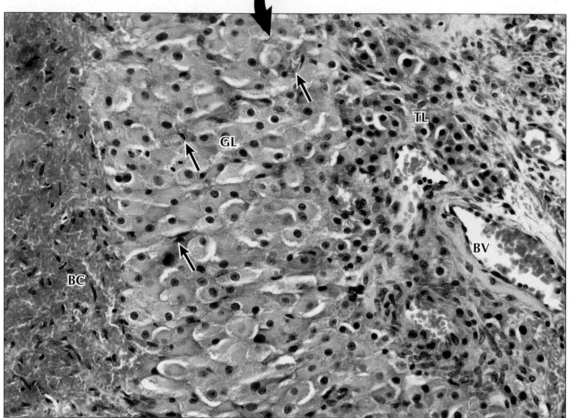

▲ **LM of part of the corpus luteum.** The large, polyhedral granulosa lutein cells (**GL**) have round nuclei and pale-staining cytoplasm. The cells encroach on a fibrin-containing blood-filled cavity (**BC**). Peripherally aggregated theca lutein cells (**TL**) are smaller and have more darkly stained nuclei than do granulosa lutein cells. Blood vessels (**BV**) are abundant peripherally; capillaries (**arrows**) invade the granulosa layer. 250×. *H&E.*

18.7 STRUCTURE AND FUNCTION OF THE CORPUS LUTEUM

After the Graafian follicle has ruptured at *ovulation* and the secondary **oocyte** is released, a temporary glandular structure—the corpus luteum (yellow body)—forms in the follicular remnant. The follicle collapses and becomes highly infolded, and its lumen fills with fibrin-containing fluid and blood. The coagulation in the antral space forms a clot that is replaced by **fibrous scar tissue.** The basement membrane separating **granulosa cells** from **theca interna cells** is broken down, and vascular invasion of the formerly avascular granulosa layer results. Luteinizing hormone from the anterior pituitary influences both granulosa and theca interna cells to undergo marked histologic changes and become

granulosa lutein and **theca lutein cells,** respectively. These increase in number and size and become polyhedral. They are lightly eosinophilic; their cytoplasm accumulates numerous lipid droplets. Both cell types have features in common with steroid-secreting cells. Granulosa lutein cells synthesize and secrete the hormone progesterone, which prepares the endometrium for *implantation* of a fertilized ovum and stimulates growth of mammary glands. Theca lutein cells synthesize and secrete estrogen. If *pregnancy* occurs, the corpus luteum persists for the first 8 weeks, after which the placenta becomes the major site for steroid hormone production. If pregnancy does not occur, the corpus luteum gradually involutes, stops producing progesterone, and forms a white scar called the corpus albicans, or white body.

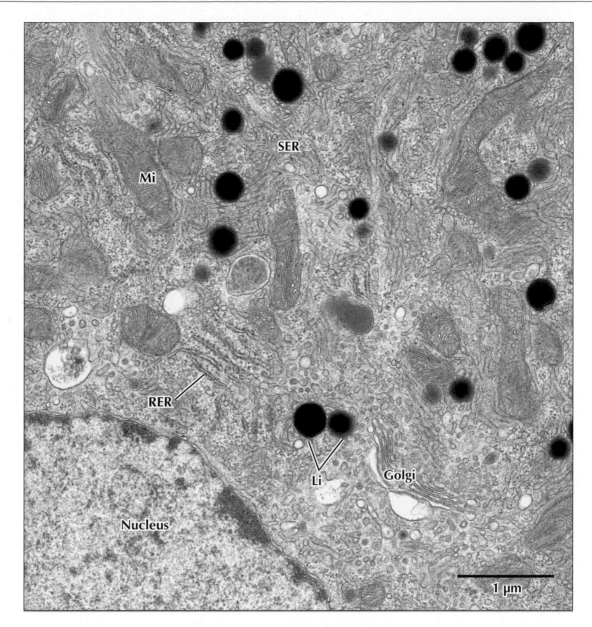

▲ **EM of part of a granulosa lutein cell from a near-term pregnant mouse.** The typical euchromatic nucleus is consistent with the cell's functionally active state. The cytoplasm is packed with various closely packed organelles. As in other steroid-secreting cells, a well-developed juxtanuclear Golgi complex and numerous round lipid droplets (**Li**) are found. The abundant SER is organized as an intercommunicating network of membrane-bound tubules and vesicles; the RER, as parallel stacks studded with ribosomes. Variably sized mitochondria (**Mi**) contain tubulovesicular cristae. 25,000×.

18.8 ULTRASTRUCTURE AND FUNCTION OF STEROID-SECRETING CELLS IN THE OVARY

Ovarian steroid-secreting cells include **theca interna, granulosa lutein,** and **theca lutein cells.** They share ultrastructural features with steroid-secreting cells in the male reproductive tract and in other organs producing steroid hormones. They have many unique structural features that facilitate acquisition of cholesterol and its conversion into steroid hormones. The plasma membrane on the cell surface has many microvilli and clathrin-coated pits that house receptors for low-density lipoprotein for cholesterol uptake. Underlying the microvilli is a narrow zone of cytoplasm with many tightly packed filaments extending into the microvilli. Steroidogenic **organelles** include **smooth endoplasmic reticulum** (SER) and abundant **mitochondria** with **tubulovesicular cristae.**

The SER consists of highly folded, radiating **cisternae** that communicate and interdigitate with each other. The SER contains enzymes involved in cholesterol synthesis and steroid hormone production. The cytoplasm also has well-developed, dispersed **Golgi complexes.** Free **ribosomes** and elements of RER are present in variable amounts for protein synthesis. **Lipid droplets** for cholesterol storage are also prominent. Most cells have a free surface with many microvilli and bordering a pericapillary space from which they are separated by a thin basal lamina. Steroidogenic cells are linked by many gap junctions, which likely provide a mechanism for coordinating hormonal activity of the cells. Nearby capillaries are typically fenestrated, with an attenuated endothelium for rapid, efficient delivery of secretory product into the circulation.

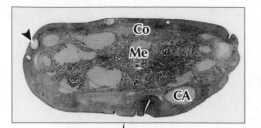

◀ **Low-magnification LM of a postmenopausal ovary.** Many pale-stained corpora albicantia (**CA**) occupy the cortex (**Co**) and extend into the medulla (**Me**). The stroma is highly cellular; many blood vessels are in the central medulla. Only a few small follicles (**arrow head**) persist close to the ovarian surface. Parts of the ovarian surface look slightly convoluted. 4×. *H&E.*

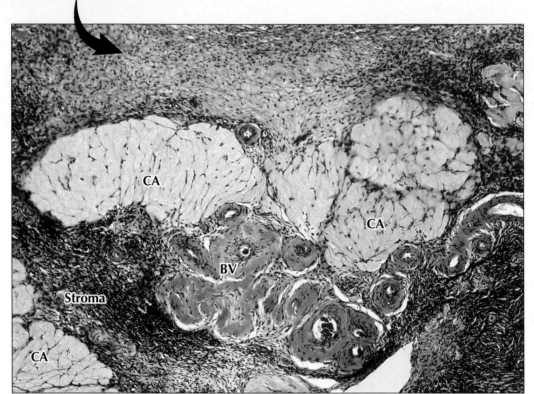

▲ **Higher magnification LM of part of a postmenopausal ovary.** The corpus albicans (**CA**) consists of dense hyaline connective tissue that forms scar tissue sharply demarcated from surrounding ovarian stroma. Many large, coiled blood vessels (**BV**) are present. Macrophages are often seen in a newly formed corpus albicans; a mature corpus albicans has convoluted borders and contains densely packed collagen fibers with occasional fibroblasts. With aging, corpora albicantia may become focally calcified. Most are resorbed and replaced by ovarian stroma, but persistent corpora albicantia are abundant in the medulla of postmenopausal ovaries. 85×. *H&E.*

18.9 HISTOLOGY OF ATRETIC FOLLICLES AND SENILE OVARIES

During the normal reproductive period, only about 400 **ovarian follicles** of the 400,000 present at birth mature fully. Beginning in fetal development and progressing to puberty, maturity, and **menopause,** most follicles, either primordial follicles or later developmental stages, degenerate. Their remnants remain in the ovary as atretic follicles. *Atresia,* or involution of follicles, first occurs in the oocyte, which shrinks and undergoes cytolysis. Degeneration of follicular cells then occurs: they become pyknotic, detach from each other, and undergo autolysis. The zona pellucida swells and may last for long periods. The theca cells become arranged in vascularized cords, degenerate, and are replaced by **connective tissue. Macrophages** in the **stroma** are abundant. Atretic follicles typically show remnants of the basal lamina between granulosa cells and theca interna that appear as thick, partially collapsed, eosinophilic glassy membranes. Masses of remaining **scar tissue,** known as corpora atretica, look similar to **corpora albicantia** but are smaller. Menopause marks the end of the reproductive period, and ovaries no longer release oocytes or produce hormones. Postmenopausal ovaries are shrunken in size and appear puckered, with a few widely scattered follicles that have not developed and many remnants of corpora lutea, which have become corpora albicantia. With aging, the stroma is denser, the tunica albuginea is thicker, and the ovarian surface epithelium is quite attenuated. A common feature of old age is the presence of large, abnormal, fluid-containing cystic follicles.

▼ **Fallopian tubes (oviducts, uterine tubes).**

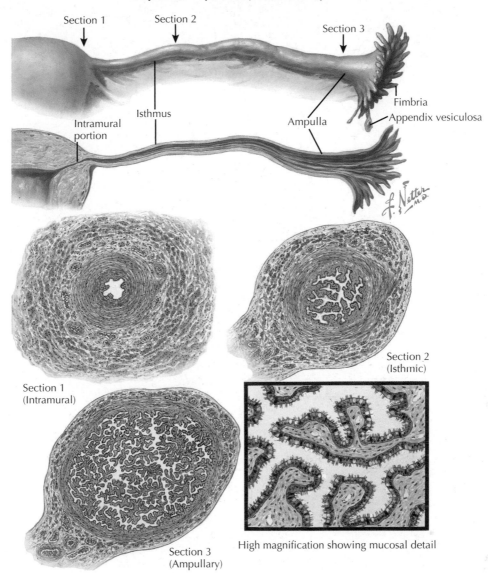

Section 1   Section 2   Section 3

Isthmus

Intramural portion

Fimbria
Appendix vesiculosa

Ampulla

f. Netter
m.d.

Section 1
(Intramural)

Section 2
(Isthmic)

Section 3
(Ampullary)

High magnification showing mucosal detail

18.10   STRUCTURE AND FUNCTION OF FALLOPIAN TUBES

Fallopian tubes (oviducts, uterine tubes) extend from the ovary to the uterus. They are 12-15 cm long and 0.7-5 cm in diameter. They develop from unfused midregions of müllerian ducts in the embryo. They are suspended by thin mesentery known as the mesosalpinx, which is derived from the broad ligament. After *ovulation,* the fallopian tube receives the oocyte and provides a suitable environment for *fertilization.* It is also where initial embryonic development normally occurs, for about 3 days before transport of the early embryo, or zygote, to the uterus. The fallopian tube has four parts. The **infundibulum** is the initial, open-ended, trumpet-shaped segment that bears fringed folds called **fimbria.** The tube opens into the peritoneal cavity, so it may allow infection to enter the abdomen. The most dilated part of the fallopian tube, which accounts for most of its length, is the **ampulla.**

It has a thin wall with complex infoldings of **mucosa.** The ampulla leads into the shortest, thick-walled segment known as the **isthmus,** which connects to the uterus. The last part, which passes through the uterine wall, is the **intramural part.**

CLINICAL POINT

Ectopic pregnancy occurs when a fertilized ovum implants in tissue outside of the uterus. The most common such site is a fallopian tube, but this type of pregnancy may occur in the ovary, abdomen, or cervix. Most cases are caused by conditions that obstruct or slow passage of a fertilized ovum through the fallopian tube to the uterus. They often result from scarring caused by prior tubal infection or surgery. About 50% of women with ectopic pregnancies have a history of *salpingitis* or *pelvic inflammatory disease.* Ectopic pregnancy usually leads to death of the embryo and severe internal hemorrhage by the mother during the second month of pregnancy.

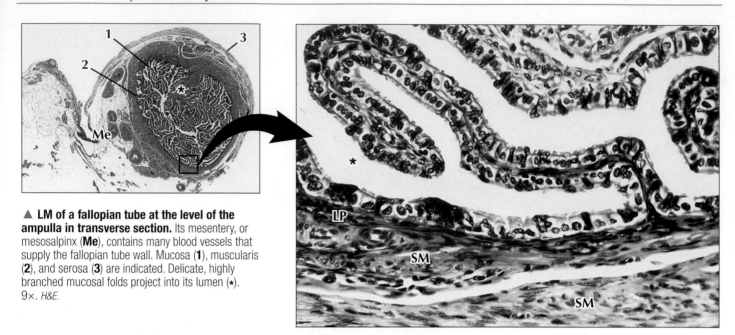

▲ **LM of a fallopian tube at the level of the ampulla in transverse section.** Its mesentery, or mesosalpinx (**Me**), contains many blood vessels that supply the fallopian tube wall. Mucosa (**1**), muscularis (**2**), and serosa (**3**) are indicated. Delicate, highly branched mucosal folds project into its lumen (*). 9×. *H&E.*

▲ **LM of part of a fallopian tube wall.** Mucosal folds projecting into the lumen (*) greatly enhance the surface area of the epithelium. Deep to the lamina propria (**LP**) are scattered smooth muscle cells (**SM**) arranged in two ill-defined layers. 250×. *H&E.*

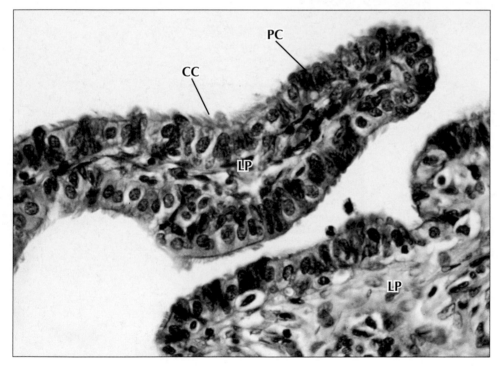

◄ **Higher magnification LM of the mucosa of a fallopian tube.** Simple columnar epithelium covering slender mucosal folds is better seen. Peg cells (**PC**) with apical blebs interspersed with ciliated cells (**CC**) rest on a delicate basement membrane. Underlying lamina propria (**LP**) is richly cellular and well vascularized. 475×. *H&E.*

18.11   HISTOLOGY AND FUNCTION OF FALLOPIAN TUBES

A fallopian tube consists of an inner **mucosa, muscularis,** and external **serosa.** The mucosa's many longitudinal folds greatly increase surface area, especially in uppermost areas of the tube. The folds decrease progressively in height and complexity toward the uterus. The lining **epithelium** is mostly **simple columnar** and a mixture of two cell types. **Ciliated cells** with spherical nuclei bear apical cilia that beat toward the uterus. The fewer nonciliated **secretory cells** are named **peg cells,** because they bulge above the surface and appear to insert into the epithelium like pegs. Changes in the height of the epithelium and relative numbers of these cell types vary regionally and according to stages of the *menstrual cycle.* During the *proliferative phase,* epithelial cells are tall and colum-nar, and ciliated cells predominate. During the *secretory phase,* the epithelium is low columnar to cuboidal, with a high number of peg cells, which synthesize and secrete glycoproteins to provide nutrients to oocytes. The chief function of ciliary motility is transport of oocytes from upper to lower ends of fallopian tubes. The fallopian tube wall contains no glands. The muscularis consists of two indistinct layers of **smooth muscle**—an inner circular and an outer longitudinal—that undergo peristaltic contractions. The serosa is loose connective tissue with an outer covering of meso-thelial cells, corresponding to visceral peritoneum. Fallopian tubes have a rich vascular supply and lymphatic drainage; the nerve supply, sympathetic and parasympathetic nerves that innervate smooth muscle, follows the vasculature.

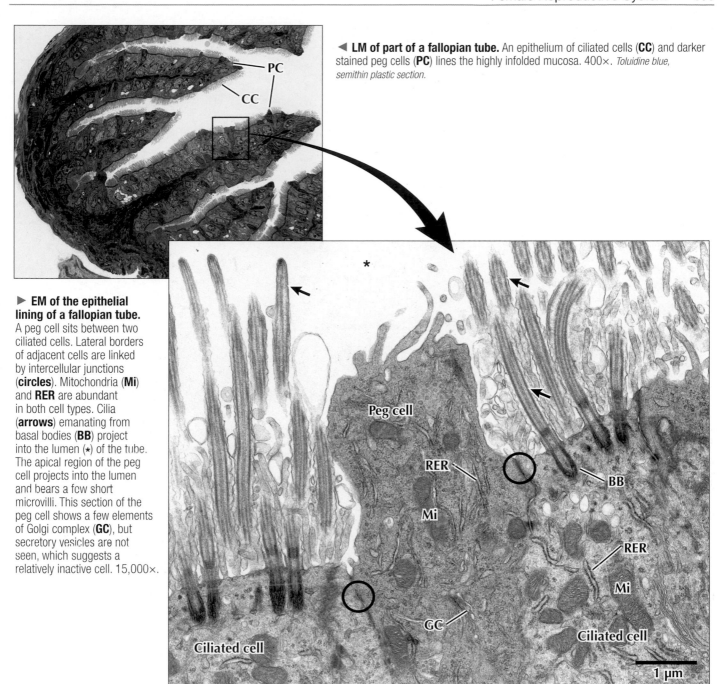

◀ **LM of part of a fallopian tube.** An epithelium of ciliated cells (**CC**) and darker stained peg cells (**PC**) lines the highly infolded mucosa. 400×. *Toluidine blue, semithin plastic section.*

▶ **EM of the epithelial lining of a fallopian tube.** A peg cell sits between two ciliated cells. Lateral borders of adjacent cells are linked by intercellular junctions (**circles**). Mitochondria (**Mi**) and **RER** are abundant in both cell types. Cilia (**arrows**) emanating from basal bodies (**BB**) project into the lumen (★) of the tube. The apical region of the peg cell projects into the lumen and bears a few short microvilli. This section of the peg cell shows a few elements of Golgi complex (**GC**), but secretory vesicles are not seen, which suggests a relatively inactive cell. 15,000×.

18.12   ULTRASTRUCTURE AND FUNCTION OF THE EPITHELIUM OF FALLOPIAN TUBES

Cells of this epithelium have function-related ultrastructural features. It was originally thought that the two cell types represented different functional states of the same cell, but now **nonciliated (peg) cells** are recognized as secretory and **ciliated cells** as involved in ciliary motility and oocyte transport. Epithelial cells in fallopian tubes, like those in the uterus, undergo cyclic changes related to phases of the *menstrual cycle*. Early in the *follicular phase*, estrogen stimulates synthetic activity of peg cells and ciliogenesis in ciliated cells. Both proliferation and functional activity of this epithelium are regulated by estrogen receptors and fallopian tube-specific transcription factors in the cells. The frequency of ciliary beat also depends on hormone levels. Actively secreting peg cells have a prominent RER, conspicuous **Golgi complex,** numerous **secretory vesicles,** a few **lysosomes,** and apical **microvilli** that amplify surface area. They produce a high-molecular-weight *glycoprotein*, which binds to the zona pellucida of oocytes in the fallopian tube. The glycoprotein likely regulates prefertilization reproductive events, including sperm capacitation and zona pellucida penetration. Ciliated cells have ultrastructural features similar to those of such cells of the respiratory tract. Cilia emanate from **basal bodies** and show a normal 9 + 2 microtubule pattern. *Kartagener syndrome*, a rare genetic disorder, is characterized by ciliary dyskinesia. Patients are often infertile, which in women is likely due to abnormal fallopian tube cilia, which are markedly reduced in number, lack the central microtubule pair, and show altered ciliary beat frequency.

▼ **Uterus and adnexa.**

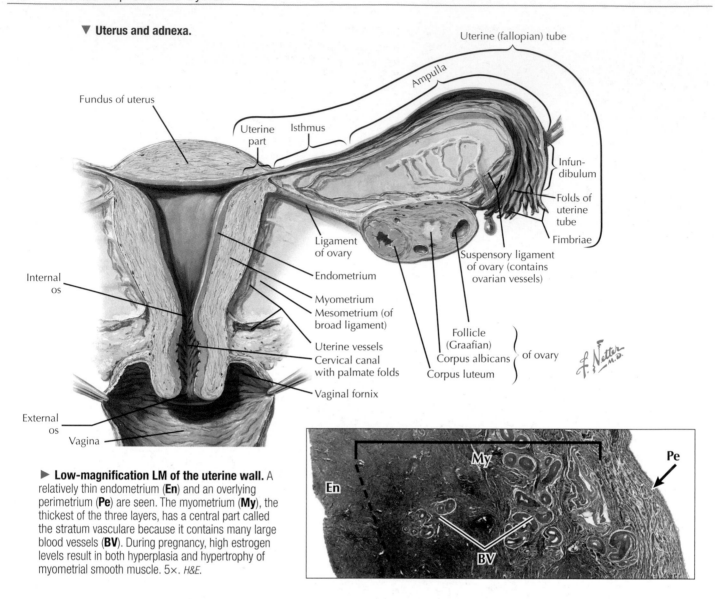

▶ **Low-magnification LM of the uterine wall.** A relatively thin endometrium (**En**) and an overlying perimetrium (**Pe**) are seen. The myometrium (**My**), the thickest of the three layers, has a central part called the stratum vasculare because it contains many large blood vessels (**BV**). During pregnancy, high estrogen levels result in both hyperplasia and hypertrophy of myometrial smooth muscle. 5×. *H&E.*

18.13 ANATOMY AND HISTOLOGY OF THE UTERUS

In the pelvis, between the urinary bladder and rectum, lies the uterus, a hollow pear-shaped organ with a thick muscular wall and a lumen lined by a mucous membrane. The expanded, upper part of the organ is the body, or **corpus. Fallopian tubes** enter the wall at the most superior, dome-shaped region, called the **fundus.** At the narrowest and most inferior part of the organ, the **cervix** opens into the **vagina.** The corpus and fundus are almost identical histologically, but the cervix shows some important structural differences. The wall of the nonpregnant uterus is about 2.5 cm thick and consists of three layers. The outer **perimetrium** is mainly connective tissue that is only partly covered in some areas by a peritoneal mesothelium constituting a serosa. The intermediate and thickest layer, the **myometrium,** consists of interconnecting bundles of **smooth muscle** separated by connective tissue. The three poorly defined layers of this smooth muscle are a function of the orientation of individual cells: inner and outer layers are mostly longitudinal, and the middle layer is obliquely circular.

The innermost **endometrium** is a specialized mucosa consisting of simple columnar epithelium, which undergoes pronounced cyclic changes during the *menstrual cycle.* It has associated simple tubular uterine glands and a highly cellular stroma, or lamina propria. Recurring changes in endometrial histology reflect the complex sequence of pituitary stimulation and ovarian response that prepare the endometrium each month for implantation and nutrition of a fertilized ovum.

CLINICAL POINT
Leiomyomas, commonly known as **fibroids,** are benign tumors of the uterus that arise as localized hyperplasia of smooth muscle cells of the myometrium. They are the most common tumors in the female pelvis, usually occurring before menopause and most likely as a result of endocrine imbalance. The single or multiple growths may be located in subserous, intramural, or submucosal sites in the uterine wall. Leiomyomas are usually completely surrounded by a connective tissue capsule. A common symptom is excessive and prolonged bleeding at menstruation.

▼ **Endometrial Blood Supply**

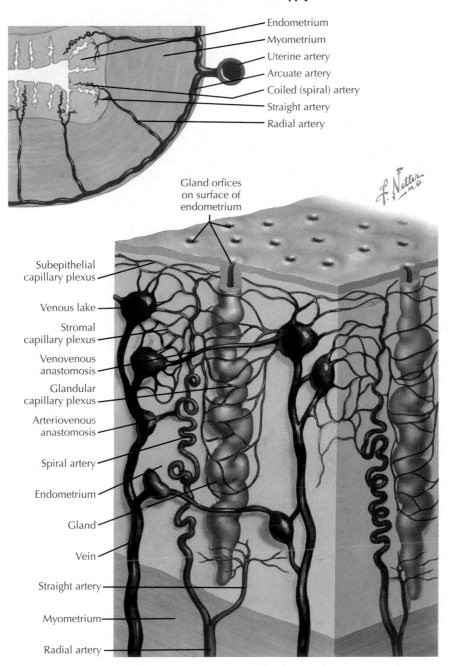

Endometrium
Myometrium
Uterine artery
Arcuate artery
Coiled (spiral) artery
Straight artery
Radial artery

Gland orfices
on surface of
endometrium

Subepithelial
capillary plexus

Venous lake

Stromal
capillary plexus

Venovenous
anastomosis

Glandular
capillary plexus

Arteriovenous
anastomosis

Spiral artery

Endometrium

Gland

Vein

Straight artery

Myometrium

Radial artery

18.14 ENDOMETRIAL BLOOD SUPPLY

The **endometrium** has a unique and dual blood supply. Knowledge of this supply has physiologic significance and provides a basis for understanding mechanisms of *menstruation.* The endometrium consists of two functional layers. The thicker, more superficial functionalis layer is most affected by menstruation; it is periodically shed and regenerated. A deeper basal layer, the stratum basale, is unaffected by hormonal variations, is not sloughed off during menstruation, and remains to aid the superficial layer regeneration. The blood supply to the two layers is from two separate sources. The **uterine artery** distributes blood to 6-10 **arcuate arteries,** which encircle the **uterus** just beneath the serosa. They, in turn, give off **radial arteries** that penetrate inward to the inner muscular layer of the **myometrium** and give

off two distinct sets of arteries, known as **basal** and **spiral arteries.** Short, straight basal arteries supply the stratum basale and maintain uninterrupted circulation. In contrast, spiral (coiled) arteries pass through the stratum basale, run parallel with uterine **glands,** and reach the endometrial surface. They drain into an extensive capillary network, which ramifies into thin-walled **venous lakes** that drain into efferent **veins.** The distal segment of spiral arteries degenerates and regenerates with each menstrual cycle. About 1 day before menstruation, intense vasoconstriction of these arteries produces ischemia and rupture of the capillaries that they supply. Uterine glands undergo necrosis; blood, uterine secretions, and tissue debris are sloughed off from the endometrium and discharged through the vagina.

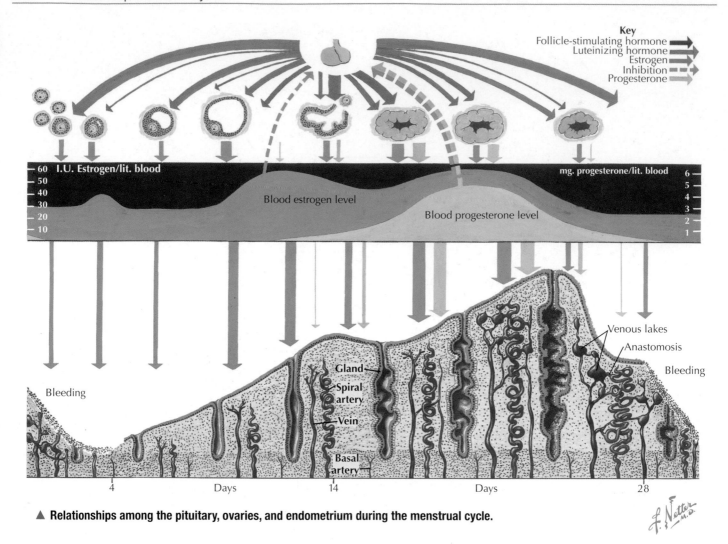

Key
Follicle-stimulating hormone
Luteinizing hormone
Estrogen
Inhibition
Progesterone

60
50
40
30
20
10

I.U. Estrogen/lit. blood

mg. progesterone/lit. blood

6
5
4
3
2
1

Blood estrogen level

Blood progesterone level

Venous lakes
Anastomosis

Bleeding

Bleeding

Gland
Spiral artery
Vein

Basal artery

4   Days   14   Days   28

▲ Relationships among the pituitary, ovaries, and endometrium during the menstrual cycle.

F. Netter M.D.

18.15 THE MENSTRUAL CYCLE: HISTOLOGIC AND HORMONAL CHANGES

The menstrual cycle is a sequence of morphologic and functional changes during the reproductive part of a woman's life that occurs every 28 days in the absence of pregnancy. The **endometrium** and **ovaries** undergo cyclic changes resulting from interplay of hormones produced by the **pituitary, ovarian follicles,** and **corpus luteum.** Phases in the cycle are **menstrual** (days 1-4); **follicular,** or **proliferative** (days 4-15); **luteal,** or **secretory** (days 15-27); and **premenstrual,** or **ischemic** (day 28). The pituitary contributes *follicle-stimulating hormone* (FSH), *luteinizing hormone* (LH), and *prolactin;* ovaries, *estrogen* and *progesterone.* Menstrual bleeding starts on day 1, with menstrual discharge a result of necrosis and shedding of the functionalis layer of the endometrium. The stratum basale is preserved to restore the endometrium during the follicular phase. At days 1-5, production of estrogen is low but that of FSH is maximal, leading to follicular growth in ovaries. The start of the menstrual cycle coincides with involution of the corpus luteum. The follicular stage involves rapid regeneration and repair of the endometrium and ovarian follicle maturation up to *ovulation,* which is induced by an LH surge and FSH. Estrogen

secretion by ovarian follicles stimulates growth of the endometrium. During the luteal stage, LH stimulates corpus luteum formation. Progesterone produced by the corpus luteum also influences development of **uterine glands** and stimulates uterine epithelial cells to accumulate glycogen and **spiral arteries** to lengthen. These marked histologic changes in the endometrium provide an optimal, receptive environment for embryo implantation.

CLINICAL POINT

Endometriosis is a common gynecologic disease in which endometrial tissue appears at unusual locations in the lower abdomen and pelvis. Diagnosis is based on laparoscopic surgical visualization, with histologic criteria used to determine disease stage and severity. It affects females between puberty and menopause but is most common between ages of 20 and 30 years. Symptoms include pelvic pain and premenstrual bleeding. Of unknown etiology, the disorder may result when endometrial cells peel off the uterine lining during the menstrual cycle and migrate via fallopian tubes to the peritoneal cavity. The condition often subsides after menopause, when estrogen stimulation declines.

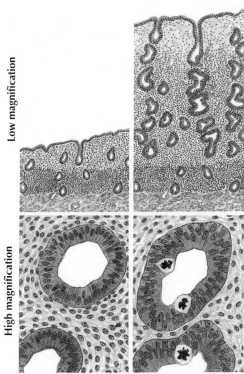

Low magnification

High magnification

Early proliferative phase   Late proliferative phase

▲ **Schematics of the endometrium during early (left) and late (right) follicular phases of the menstrual cycle.** In the former, the endometrium is relatively thin, and glands are simple and straight. In the late phase, the thicker endometrium shows marked growth in glands and stroma. Uterine glands appear more convoluted, and mitoses are often seen at higher magnification. This phase is one of maximum regeneration in both epithelium and surrounding stroma.

F. Netter M.D.

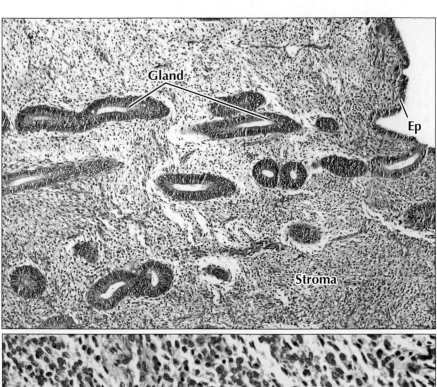

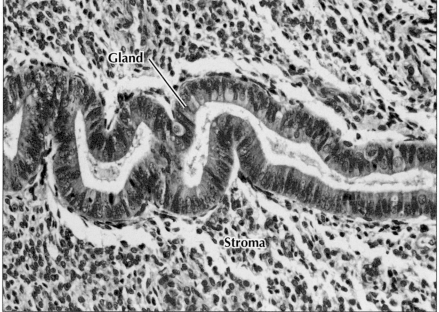

▲ **LMs of the endometrium during the early follicular phase at low magnification (Above) and late follicular phase at higher magnification (Below).** Uterine glands first appear straight and gradually become more tortuous as they reach the epithelial surface (**Ep**). Surrounding stroma is highly cellular. **Above:** 75×; **Below:** 280×. *H&E.*

18.16 HISTOLOGY OF THE ENDOMETRIUM: FOLLICULAR PHASE

This phase of the menstrual cycle is also called the *proliferative* or *estrogenic phase,* as it occurs during development of a Graafian follicle and depends on estrogen. It begins just after *menstruation* and ends 1 or 2 days after *ovulation.* Rapid regeneration of the **endometrium** begins from the narrow zone left after menstruation. The epithelium in the basal portions of the **uterine glands** replicates and grows to cover the raw mucosal surface. Numerous **mitoses** are seen in **columnar epithelial cells** of the glands, and **connective tissue cells** in the **stroma** multiply and rebuild the lamina propria. Uterine glands lengthen and become closely packed. They are at first simple and straight and lead directly from the base to the mucosal surface. Spiral arteries also grow from the stratum basale into more superficial regenerated tissue. In the **late follicular phase,** both glands and stroma show marked growth. Glands become tortuous and begin to show corkscrew convolutions. Stromal cells are separated by edematous fluid, mitoses are frequent, and epithelium is higher and more columnar, with nuclei being randomly placed. During the follicular phase, the endometrium thickens from about 0.5 mm to 2-3 mm.

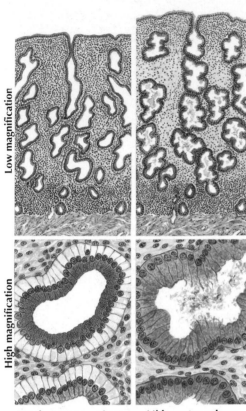

Early secretory phase Midsecretory phase

▲ **Schematic of the endometrium during early secretory (left) and midsecretory (right) phases of the menstrual cycle.** In the early phase and under the influence of progesterone, endometrial stroma shows less edema. Epithelial cells of the glands have round nuclei, with pale-staining basal cytoplasm due to glycogen deposits. In the later phase, glands have a distinctive saw-toothed appearance, and glandular epithelial cells are tall columnar with apically located glycogen. Secretions form bubbles at luminal margins and are discharged into the glandular lumen.

f. Netter M.D.

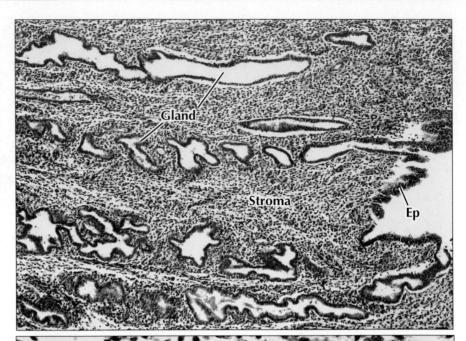

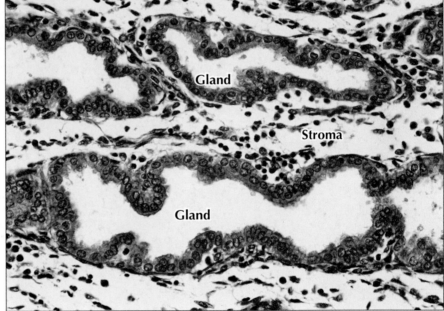

▲ **LMs of the endometrium during the secretory phase of the cycle at low (Above) and higher (Below) magnification.** Uterine glands are highly tortuous and have a serrated outline in section. They open onto the epithelial surface (**Ep**). Surrounding stroma is highly cellular. **Above:** 75×; **Below:** 280×. *H&E.*

18.17 HISTOLOGY OF THE ENDOMETRIUM: LUTEAL PHASE

This phase, also called the *progestational* or *secretory phase*, begins just after *ovulation* and ends on days 26-27 of the *menstrual cycle*. At 2-3 days after ovulation, **epithelial cells** of the **glands** and **mucosal surface** show early signs of secretory activity induced by progesterone. The **endometrium** shrinks slightly as **edema** in superficial layers is lost. At first, the round **nuclei** of epithelial cells are uniformly in line with the middle of each cell. **Glycogen** accumulates in basal areas of the cells, and mitoses are less common than in the preceding proliferative phase. On days 21-25, active secretion occurs, and glycogen is seen more apically in the epithe-

lial cells. *Hypertrophy* of uterine glands plus increased edema eventually expands endometrial thickness to a maximum of 4 mm or more. Uterine glands appear distinctively jagged. Rounded nuclei are now basal in location. Secretions, which are thick and mucoid and have a high glycogen and glycoprotein content, discharge into the glandular lumen and form bubbles at luminal margins of the epithelial cells. Cells in the **stroma** become greatly enlarged and pale staining, and glands are widely dilated. Spiral arteries extend to nearly the surface of the endometrium. If pregnancy occurs, stromal cells become decidual cells, which store lipid and glycogen.

▼ Low- and high-power colposcopic views of the normal transformation zone.

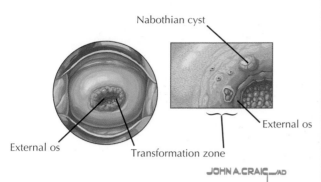

Nabothian cyst

External os

External os

Transformation zone

JOHN A.CRAIG—AD

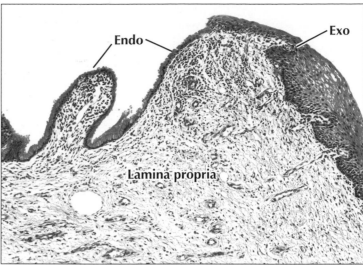

Endo

Exo

Lamina propria

▲ **Low-magnification LM of the mucosa of the uterine cervix.** The simple epithelium of the endocervix (**Endo**) is highly folded and continuous with stratified epithelium of the exocervix (**Exo**). Underlying lamina propria is richly cellular. 96×. *H&E.*

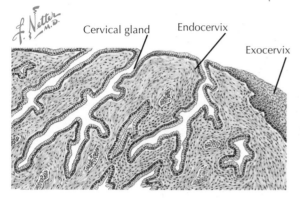

Cervical gland

Endocervix

Exocervix

▲ Schematic of the cervical squamocolumnar junction.

▶ **Higher magnification LM of the cervical squamocolumnar junction.** The endocervix (**Endo**) is lined by simple columnar epithelium with tall mucus-secreting cells. The epithelium abruptly changes to a nonkeratinized stratified squamous type in the exocervix (**Exo**). 290×. *H&E.*

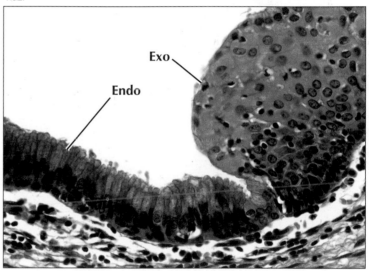

Exo

Endo

18.18 HISTOLOGY OF THE CERVIX

The cervix is the inferior, cylindrical tapering end of the uterus that consists of two anatomic regions. The upper part—the cervical canal—begins at the uterine isthmus and is about 3 cm long. It extends downward into the upper part of the vagina, known as the portio vaginalis. The cervical canal is lined by **mucous membrane** known as **endocervix.** The portio vaginalis is lined by the **exocervix,** which is continuous with the mucosal lining of the vagina. The endocervix is lined by mucus-secreting **simple columnar epithelium** that is arranged as deep compound furrows. The epithelium has glandular invaginations that are large and more branched than those in the body of the uterus and that secrete mucus. The glands sometimes become occluded and dilate, so follicles known as **nabothian cysts** form. The cervical epithelium does not change appreciably during the *menstrual cycle,* but minor changes associated with the amount, nature, and consistency of cervical mucus can be used to determine the timing of each cycle. An abrupt change in the epithelium occurs at the **external os**—

from simple columnar to **nonkeratinized stratified squamous.** This area, known as the **transformation zone,** is subject to tumor formation and is the site of most *cervical carcinomas.*

CLINICAL POINT

Cervical cancer is the second most common cancer in women and the leading cause of cancer-related death in women in underdeveloped countries. Routine cytologic screening via the *Papanicolaou (Pap) smear* can detect premalignant disease and has markedly reduced its incidence in North America. Of cervical carcinomas, 80%-90% develop as **squamous cell carcinomas** at the squamocolumnar junction; 10%-15% develop in glandular surface cells as **adenocarcinomas.** An abnormal precancerous change known as *cervical intraepithelial neoplasia* may progress to squamous intraepithelial *dysplasia,* which may develop into *carcinoma in situ* or *invasive carcinoma.* Treatment depends on stage of disease and includes surgery, radiation, and chemotherapy.

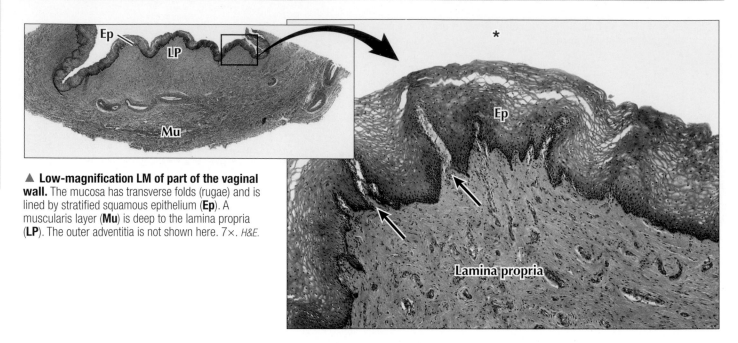

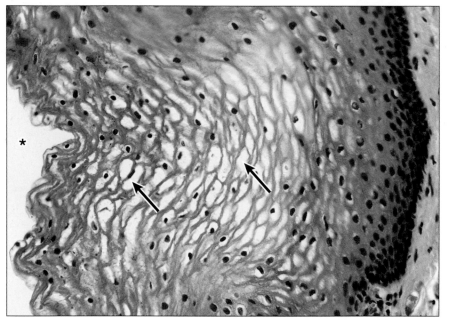

▲ **Low-magnification LM of part of the vaginal wall.** The mucosa has transverse folds (rugae) and is lined by stratified squamous epithelium (**Ep**). A muscularis layer (**Mu**) is deep to the lamina propria (**LP**). The outer adventitia is not shown here. 7×. *H&E.*

▲ **Low-magnification LM of the vaginal mucosa.** Thick stratified squamous epithelium (**Ep**), which lacks glands, lines the vaginal lumen (✱). Connective tissue papillae (**arrows**) project into the epithelium. Deeper in the lamina propria lies highly vascular, dense irregular connective tissue. 65×. *H&E.*

◀ **Higher magnification LM of the vaginal mucosa.** The multilayered stratified squamous epithelium responds to hormones and undergoes cyclic changes during the menstrual cycle. Small, round basal cells rest on the basement membrane (to the right); cells gradually become flattened and retain their nuclei as they approach the surface (to the left) and the vaginal lumen (✱). Cell maturation is marked by glycogen accumulation, which causes cytoplasm of the epithelial cells to appear clear (**arrows**). Superficial cells contain some keratin, but they normally do not show gross cornification in women of reproductive age. 300×. *H&E.*

18.19 HISTOLOGY OF THE VAGINA

The vagina is a distensible fibromuscular tube that connects the cervix of the uterus to the exterior of the body. It serves as the female organ of copulation and at final stages of pregnancy, the birth canal. Its wall has three layers: **mucosa, muscularis,** and **adventitia.** The mucosa consists of prominent **nonkeratinized stratified squamous epithelium,** 150-200 μm thick, and an underlying **lamina propria.** The vagina has no glands, with mucus for surface lubrication and protection being derived from **mucous glands** in the cervix. The transverse folds, or **rugae,** of the mucosa are prominent in the relaxed vagina. Under normal conditions, **surface cells** of the **epithelium** retain their **nuclei,** and their **cytoplasm** appears washed out because the cells store variable amounts of **glycogen.** Near the time of ovulation, estrogen stimulates an increased glycogen content. When the cells are shed, they discharge glycogen into the vaginal lumen. The highly cellular lamina propria contains an extensive venous plexus that becomes engorged with blood during sexual stimulation. Two ill-defined layers of smooth muscle make up the muscularis, which is continuous with the myometrium. The inner layer is oriented circularly; the outer layer is usually thicker and more longitudinal. A sphincter of skeletal muscle encircles the vaginal entrance. The outermost adventitia is a dense irregular connective tissue with abundant elastic fibers and an extensive vascular and nerve supply.

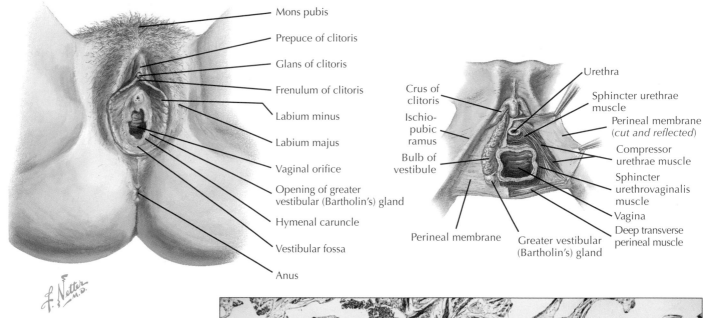

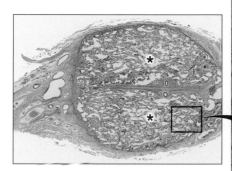

▲ **Low-magnification LM of the clitoris in transverse section.** The organ comprises two corpora cavernosa (✱). They contain erectile tissue, which accounts for the spongy appearance. 3×. *H&E.*

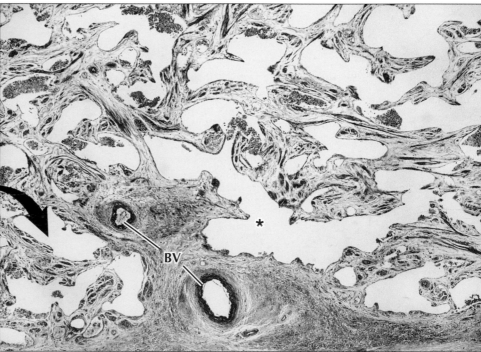

▲ **Higher magnification LM of erectile tissue of the clitoris.** An anastomotic network of many thin-walled vascular channels (✱) makes up the erectile tissue. Surrounding connective tissue contains blood vessels (**BV**) with thicker walls. 30×. *H&E.*

18.20 ANATOMY AND HISTOLOGY OF THE EXTERNAL GENITALIA

The external genitalia, or vulva, are the labia majora and minora, clitoris, vestibule, vaginal orifice, and vestibular glands. Homologous to the male scrotum, labia majora are folds of skin, covered by heavily pigmented epithelium, with hair follicles and sebaceous and sweat glands. Labia minora are folds of mucosa covered by deeply pigmented stratified squamous epithelium with underlying loose, vascularized connective tissue. Superficial cells of the epithelium are markedly keratinized. Sebaceous glands open to the surface and lack hair follicles. Homologous to corpora cavernosa of the penis, the clitoris is about 2 cm long and has two crura containing erectile tissue that end as a rudimentary glans clitoris. Unlike the penis, the clitoris lacks a corpus spongiosum. A dense connective tissue capsule with an intervening, incomplete septum covers the crura. Erectile tissue of the clitoris consists of a plexus of thin-walled venous channels that distend during sexual stimulation. Loose connective tissue and isolated smooth muscle cells are associated with these channels. Many nerve fascicles are in the connective tissue; the mucous membrane that covers the clitoris externally contains many sensory nerve endings. The vagina and urethra open into the vestibule, which is lined by stratified squamous epithelium. Near the clitoris and urethra, several minor vestibular glands (which resemble male glands of Littre) secrete mucus. Two larger tubuloalveolar glands, the major vestibular glands (of Bartholin), open on the inner surface of the labia minora. They resemble male bulbourethral glands.

▼ **Development of the placenta and fetal membranes.**

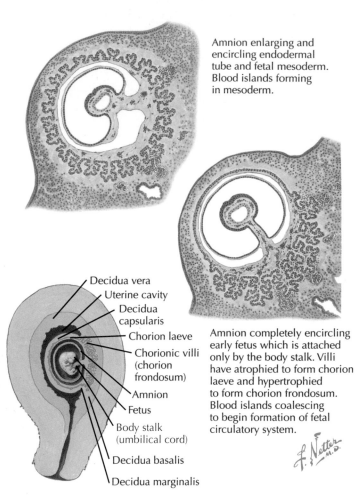

Amnion enlarging and encircling endodermal tube and fetal mesoderm. Blood islands forming in mesoderm.

Amnion completely encircling early fetus which is attached only by the body stalk. Villi have atrophied to form chorion laeve and hypertrophied to form chorion frondosum. Blood islands coalescing to begin formation of fetal circulatory system.

f. Netter
M.D.

Decidua vera
Uterine cavity
Decidua capsularis
Chorion laeve
Chorionic villi (chorion frondosum)
Amnion
Fetus
Body stalk (umbilical cord)
Decidua basalis
Decidua marginalis

Early fetal development and membrane formation in relation to uterus.

▶ **Panoramic LM of part of the placenta at low magnification.** Its spongy architecture is due to many closely packed chorionic villi and blood-filled intervillous spaces. 5×. *H&E.*

▼ **Placenta: form and structure.**

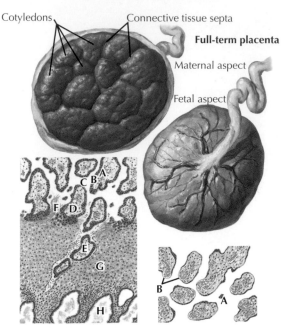

Cotyledons   Connective tissue septa

Full-term placenta
Maternal aspect
Fetal aspect

Section through deep portion of placenta—early gestation (A) Villus, (B) trophoblast, (C) intervillous space, (D) anchoring villus, (E) villus invading blood vessel, (F) fibrinoid degeneration, (G) decidua basalis, (H) gland.

Appearance of placental villi at term (A) Syncytial cell mass becoming trophoblastic embolus, (B) fetal blood vessel endothelium against a thinned syncytiotrophoblast, where they share a basal lamina. The cytotrophoblast has disappeared.

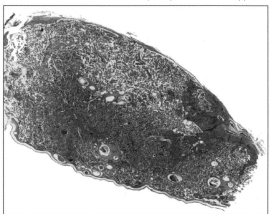

18.21   STRUCTURE AND FUNCTION OF THE PLACENTA

The placenta is a transitory composite structure with both **fetal** and **maternal** components. It develops in pregnancy in close association with uterine endometrium. The disc-shaped organ is 15-25 cm in diameter and 2-3 cm thick; it weighs 400-600 g at term. When viewed on the maternal side, it has 15-20 lobules, or cotyledons. The placenta serves many critical functions related to physiologic exchanges between mother and developing embryo or fetus, such as exchange of gases, electrolytes, and metabolites between maternal and fetal blood. Fetal waste products are excreted into maternal blood. Maternal antibodies are transmitted to the fetus, and the placenta produces several hormones including estrogens, progesterone, and human chorionic gonadotropin.

The maternal component of the placenta is the **decidua basalis** of the endometrium, which is the modified stratum basale in which the embryo is implanted. The fetal component, formed from the chorionic sac surrounding the embryo, consists of the chorionic plate and its branching **chorionic villi** that extend from the chorion like branches of a tree. The tips of the villi are attached to the decidua and, by 6 weeks, branches are formed with free tips, which create a villous spongework. **Intervillous spaces** contain maternal blood. Many chorionic villi end freely; others fuse with the decidua as anchoring elements. The villi provide a large surface area in contact with maternal blood for nutrient exchange. Fetal blood and maternal blood are close to each other but follow independent courses and do not mix, being separated by an efficient placental barrier.

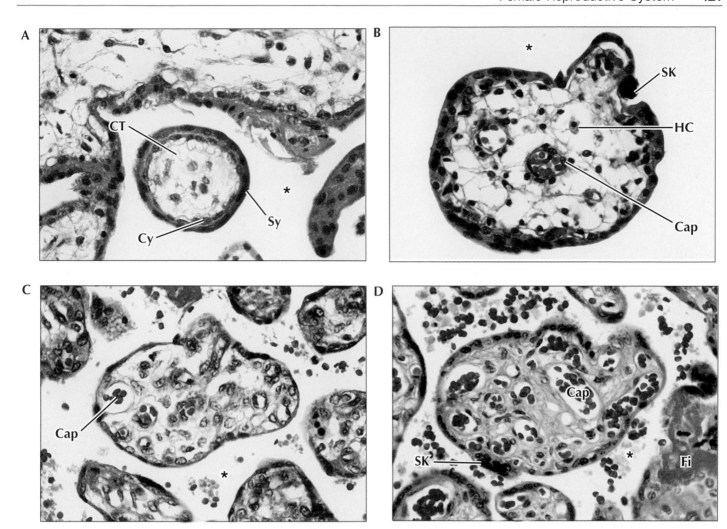

▲ **LMs of chorionic villi at different stages of placental development in transverse section.** At 8 weeks (**A**), placental villi are narrow and covered by two distinct cell layers. Outer syncytiotrophoblast (**Sy**) and inner cytotrophoblast (**Cy**) layers surround a core of mesenchymal connective tissue (**CT**) in which fetal vasculature will develop. Intervillous spaces (✱) are shown. By 12 weeks (**B**), the double trophoblast cell layer is less apparent, and reduced numbers of cytotrophoblasts appear singly, not as a continuous layer. Thin-walled fetal capillaries (**Cap**) are prominent, most lying in the center of each villus. In the stroma, Hofbauer cells (**HC**)—large pale-stained cells with eccentric nuclei—are more numerous in late pregnancy and serve as phagocytes. By 20 weeks (**C**) and at term (**D**), the many fetal capillaries with enlarged lumina are more peripherally located, lying close to the syncytiotrophoblast layer. Maternal blood fills intervillous spaces (✱). Syncytial knots (**SK**) and patches of fibrinoid substance (**Fi**) are common and increase progressively during the last trimester. 380×. *H&E.*

18.22 HISTOLOGY OF THE PLACENTA

Chorionic villi are the fundamental units of the placenta. Each villus is formed from two epithelial cell layers derived from the **trophoblast** of the embryo, which are closely associated with extraembryonic connective tissue. An inner single layer of **cytotrophoblasts**, or Langhans cells, consists of cuboidal epithelial cells with light-staining cytoplasm and distinct cell boundaries. They give rise to a continuous superficial layer of larger **syncytiotrophoblasts**, which stain darker and have ill-defined cell boundaries. Trophoblast cell layers initially form proliferating villous cords that invade the endometrium and destroy the walls of coiled arterioles and venules of the endometrial **stroma**. Extravasated **maternal blood** creates irregular **intervillous spaces** in eroded decidual tissue, circulates in these spaces, and bathes the chorionic villi. The core of each villus consists of loose mesenchymal **connective tissue** containing **fetal capillaries,** fibroblasts, and isolated smooth muscle cells. Macrophages, known as **Hofbauer cells,** are also present in villi and become more numerous during gestation. In the second half of pregnancy, cytotrophoblasts gradually disappear, and a thin layer of multinucleated syncytiotrophoblasts remains on villi surfaces. In the third trimester, local bulges of syncytiotrophoblast nuclei, called **syncytial knots,** are common. Fetal capillaries in the stroma of each villus receive blood from umbilical arteries and drain into venules that deliver blood to umbilical veins.

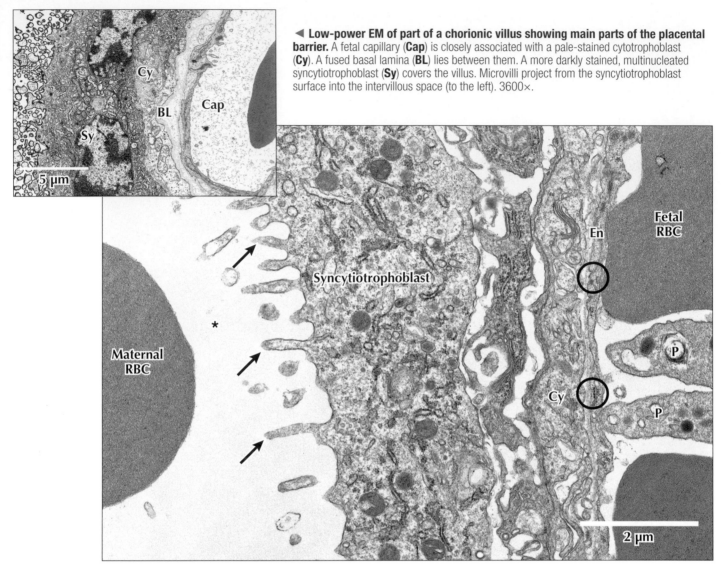

◄ **Low-power EM of part of a chorionic villus showing main parts of the placental barrier.** A fetal capillary (**Cap**) is closely associated with a pale-stained cytotrophoblast (**Cy**). A fused basal lamina (**BL**) lies between them. A more darkly stained, multinucleated syncytiotrophoblast (**Sy**) covers the villus. Microvilli project from the syncytiotrophoblast surface into the intervillous space (to the left). 3600×.

▲ **Higher power EM of the placental barrier in late pregnancy.** The lumen of a fetal capillary (to the right) contains erythrocytes (**Fetal RBC**) and platelets (**P**). It is lined by an attenuated, continuous endothelium (**En**) with tight junctions (**circles**). Short, stubby microvilli (**arrows**) project from the syncytiotrophoblast surface into the intervillous space (∗), which is bathed with maternal blood and contains an RBC. Syncytiotrophoblast cytoplasm contains many closely packed organelles including mitochondria, assorted vesicles, and SER and RER. Part of a cytotrophoblast (**Cy**) and its thin basal lamina are also seen. 15,000×.

18.23 ULTRASTRUCTURE AND FUNCTION OF THE PLACENTAL BARRIER

The placental barrier separates **fetal** and **maternal blood** and is the site of *fetal-maternal exchange* of substances. It consists of the **continuous endothelium** of the **fetal capillary** and its **basal lamina,** a layer of **cytotrophoblasts** and its adjacent basal lamina, and a layer of **syncytiotrophoblasts** exposed to maternal blood. All substances that cross this barrier for gas exchange, waste elimination, and transport of electrolytes, glucose, and other substances traverse syncytiotrophoblasts. Syncytiotrophoblasts perform many functions, such as undertaking passive and facilitative diffusion, active transport, receptor-mediated endocytosis of immunoglobulins, and exocytosis for secretion. These multinucleated cells have ultrastructural features in common with secretory, metabolically active, and absorptive epithelia. Their plasma membranes in contact with maternal blood have **apical microvilli** that amplify surface area. Their **cytoplasm** contains numerous **organelles,** including **mitochondria, lysosomes, secretory vesicles,** and SER and RER. Pinocytotic vesicles and multivesicular bodies abound for active transport. Features typical of steroid-secreting cells include SER, lipid droplets, and Golgi complexes for synthesis and release of progesterone and estrogens. RER and ribosomes function in protein synthesis and secretion of hormones such as chorionic gonadotropin and placental lactogen. Syncytiotrophoblasts arise from cytotrophoblasts, which have a normal complement of organelles. Their plasma membranes interdigitate with those of neighboring cytotrophoblasts and possess **desmosomes** at lateral margins of adjacent cells and at surfaces in contact with syncytiotrophoblasts.

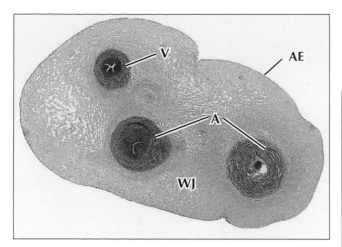

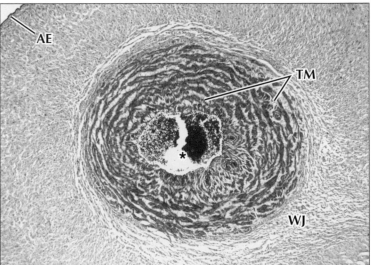

◄ **Low-magnification LM of the umbilical cord.** Wharton's jelly (**WJ**) surrounds two umbilical arteries (**A**) and one umbilical vein (**V**). The vein here is constricted, but in the relaxed state its lumen is usually larger than that of the arteries. The outer aspect of the cord is enveloped by amniotic epithelium (**AE**), which is better resolved at higher magnification (**to the right**). 7.5×. *H&E.*

▲ **The umbilical artery in transverse section.** Blood fills its lumen (∗). Two layers of smooth muscle make up its tunica media (**TM**), an outer circular coat and a thicker internal layer of longitudinally oriented muscle. The adventitia, which is a normal feature of most arteries, is replaced by mucous connective tissue of Wharton's jelly (**WJ**). The amniotic epithelium (**AE**) is shown. 30×. *H&E.*

▲ **The umbilical vein in transverse section.** The large lumen (∗) is not filled with blood in this section. The tunica intima (**TI**) contains an endothelium and underlying internal elastic lamina. The prominent tunica media (**TM**) contains an interlacing network of circular smooth muscle cells. Wharton's jelly (**WJ**) surrounds the vessel. 30×. *H&E.*

18.24 HISTOLOGY OF THE UMBILICAL CORD

The tortuous umbilical cord connects the fetus to the placenta—attached centrally or eccentrically—and at term is an average 55 cm long. It contains two **umbilical arteries** and **one umbilical vein** coiled around each other in **Wharton's jelly,** a matrix of embryonic **connective tissue** that has a mucous consistency. This extracellular matrix has an interlacing network of delicate collagen fibers and is rich in hyaluronic acid and chondroitin sulfate. It contains stellate or fusiform cells that resemble mesenchymal cells but lacks other blood vessels, lymphatics, and nerve fibers. Via special staining techniques, small autonomic nerves may be seen in the proximal end of the cord. A single layer of cuboidal epithelium, which is derived from the lining of the amniotic cavity and is known as **amniotic epithelium,** covers the cord. This epithelium is protective and secretes amniotic fluid. Umbilical arteries carry deoxygenated blood from the fetus to the chorion. Blood pressure is relatively low in these vessels, so their **tunica media** is usually not as thick as that in typical adult arteries. Umbilical arteries lack an **internal elastic lamina** and have a double-layered coat of **smooth muscle** composed of an interlacing network of cells. The umbilical vein delivers oxygenated blood to the fetus. It has a thick, single layer of circular smooth muscle but lacks valves or vasa vasorum. Some cords contain remnants of embryonic allantois and primitive yolk sac.

CLINICAL POINT

Umbilical cord blood **stem cell transplants** are less prone to rejection than bone marrow or peripheral blood stem cells. This is because the cells do not yet have antigenic features that can be recognized by a recipient's immune system. Because of this lack of well-developed immune cells, there is less chance that transplanted cells will attack the recipient's body, a condition called *graft-versus-host disease.* Both the versatility and availability of these cells make them a potent resource for transplant therapies.

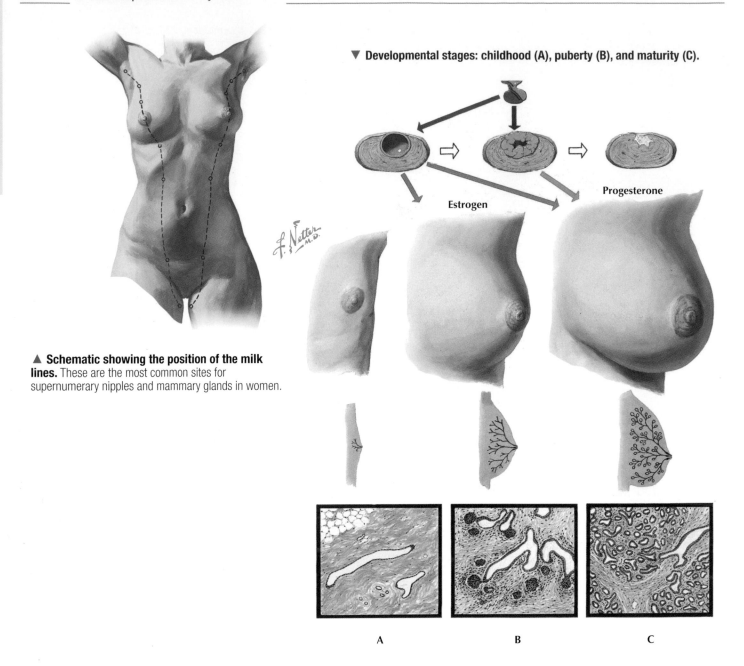

▼ Developmental stages: childhood (A), puberty (B), and maturity (C).

Estrogen

Progesterone

▲ **Schematic showing the position of the milk lines.** These are the most common sites for supernumerary nipples and mammary glands in women.

A   B   C

18.25 DEVELOPMENT AND FUNCTION OF MAMMARY GLANDS

Paired mammary glands are modified *apocrine sweat glands* with a cutaneous origin. Present in both males and females, they consist of *parenchyma,* which is formed from ducts, and connective tissue *stroma.* Parenchyma derives embryonically from *surface ectoderm;* stroma arises from surrounding *mesenchyme.* The 6-week embryo has two ventral ridge-like thickenings of epidermis, the **mammary (milk) lines,** extending from axillae to the inguinal area. The major part of each ridge disappears almost immediately, but one pair remains in the pectoral area and penetrates the mesenchyme. Then, 15-25 solid epithelial cords develop from each and are later canalized to form future *lactiferous ducts.* Mesenchyme gives rise to loose connective tissue around each duct. Denser connective tissue forms septa between them to divide the gland into *lobes.* Childhood gland structure is rudimentary and alike in both sexes. At puberty, glands in girls grow and undergo structural changes directly influenced by ovarian hormones (estrogen and progesterone). They are not fully formed and functional, however, until pregnancy and lactation. In pregnancy, terminal ends of ducts develop into hollow, sac-like *secretory alveoli,* which are lined by *simple cuboidal epithelium.* Women who give birth have highly specialized *exocrine glands* that synthesize and secrete milk. Prolactin, human placental lactogen, estrogen, and progesterone in the presence of prolactin from the anterior pituitary result in milk production; oxytocin from the posterior pituitary induces milk release.

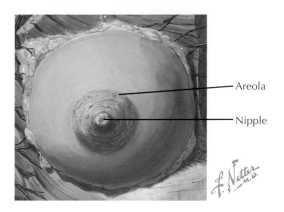

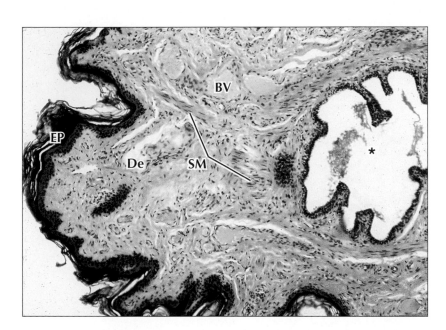

▶ **LM of a nipple.** Stratified squamous epithelium (**EP**) covers the wrinkled surface. The dermis (**De**) contains many small blood vessels (**BV**) and bundles of smooth muscle (**SM**). A lactiferous duct (∗) with a highly folded wall is seen (its connection to the surface is not in the plane of section). 120×.

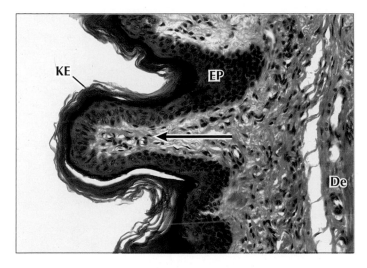

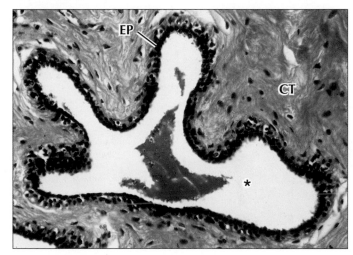

▲ **LM of the surface of a nipple.** Stratified squamous epithelium (**EP**), which makes up epidermis of thin skin, is invested externally by keratin (**KE**). A vascularized dermal papilla (**arrow**) invaginates deeply into epithelium. Deeper parts of dermis (**De**) are made of dense irregular connective tissue. 320×.

▲ **LM of a lactiferous duct.** The wall is highly corrugated; the lumen (∗) holds a flocculent eosinophilic precipitate (milk components). Stratified epithelium (**EP**) made of a double layer of cuboidal cells lines the duct, around which is dense irregular connective tissue (**CT**). 320×.

18.26 HISTOLOGY AND FUNCTION OF NIPPLES AND AREOLAE

The nipple, a pointed protuberance that extends a few millimeters from the breast, is surrounded by the areola, a deeply pigmented circular area of skin in the center of the breast. The areola, 1.5-2.5 cm in diameter, surrounds the nipple and contains *sweat glands, sebaceous glands,* and small *areolar glands of Montgomery,* which are modified **apocrine sweat glands** that cause surface elevations and lubricate the **epidermis.** Covering the nipple and areola is **thin skin,** which consists of **keratinized stratified squamous epithelium** continuous with that over the rest of the breast. The **dermis** projects deeply into epithelium and forms very high, irregular **dermal papillae. Capillaries** in richly vascularized papillae carry blood close to the epithelial surface, so the areola is dark

pink. Darker pigmentation that occurs at puberty and during pregnancy is due to stimulatory effects of ovarian hormones on epidermal melanocytes. **Connective tissue** of the dermis is richly endowed with elastic fibers. Deep dermal layers have **smooth muscle** bundles arranged circularly and longitudinally. Contracted, they elevate the nipple during suckling, which is a reflex regulated by sensory nerve fibers. The many sensory nerves in the nipple skin also influence release of *oxytocin* from the pituitary in the *milk ejection reflex.* Many **lactiferous ducts** cross the nipple and drain into the tip. Deep in the nipple, ducts are lined by a double layer of **stratified cuboidal epithelium,** but as they reach external orifices, they are lined by keratinized stratified squamous epithelium.

19

EYE AND ADNEXA

▼ **Horizontal section.**

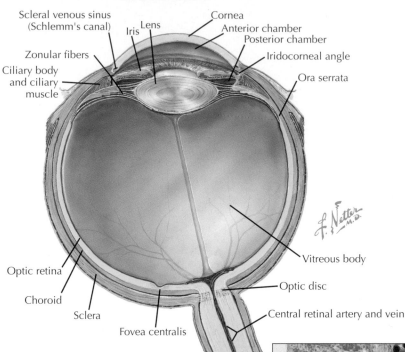

Scleral venous sinus
(Schlemm's canal)
Iris   Lens
Cornea
Anterior chamber
Posterior chamber
Zonular fibers
Iridocorneal angle
Ciliary body
and ciliary
muscle
Ora serrata

Optic retina
Choroid
Sclera
Fovea centralis

Vitreous body
Optic disc
Central retinal artery and vein

▼ **Horizontal section of the eyeball showing its main parts.** The section passes between anterior and posterior poles. 2×. *H&E.*

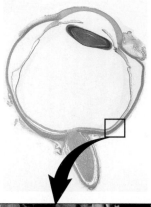

► **Light micrograph (LM) showing the three layers of the eye.** The multilayer inner retina contains a large blood vessel (**BV**). The middle choroid is highly pigmented and vascular. The outer sclera is dense fibrous connective tissue. 250×. *H&E.*

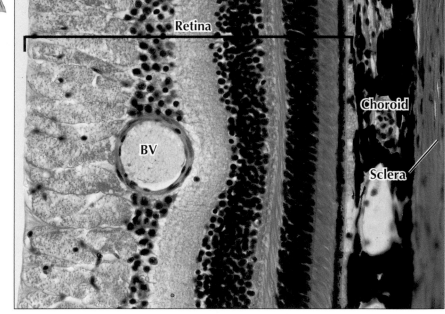

Retina

Choroid

BV

Sclera

19.1 OVERVIEW

Eyes are complex, paired *photoreceptor organs.* Each is roughly spherical, about 2.5 cm in diameter. Eyes communicate with the brain via the *optic (II) cranial nerve.* They develop as an outgrowth of the brain, mostly from *neuroectoderm,* and from *surface ectoderm* and *mesoderm,* which give rise to adnexa. The wall has three concentric coats. The mainly protective outer fibrous layer consists of an opaque **sclera** posteriorly and a transparent **cornea** anteriorly. The middle vascular coat, or **uvea,** comprises **choroid, ciliary body,** and **iris.** The inner layer, the **retina,** consists of a small nonneural region, anteriorly. At the **ora serrata,** it becomes the neural retina, posteriorly. The multilayer neural retina contains specialized *photoreceptors* and other retinal cells. Optic nerve fibers from the retina exit posteriorly at the **optic disc** (**blind spot**). Three interior ocular chambers are the small **anterior** and **posterior chambers,** containing transparent fluid—*aqueous humor*—and the main chamber, the **vitreous body.** It is behind the **lens** and ciliary body and holds a transparent, semisolid gel rich in hyaluronic acid, which cushions the retina against shock and vibration. Descriptive terms for the eye can be confusing. Outer (or external) means the eye's exterior; inner (or internal) applies to more central areas in the bulb. The *anatomic (optical) axis* refers to a line between anterior and posterior poles, through the center of the cornea. The *visual axis* joins the center of the pupil through the posterior part of the lens and the **fovea centralis,** the site of sharpest visual acuity in the retina. The eyeball sits in the bony *orbital socket,* which contains *adipose tissue,* nerves, blood vessels, and three sets of *skeletal (extraocular) muscles.*

▼ Eye development

Optic vesicle

Surface ectoderm
Neuroectoderm (forebrain)
Mesenchyme
Optic cup
Lens placode

Optic stalk
Optic cup

Early eye develops as neuroectodermal outpouching (optic vesicle) of primitive forebrain and thickening (**clear arrow**) of adjacent surface ectoderm (lens placode)

Lens vesicle
Hyaloid artery
Internal carotid artery

Lens placode invaginates to form the lens vesicle. The optic vesicle invaginates (**clear arrow**) to form a double layered optic cup that surrounds the lens vesicle and hyaloid vessels

Eyelid primordia

Mesenchymal condensation forms outer layers of globe (cornea and sclera)
Hyaloid artery
Inner layer of optic vesicle (visual retina)
Outer layer of optic vesicle (pigmented retina [epithelium])

Anterior chamber

Hyaloid vessels regress prior to birth

Fusion of visual retina and pigmented retinal epithelium

Orbicularis oculi (2nd pharyngeal arch)
Conjunctiva (surface ectoderm)
Corneal epithelium (surface ectoderm)
Cornea (mesenchyme)
Anterior chamber
Lens (surface ectoderm)
Iris (neuroectoderm)
Visual retina (neuroectoderm)
Pigmented retina (epithelium) (neuro-ectoderm)

Extraocular muscles (preotic somitomeres)
Sclera (mesenchyme)
Choroid (mesenchyme)

Optic nerve (neuroectoderm)

JOHN A. CRAIG—MD

19.2 DEVELOPMENT OF THE EYE

In the 4-week embryo, bilateral projections of **neuroectoderm** from the developing forebrain (diencephalon) become the **optic vesicles.** An **optic stalk** attaches each vesicle to the wall of the primitive brain. Optic vesicles induce overlying **surface ectoderm** to thicken and become the **lens placode.** A condensation of **mesenchyme** is interposed between the optic vesicle and lens placode. The hollow optic vesicle then invaginates onto itself, as if the side of a balloon is compressed, and becomes cup shaped with two layers. The inner layer of this **optic cup,** destined to be the *neural retina,* undergoes proliferation and stratification. The outer layer remains as simple epithelium and gives rise to **retinal pigment epithelium.** The potential space, or cleft, between the two layers may be the site of *retinal detachment.* Mesenchyme inside the optic cup invagination gives rise to the *vitreous body.* The inferior surface of the optic vesicle has a fissure that encloses **hyaloid vessels** and nerve fibers that will form the *optic nerve.* Proximal parts of hyaloid vessels become the retina's central vessels; distal parts supply the lens before they regress. A condensation of head mesenchyme around the optic cup gives rise to the middle vascular layer (**uvea**) and outer supportive layer (**sclera**). The sclera (dense connective tissue) is continuous with *dura mater* around the developing brain. The lens placode bulges inward to become the *lens vesicle,* which then separates from corneal epithelium to become the biconvex **lens.** The inner substance of the cornea also arises from mesenchyme, but the anterior surface is epithelium derived from ectoderm. The anterior chamber develops as a space in the mesenchyme. **Ciliary body** and **iris** also develop from mesenchyme. **Extraocular muscles** arise from mesoderm of *preoptic somites.*

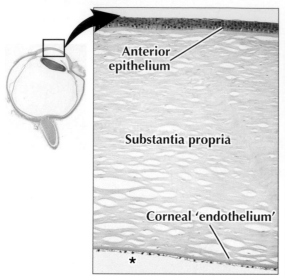

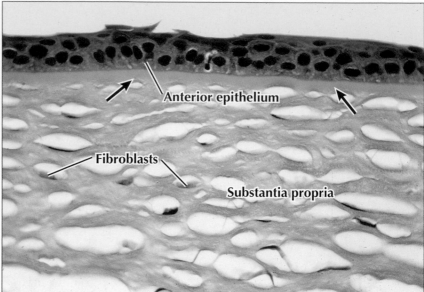

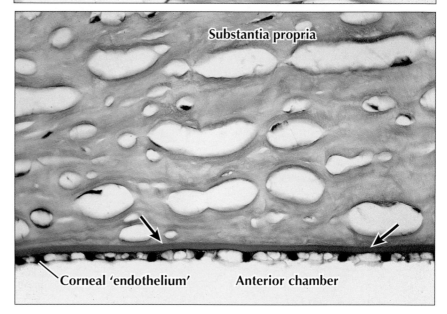

▲ **LM of the cornea at low magnification.** The anterior epithelium overlies the substantia propria. The posterior corneal endothelium contacts the anterior chamber (∗). 45×. *H&E.*

▼ **LM of the anterior cornea.** Nonkeratinized stratified squamous epithelium rests on Bowman's membrane (**arrows**). The substantia propria contains collagen fibers with occasional fibroblasts; clear areas are fixation artifacts. 400×. *H&E.*

▶ **LM of the posterior cornea.** The corneal endothelium—simple cuboidal epithelium—rests on Descemet's membrane (**arrows**). 400×. *H&E.*

19.3 HISTOLOGY AND FUNCTION OF THE CORNEA

The cornea—dense connective tissue with a layer of epithelium on both sides—is about 0.5 mm thick, 11.5 mm in diameter, transparent, and resistant to deformation. It occupies one-fifth of the ocular surface, with its radius of curvature less than that of the rest of the eyeball. Its anterior surface is **nonkeratinized stratified squamous epithelium,** about 50 μm thick and consisting of 3-6 layers of cells, except near the periphery, where it is 8-10 layers. Basal cells are polygonal, but the most superficial cells, which retain nuclei, are flattened. The epithelium continuously replicates, and it regenerates in response to wear and tear. Its rich sensory nerve supply (from the ophthalmic branch of cranial nerve V) is sensitive to touch and pain. A layer of tears lubricates the anterior surface. Deep to the epithelium is **Bowman's membrane**—a prominent basement membrane, 8-15 μm thick—that binds epithelium to underlying connective tissue. The thick central region, the **substantia propria,** contains 60-70 layers of **type I**

collagen fibers, which are uniform in diameter and embedded in a proteoglycan-rich extracellular matrix. A unique pattern of collagen fibers—regularly arranged, parallel in each layer and at right angles in successive layers—contributes to transparency of the cornea. **Simple cuboidal epithelium**—misnamed **corneal endothelium**—lines the posterior surface. Its basement membrane (10-12 μm thick) is **Descemet's membrane.** Its free (apical) surface is directly exposed to *aqueous humor* in the **anterior chamber.** Being avascular, the cornea is immunologically privileged and a good candidate for transplants. Most of it relies on diffusion of oxygen and nutrients from aqueous humor. The boundary between cornea and *sclera* (white of the eye) is an abrupt transitional zone, the *limbus,* where mucous membranes covering the sclera (*bulbar conjunctiva*) and underside of the eyelid (*palpebral conjunctiva*) join the anterior corneal epithelium. The sclera, about 0.5 mm thick and four-fifths of the surface area, consists of dense fibrous connective tissue.

▼ **Anterior segment of the eye.**

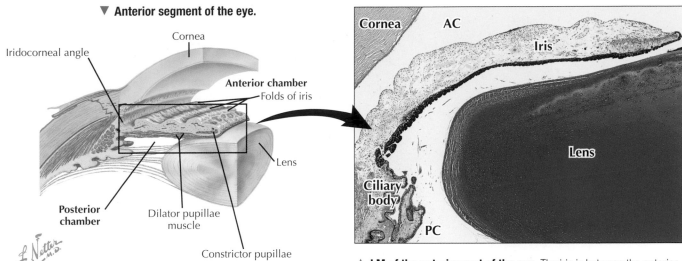

▲ **LM of the anterior part of the eye.** The iris is between the anterior (**AC**) and posterior (**PC**) chambers, and thus between the cornea and lens. Its root is continuous with the ciliary body. 20×. *H&E.*

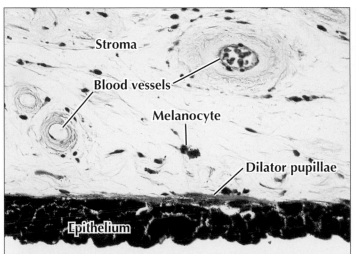

▲ **LM of the core of the iris.** The dilator pupillae muscle forms the inner layer of the heavily pigmented epithelium that covers the posterior surface. The stroma—loose connective tissue—contains many blood vessels, flattened fibroblasts, and melanocytes. 380×. *H&E.*

▲ **LM of the iris close to the pupillary margin.** A double layer of heavily pigmented epithelium is in contact with the posterior chamber. A band of circumferential smooth muscle makes up constrictor pupillae. The anterior surface lacks an epithelial lining. 380×. *H&E.*

19.4 HISTOLOGY AND FUNCTION OF THE IRIS

The iris—a circular diaphragm, 10-12 mm in diameter—is the most anterior part of the *uvea* and separates **anterior** and **posterior chambers.** Its free end is suspended in aqueous humor between the **cornea** and **lens;** its root is continuous with the **ciliary body.** Its central adjustable aperture is the *pupil,* whose opening and thus the amount of light reaching the retina, it regulates. Its anterior surface, which contacts the anterior chamber, has, instead of epithelium, a discontinuous layer of stromal cells: a mixture of **fibroblasts** and pigment-containing **melanocytes.** Spaces between the cells allow fluid from aqueous humor to percolate into the **stroma.** The stroma is richly vascularized, and most **vessels** have a corkscrew shape to adjust for length changes in the iris. The number of melanocytes in the stroma and the amount of *melanin* in their cytoplasm mostly determine eye color. A double layer of pigmented **cuboidal epithelium,** continuous with that of the ciliary body, covers the posterior surface. The superficial layer of these cells is in contact with aqueous humor in the posterior chamber. The inner layer is made of *myoepithelial cells,* which form the **dilator pupillae muscle.** Basal processes of these cells have abundant *contractile filaments.* Postganglionic nerve fibers of the *sympathetic nervous system* stimulate the cells to contract, which causes pupil dilation. In the stroma, near the pupillary margin, lies the involuntary **constrictor pupillae muscle,** a flat ring of circumferential smooth muscle, about 0.75 μm in diameter, that reduces pupillary diameter by contraction. Postganglionic nerve fibers of the *parasympathetic nervous system* innervate it. Both dilator and constrictor muscles derive from *neuroectoderm.*

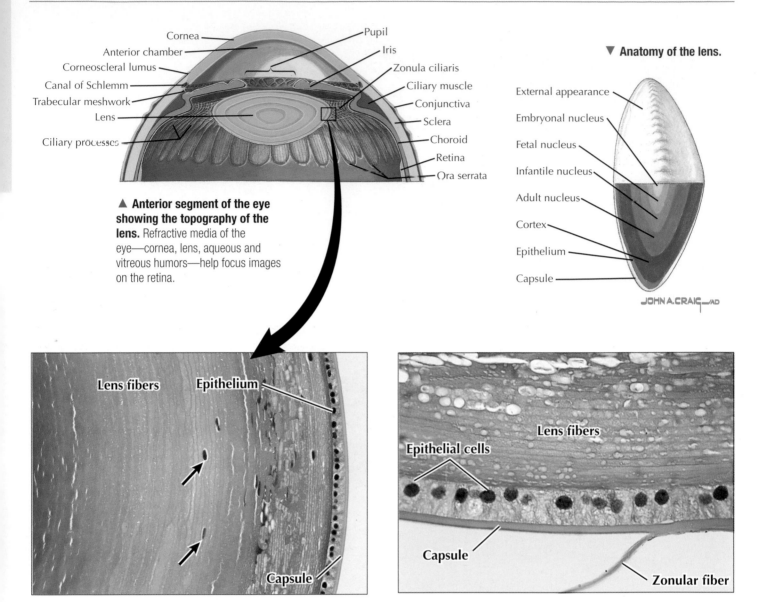

Cornea
Anterior chamber
Corneoscleral lumus
Canal of Schlemm
Trabecular meshwork
Lens
Ciliary processes

Pupil
Iris
Zonula ciliaris
Ciliary muscle
Conjunctiva
Sclera
Choroid
Retina
Ora serrata

▲ **Anterior segment of the eye showing the topography of the lens.** Refractive media of the eye—cornea, lens, aqueous and vitreous humors—help focus images on the retina.

▼ **Anatomy of the lens.**

External appearance
Embryonal nucleus
Fetal nucleus
Infantile nucleus
Adult nucleus
Cortex
Epithelium
Capsule

JOHN A. CRAIG—AD

Lens fibers Epithelium

Capsule

▲ **LM of the equator of the lens from the eye of an adult.** A thin, lightly eosinophilic outer capsule covers the lens. Underlying simple cuboidal epithelium forms a mitotically active germinal zone. The rest of the lens is made of concentric, transparent refractile fibers, most lacking nuclei (**arrows**). 250×. *H&E.*

Lens fibers
Epithelial cells
Capsule
Zonular fiber

▲ **LM showing details of the lens from a child's eye at high magnification.** One row of simple cuboidal epithelial cells with round nuclei rests on an external capsule. These cells serve as progenitors for new lens fibers. Zonular fibers from the ciliary body attach to the capsule. 500×. *H&E.*

19.5 HISTOLOGY AND FUNCTION OF THE LENS

The lens is an elastic, biconvex avascular structure between the **iris** and **vitreous body.** It is about 10 mm in diameter and 3.5-5 mm wide. It is held in a fairly fixed position by **zonular fibers** (from the ciliary body) and the vitreous body behind it. Tensile forces in the lens cause its roughly globular shape. Its elasticity diminishes with age, which restricts its limit of focus. **Lens fibers,** the main cells of the lens, are elongated columnar epithelial cells with distinctive cytoplasmic proteins *(crystallins), filensin interme-*diate filaments, and a degenerated nucleus. Enveloping the lens is a homogeneous **capsule** that corresponds to a thick **basement membrane** containing a network of collagen fibrils. Underneath it, the anterior half of the lens has a **simple cuboidal (lens) epithelium,** the germinal zone. The lens epithelial cells in the equator undergo mitosis and differentiation throughout life. They elongate, accumulate protein, and lose nuclei. The posterior half of the lens lacks an epithelium. Like the cornea, the lens depends on diffusion of *aqueous humor* for nutrition.

▼ The developing lens before birth showing orientation of lens fibers.

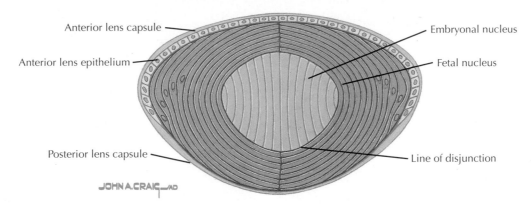

Anterior lens capsule — Embryonal nucleus

Anterior lens epithelium — Fetal nucleus

Posterior lens capsule — Line of disjunction

JOHN A. CRAIG—AD

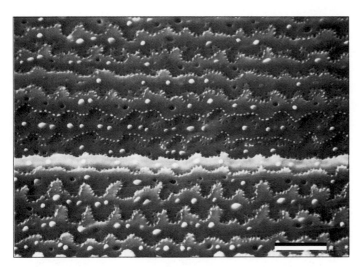

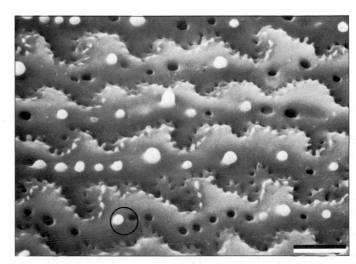

▲ **Scanning electron micrographs (SEMs) showing mature lens fibers at low (Left) and high (Right) magnification.** Interlocked processes of adjacent lens fibers have a zigzag pattern. These processes, like a ball and socket (**circle**), hold upper and lower surfaces of fibers together. **Left:** 1500×; **Right:** 6000×. *(Courtesy of Dr. M. J. Hollenberg)*

19.6 ULTRASTRUCTURE OF LENS FIBERS

Lens fibers are difficult to appreciate by light microcopy, mostly because of tight packing and high density, which lead to preparation artifacts in conventional sections. Scanning electron microscopy of the lens after freeze fracturing shows that fibers are hexagonal prisms about 10 μm long, 10 μm wide, and 2 μm thick. Most fibers are in rows, arranged concentrically and parallel to the lens surface. Adjacent lens fibers have complex **interlocking cytoplasmic processes** with many *intercellular junctions* and ball and socket interdigitations. Lens transparency is due to the regular arrangement of the fibers and the balance of its chemical constituents. Lens fibers develop in successive waves from the embryonic period through adulthood. Ellipsoidal zones called **fetal, infantile, and adult nuclei** surround an **embryonal nucleus,** the earliest fibers. Lens fiber elaboration continues throughout life in the equatorial region by deposition of new fibers in the peripheral cortex. Lines of disjunction at interfaces of various generations of lens fibers are useful anatomic landmarks that allow clinicians to estimate onset and progression of pathologic changes. Because the lens capsule is impermeable to most substances, lens fiber metabolism is isolated from foreign antigens and exterior cells throughout life.

CLINICAL POINT

Cataracts are opacities of the crystalline lens whose cause may be diabetes, genetic disorders, toxins, or aging. Clefts first appear between lens fibers, and then degenerated material collects in the spaces. Increased osmotic pressure causes the damaged lens to imbibe water and swell, which may obstruct the pupil and cause **glaucoma.** Compressed lens fibers in the lens center usually harden with age and may become brown or black. The lens can be surgically removed and replaced by a prosthetic, which can restore normal function and allow focusing of light on the retina.

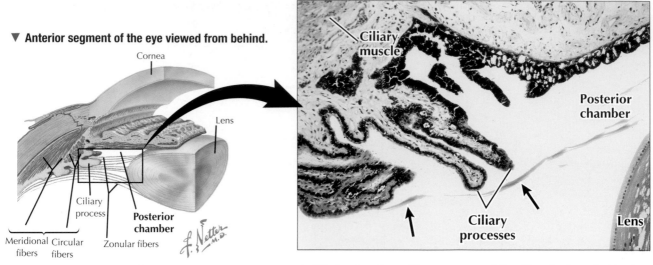

▼ Anterior segment of the eye viewed from behind.

Cornea

Lens

Ciliary process

Posterior chamber

Meridional fibers   Circular fibers   Zonular fibers

Ciliary muscle

f. Netter M.D.

▲ **LM showing finger-like processes of the ciliary body projecting into the posterior chamber.** Zonular fibers (**arrows**) anchor the lens equator to the epithelium of the processes. Part of the ciliary muscle—the smooth muscle of accommodation—is seen. 60×. *H&E.*

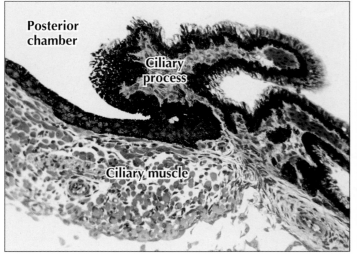

▲ **LM of part of the ciliary body.** Double-layered epithelium lines a ciliary process projecting into the posterior chamber. Ciliary smooth muscle cells form most of the ciliary body. 350×. *Toluidine blue, plastic section.*

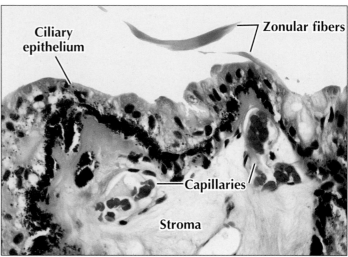

▲ **LM of the ciliary epithelium.** A layer of nonpigmented cells covers a deeper layer of pigmented cells. Underlying stroma contains many capillaries. Zonular fibers in the posterior chamber attach to the epithelium. 400×. *H&E.*

19.7   HISTOLOGY AND FUNCTION OF THE CILIARY BODY

The ciliary body, the specialized anterior part of the uvea, has main functions of *accommodation* and production of *aqueous humor.* It extends from the *corneoscleral* junction to the **ora serrata** of the *retina.* This wedge-shaped fibromuscular ring anchors and suspends the lens by **zonular fibers,** which allow changes in lens shape for accommodation. The inner surface of the ciliary body has 70-80 radiating folds, or **ciliary processes,** covered by a double-layered cuboidal **ciliary epithelium.** The outer layer contains melanin and is in contact with a richly vascularized connective tissue. This epithelial layer is a rostral continuation of retinal pigment epithelium. The inner nonpigmented epithelial layer—a continuation of the neural retina—is made of simple cuboidal to columnar cells. These ion-transporting cells modify plasma filtrate from capillaries in ciliary body processes that is then secreted as aqueous humor into the **posterior chamber.** Deep in the ciliary body is the mesenchymally derived **ciliary muscle,** which consists of three groups of smooth muscle cells. They pull in radial, circular, and meridional directions. Contraction of this muscle eases tension on zonular fibers, which allows the lens to become more convex, thereby altering its refractive power to accommodate for near vision.

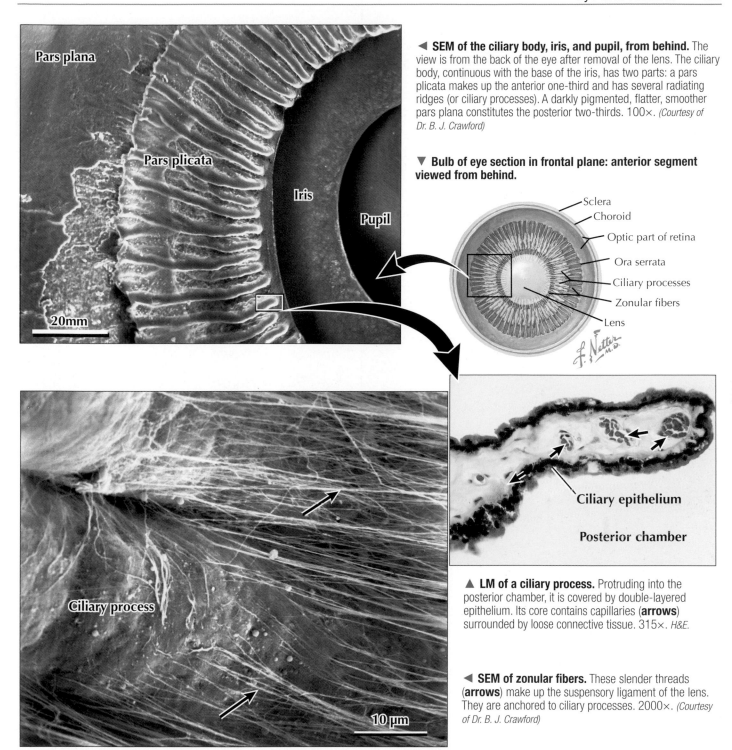

◄ **SEM of the ciliary body, iris, and pupil, from behind.** The view is from the back of the eye after removal of the lens. The ciliary body, continuous with the base of the iris, has two parts: a pars plicata makes up the anterior one-third and has several radiating ridges (or ciliary processes). A darkly pigmented, flatter, smoother pars plana constitutes the posterior two-thirds. 100×. *(Courtesy of Dr. B. J. Crawford)*

▼ **Bulb of eye section in frontal plane: anterior segment viewed from behind.**

Sclera
Choroid
Optic part of retina
Ora serrata
Ciliary processes
Zonular fibers
Lens

Pars plicata

Iris

Pupil

20mm

Ciliary epithelium

Posterior chamber

▲ **LM of a ciliary process.** Protruding into the posterior chamber, it is covered by double-layered epithelium. Its core contains capillaries (**arrows**) surrounded by loose connective tissue. 315×. *H&E.*

Ciliary process

◄ **SEM of zonular fibers.** These slender threads (**arrows**) make up the suspensory ligament of the lens. They are anchored to ciliary processes. 2000×. *(Courtesy of Dr. B. J. Crawford)*

10 µm

19.8 SCANNING ELECTRON MICROSCOPY OF THE CILIARY BODY AND ZONULAR FIBERS

This technique is useful as it provides three-dimensional views of the eye's interior to help understanding of the surface morphology of component parts. Zonular fibers of the suspensory ligament are not well visualized in conventional histologic sections, so their radial pattern and manner of attachment to the **ciliary body** are best appreciated in a scanning electron micrograph. Three-dimensional anatomy of ridges and intervening grooves making up the ciliary body are also dramatically highlighted. Zonular

fibers are delicate **collagen fibers** that radiate from the equatorial part of the *lens capsule* to insert into the ciliary body's inner surface and the grooves between ciliary processes. When the *ciliary muscle* contracts, the ciliary body and choroid are directed forward and centrally, thus relaxing normal tension on zonular fibers. The lens thickens and becomes more convex when tension on its capsule is reduced. This process, named *accommodation*, allows the eye to focus on close objects. When the ciliary muscle relaxes, greater tension is exerted on the lens, which becomes flattened and less convex. Distant objects can then be focused more clearly.

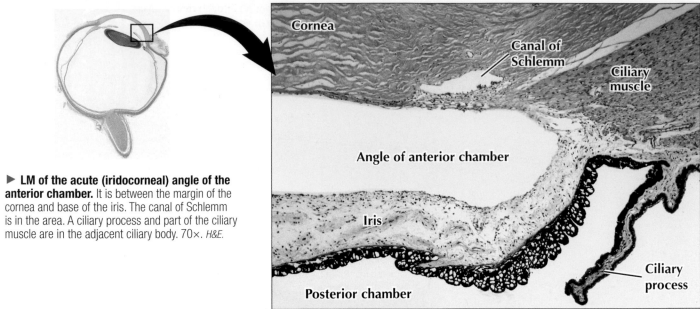

▶ **LM of the acute (iridocorneal) angle of the anterior chamber.** It is between the margin of the cornea and base of the iris. The canal of Schlemm is in the area. A ciliary process and part of the ciliary muscle are in the adjacent ciliary body. 70×. *H&E.*

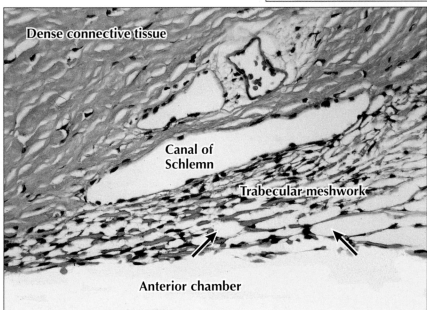

◀ **LM of the aqueous outflow apparatus.** At the acute angle of the anterior chamber, spaces of Fontana (**arrows**) and a trabecular meshwork occupy connective tissue. They are near the thin-walled canal of Schlemm, which is lined by endothelium. Fluid drained by this canal passes into the venous circulation. 360×. *H&E.*

19.9   HISTOLOGY OF THE CANAL OF SCHLEMM AND DRAINAGE OF AQUEOUS HUMOR

Aqueous humor produced in ciliary processes first enters the **posterior chamber.** It circulates around the pupillary aperture, enters the **anterior chamber,** and reaches the **iridocorneal angle (acute angle of the anterior chamber),** which contains the aqueous outflow apparatus. This **trabecular meshwork** of loose **connective tissue,** which contains collagen and elastic fibers, encloses labyrinthine spaces (**of Fontana**) that communicate with the anterior chamber. Anterior and lateral to the spaces is the **canal of Schlemm,** which drains aqueous humor that filters through the spaces. A discontinuous *basement membrane* surrounds this flattened, thin-walled channel (about 400 μm in diameter), lined by **endothelium.** The canal is the main exit route from the anterior chamber for aqueous humor, which courses around the corneal circumference to drain into a plexus of *episcleral veins* that leaves the eye and delivers the fluid to the venous circulation.

CLINICAL POINT

The dense connective tissue of the sclera and cornea become more fibrous with age, and obstruction of the canal of Schlemm may lead to **glaucoma,** a common condition involving abnormally increased intraocular pressure. Untreated, it leads to visual impairment and blindness. Two main forms—**primary open-angle** and **closed-angle**—are caused by impaired outflow of aqueous humor from the anterior chamber. The ciliary body continues to produce aqueous humor, so increased pressure in the eye from normal levels (10-20 mm Hg) to above 25 mm Hg causes deterioration of the optic disc and degeneration of retinal ganglion cells.

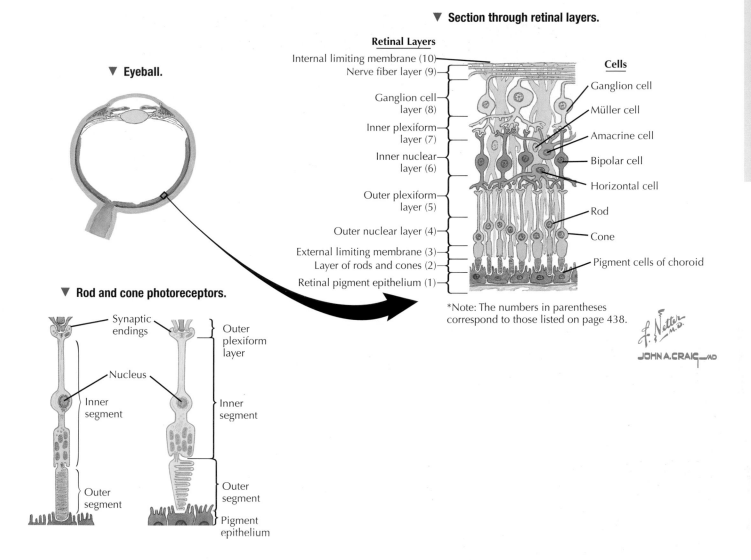

▼ Section through retinal layers.

Retinal Layers

Internal limiting membrane (10)
Nerve fiber layer (9)
Ganglion cell layer (8)
Inner plexiform layer (7)
Inner nuclear layer (6)
Outer plexiform layer (5)
Outer nuclear layer (4)
External limiting membrane (3)
Layer of rods and cones (2)
Retinal pigment epithelium (1)

Cells

Ganglion cell
Müller cell
Amacrine cell
Bipolar cell
Horizontal cell
Rod
Cone
Pigment cells of choroid

*Note: The numbers in parentheses correspond to those listed on page 438.

▼ Eyeball.

▼ Rod and cone photoreceptors.

Synaptic endings
Outer plexiform layer
Nucleus
Inner segment
Inner segment
Outer segment
Outer segment
Pigment epithelium

19.10 STRUCTURE AND FUNCTION OF THE RETINA

The retina, in the posterior segment of the eye, has two parts derived from separate layers of the embryonic optic cup. The outer is the **retinal pigment epithelium** (RPE). The inner, stratified layer—the **neural retina**—contains three sets of modified neurons (**photoreceptors, bipolar cells,** and **ganglion cells**) that are linked in series by **synapses.** They are cross-linked by association neurons (*amacrine* and *horizontal cells*) and supported by *glial cells* (**Müller cells** and *astrocytes*). Photoreceptors (**rods** and **cones**) are polarized, primary sensory cells. Their light-sensitive parts—the **outer segments**—face the RPE, and light must cross all layers of the retina before reaching rods and cones. These cells in turn synapse with bipolar neurons, which synapse with multipolar ganglion cells. Nerve fibers emanating from them form the *optic nerve (cranial nerve II)* and leave the eyeball. They conduct impulses that stimulate the *visual (occipital) cortex* of the brain. Rods and cones are structurally similar—each has **outer** and **inner segments** connected by a slender stalk—but their outer segments differ in shape and the type of *visual pigment.* Outer segments consist of parallel *membranous discs.* Visual pigments are incor-

porated in disc membranes, which undergo a steady daily turnover, being progressively shed at the outer segment tips and then phagocytosed by adjacent RPE cells. Rods are narrow, cylindrical cells for dim light perception that produce visual images in shades of gray. Cones are larger, shorter, conical cells that are used for color perception and fine visual acuity. The retina has more than 12×10^6 photoreceptors. Rods outnumber cones by a ratio of about 15 : 1.

CLINICAL POINT

In **retinal detachment,** a common cause of blindness, neural retina separates from RPE. During fetal development, the space between the two layers disappears when they become apposed, but they may separate if fluid (such as vitreous, blood, or exudate) accumulates in the potential space. Photoreceptors and RPE usually act as a unit, but if they separate, oxygen and nutrients reaching the outer retina from the choroid must diffuse across a greater distance. Photoreceptor degeneration results. Retinal detachment may occur in *diabetic retinopathy* and intraocular *infection.* Laser treatment has greatly improved the prognosis for this condition.

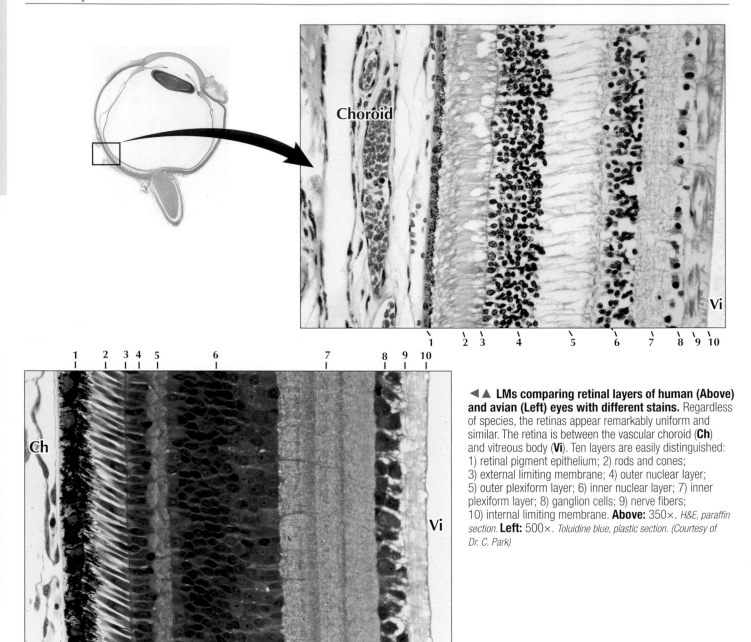

▲▲ **LMs comparing retinal layers of human (Above) and avian (Left) eyes with different stains.** Regardless of species, the retinas appear remarkably uniform and similar. The retina is between the vascular choroid (**Ch**) and vitreous body (**Vi**). Ten layers are easily distinguished: 1) retinal pigment epithelium; 2) rods and cones; 3) external limiting membrane; 4) outer nuclear layer; 5) outer plexiform layer; 6) inner nuclear layer; 7) inner plexiform layer; 8) ganglion cells; 9) nerve fibers; 10) internal limiting membrane. **Above:** 350×. *H&E, paraffin section.* **Left:** 500×. *Toluidine blue, plastic section. (Courtesy of Dr. C. Park)*

19.11   HISTOLOGY OF THE RETINA

The retina has an outer surface next to the highly vascular **choroid** and an inner surface in contact with the **vitreous body.** A highly ordered, multilayered structure, it is about 0.5 mm thick. From outside to inside, 10 distinct layers are usually seen in histologic sections. 1) The **retinal pigment epithelium** consists of one layer of melanin-rich cuboidal cells. Separated from the choroid by Bruch's basement membrane, they are between the choroid and outer tips of photoreceptors. 2) A **layer of rods and cones,** arranged in parallel, is a prominent, fibrillar layer that comprises the outer photoreceptor segments. 3) An **external limiting membrane** is the line formed by junctional complexes between photoreceptors and supportive (Müller) cells. 4) An **outer nuclear layer** marks the middle nucleated parts of rods and cones, which are arranged in palisade manner. 5) The **outer plexiform layer,** a

lightly stained zone, represents synaptic areas between photoreceptors and dendrites of bipolar cells. 6) An **inner nuclear layer** contains mostly cell bodies of bipolar cells, other associated neurons, and nuclei of Müller cells. 7) An **inner plexiform layer** is a relatively thick synaptic region, mostly between bipolar cells and ganglion cells, that also holds amacrine cell processes spreading laterally as interconnecting neurons. 8) The **ganglion cell layer** contains cell bodies of multipolar ganglion cells. Their dendrites branch in the inner plexiform layer, and their axons enter the next layer. 9) The **nerve fiber layer** comprises ganglion cell axons, about 1 million in each retina, that course radially toward the optic nerve. 10) An **internal limiting membrane,** the thin basal lamina of Müller cells, marks the boundary between neural retina and vitreous body.

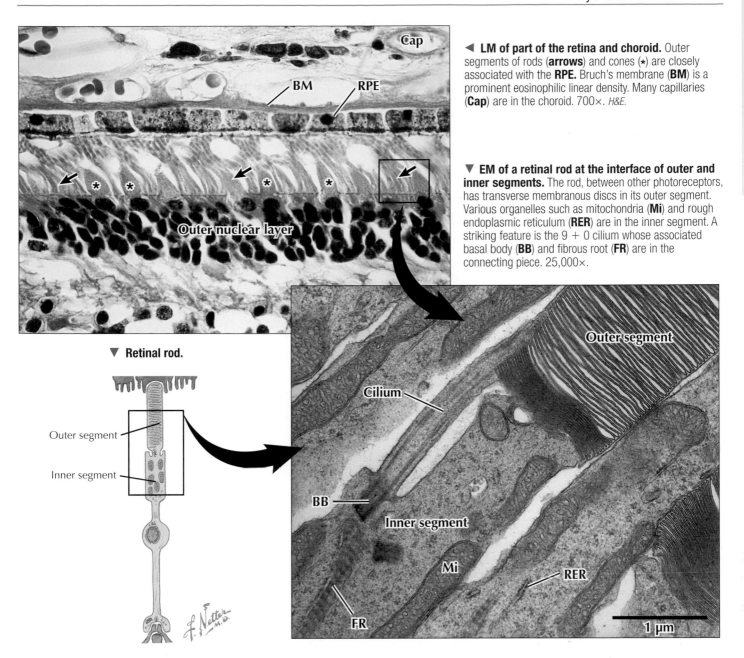

◀ **LM of part of the retina and choroid.** Outer segments of rods (**arrows**) and cones (⋆) are closely associated with the **RPE**. Bruch's membrane (**BM**) is a prominent eosinophilic linear density. Many capillaries (**Cap**) are in the choroid. 700×. *H&E.*

▼ **EM of a retinal rod at the interface of outer and inner segments.** The rod, between other photoreceptors, has transverse membranous discs in its outer segment. Various organelles such as mitochondria (**Mi**) and rough endoplasmic reticulum (**RER**) are in the inner segment. A striking feature is the 9 + 0 cilium whose associated basal body (**BB**) and fibrous root (**FR**) are in the connecting piece. 25,000×.

▼ **Retinal rod.**

19.12 HISTOLOGY AND ULTRASTRUCTURE OF RETINAL PHOTORECEPTORS

Rods and **cones** are elongated, polarized cells oriented parallel to each other, with their **outer segments** toward the RPE. Their opposing ends synapse with bipolar cells and other retinal neurons. Rods, about 120 µm long and 2 µm in diameter, have long, thin **inner segments;** cones, about 75 µm long and 5 µm wide, normally have a broader base. Outer segments of rods are cylindrical, and those of cones are more conical. Outer segments of both are modified cilia and are characterized by many parallel stacks of **membranous discs.** These segments are connected to inner segments by a thin stalk (connecting piece), which has a **9 + 0 cilium** with associated **basal body** and **fibrous root** that extends down from the basal body. The inner segment has many **organelles** consistent with its role in protein synthesis. The many **mitochon-** dria in this area are elongated and show well-developed internal cristae to produce ATP and thus meet high-energy demands of these cells.

CLINICAL POINT

Retinoblastoma, the most common intraocular *malignancy* in infants and children, is so named because most cells in the tumor resemble undifferentiated embryonic retinal cells called retinoblasts. It is caused by a mutation in the long arm of chromosome 13 (13q14), which leads to an abnormal or absent *tumor suppressor gene.* The normal function of this *retinoblastoma gene (RB1),* the first human cancer suppressor gene to be completely characterized, is to suppress cell growth. Surgical removal of the tumor and enucleation (removal of the eye) are common treatments, but new chemotherapy agents that can cross the blood-ocular barrier, combined with laser and cryotherapy, provide favorable results.

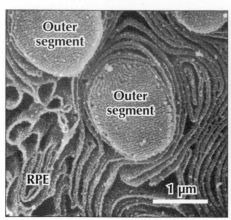

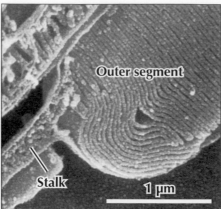

◄ **High-resolution SEM (HRSEM) showing interdigitations between photoreceptor outer segments and apical membranes of RPE cells (Left).** Apical folds extending from the surface of the **RPE** surround rod **outer segments,** fractured across their long axis. 14,000×. *(Courtesy of Dr. M. J. Hollenberg)*

◄ **HRSEM of a retinal rod (Right).** It is polarized with a slender **stalk** and an **outer segment,** which has flattened membranous discs. The inner segment is not in view. 27,500×. *(Courtesy of Dr. M. J. Hollenberg)*

► **EM showing the disposition of membranous discs in a rod outer segment.** The discs (**arrows**), oriented at right angles to the long axis of the cell, are stacked on top of each other like lamellae. They are the photosensitive part of the **outer segment.** The **cilium** of the rod contains microtubules. 40,000×.

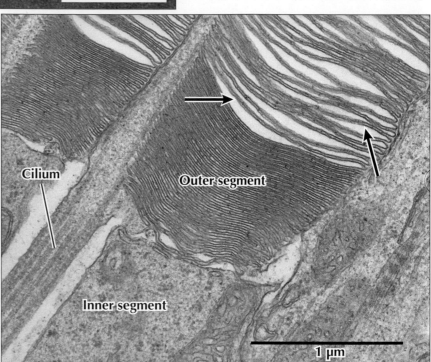

19.13 ULTRASTRUCTURE AND FUNCTION OF MEMBRANOUS DISCS

Photoreceptor discs are flattened, bilaminar, transverse saccules of *plasma membrane,* about 1 μm in diameter, that are enclosed with an extension of this membrane. They contain *visual pigments—rhodopsin* in rods and *iodopsin* in cones—that absorb light and trigger the visual response. They are transmembrane glycoproteins, which are synthesized in **inner segments,** transported through connecting stalks to **outer segments,** and incorporated into newly formed discs. Discs form via repeated invaginations of plasma membrane at the ciliary connection zone; each is made of two opposing membranes with a narrow intervening space. They eventually pinch off from the cell surface. Discs in rods move from base to tip in a centrifugal manner, are cast off at the outermost tips, and are phagocytosed by RPE. Rods hold 600-1000 discs. Outer segments of rods are continuously renewed every 10-14 days, but no evidence exists for replacement of discs in cones, even though visual pigments are constantly replenished. Membranous discs in rods are not continuous with plasma membrane, but those in cones often connect with it. The retina contains one type of rod, which responds to low-intensity light, and three types of retinal cones with selective sensitivities to blue, green, and red wavelengths. The cones cannot be distinguished morphologically, however.

CLINICAL POINT

A group of genetic diseases, called **retinitis pigmentosa** (RP), leads to progressive visual loss. Diverse forms have been mapped to changes in different chromosomes. In one RP subtype, an amino acid alteration in rhodopsin leads to photoreceptor cell death and hypertrophy or atrophy of RPE. In this subtype, changes in RPE cells are likely due to a greatly increased workload in the turnover of photoreceptor outer segments. Patients have problems with *night vision,* which progresses to *tunnel vision* and loss of visual acuity and color discrimination. High daily doses of antioxidants such as vitamin A may help slow disease progression.

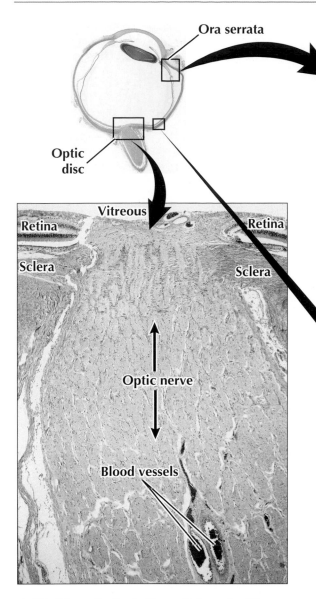

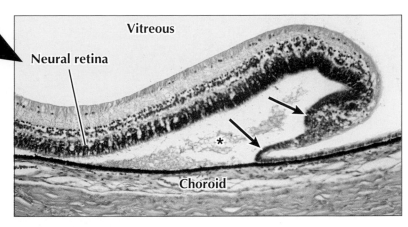

▲ **LM of the ora serrata.** This ragged margin between neural (**left**) and non-neural (**right**) parts of the retina shows an abrupt line of transition (**arrows**). The retina attaches loosely to the choroid in this area, so the inner layer has detached from the outer pigmented layer. This separation (∗) is a common artifact of preparation but is a useful landmark because it also shows the site of clinical retinal detachment. 100×. *H&E.*

▲ **LM of the optic disc in the posterior pole of the eyeball.** This site of exit of the optic nerve penetrates the sclera. The optic nerve (**arrows**), sectioned longitudinally, contains converging unmyelinated ganglion cell axons, which become myelinated nerve fibers. Branches of central retinal vessels pass through the disc and travel in the optic nerve. 25×. *H&E.*

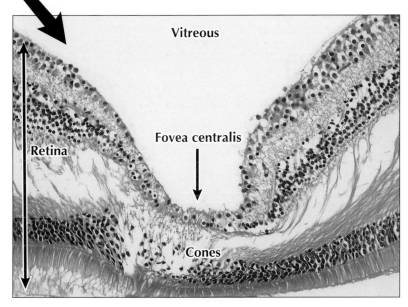

▲ **LM of the fovea centralis of the macula lutea.** This retinal depression is the site of highest visual acuity. This area shows markedly attenuated retinal layers and no blood vessels, with almost all photoreceptors being tightly packed cones. 300×. *H&E.* (Courtesy of Dr. V. White)

19.14 REGIONAL SPECIALIZATIONS OF THE RETINA

Specialized areas of the retina with regional variations in structure are the **ora serrata, optic disc, macula lutea,** and **fovea centralis.** The ora serrata, a dentate wavy line at the posterior border of the ciliary body, delineates neural from nonneural (ciliary) parts of the retina. It marks an abrupt reduction in multiple layers of most of the retina to two layers in the ciliary part. The main expanse of the retina extends from the ora serrata to the **optic disc,** the head of the **optic nerve.** Also called the *blind spot* because it lacks photoreceptors and is insensitive to light, this small, disc-shaped area (1.5-1.8 mm in diameter) is about 3 mm toward the nasal aspect of the posterior pole of the eye. In this area, optic nerve fibers, which begin as unmyelinated axons of retinal ganglion cells, enter the optic nerve and become myelinated. Unlike the retina, which is red when viewed with the ophthalmoscope, the optic disc is pink because of relatively poor vascularization. The yellow of the macula lutea, a circular area (about 3 mm in diameter), is due to accumulated *xanthophyll* pigment in ganglion and bipolar cells. In the center of the macula is a small depression—the fovea centralis, about 1.5 mm in diameter, with a markedly thinner retina (to about 0.1 mm). It has the highest concentration of cones and is directly in line with the visual axis.

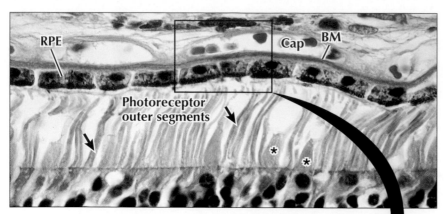

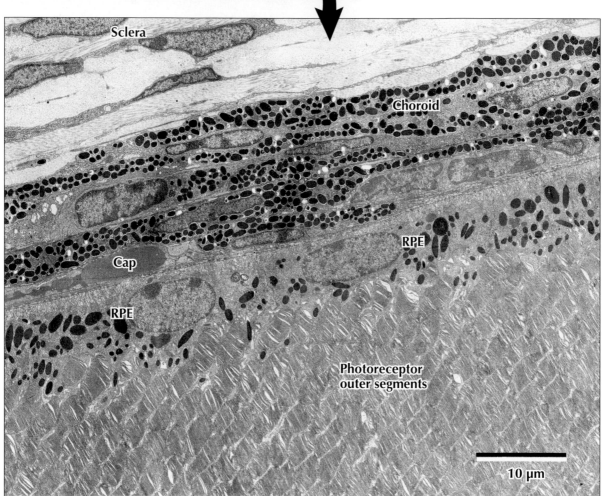

19.15   ULTRASTRUCTURE AND FUNCTION OF THE SCLERA, CHOROID, AND OUTER RETINA

The sclera, a dense regular connective tissue resembling that of ligaments and tendons, provides rigid structural support for the eyeball. It consists of regularly arranged, interwoven collagen fibrils with interspersed fibroblasts. The choroid is a highly vascular loose connective tissue with many melanin-containing cells. A large network of **capillaries** in its **choriocapillaris** layer supplies the outer retina with nutrients and oxygen by diffusion. **Bruch's membrane,** which abuts the choroid, is the basement membrane of the RPE, a layer of cuboidal epithelial cells. To increase surface area, their basal *plasma membranes* are highly infolded—a feature of ion-transporting cells. *Intercellular junctions* link lateral borders of adjacent cells, which contributes to a *blood-retinal barrier.* **Melanin granules,** which are usually larger and more oval than those in other pigmented cells, respond to light by migrating toward the tips of **photoreceptors** to protect them from excessive light and increase visual discrimination. RPE cells also have many *lysosomes,* and apical cell surfaces are studded with **microvilli,** which interdigitate with outer photoreceptor segments. One euchromatic nucleus with a prominent nucleolus indicates highly active cells. Various organelles such as a juxtanuclear **Golgi complex,** *smooth* and *rough endoplasmic reticulum,* and **mitochondria** pack the polarized cytoplasm. The main function of these cells is to phagocytose photoreceptor outer segments, which are continuously shed in a renewal process. RPE cells also store *vitamin A,* a *rhodopsin* precursor.

▼ **Intrinsic arteries and veins of the eye.**

Canal of Schlemm
Minor arterial circle of iris
Major arterial circle of iris
Blood vessels of ciliary body
Conjunctival vessels
Anterior ciliary artery and vein
Muscular artery and vein
Extrinsic eye muscle
Long posterior ciliary artery
Vorticose vein
Episcleral artery and vein
Retinal artery and vein
Long posterior ciliary artery
Short posterior ciliary arteries
Central retinal artery and vein

▼ **Ophthalmoscopic view of retinal blood vessels.**

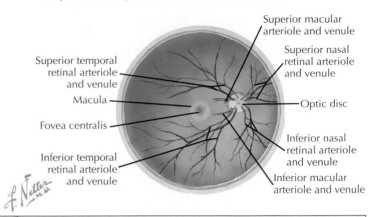

Superior macular arteriole and venule
Superior nasal retinal arteriole and venule
Superior temporal retinal arteriole and venule
Optic disc
Macula
Fovea centralis
Inferior nasal retinal arteriole and venule
Inferior temporal retinal arteriole and venule
Inferior macular arteriole and venule

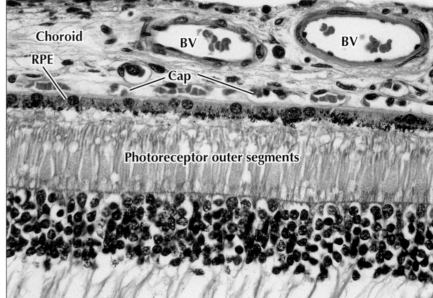

Choroid
RPE
BV
BV
Cap
Photoreceptor outer segments

▶ **LM of the junction of the choroid and the outer neural retina.** A network of many small blood vessels (**BV**) and capillaries (**Cap**) is in the choriocapillaris (**above**). Oxygenated blood from them diffuses across the **RPE** to provide nutrients to photoreceptors. 460×. *H&E.*

19.16 BLOOD SUPPLY TO THE RETINA

The retina receives oxygenated blood from two separate, independent branches of the *ophthalmic artery—ciliary* and *central arteries*. The layer of rods and cones lacks blood vessels; arterioles from branches of the ciliary artery give rise to **fenestrated capillaries,** which occur only in the **choriocapillaris** layer of the **choroid.** Oxygen and nutrients from them diffuse across the RPE for metabolic needs of photoreceptor cells in outer nuclear and outer plexiform layers. At the *optic disc,* central artery branches enter the retina with the *optic nerve* and drain into arterioles that form a large plexus of **tight capillaries** in inner retinal layers. They supply oxygen and nutrients to all cells in the retina except rods and cones. They are lined by an **endothelium** with many **tight junctions,** associated **pericytes,** and an unusually thick **basement membrane.** Processes of **Müller cells** are in close contact with retinal capillary walls. These features contribute to a tight permeability barrier in the inner retina—the **blood-retinal barrier—** similar to the blood-brain barrier. Tight junctions between RPE cells in the outer retina form another permeability barrier and limit access of high-molecular-weight substances from choroid capillaries. Postcapillary venules drain blood from retinal capillaries and join at right angles with larger veins in the nerve fiber layer. Branches of the *central retinal vein* exit the eye, via the optic disc, with the central artery.

CLINICAL POINT

Persons with **type 1** or **type 2 diabetes** are at risk of **diabetic retinopathy,** a major cause of adult blindness in developed countries that is due to pathologic changes in walls of retinal blood vessels. Initial changes involve microaneurysms, or outpocketings, which lead to hemorrhage and fluid leakage into the retina. Reduced blood flow and edema may then compromise vision. More advanced stages lead to proliferation of abnormal blood vessels into the retina, optic disc, and vitreous, accompanied by capillary closure. *Retinal detachment, glaucoma,* and *blindness* can result. Scatter laser surgery helps shrink abnormal blood vessels in proliferative retinopathy.

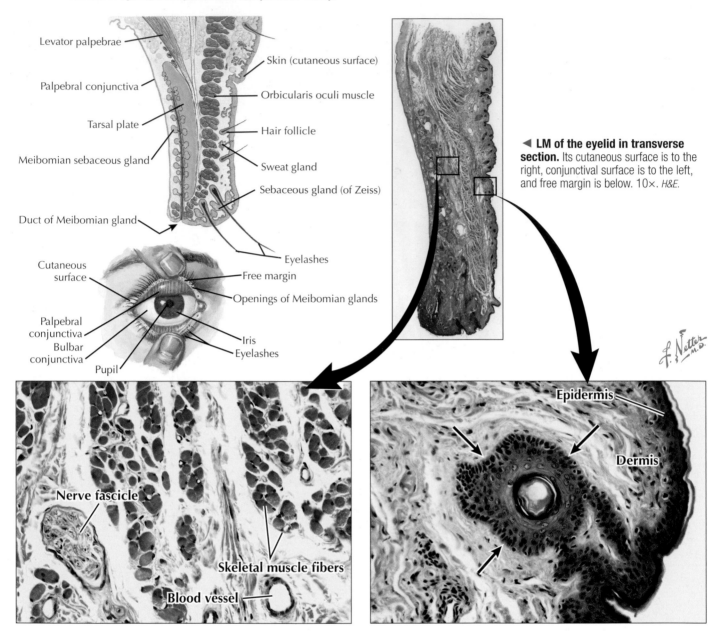

▼ Section of eyelid, and eyelid retracted (anterior view).

Levator palpebrae

Palpebral conjunctiva

Tarsal plate

Meibomian sebaceous gland

Duct of Meibomian gland

Skin (cutaneous surface)

Orbicularis oculi muscle

Hair follicle

Sweat gland

Sebaceous gland (of Zeiss)

Cutaneous surface

Palpebral conjunctiva

Bulbar conjunctiva

Pupil

Eyelashes

Free margin

Openings of Meibomian glands

Iris

Eyelashes

◄ **LM of the eyelid in transverse section.** Its cutaneous surface is to the right, conjunctival surface is to the left, and free margin is below. 10×. *H&E.*

Nerve fascicle

Skeletal muscle fibers

Blood vessel

Epidermis

Dermis

▲ **LMs of different parts of the eyelid.** A richly innervated skeletal muscle in the eyelid core is the orbicularis oculi (**Left**). Skeletal muscle fibers are arranged as irregular bundles. Nerve fascicles and blood vessels are in the connective tissue. The cutaneous surface (**Right**) consists of thin epidermis made of keratinized stratified squamous epithelium and underlying dermis. A hair follicle (arrows), sectioned transversely, is close to the surface. **Left:** 220×; **Right:** 300×. *H&E.*

19.17 STRUCTURE AND FUNCTION OF EYELIDS: CUTANEOUS SURFACE AND CORE

The eyelid covers the eyeball anteriorly, helps keep it moist, and protects it from physical injury and excessive light. **Thin skin** covers the eyelid externally; a **mucous membrane,** the **palpebral conjunctiva,** internally. A dense internal plate of fibrous **connective tissue**—the **tarsal plate**—provides rigidity and contains large **Meibomian sebaceous glands.** Keratinized stratified squamous epithelium, which is similar to that of the rest of the face, covers the skin surface. Underlying **dermis** is loose, highly cellular con-

nective tissue with **sweat glands, sebaceous glands,** and **hair follicles.** Free edges of the eyelids have slightly curved eyelashes, each of which has associated sebaceous glands (of Zeiss). The hair has no arrector pili muscle, however. Between eyelash follicles are openings of **apocrine sweat glands** (of Moll). Concentrically arranged **skeletal muscle fibers** of the **orbicularis oculi** (that closes the lid) and the **superior levator palpebrae** (that raises the lid) are in subdermal connective tissue. Small bundles of smooth muscle cells—*Müller's muscle*—are in both upper and lower eyelids.

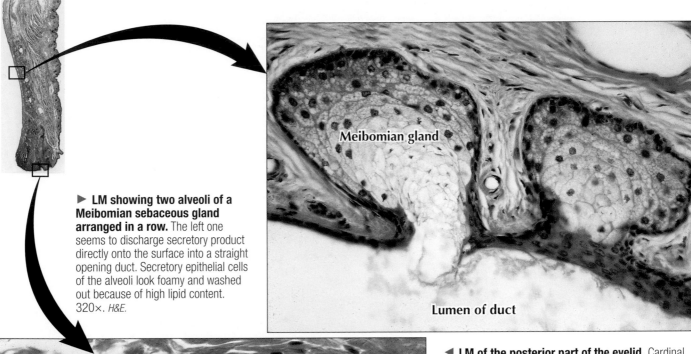

► **LM showing two alveoli of a Meibomian sebaceous gland arranged in a row.** The left one seems to discharge secretory product directly onto the surface into a straight opening duct. Secretory epithelial cells of the alveoli look foamy and washed out because of high lipid content. 320×. *H&E.*

Meibomian gland

Lumen of duct

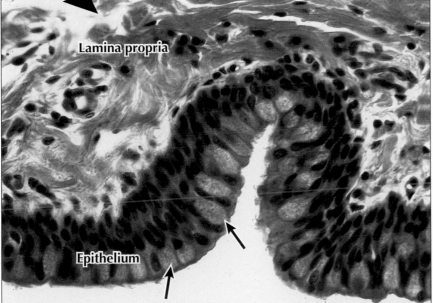

Lamina propria

Epithelium

◄ **LM of the posterior part of the eyelid.** Cardinal features of palpebral conjunctiva are seen. Many mucus-secreting goblet cells (**arrows**) make up the epithelium of this mucous membrane. Mucus here provides a protective layer on the exposed surface of the eye. The lamina propria is vascularized connective tissue, which may swell during infection. 420×. *H&E.*

▼ **Conjunctivitis.**

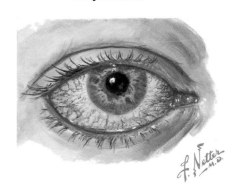

19.18 STRUCTURE OF EYELIDS: FREE MARGIN AND CONJUNCTIVAL SURFACE

The free lid margin marks the transition between **skin** and **mucous membrane.** Posterior to the row of eyelashes are openings for **Meibomian sebaceous glands,** which discharge an oily lubricant onto the free outer lid margin. This secretion prevents edges of opposing eyelids from adhering and tears from evaporating. The **palpebral conjunctiva,** a transparent **mucous membrane,** is made of **stratified columnar epithelium,** two or three cells thick. It contains many mucus-secreting **goblet cells** that lubricate the corneal epithelium. The palpebral epithelium rests on richly vascularized dense **connective tissue** replete with elastic fibers and lymphocytes. The conjunctiva is subject to reversible congestion and swelling. The palpebral conjunctiva of the eyelid is continu-ous with the *bulbar conjunctiva,* which reflects over the front of the eyeball.

CLINICAL POINT

Because of their external surface location, eyelids and conjunctiva are subject to injury and common diseases. *Bacterial* and *viral infections* and *allergic responses* often lead to **conjunctivitis**—inflammation of the bulbar or palpebral conjunctiva. Also, obstruction and resultant infection of Meibomian sebaceous glands in the eyelid form a hard, painless, nodular swelling under the palpebral conjunctiva called a **chalazion.** It is characterized histologically by chronic inflammation in the lamina propria around clear spaces previously filled with lipid from the affected gland. Many polymorphonuclear leukocytes, plasma cells, and lymphocytes may also be seen.

▼ Lacrimal apparatus.

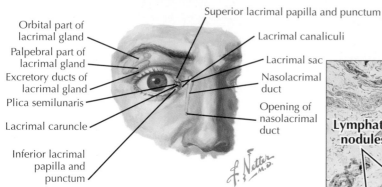

Superior lacrimal papilla and punctum

Orbital part of
lacrimal gland

Palpebral part of
lacrimal gland

Excretory ducts of
lacrimal gland

Plica semilunaris

Lacrimal caruncle

Inferior lacrimal
papilla and
punctum

Lacrimal canaliculi

Lacrimal sac

Nasolacrimal
duct

Opening of
nasolacrimal
duct

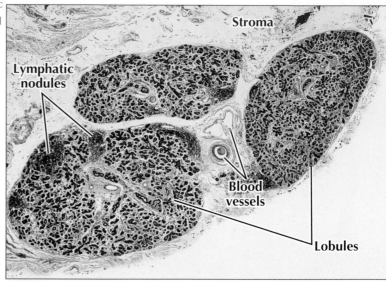

Stroma

Lymphatic
nodules

Blood
vessels

Lobules

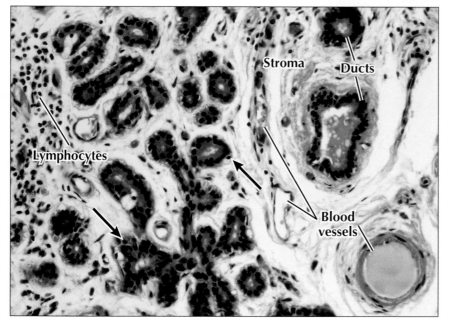

Lymphocytes

Stroma

Ducts

Blood
vessels

▲ **LM showing three lobules in a lacrimal gland.**
Thin connective tissue septa separate them. Blood
vessels, nerves, lymphatics, and excretory ducts travel in
the septa. In adults, the stroma usually has various
amounts of lymphatic tissue. Lymphocytes are loosely
scattered in the stroma or are in lymphatic nodules.
26×. *H&E.*

◀ **LM of part of a lacrimal gland at high
magnification.** The parenchyma consists of secretory
acini (**arrows**) lined by simple cuboidal to columnar
epithelium. Stratified cuboidal epithelium forms excretory
ducts in the stroma, which also contains many
lymphocytes (some of which become antibody-producing
plasma cells) and small blood vessels. 360×. *H&E.*

19.19 STRUCTURE AND FUNCTION OF LACRIMAL GLANDS

The paired lacrimal glands produce *tears,* which moisten and
lubricate the anterior surface of the cornea and conjunctiva of the
orbit and protect against bacterial infection via *lysozyme,* a bactericidal enzyme. Each gland, in the superior temporal part of the
orbit, has the size and shape of an almond. Its two major parts—
orbital and *palpebral*—drain via 10-12 small ducts into the *conjunctival sac.* The **lacrimal drainage apparatus** consists of the
conjunctival sac and **nasolacrimal duct,** which collect tears and
drain them into the *nasal cavity.* A thin connective tissue *capsule*
surrounds the compound *tubuloacinar* exocrine gland externally
and sends in delicate **septa** that divide it into irregular **lobules.**

Like the parotid, it is a purely **serous gland.** The **parenchyma**
consists of **secretory acini** that drain into a highly branched excretory **duct system.** The height of serous secretory cells of the acini
varies with function. Cells discharge the product, which has a high
concentration of K⁺ and Cl⁻ ions, into centers of the acini. *Myoepithelial cells,* which are hard to see by light microscopy, surround
the bases of the acini. They help expel lacrimal secretions into the
duct system, which drains into the conjunctiva. Simple cuboidal
epithelium lines the smallest ducts; double-layered epithelium
lines larger ones. **Lymphocytes,** plasma cells, and **blood vessels**
abound in the loose **connective tissue stroma.** Innervation of the
gland is by *parasympathetic nerve fibers* (stimulate secretion) and
sympathetic nerve fibers (inhibit it).

20

SPECIAL SENSES

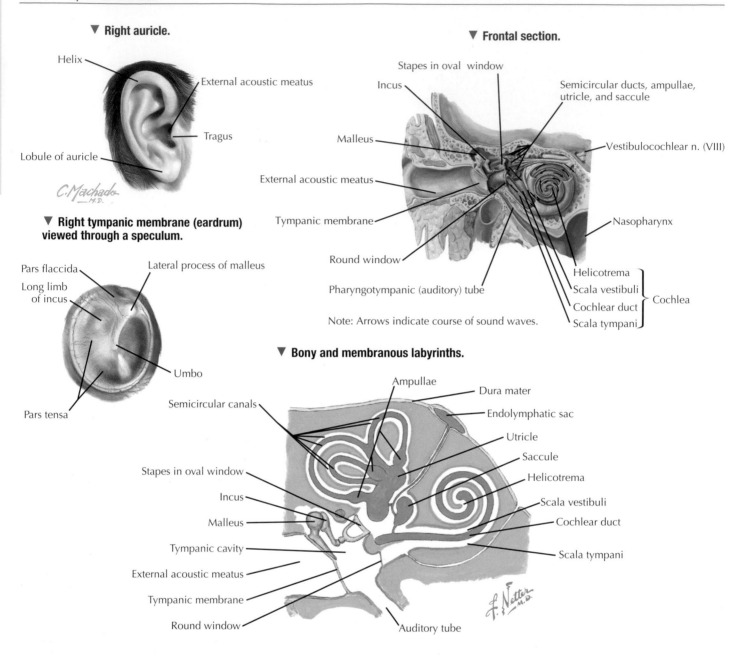

▼ **Right auricle.**

Helix

External acoustic meatus

Tragus

Lobule of auricle

C. Machado
M.D.

▼ **Right tympanic membrane (eardrum) viewed through a speculum.**

Pars flaccida

Lateral process of malleus

Long limb of incus

Umbo

Pars tensa

▼ **Frontal section.**

Stapes in oval window

Incus

Semicircular ducts, ampullae, utricle, and saccule

Malleus

Vestibulocochlear n. (VIII)

External acoustic meatus

Tympanic membrane

Nasopharynx

Round window

Helicotrema

Pharyngotympanic (auditory) tube

Scala vestibuli

Cochlear duct   } Cochlea

Note: Arrows indicate course of sound waves.

Scala tympani

▼ **Bony and membranous labyrinths.**

Ampullae

Dura mater

Semicircular canals

Endolymphatic sac

Utricle

Saccule

Stapes in oval window

Helicotrema

Incus

Scala vestibuli

Malleus

Cochlear duct

Tympanic cavity

Scala tympani

External acoustic meatus

Tympanic membrane

Round window

Auditory tube

F. Netter
M.D.

20.1   OVERVIEW

Sense organs include the **ear, olfactory mucosa, taste buds, cutaneous receptors, interoceptors** (monitor the internal environment), **proprioceptors** in muscles, tendons, and joints, and eye. Specialized receptor organs in ears sense hearing and balance. The ear has three parts: external, middle, and inner (labyrinth). The **external ear,** consisting of the **auricle** (**pinna**) and **external acoustic meatus,** conducts sound waves from the external environment to the **tympanic membrane (eardrum).** The **middle ear** (**tympanic cavity**) is an air-filled cavity in the petrous temporal bone that transforms sound waves into mechanical vibrations. Lined by a mucous membrane, it contains three **auditory ossicles** and communicates with the nasopharynx via the **auditory (eustachian) tube.** The **inner ear** has special receptors for hearing and maintenance of equilibrium. The **bony labyrinth** in the inner ear contains *perilymph,* which surrounds the *endolymph*-filled **membranous labyrinth.** The bony labyrinth—a series of communicating channels hollowed out in the petrous temporal bone—consists of a vestibule that houses the **saccule, utricle, semicircular canals,** and **cochlea.** The membranous labyrinth is lined by epithelium, which is modified in parts containing nerve endings. Specialized sensory areas are **cristae ampullaris** of the semicircular canals (detect angular acceleration), **maculae** of the utricle and saccule (respond mostly to gravity and linear movement of the head), and **organ of Corti** of the cochlea (responds to sound). Despite some differences, all three receptors conform to a similar histologic plan: receptor (sensory) *hair cells, supporting cells, afferent nerve endings* at the bases of hair cells connected to a *ganglion,* and a gelatinous *glycoprotein coat* in contact with endolymph and associated with "hairs" *(stereocilia)* of the hair cells. In the inner ear, vibrations are transduced by hair cells into specific nerve impulses via the *vestibulocochlear cranial nerve* (VIII).

▼ **Primordia of the external, middle, and inner ear.**

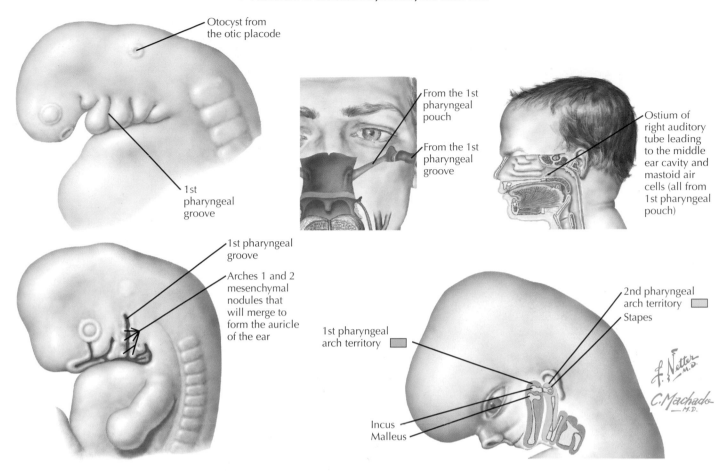

20.2 DEVELOPMENT OF THE EAR

The pharynx of the 4-week embryo shows several segmented lateral outpouchings called **pharyngeal** (or **branchial**) **pouches,** with intervening **pharyngeal clefts** (or **grooves**), which make the neck region look furrowed. The first pharyngeal cleft (between the first and second pouches) deepens and gives rise to the *external acoustic meatus.* The *ectoderm* of the first pharyngeal cleft grows inward and fuses with *endoderm* that lines the first pharyngeal pouch to form the *tympanic membrane.* At the same time, bilateral ectodermal thickenings—**otic placodes**—arise on the surface at the level of the hindbrain. Each placode invaginates, separates from the surface, and gives rise to a small saccule called the **otocyst.** With continued growth, it develops into the *membranous labyrinth* of the inner ear. Then, coiling of the otocyst, accompanied by a series of complex constrictions and outgrowths, gives rise to the *saccule, utricle,* three *semicircular canals,* and *cochlea.* The *endolymphatic duct* develops as a medial tubular outgrowth of the utricle. By the second trimester, the characteristic form and anatomic parts of the inner ear are established. Surrounding *mesenchyme* differentiates into *hyaline cartilage,* which is replaced via *endochondral ossification* to form the *bony labyrinth.* The three small middle ear ossicles (**malleus, incus,** and **stapes**) originate from cartilage of the first two pharyngeal pouches: the malleus

and incus from cartilage of the first pouch; the stapes, from cartilage of the second pouch. Bone soon replaces cartilage, and the three ossicles form a chain united by small *synovial joints.* They will transmit vibrations from the tympanic membrane to the inner ear. Vibrations are then transmitted to the fluid-filled membranous labyrinth and then the organ of Corti, where hair cells are stimulated for sound reception. The *tympanic cavity, auditory tube,* and *mastoid air cells* arise from endoderm of the first pharyngeal pouch; the **auricle,** from mesenchyme of the first and second pharyngeal pouches.

CLINICAL POINT

The most serious ear disorders are those of the inner ear that lead to **deafness.** *Congenital deafness* may be acquired by intrauterine infection with neurotrophic viruses such as *German measles (rubella) virus* and *cytomegalovirus* or parasites such as *Toxoplasma (toxoplasmosis).* In *congenital rubella syndrome,* rubella virus affects the embryo, especially at 7-8 weeks, and causes atrophy or serious damage to the organ of Corti. Inherited congenital deafness disorders are usually autosomal recessive and lead to defective neural connections or faulty development of cochlear hair cells.

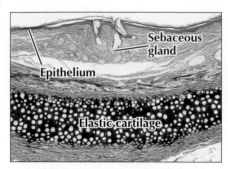

▲ **Light micrograph (LM) of the outer part of the external acoustic meatus.** Keratinized stratified squamous epithelium lines the meatus, which has associated sebaceous glands draining to the surface and elastic cartilage in the wall. 45×. *Masson trichrome.*

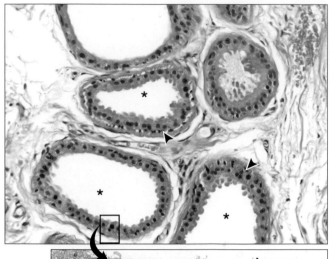

◀ **LM of part of a ceruminous gland in the external acoustic meatus.** A layer of secretory cells lines coiled tubular alveoli with wide lumina (★). The waxy cerumen, produced partly by these cells, lowers bacterial levels in the external ear and traps foreign particles. Myoepithelial cells (**arrowheads**) are at the base of the glandular epithelium. 200×. *H&E. (Courtesy of Dr. M. Stockelhuber)*

▶ **Electron micrograph (EM) of part of a ceruminous gland.** Secretory cells with rounded apical protrusions that line the lumen have spherical euchromatic nuclei and many cytoplasmic organelles such as mitochondria (**Mi**). Multiple residual bodies are a prominent feature. Myoepithelial cell processes are at the basal aspect of the epithelium. 3430×. *(Courtesy of Dr. M. Stockelhuber)*

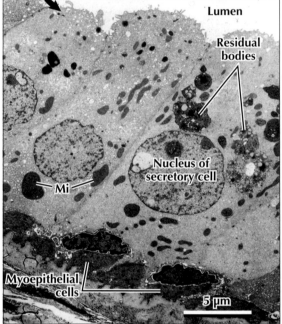

20.3 HISTOLOGY AND ULTRASTRUCTURE OF THE EXTERNAL ACOUSTIC MEATUS

The external acoustic meatus, a resonator for sound, is an S-shaped tubular cul-de-sac about 2.5 cm long. The outer two-thirds has **elastic cartilage** in the wall, which is continuous with that of the auricle. A thin layer of skin continuous with that of the *epidermis* of the auricle lines the meatus. Thin skin also lines the inner osseous part, which is a tunnel through temporal bone. It consists of **keratinized stratified squamous epithelium** and dense collagenous connective tissue of the *dermis.* Associated with the epithelium of the cartilagenous part are *hair follicles,* **sebaceous glands,** and **ceruminous glands.** Secretions from both glands contribute to yellowish **earwax (cerumen).** Ceruminous glands—branched, highly coiled tubuloalveolar glands—are modified *apocrine sweat glands* consisting of cuboidal **secretory cells** that face the glandular lumen and a deeper layer of **myoepithelial cells.** Secretory cell cytoplasm contains **residual bodies** and *pigment granules.* Gland excretory ducts open directly onto the skin surface or into a hair follicle. Lipid-rich cerumen has both hydrophobic and acidic properties to protect against pathogens and infection by stopping water from entering the skin and causing maceration. It also contains bacterial *lysozyme.* The external acoustic meatus keeps temperature and humidity relatively constant to protect the eardrum and preserve its elasticity. The *tympanic membrane,* which separates the external acoustic meatus from the tympanic cavity, is a thin layer of dense fibrous connective tissue covered externally by thin skin and internally by thin mucous membrane.

CLINICAL POINT

Acute otitis externa, commonly called *swimmer's ear,* is inflammation, often with infection, of the external ear. The usual cause is infection with bacteria (*Pseudomonas aeruginosa* or *Staphylococcus aureus*) and less often fungus. Hot, humid climates, excessive moisture, and swimming in contaminated waters are predisposing factors. Because the epidermis of the external auditory meatus is richly innervated with sensory nerves, progressive inflammation and edema lead to mild or severe ear pain *(otalgia);* blockage (stenosis) of this canal may lead to *conductive deafness.* Topical antibiotics and steroids are usual treatments.

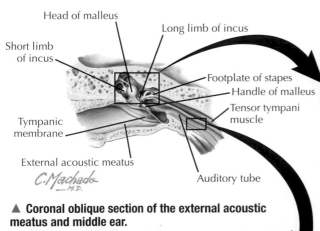

Head of malleus
Short limb of incus
Long limb of incus
Footplate of stapes
Handle of malleus
Tensor tympani muscle
Tympanic membrane
External acoustic meatus
C. Machado M.D.
Auditory tube

▲ Coronal oblique section of the external acoustic meatus and middle ear.

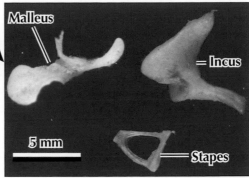

Malleus
Incus
5 mm
Stapes

◀ **The adult malleus, incus, and stapes.** Connected by typical synovial joints, they normally reach their full size in the late fetal period.

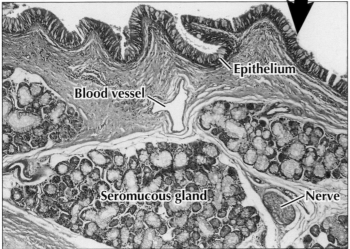

Epithelium
Blood vessel
Seromucous gland
Nerve

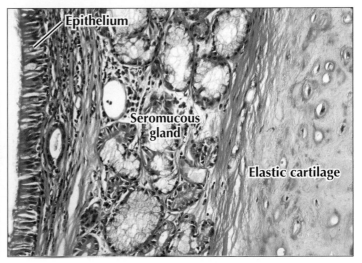

Epithelium
Seromucous gland
Elastic cartilage

▲ **LM of the auditory tube.** Pseudostratified epithelium lines the lumen. Blood vessels, mixed seromucous glands, and a nerve fascicle are in the connective tissue. 60×. *H&E.*

▲ **LM of the auditory tube at higher magnification.** Pseudostratified epithelium lines the tube. Seromucous glands and elastic cartilage are in the connective tissue. 200×. *H&E.*

20.4 HISTOLOGY AND FUNCTION OF THE MIDDLE EAR AND AUDITORY TUBE

The middle ear is an air space in temporal bone that is lined by mucous membrane consisting of, in most areas, simple cuboidal epithelium. Its lateral wall is the **tympanic membrane;** its medial wall contains the *vestibular (oval)* and *cochlear (round) windows.* Three **auditory ossicles** extend across the tympanic cavity. The **malleus** is shaped like a hammer, and its handle directly attaches to the tympanic membrane. The malleus head articulates with the anvil-shaped **incus,** which, in turn, articulates with the stirrup-shaped **stapes.** The base (footplate) of the stapes transmits vibrations to the oval window. Two skeletal muscles insert into the ossicles in the middle ear and contract in response to sounds. The **tensor tympani** (innervated by cranial nerve V) inserts into the malleus handle and adjusts tympanic membrane tension. The *stapedius* (innervated by cranial nerve VII) attaches to the neck of the stapes and dampens its oscillatory vibrations. The **auditory (Eustachian) tube,** 3-4 cm long, consists of bony and cartilaginous parts and connects tympanic cavity with nasopharynx. Most of its medial wall near the pharynx contains **elastic cartilage,** which is J-shaped in transverse section. Mostly **pseudostratified ciliated columnar epithelium** with **goblet cells** lines its lumen. As part of the mucociliary system of the middle ear, cilia beat synchronously toward the pharynx. The auditory tube is normally ventilated three or four times per minute, as it opens with swallowing, to allow equalization of pressure between the middle ear and pharynx. Impaired tube patency leads to relative negative pressure in the middle ear. Underlying connective tissue contains mixed **seromucous glands** and various amounts of *lymphatic tissue.* At the opening of the auditory tube with the pharynx, aggregates of *lymphoid nodules* form the *tubal tonsil.*

CLINICAL POINT

Otitis media is inflammation of the middle ear. Persistent, severe earache is an initial sign; hearing loss may occur. Common in young children, it is often caused by migration of pathogens or microorganisms from the nasopharynx to the middle ear via the auditory tube. It may also be due to an inflammatory process in the nasopharynx, allergy, hypertrophic adenoids, or benign or malignant tumors. Contributing is obstruction of the auditory tube by inflammation and mucosal edema. Dysfunction of this tube limits its ability to drain middle ear secretions.

▼ **Membranous labyrinth within the bony labyrinth.**

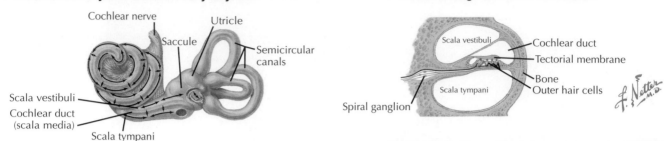

▼ **Section through the turn of the cochlea.**

► **LM of one of the turns of the cochlea in the inner ear showing the organ of Corti.** Cochlear hair cells and supporting cells sit on the basilar membrane (**BM**). Tips of hair cell stereocilia insert in the tectorial membrane (**arrowhead**). Stria vascularis (**SV**) produces endolymph of the cochlear duct (∗). Scalae tympani and vestibuli contain perilymph. Reissner's membrane (**RM**) separates cochlear duct from scala vestibuli. Afferent nerve fibers in the base of the organ have cell bodies in the spiral ganglion where their proximal axons form the auditory part of cranial nerve VIII. 90×. *H&E.*

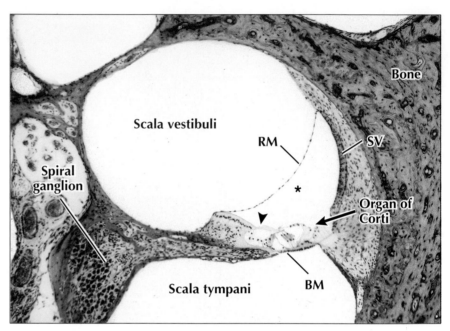

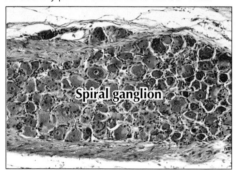

◄ **LM of the spiral ganglion.** Located in the modiolus of the bony labyrinth, it contains cell bodies of bipolar neurons of the auditory nerve. Dendrites of these neurons emanate from the organ of Corti, where they synapse with cochlear hair cells. Bipolar neuron axons enter the brainstem to end in the cochlear nuclei of the medulla. 130×. *H&E.*

20.5 HISTOLOGY AND FUNCTION OF THE COCHLEA

The cochlea, a spiral canal shaped like a snail shell, is embedded in temporal bone. It forms $2^{3}/_{4}$ turns from base to apex, is 30-35 mm long, and has a lumen with three compartments: **scala media (cochlear duct), scala vestibuli,** and **scala tympani.** The cochlear duct is filled with *endolymph; perilymph* fills the other two scalae. The scalae vestibuli and tympani communicate through the *helicotrema,* a small opening at the cochlear apex. The cochlear duct is a triangular space in transverse section. Its lateral border makes up the *stria vascularis*—a richly vascularized *pseudostratified epithelium* that secretes endolymph. **Reissner's (vestibular) membrane,** which marks the roof of the cochlear duct, consists of two layers of **simple squamous epithelium** and delineates cochlear duct from scala vestibuli. A thicker **basilar membrane** forms the floor of the cochlear duct and separates it from scala tympani. Superimposed on the basilar membrane is highly specialized epithelium—the **organ of Corti**—that consists of **hair cells** and **supporting cells.** Cochlear hair cells are specialized audi-tory receptor cells. They have apical **stereocilia** whose tips are embedded in the gelatinous **tectorial membrane.** Arising from the base of the organ of Corti are **afferent nerve fibers** that synapse with bases of hair cells. Nerve fibers converge toward the **spiral ganglion,** which contains cell bodies of neurons of the cochlear part of *cranial nerve VIII.* These bipolar neurons send axons to the brain's *auditory cortex.*

CLINICAL POINT

Deafness (hearing loss), a common condition often related to advancing age, takes one of two forms. **Conductive hearing loss** is due to a lesion in the external auditory canal or middle ear; **sensorineural hearing loss** is caused by a lesion in the cochlea or cochlear division of cranial nerve VIII. To distinguish the two types clinically, hearing by air or bone conduction is tested via a vibrating tuning fork and audiometry. Presenting an acoustic stimulus in air tests for the conductive type. Placing a tuning fork in contact with the skull tests for the sensorineural type, which accounts for 90% of all cases of deafness.

▼ **Organ of Corti.**

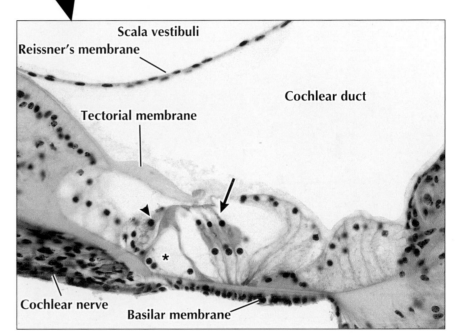

▲ **LM showing the organ of Corti at low magnification.** 80×. *H&E.*

Hair cells
Inner   Outer
Tectorial membrane
Stereocilia
Basilar membrane
Supporting cells
Afferent nerve fibers
Efferent nerve fibers
Spiral ganglion

Scala vestibuli
Reissner's membrane
Cochlear duct
Tectorial membrane
Cochlear nerve
Basilar membrane

▶ **LM of the organ of Corti at high magnification.** On the sides of the inner tunnel (∗), three rows of outer hair cells (**arrow**) and a row of inner hair cells (**arrowhead**) rest on the basilar membrane. Apical stereocilia of outer hair cells protrude into the tectorial membrane. A thin, slanting Reissner's (vestibular) membrane separates perilymph in the scala vestibuli from endolymph in the cochlear duct. Dendrites of the cochlear nerve travel from the organ of Corti toward the spiral ganglion, which houses cell bodies of these bipolar neurons. 200×. *H&E.*

20.6 HISTOLOGY OF THE ORGAN OF CORTI

The organ of Corti in the **cochlear duct** is exquisitely designed for its role in auditory sensation. Lying on the **basilar membrane,** it is composed of hair cells, which have a complex organization, with several types of columnar **supporting cells.** Hair cells are arranged segmentally in two groups on the sides of an inner tunnel. A group of typically rounded **inner hair cells** is in one row; a group of **outer hairs cells,** usually more cylindrical, forms three rows. Ultrastructural criteria identify two different types of hair cells (I and II). Hair cells are polarized and bear apical **stereocilia** that project into the lumen of the endolymph-filled cochlear duct. Bases of hair cells are embedded in recesses formed by neighboring supporting cells that are rich in cytoskeletal components. Synapsing with these bases are **afferent** and **efferent nerve terminals** of **cranial nerve VIII.** Also, some supporting cells at the outer part of the organ of Corti produce the **tectorial membrane,** into which tips of stereocilia of the tallest outer hair cells project. The tectorial membrane, a gelatinous, resilient cuticular sheet that extends over

hair cells, is made of glycoprotein in which are embedded 4-nm *microfilaments* made of a protein that resembles *keratin. Endolymph* in the cochlear duct is like intracellular fluid, but *perilymph* in adjacent scalae vestibuli and tympani is chemically more similar to extracellular or cerebrospinal fluid.

CLINICAL POINT

Because a rigid bony canal encloses the membranous labyrinth of the inner ear, control of ionic balance and pressure equilibration between perilymph and endolymph is critical. Increased pressure in endolymph may lead to **Ménière's disease** (**endolymphatic hydrops**). Characteristic distention and distortion of the membranous labyrinth may lead to degeneration of receptor hair cells in both vestibule and cochlea. Patients show malfunction in both parts of the inner ear with recurrent episodes of *vertigo* (dizziness), *tinnitus* (ringing), and low-frequency *deafness.* The cause of the disease is unknown.

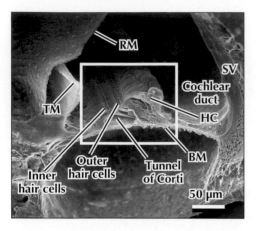

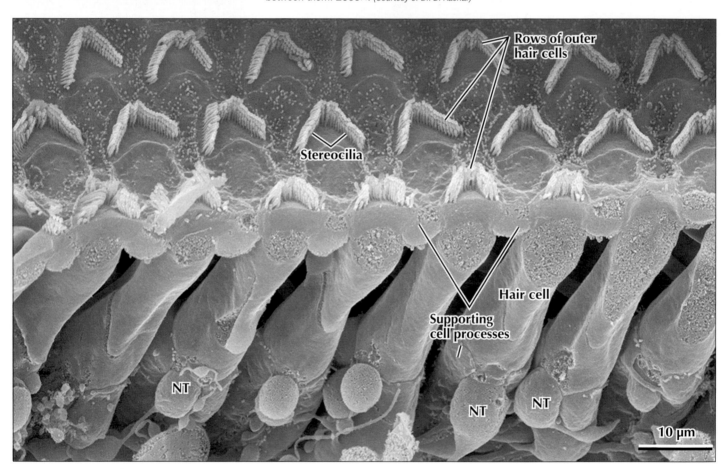

◀ **Scanning electron micrograph (SEM) of the mouse organ of Corti.** Stria vascularis (**SV**) and basilar (**BM**) and Reissner's (**RM**) membranes delineate the cochlear duct. The tectorial membrane (**TM**) is peeled back to expose rows of inner and outer hair cells. Inner hair cells are the primary auditory receptors; outer hair cells amplify low-intensity sounds. A small inner tunnel (of Corti) between them is bounded by supporting cell processes. Outer supporting cells of the organ of Corti are named Hensen's cells (**HC**). 180×. *(Reprinted with permission, Pompeia C, Hurle B, Belvamseva I, et al: Gene expression profile of the mouse organ of Corti at the onset of hearing. Genomics 83 (6) 1000-1011, 2004. Elsevier.)*

▼ **SEM showing three rows of outer hair cells in the guinea pig organ of Corti.** V- or W-shaped clusters of stereocilia project from apical cell surfaces. Tips of the longest stereocilia are usually embedded in the tectorial membrane, but the membrane was peeled back during the SEM preparation. The cells are cylindrical with rounded lower ends, which contact nerve terminals (**NT**). Hair cells are slanted relative to the surface of the organ of Corti, and supporting cell processes are between them. 2000×. *(Courtesy of Dr. B. Kachar)*

20.7 ULTRASTRUCTURE AND FUNCTION OF COCHLEAR HAIR CELLS

About 15,000 hair cells rest on the **basilar membrane** in each **organ of Corti.** Some 3500 of them are inner hair cells; the rest are outer hair cells. Cochlear hair cells reside in cup-like depressions of two types of **supporting cells**—phalangeal and pillar—that help hold the hair cells in position. Supporting cells have a well-developed cytoskeleton and are linked to hair cells by intercellular junctions. Afferent and efferent fibers of the cochlear nerve form **synapses** at bases of hair cells. A graduated array of 100-200 cross-linked **stereocilia,** of various lengths, extends from apical hair cell surfaces. The stereocilium interior contains a dense bundle of actin filaments, for stiffness and rigidity. Vestibular hair

cells have one kinocilium and several stereocilia, but cochlear hair cells have a kinocilium that disappears shortly after birth. Stereocilia of inner hair cells appear as U-shaped bundles; those of outer hairs cells show V- or W-shaped pattern. Hair cells are biologic strain gauges that function as mechanoelectric transducers. Upward displacement of the basilar membrane as it vibrates in response to sound waves causes stereocilia to pivot at their bases. Mechanically gated cation channels at tips of stereocilia then open, and influx of K^+ ions causes depolarization. This leads to opening of voltage-gated Ca^{2+} channels at hair cell bases. Release of neurotransmitter at the basal synapse then stimulates adjacent nerve fibers of the cochlear nerve to elicit action potentials, which transmit information to the central nervous system.

▼ **Membranous labyrinth.**

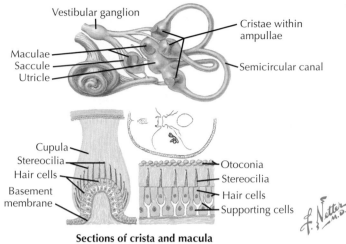

Vestibular ganglion
Cristae within ampullae
Maculae
Saccule
Utricle
Semicircular canal

Cupula
Stereocilia
Hair cells
Basement membrane
Otoconia
Stereocilia
Hair cells
Supporting cells

F. Netter m.d.

Sections of crista and macula

▼ **Structure and innervation of hair cells.**

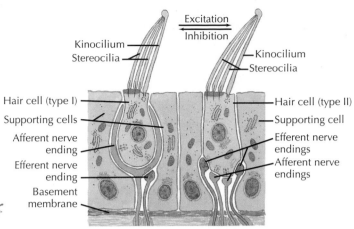

Excitation
Inhibition
Kinocilium
Stereocilia
Kinocilium
Stereocilia
Hair cell (type I)
Hair cell (type II)
Supporting cells
Supporting cell
Afferent nerve ending
Efferent nerve endings
Efferent nerve ending
Afferent nerve endings
Basement membrane

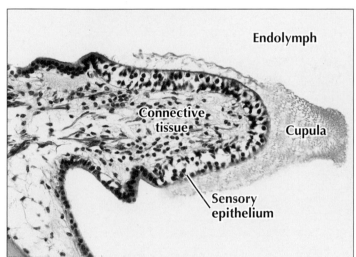

Endolymph
Connective tissue
Cupula
Sensory epithelium

▲ **LM of the crista ampullaris.** A cone-shaped cupula forms a cap over the crest of sensory epithelium, which consists of hair cells and supporting cells. Apical stereocilia of hair cells normally insert into the cupula but are not well preserved because of preparation artifact. The loose connective tissue contains nerve fibers, which are dendrites of the vestibular part of cranial nerve VIII. 225×. *H&E.*

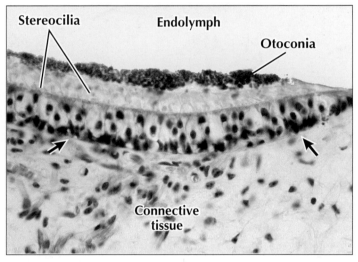

Stereocilia
Endolymph
Otoconia
Connective tissue

▲ **LM of the macula.** Its epithelium comprises apical hair cells and basal supporting cells. They rest on an ill-defined basement membrane (**arrows**) and underlying connective tissue. Each hair cell has many apical projections—multiple stereocilia and one kinocilium. These surface specializations insert into the overlying otolithic membrane, which contains calcium carbonate-rich otoconia. 420×. *H&E.*

20.8 HISTOLOGY OF VESTIBULAR RECEPTORS: CRISTA AMPULLARIS AND MACULA

The vestibular part of the **membranous labyrinth** comprises three **semicircular canals,** an ellipsoidal **utricle,** and spherical **saccule.** The canals lie at right angles to each other in three planes; each has an ampullated end. The vestibular receptor areas in the utricle and saccule are in the macula; the crista ampullaris is the equivalent receptor area in the canals. The crista, a prominent crest of **sensory epithelium** with underlying **connective tissue,** responds to angular acceleration and, like the organ of Corti, has two types of **hair cells** as well as **supporting cells.** Hair cells are best appreciated by electron microscopy. Flask-shaped **type I cells** are innervated at the base by a cup-like **afferent nerve terminal.** They resemble inner hair cells of the organ of Corti. More elongated **type II cells** are in contact with several small, punctate afferent and **efferent nerve terminals.** The free surface of hair cells in the crista has a nonmotile **kinocilium** and many (40-80) **stereocilia.** Stereocilia are embedded in an extracellular glycoprotein coat, the **cupula,** which is surrounded by **endolymph.** The crista is perpendicular to the long axis of each semicircular canal and responds to angular acceleration. Maculae of the utricle and the saccule conform to the same histologic plan but have different senses—linear acceleration and gravity. Their sensory epithelium has two types of hair cells and supporting cells, all resting on a basement membrane. A macula hair cell has one kinocilium and many stereocilia that project into the gelatinous **otolithic membrane.** Calcium carbonate crystals make up the **otoconia,** which are suspended on top of the otolithic membrane. Macula hair cells are innervated at their bases by both afferent and efferent nerve fibers of the vestibular part of *cranial nerve VIII.*

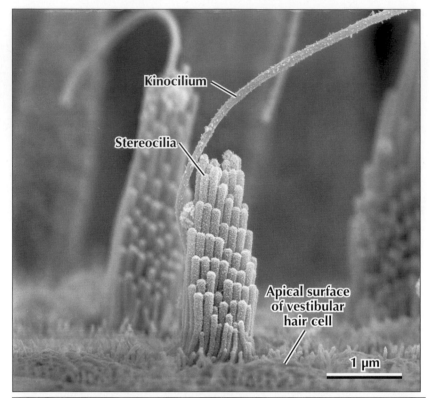

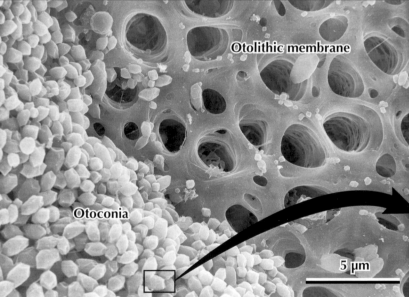

◀ **SEM showing surface specializations of rodent vestibular hair cells.** Rows of closely packed stereocilia, with longitudinal actin filaments, ascend stepwise in height (from front to back) from each cell. One long kinocilium is at the tall edge of the stereocilia bundle. Markedly longer than the tallest stereocilia, it may be 80 μm long in some species. It arises from a basal body in apical cytoplasm; its central core has a 9+2 arrangement of microtubules. 20,000×. *(Reprinted with permission, The Journal of Cell Biology 2004, 164: 887–897. The Rockefeller University Press.)*

▶ **SEM of normal mouse utricular macula.** Otoconia (to the left) aid in sensing linear acceleration and gravity. The porous structure (to the right) is the gelatinous layer of the otolithic membrane. Bundles of apical stereocilia (not in view) normally project from individual hair cells into the otolithic membrane holes. 5000×. *(Reprinted with permission, Everett L, et al: Targeted disruption of mouse Pds provides insight about the inner-ear defects encountered in Pendred syndrome. Human Molecular Genetics 10(2)153-161, 2001.)*

▼ **SEM of an otoconium of a pendrin-deficient knockout mouse at high magnification.** Its multifaceted surface contour is clear. Otoconia, produced by supporting cells in the epithelium of the macula, are abnormally enlarged in pendrin-deficient disorders that affect Cl⁻ ion transport of this epithelium. 50,000×. *(Courtesy of Dr. B. Kachar)*

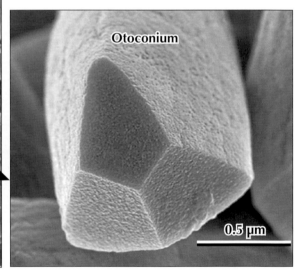

20.9   ULTRASTRUCTURE AND FUNCTION OF VESTIBULAR HAIR CELLS

Vestibular hair cells have ultrastructural features in common with those of the cochlea, but a few features set them apart. Vestibular cells have 40-80 **stereocilia** that project from **apical surfaces.** Graded in length, they are organized in a step-like fashion. Like those in the cochlea, stereocilia play a role in mechanotransduction. Unlike those of cochlear hair cells, stereocilia of vestibular hair cells progressively lengthen toward one pole of the cell that has one nonmotile **kinocilium** with a 9 + 2 microtubule pattern. The other stereocilia are modified microvilli with tightly packed actin filaments to provide rigidity. Stereocilia are connected by thin filamentous tip links, which maintain cohesion and engage in transduction. When stereocilia bend in the direction of the kinocilium, gated ion channels in their plasma membranes open, which triggers membrane depolarization by entering K⁺ ions. After release of the neurotransmitter *glutamate* from a hair cell, the sensory nerve fiber contacting that cell increases its firing rate. Opposite displacement causes ion channel closure, membrane hyperpolarization, and reduced neuronal firing frequency. In the **macula** of the saccule and utricle, **otoconia** embedded in the **otolithic membrane** are denser than endolymph. Gravity thus causes a shear motion of the otolithic membrane relative to hair cells, which excites or inhibits them. Otoconia contain a dense filamentous core of the protein otoconin-90, which is linked to an outer cortex of calcium carbonate-rich microcrystals.

▼ **Distribution of olfactory epithelium (blue area).**

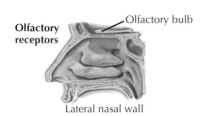

Olfactory receptors

Olfactory bulb

Cribriform plate of ethmoid bone

Lateral nasal wall

Septum

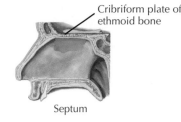

▼ **Section through olfactory mucosa.**
(Olfactory basal cells are omitted.)

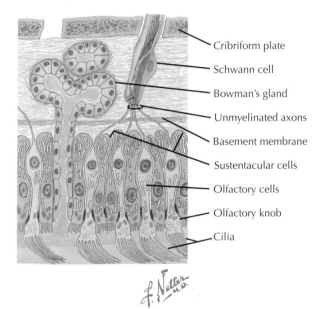

- Cribriform plate
- Schwann cell
- Bowman's gland
- Unmyelinated axons
- Basement membrane
- Sustentacular cells
- Olfactory cells
- Olfactory knob
- Cilia

f. Netter.

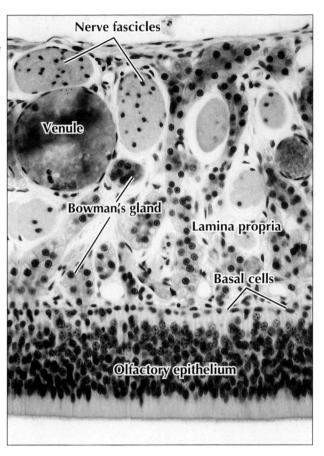

Nerve fascicles

Venule

Bowman's gland

Lamina propria

Basal cells

Olfactory epithelium

▲ **LM of the olfactory mucosa.** Several nuclear layers in the epithelium correspond to layers of three main cell types. Nuclei of supporting cells are closest to the surface; those of bipolar receptor cells are in the middle. Small rounded basal cells form one layer in the deepest part of the epithelium and rest on a thin basement membrane. Unmyelinated nerve fascicles, thin-walled venules, and Bowman's glands predominate in the lamina propria. 300×. *H&E.*

20.10 HISTOLOGY AND FUNCTION OF OLFACTORY MUCOSA

Olfactory mucosa is a *mucous membrane* that is highly specialized for smell. It is found in the roof of the nasal cavity, superior concha, and upper part of the nasal septum; its total surface area is about 50 mm². It is lined by **olfactory epithelium**—an unusually thick (75-100 µm high) pseudostratified epithelium—that consists of three cell types: **olfactory cells, sustentacular (supporting) cells,** and **basal cells.** Olfactory cells, slender **bipolar neurons** spanning the width of the epithelium, are receptor cells that bind odoriferous substances and convert them to nerve impulses. They are the only neurons in the body with direct exposure to a body surface. The *apical dendrite* of each cell ends as a bulbous **olfactory knob,** which extends above the epithelial surface. The dendrite leads to a nucleated cell body, in middle to deep regions of the epithelium. Many **nonmotile cilia** that lie along the epithelial surface emanate from an olfactory knob and increase surface area for odor detection. One **basal axon** from the cell exits the epithelium by piercing the **basement membrane.** In the **lamina propria,** the unmyelinated axon converges with others to form **nerve fascicles.** They course through the cribriform plate of the ethmoid bone to end in the **olfactory bulb.** Nerve fibers

originating in this area form the *olfactory nerve (cranial nerve I).* The other spherical nuclei in the epithelium belong to supporting cells; they often have pigment and stubby apical microvilli, which make the surface look striated. One row of small rounded nuclei next to the ill-defined basement membrane is of basal cells. The lamina propria is loose, highly vascular connective tissue containing many thin-walled **blood vessels** and branched *tubuloalveolar glands* (of *Bowman*), which take serous secretions via ducts to the mucous membrane surface.

CLINICAL POINT

Viral infection of the olfactory mucosa related to the common cold may lead to **anosmia** (loss of sense of smell). It may be partial or complete and may become permanent in chronic infection of the mucous membrane (as in *rhinitis*). Proximity of olfactory bipolar neurons to an outside body surface makes them subject to infection and injury. Causes of permanent anosmia include fractures of the anterior cranial fossa, cerebral tumors of frontal lobes, and lesions of olfactory nerves. Permanent damage to the olfactory mucous membrane may occur after long exposure to neurotoxic industrial odors.

▼ **Tongue.**

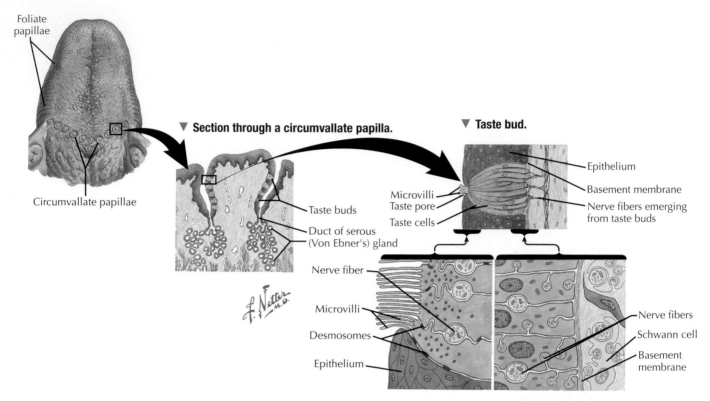

▼ **Section through a circumvallate papilla.**

Foliate papillae

Circumvallate papillae

Taste buds

Duct of serous (Von Ebner's) gland

▼ **Taste bud.**

Microvilli
Taste pore
Taste cells

Epithelium
Basement membrane
Nerve fibers emerging from taste buds

Nerve fiber
Microvilli
Desmosomes
Epithelium

Nerve fibers
Schwann cell
Basement membrane

▲ **Detail of a taste pore.** ▲ **Detail of the base of receptor cells.**

▶ **LM of a circumvallate papilla in the tongue.**
Nonkeratinized stratified squamous epithelium covers the papilla, whose core is loose connective tissue—the lamina propria. Several taste buds (**arrows**) are embedded in the epithelium along lateral margins of the papilla. 80×. *H&E.*

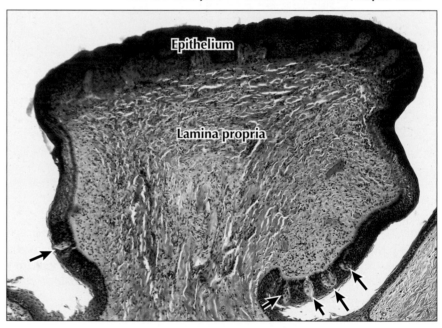

20.11 STRUCTURE AND DISTRIBUTION OF TASTE BUDS

The organs of taste consist of many ovoid taste buds, about 50 μm in diameter, that are modified epithelial cells in the surface epithelium. Pale-staining areas, they are widely distributed in **fungiform, foliate,** and **circumvallate papillae** of the **stratified squamous epithelium** on the dorsal aspect of the **tongue.** The anterior surface and lateral margins of the tongue contain 200-300 mushroom-shaped fungiform papillae, each containing 3-5 taste buds. Multiple leaf-shaped foliate papillae are on the lateral sides of the posterior part of the tongue; each contains 100-150 taste buds. Most taste buds are in lateral grooves of the 8-12 circumvallate papillae at the junction of the dorsum and base of the tongue. The wall of each circumvallate papilla holds 200-250 taste buds. The total number of taste buds in the human tongue is about 5000, but their number decreases with age. Variable numbers of taste buds are also found on the *soft palate, pharynx,* and *epiglottis.*

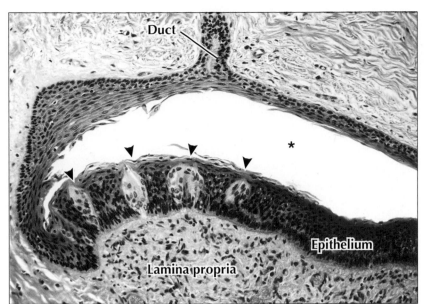

◀ **LM of the sulcus (∗) of a circumvallate papilla.** Four taste buds (**arrowheads**) appear as pale, ovoid bodies within stratified squamous epithelium of the tongue. The duct of a serous gland of von Ebner delivers watery secretions to the sulcus to cleanse the taste buds. A thin basement membrane separates bases of taste buds from lamina propria. 150×. *H&E.*

▶ **LM of a taste bud in the epithelium of the oral mucosa at high magnification.** Several pale cells in the taste bud are oriented vertically and extend upward toward the taste pore (**arrow**), which opens to the surface. Small, round basal cells are stem cells for other cells in the taste bud. The basement membrane (**arrowheads**) is indicated. Afferent nerve fibers innervating the taste bud are not seen well with standard stains and need special techniques for elucidation. 720×. *H&E.*

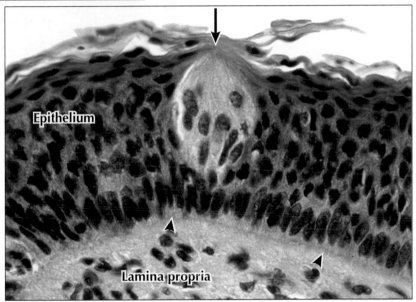

20.12 HISTOLOGY AND FUNCTION OF TASTE BUDS

Taste buds are ovoid to barrel-shaped clusters of pale-staining cells lying vertically in stratified squamous epithelium. They extend from basement membrane to the free surface. Each taste bud has 50-75 cells, whose arrangement resembles segments of a citrus fruit. About 20-40 cells are slender, spindle-shaped **taste (gustatory) cells** that are **chemoreceptors.** Nuclei of these cells are ovoid to columnar and are centrally located. These cells are mixed with several types of tall **supporting (sustentacular) cells** that resemble staves of a barrel. At the base are small rounded **basal cells,** resting on a basement membrane. These undifferentiated cells with mitotic potential and a turnover rate of about 10-14 days give rise to all other cells in the taste bud. Each taste bud communicates at its apex with the oral cavity via a **taste pore,** into which long apical **microvilli** of the elongated cells project. Molecules gain access to taste receptor cells at the pore; four classes of taste are recognized: sweet, salt, sour, and bitter. Unlike olfactory receptor cells, which are primary receptor neurons in olfactory mucosa, taste cells are epithelial cells that are contacted by **synapses** at their basal aspect by **afferent nerve fibers.** Nerves are difficult to see in routine sections, so special staining methods and electron microscopy are needed to elucidate taste bud innervation.

CLINICAL POINT

Hypogeusia—reduced sense of taste—or a strongly metallic, bitter, or sweet taste may adversely affect quality of life. Oral infections (e.g., *gingivitis*), dental appliances (e.g., dentures), oral surgical procedures, and radiation of the head and neck can interfere with taste. Influenza, the common cold, vitamin deficiencies, and anesthetic agents affect taste buds. Antibiotics and antihypertensive drugs commonly cause excessive dryness of the oral cavity, which often changes taste. *Viral Bell's palsy,* which alters impulse conduction in cranial nerve VII to the central nervous system, may also affect taste. Taste deficits in the elderly have been implicated in weight loss, impaired immunity, and malnutrition.

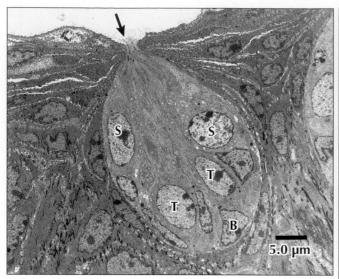

▲ Low-magnification EM of a taste bud. Taste cells (**T**) and supporting cells (**S**) have apical microvilli that project into the taste pore (**arrow**). The lower basal cells (**B**), resting on the basement membrane, are replacement cells for non-neural epithelial cells of the taste bud. 1600×.

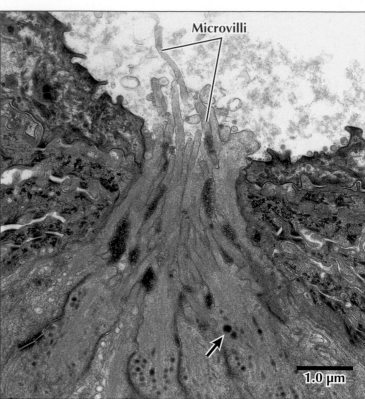

▲ EM showing apical microvilli of taste and supporting cells of a taste bud. Microvilli project into the taste pore and provide greatly increased surface area for secretion of material into the pore. Finger-like projections of plasma membrane, microvilli of taste cells are specialized for chemoreception. Supporting cells have small apical secretory vesicles (**arrow**) that release serous secretory product into the pore. 14,000×.

◄ EM showing afferent nerve terminals at the base of the taste bud. Nerve terminals contain synaptic vesicles, penetrate the basement membrane (**arrowheads**), and snake around taste cells to end in synaptic contact with them. 7500×.

20.13 ULTRASTRUCTURE OF TASTE BUDS

Apical ends of **taste cells** bear prominent **microvilli** that converge into a small **taste pore** open to the *oral cavity*. Chemicals in solution diffuse through the pore to contact **plasma membranes** of microvilli, which contain taste receptors that respond to molecules on the surface. Unmyelinated **afferent nerves** enter the taste bud at its inferior pole. After winding around the taste cells, they end close to basal and lateral plasma membranes of the taste cells. Chemical stimuli received by taste cells are transduced into electri-

cal impulses, which are transmitted to *synapses* formed with afferent fibers. Neurotransmitters released from *synaptic vesicles* in taste cells stimulate afferent nerve terminals. The sense of taste is mediated by nerve fibers of three *cranial nerves: facial* (VII), *glossopharyngeal* (IX), and *vagus* (X). Their central connections end in the nucleus of the tractus solitarius in the *brainstem*. Central neural pathways cross the pons, ascend to the thalamus, and end in the *cerebral cortex* insula.

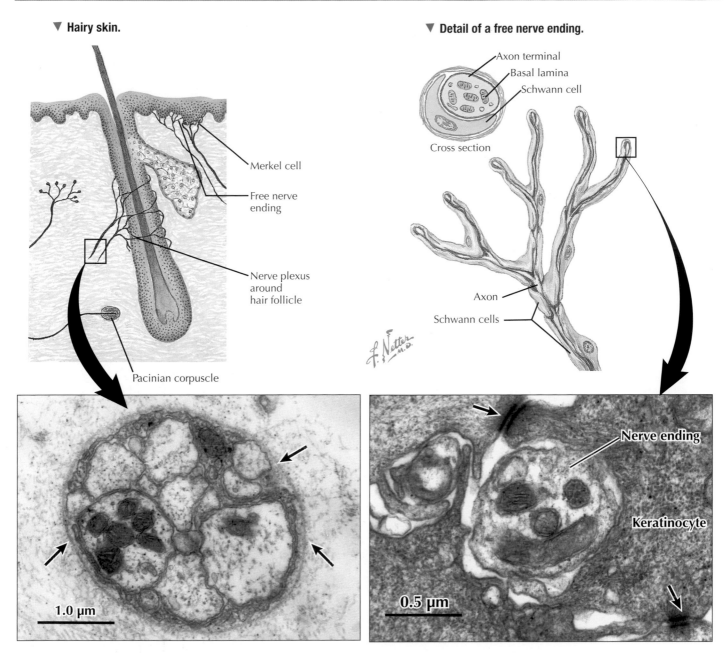

▼ **Hairy skin.**

Merkel cell

Free nerve ending

Nerve plexus around hair follicle

Pacinian corpuscle

▼ **Detail of a free nerve ending.**

Axon terminal

Basal lamina

Schwann cell

Cross section

Axon

Schwann cells

Nerve ending

Keratinocyte

1.0 μm

0.5 μm

▲ **EM of a group of unmyelinated nerve fibers in the dermis, close to the junction with the epidermis.** They contain mitochondria, neurofilaments, and microtubules and are invested by Schwann cell processes and an external (basal) lamina (**arrows**). The fibers lose their external covering and end freely in the epidermis. 20,000×.

▲ **EM of a free intraepidermal nerve ending.** It lacks a Schwann cell covering. Epidermal keratinocytes, which are linked by desmosomes (**arrows**), surround it. The nerve ending contains microtubules, neurofilaments, and many mitochondria sectioned in different planes. 40,000×.

20.14 STRUCTURE AND FUNCTION OF CUTANEOUS SENSORY RECEPTORS

Sensory nerve terminals, which act as *mechanoreceptors,* are widespread in the body and are classified histologically as *unencapsulated (naked) nerve endings* or more complicated *encapsulated receptors.* They monitor mechanical stimuli such as touch, vibration, pressure, pain, and temperature. Unencapsulated sensory nerves in the epidermis and mucous membranes take two forms: **free nerve endings** and **Merkel cell-neurite complexes.** Free nerve endings are terminal branches of afferent nerve fibers with a relatively simple microscopic structure. Ending freely among epithelial cells without any structural specialization, they act as nociceptors or respond to thermal stimuli. They consist of unmyelinated axons (1 μm or less in diameter), which lose their *myelin sheath* and **Schwann cells** before contacting epithelial cells. The cytoplasm of each nerve fiber contains mitochondria, microtubules, neurofilaments, and clear membrane-bound (60-nm) vesicles. Merkel cell-neurite complexes—slowly adapting touch receptors—consist of enlarged terminal endings of afferent nerve fibers, which form synaptic contacts with **Merkel cells** that have distinctive dense core vesicles. More elaborate encapsulated receptors in the skin are *Meissner's corpuscles.* These fast-adapting mechanoreceptors detect moving touch. Deeper subcutaneous regions contain larger **Pacinian corpuscles,** which have an unmistakable morphologic appearance. They respond to deep pressure and vibratory stimuli.

▼ **Detail of a Merkel cell-neurite complex.**

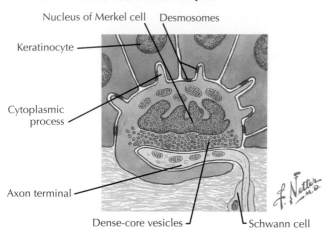

Nucleus of Merkel cell — Desmosomes

Keratinocyte

Cytoplasmic process

Axon terminal

Dense-core vesicles — Schwann cell

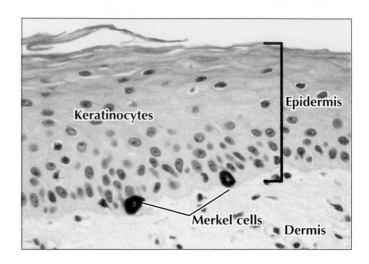

Keratinocytes

Epidermis

Merkel cells — Dermis

◀ **LM of Merkel cells in the epidermis of thick skin.** Merkel cells, not seen by usual histologic methods, require special stains. With a monoclonal antibody (CAM 5.2) to cytokeratin, they stain immunocytochemically and are easily distinguished from other cells. Two Merkel cells are seen here in the basal epidermal layer, close to the junction with the dermis. Their cytoplasm stains brown. Except for other nuclei, which stain blue, surrounding keratinocytes lack staining. 360×. *CAM 5.2, diaminobenzidine, hematoxylin. (Courtesy of Dr. M. Martinka)*

▶ **EM of part of a Merkel cell-neurite complex at high magnification.** The cell is in contact with two expanded nerve terminals. Finger-like cytoplasmic extensions (**arrows**) of the cell interdigitate with keratinocytes. Membrane-bound dense core vesicles lie close to the contact site between the cell and nerve terminal. Small clear cytoplasmic vesicles fill the axoplasm of the nerve terminals. 22,000×.

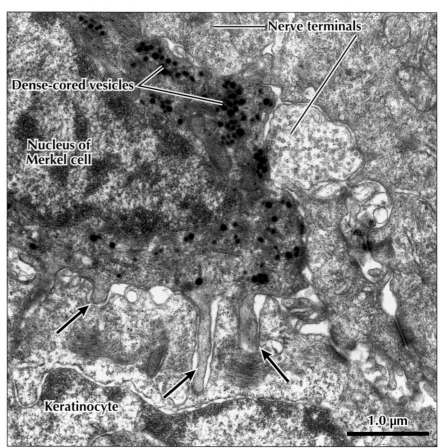

Nerve terminals

Dense-cored vesicles

Nucleus of Merkel cell

Keratinocyte

1.0 µm

20.15 ULTRASTRUCTURE AND FUNCTION OF MERKEL CELL-NEURITE COMPLEXES

Merkel cells are neural crest-derived, ellipsoidal cells found in glabrous and hairy skin as well as some mucous membranes. They express various substances such as neuron-specific proteins, cytokeratin 20, amines, chromogranins, and villin. Best seen by immunocytochemistry or electron microscopy, they are 9-16 µm in diameter and usually have one large lobulated nucleus. Each cell has many finger-like **cytoplasmic processes** that interdigitate with slight invaginations of adjacent **keratinocytes. Desmosomes** link cells to keratinocytes. Merkel cell cytoplasm contains abundant **filaments,** oriented in different directions, that extend into the cytoplasmic processes. Many electron-dense **membrane-bound vesicles** (80-100 nm in diameter), a prominent feature of the cells, normally accumulate in cytoplasm near the junction with afferent nerve terminals. At these sites, the **plasma membrane** of a Merkel cell is apposed to the cell membrane of the **nerve terminal,** with areas of synaptic specialization that appear as membrane-associated densities. Immunocytochemistry shows **dense core vesicles** of Merkel cells to possess substances that may act as neurotransmitters or neuromodulators. As mechanoreceptors, Merkel cells respond to punctate pressure and bending of hairs and transform mechanical signals into action potentials in the nerve terminals.

▼ **Thick (glabrous) skin.**

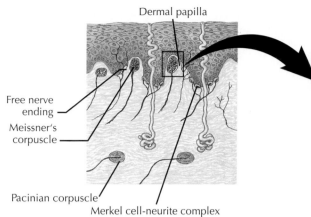

Dermal papilla

Free nerve ending

Meissner's corpuscle

Pacinian corpuscle

Merkel cell-neurite complex

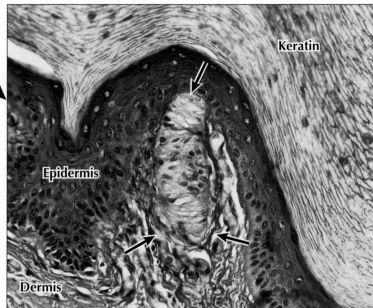

Keratin

Epidermis

Dermis

▶ **LM of Meissner's corpuscle (arrows) in thick skin.** Parallel stacks of thin capsular lamellae characterize these receptors. Overlying epidermis is keratinized stratified squamous epithelium; underlying dermis is loose connective tissue. 300×. *H&E.*

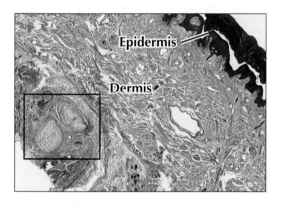

Epidermis

Dermis

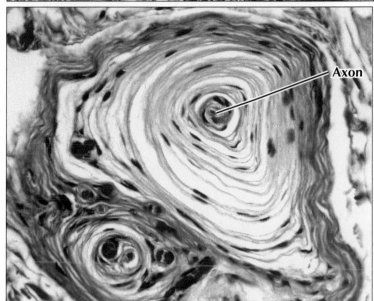

Axon

▲ **LM of thick skin.** Two Pacinian corpuscles are deep in the dermis in subcutaneous connective tissue. 25×. *H&E.*

▶ **LM of a Pacinian corpuscle in transverse section.** The capsule is made of multiple concentric lamellae that enclose one unmyelinated axon in the receptor core. 300×. *H&E.*

20.16 HISTOLOGY AND FUNCTION OF MEISSNER'S AND PACINIAN CORPUSCLES

Meissner's and Pacinian corpuscles are rapidly adapting *encapsulated mechanoreceptors* in dermal papillae of thick skin in fingertips, palms of the hands, and soles of the feet; Pacinian corpuscles also occur in mesenteries, periosteum of bone, genital organs, and near tendinous insertions of muscles and joint capsules. Sensitive to fine tactile stimuli, Meissner's corpuscles are elliptical, with diameters of about 150 µm and long axes perpendicular to the skin surface. One **myelinated nerve fiber** loses its myelin sheath as it enters the receptor. It then branches repeatedly and winds spirally through multiple transverse stacks of specialized connective tissue cells, the **perineurial cells.** These cells are arranged as a layered stack at right angles to the long axis of the receptor. They aid transduction of mechanical stimuli into initiation of a nerve

impulse. A thin, fibrous **connective tissue** coat encloses the receptor externally. Pacinian corpuscles, which respond to pressure, vibration, and gross tactile stimuli, are among the largest encapsulated receptors, with wide distribution in the body, usually deep in subcutaneous connective tissue of skin. These bulbous, elliptical corpuscles vary in size (up to 1 µm in diameter) and complexity and occur singly or in groups. The capsule comprises multiple, onion-like concentric **lamellae** of flattened perineurial cells that are continuous with the *perineurium* of the nerve that ends in the capsule. They resemble capsular cells of *muscle spindles* and *Golgi tendon organs.* One myelinated sensory axon loses its myelin as it enters one pole of the capsule and immediately ends in the receptor. The capsule isolates receptor contents from the extracellular space and is a mechanical filter that modifies stimuli before they reach sensory nerve endings.

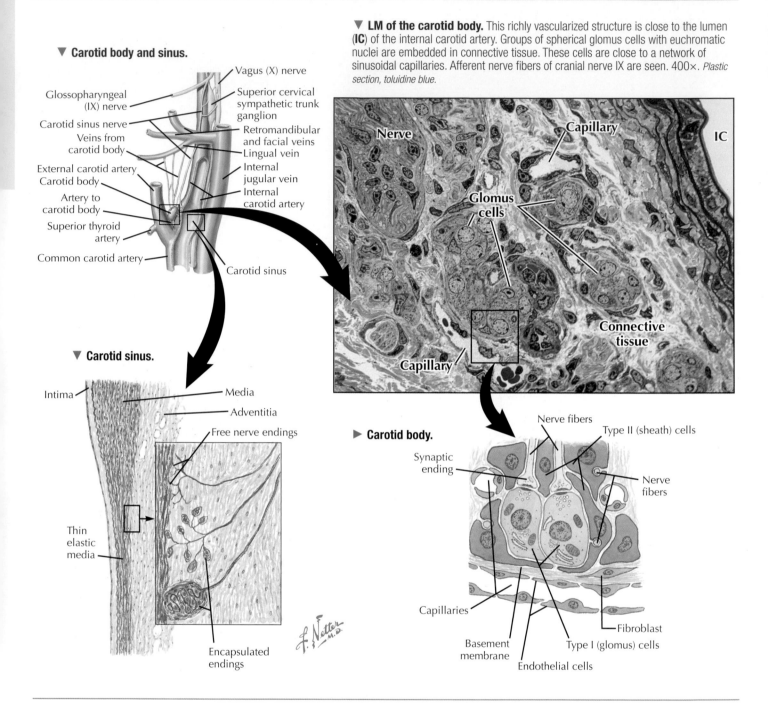

▼ **Carotid body and sinus.**

Glossopharyngeal (IX) nerve

Vagus (X) nerve

Superior cervical sympathetic trunk ganglion

Carotid sinus nerve

Veins from carotid body

Retromandibular and facial veins

Lingual vein

External carotid artery

Carotid body

Internal jugular vein

Internal carotid artery

Artery to carotid body

Superior thyroid artery

Common carotid artery

Carotid sinus

▼ **LM of the carotid body.** This richly vascularized structure is close to the lumen (**IC**) of the internal carotid artery. Groups of spherical glomus cells with euchromatic nuclei are embedded in connective tissue. These cells are close to a network of sinusoidal capillaries. Afferent nerve fibers of cranial nerve IX are seen. 400×. *Plastic section, toluidine blue.*

Nerve

Capillary

IC

Glomus cells

Connective tissue

Capillary

▼ **Carotid sinus.**

Intima

Media

Adventitia

Free nerve endings

Thin elastic media

Encapsulated endings

▶ **Carotid body.**

Nerve fibers

Type II (sheath) cells

Synaptic ending

Nerve fibers

Capillaries

Fibroblast

Basement membrane

Type I (glomus) cells

Endothelial cells

20.17 STRUCTURE AND FUNCTION OF INTEROCEPTORS: CAROTID BODY AND SINUS

Carotid and aortic bodies contain **chemoreceptors.** The carotid body is a lenticular encapsulated structure (0.5-5 mm in diameter) at the division of the carotid artery into external and internal branches. Classified as a **parasympathetic paraganglion,** with its own separate arterial and venous circulation, it contains groups of chemoreceptor cells close to many **sinusoidal capillaries.** These cells respond to increased CO_2, reduced O_2, and raised H^+ levels in arterial blood. **Type II (sheath) cells** surround clusters of **type I (glomus) cells,** whose cytoplasm contains many membrane-bound **dense core vesicles** (60-120 nm in diameter). **Dendrites** of **afferent nerve fibers** of **cranial nerve IX** synapse with the chemoreceptor cells; acetylcholine and catecholamines (such as dopa-

mine) are neurotransmitters. These receptor cells monitor changes in blood pH, O_2 tension, and CO_2 in arterial blood to maintain normal physiologic levels. Efferent nerve fibers from the carotid body become myelinated and travel to the medulla's respiratory center, where they effect increased respiration and heart rates. The aortic body comprises two groups of cell aggregates in connective tissue between the aorta and pulmonary artery. They resemble chemoreceptors in the carotid body. The carotid sinus, a thin-walled dilated part of the internal carotid artery, contains **free** and **encapsulated nerve endings** that are sensitive to stretch. Innervated by afferent nerve fibers of cranial nerve IX, these *baroreceptors* inform the central nervous system about changes in blood pressure in the carotid artery. Baroreceptors are also found in other large elastic arteries and act to maintain blood pressure within normal physiologic limits.

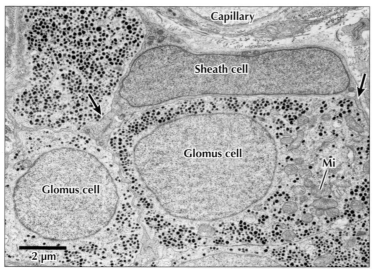

◀ **EM of part of a carotid body.** Glomus cells have many dense core vesicles, mitochondria (**Mi**), and a round euchromatic nucleus. Sheath (type II) cell nuclei stain darker and are elongated. Processes (**arrows**) of sheath cells partially invest glomus cells. Part of a fenestrated capillary is above. 6100×. *(Courtesy of Dr. J. T. Hansen)*

▼ **EM showing a synapse between a glomus cell and a nerve terminal.** Abundant dense core vesicles are in the glomus cell cytoplasm. Its rounded nucleus is euchromatic. The nerve terminal contains many small clear vesicles. Mitochondria (**Mi**) appear in both the cell and terminal. The process of a sheath cell is next to the nerve terminal above. Synaptic areas in the rectangles show apposition of plasma membranes of the cell and terminal, where a small cleft appears between the two cells. 16,900×.

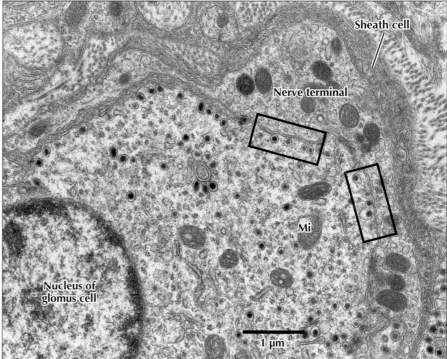

20.18   ULTRASTRUCTURE AND FUNCTION OF A CAROTID BODY

Ultrastructural organization of the carotid body is consistent with a role as a *chemoreceptor*. **Glomus cells**—the main parenchymal cells—are thought to be paraneurons, which likely derive from *neural crest ectoderm*. A distinctive feature of these cells is abundant membrane-bound **dense core vesicles** that store several substances, such as *serotonin, epinephrine, norepinephrine, neurotensin, bombesin, dopamine,* and *enkephalins*. Several types of glomus cells have been described on the basis of vesicle size, numerical density, and shape. Many visceral afferent **unmyelinated axons** synapse directly with glomus cells. At these sites, a narrow **synaptic cleft** sits between the nerve terminal and glomus cell. Nerve terminals contain many spherical vesicles, most with a clear center. An extensive network of **sinusoidal fenestrated capillaries,** which derive from branches of the external carotid artery, supplies the carotid body. Loose connective tissue *stroma* of the carotid body contains supportive **sheath (type II) cells,** which closely resemble glial cells. Processes of these cells partially ensheath glomus cells and **afferent nerve terminals.**

CLINICAL POINT

Carotid bodies usually undergo *involution* with aging. They may show diffuse lymphocyte infiltration, reduced number of glomus cells, proliferation of supporting cells, and accumulated fibrous connective tissue. People who become acclimatized to living at high altitudes have enlarged carotid bodies because of hyperplasia of glomus cells in response to stimulation by **hypoxia.** People living at such altitudes show a high incidence of carotid body tumors, named **chemodectomas.** Other disorders may also affect carotid bodies: **pulmonary emphysema** and **systemic hypertension** promote sheath cell hyperplasia and glomus cell atrophy.

▼ Muscle and joint receptors.

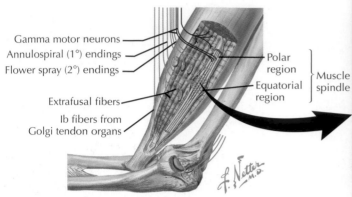

Gamma motor neurons
Annulospiral (1°) endings
Flower spray (2°) endings
Polar region
Equatorial region
Muscle spindle
Extrafusal fibers
Ib fibers from Golgi tendon organs

f. Netter M.D.

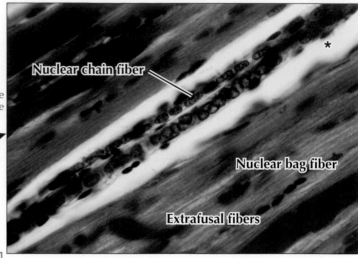

Nuclear chain fiber

Nuclear bag fiber

Extrafusal fibers

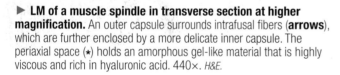

Extrafusal muscle fibers

Muscle spindle

▲ **LM of a muscle spindle in longitudinal section.** A periaxial space (*) surrounds thick nuclear bag and thin nuclear chain fibers. The spindle parallels the longitudinal axis of extrafusal fibers around it. Special staining methods are needed to show the complex innervation of intrafusal fibers. 340×. *H&E.*

▲ **LM of a muscle spindle in transverse section.** An outer capsule encloses a fluid-filled periaxial space (*) and surrounds several small intrafusal fibers (**arrowheads**). Larger, more numerous extrafusal fibers are outside the spindle capsule and make up most of the muscle. 110×. *H&E.*

▶ **LM of a muscle spindle in transverse section at higher magnification.** An outer capsule surrounds intrafusal fibers (**arrows**), which are further enclosed by a more delicate inner capsule. The periaxial space (*) holds an amorphous gel-like material that is highly viscous and rich in hyaluronic acid. 440×. *H&E.*

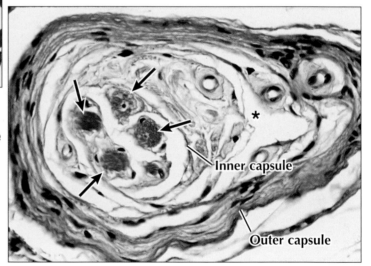

Inner capsule

Outer capsule

20.19   HISTOLOGY AND FUNCTION OF MUSCLE SPINDLES

Muscle spindles are *encapsulated sensory receptors* found in almost every skeletal muscle in the body but are most numerous in muscles needed for fine discriminative control. As part of the monosynaptic stretch reflex, they monitor changes in length of the whole muscle. They contain two types of modified skeletal muscle fibers: **nuclear bag** and **nuclear chain intrafusal fibers;** special techniques can show two types of bag fibers (*dynamic bag$_1$* and *static bag$_2$*). They parallel surrounding **extrafusal muscle fibers** that make up the bulk of the muscle. The fusiform intrafusal fibers have a central—**equatorial**—noncontractile region (innervated by *sensory nerve terminals*); and two distal—**polar**—regions

(innervated by **gamma motor nerves**), striated and contractile. When the muscle is stretched, the equatorial part of the intrafusal fiber is also stretched. This mechanically distorts sensory endings, thereby activating stretch-sensitive ion channels that trigger nerve impulses, which are conveyed to the spinal cord. Each spindle has 2-12 intrafusal fibers, on which two types of motor nerve endings and two kinds of sensory endings terminate: **primary** (**Ia,** or **annulospiral**) sensory endings arise from one myelinated nerve, which enters the spindle capsule to wrap around intrafusal fibers in an annulospiral design. **Secondary** (**IIa,** or **flower spray**) sensory endings arise from several small myelinated nerve fibers that end mostly on nuclear chain fibers on both sides of the primary endings.

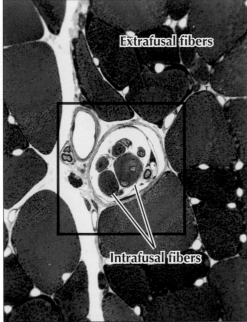

Extrafusal fibers

Intrafusal fibers

◄ ▼ **LM and EM of a muscle spindle in the equatorial region.** A thin inner capsule and periaxial space (★) surround two nuclear chain (**NC**) fibers and **bag₁** and **bag₂** intrafusal fibers. Small sensory terminals (**arrowheads**) end on the fibers. A mast cell (**MC**), nerve fascicle, and venule abut the multilayer outer capsule surrounding the receptor. Extrafusal muscle fibers are in view. **LM:** 740×. *Toluidine blue, plastic section.* **EM:** 3100×.

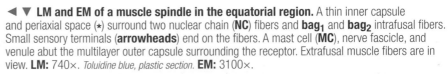

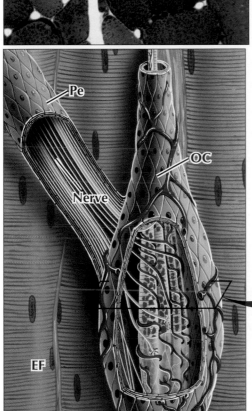

Pe

OC

Nerve

EF

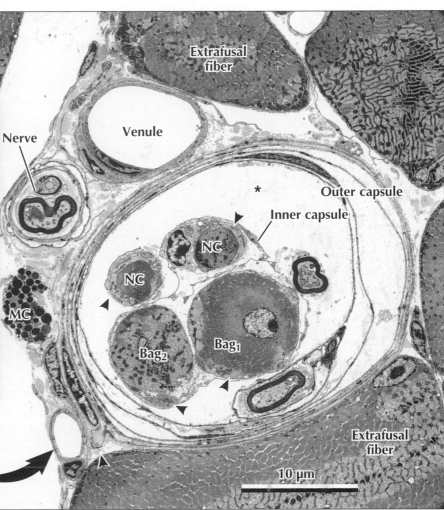

Extrafusal fiber

Nerve

Venule

*

Outer capsule

Inner capsule

NC

NC

MC

Bag₂

Bag₁

Extrafusal fiber

10 µm

◄ **Longitudinal schematic of a muscle spindle.** Innervation of nuclear bag (green) and chain (blue) fibers in the equator is seen. The outer capsule (**OC**) is continuous with the perineurium (**Pe**) of the incoming nerve. Blood vessels abut the outer capsule surface, and extrafusal fibers (**EF**) are indicated. *(Courtesy of Dr. P. R. Dow)*

20.20 ULTRASTRUCTURE AND FUNCTION OF MUSCLE SPINDLES

A multilayer **outer capsule** made of flattened perineurial cells covers the muscle spindle and a fluid-filled **periaxial space**. The capsule is continuous with the *perineurium* of afferent and efferent nerves innervating intrafusal fibers. This selective barrier, like the *blood-brain barrier,* sequesters a receptor from the external milieu. A single-layer **inner capsule** invests the thin **nuclear chain** and more robust **nuclear bag fibers. Sensory nerve terminals** at equatorial regions of fibers sit on the fiber surface and wrap around as either *primary* or *secondary endings.* Usually, primary endings respond to degree and rate of a muscle stretch; secondary endings respond to degree of stretch. Motor nerve supply to intrafusal fibers is at more distal polar regions. The *gamma nerve fibers* are either static or dynamic, depending on their physiologic effect on intrafusal fibers and pattern of innervation. Dynamic fibers innervate **bag₁ fibers;** static fibers innervate the nuclear chain and **bag₂ fibers.** They regulate the sensitivity of intrafusal fibers to stretch by increasing tension in equatorial regions. Muscle spindles contribute to control of posture, muscle tone, position sense, and movement.

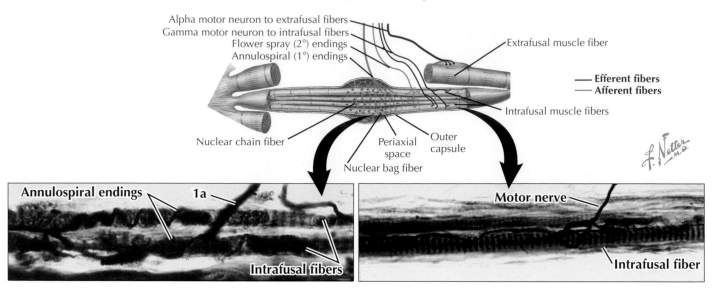

▼ **Details of muscle spindle.**

Alpha motor neuron to extrafusal fibers
Gamma motor neuron to intrafusal fibers
Flower spray (2°) endings
Annulospiral (1°) endings

Extrafusal muscle fiber

—— **Efferent fibers**
—— **Afferent fibers**

Intrafusal muscle fibers

Nuclear chain fiber

Periaxial space   Outer capsule

Nuclear bag fiber

Annulospiral endings   1a

Intrafusal fibers

Motor nerve

Intrafusal fiber

▲ **LMs of sensory and motor innervation in different parts of a muscle spindle.** Silver-impregnated nerve fibers appear black. In the equatorial region (**Left**), two primary endings are supplied by one large afferent nerve fiber (**1a**). The nerve endings wrap around the nucleated noncontractile parts of intrafusal fibers. In the polar area (**Right**), a motor nerve has a trail-like ending on the striated (contractile) part of an intrafusal fiber. 400×. *Bielschowsky's silver.*

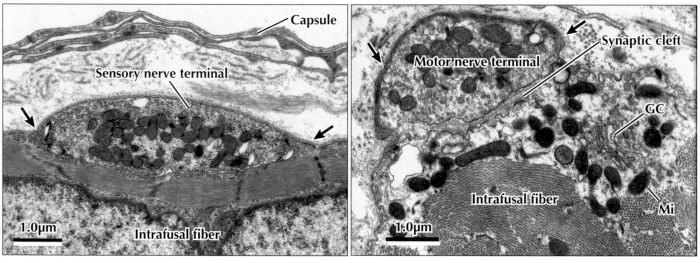

Capsule

Sensory nerve terminal

1.0μm   Intrafusal fiber

Motor nerve terminal   Synaptic cleft

GC

Mi

Intrafusal fiber

1.0μm

▲ **EM of a sensory nerve terminal on an intrafusal muscle fiber.** The terminal contains many mitochondria, cytoplasmic vesicles, and neurofilaments. It sits in a shallow depression on the fiber surface. Nerve and muscle share a continuous basal lamina (**arrows**). Processes of the inner capsule isolate the intrafusal fiber and sensory nerve from the external milieu. 13,000×.

▲ **EM of a motor endplate on an intrafusal fiber.** The axon contacts a slightly infolded sarcolemma of the muscle fiber. A Schwann cell process (**arrows**) covers the axon terminal, which shows mitochondria and synaptic vesicles. The synaptic cleft contains a thin basal lamina. Muscle fiber cytoplasm contains a Golgi complex (**GC**) and many mitochondria (**Mi**). 14,000×.

20.21   INNERVATION OF MUSCLE SPINDLES

Special staining methods and electron microscopy help elucidate the complex innervation of muscle spindles. **Motor** and **sensory nerves** penetrate the capsule, lose myelin sheaths, and end on specific parts of **intrafusal fibers**. Small motor nerves, also named **gamma efferents,** end as *neuromuscular junctions* in polar contractile regions of intrafusal fibers as either discrete **plate-like endings** or more diffuse **trail-like endings**. Both types of motor endings release the *neurotransmitter acetylcholine.* Stimulation of intrafusal fibers by motor nerves elicits contraction, thereby stretching equatorial regions of muscle fibers and their sensory

endings. Two types of sensory endings—**primary** and **secondary**—supply equatorial areas of intrafusal fibers, but electron microscopy has shown no essential fine structural differences between them. Sensory terminals lie apposed to muscle fibers with no intervening **basal lamina** or outer **Schwann cell** covering. These terminals are packed with **mitochondria, neurofilaments,** and **vesicles**. Stretching causes endings to deform, which leads to mechanoelectric transduction and a train of action potentials in the nerve that travels back to the spinal cord for the monosynaptic stretch reflex.

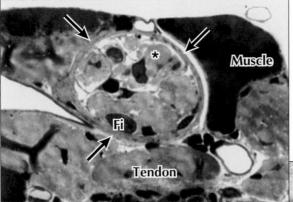

◀ **LM of a Golgi tendon organ in transverse section.** It is near the muscle-tendon junction. A capsule (**arrows**) encloses fibroblasts (**Fi**) and their processes that support collagen fiber bundles (∗). This magnification does not show sensory nerve terminals. 930×. *Toluidine blue, plastic section.*

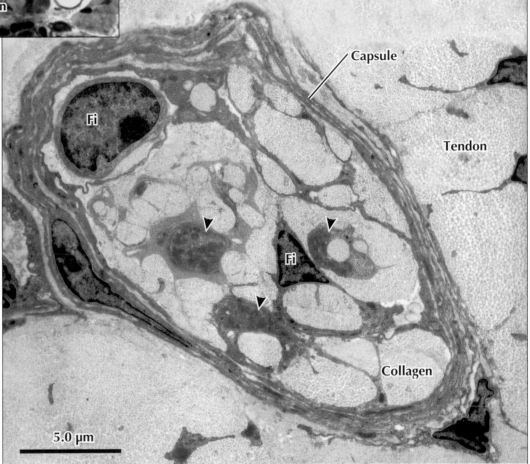

▲ **EM of a Golgi tendon organ in transverse section.** Its multilayer outer capsule, whose ultrastructure is similar to that of a muscle spindle capsule, surrounds collagen fiber bundles. Branching processes of fibroblasts (**Fi**) intertwine in the receptor and are close to sensory nerve terminals (**arrowheads**), which appear as knob-like swellings. The tendon contains closely packed collagen fibers mixed with tendon fibroblasts. 5400×.

20.22 ULTRASTRUCTURE AND FUNCTION OF GOLGI TENDON ORGANS

Golgi tendon organs are encapsulated **sensory nerve terminals** along muscle-tendon boundaries of skeletal muscles. These *slowly adapting mechanoreceptors* respond to mechanical forces during stretch and active muscle contraction. Each receptor is innervated by one *myelinated (1b) nerve fiber* that penetrates the capsule and branches into unmyelinated sensory nerve terminals close to encapsulated **collagen fiber bundles.** Each sensory ending in a receptor is replete with **mitochondria, neurofilaments,** and **cytoplasmic vesicles.** The **outer capsule** is morphologically similar to

that of a muscle spindle and is continuous with the *perineurium* over its nerve supply. Unlike muscle spindles, Golgi tendon organs do not have separate motor nerves. Golgi tendon organs are biologic transducers that monitor tension produced mostly by tendon stretching. Tension on the capsule in the longitudinal direction exerts pressure on collagen fiber bundles in the receptor, which, in turn, deforms sensory nerve endings and stimulates them to generate action potentials. Golgi tendon organs provide afferent feedback to the central nervous system for reflex regulation of motor activity, and they reduce excessive tension on the muscle at its tendinous insertion.

Appendix
STAINING METHODS AND TECHNIQUES

The combination **hematoxylin and eosin (H&E)** is one of the most popular conventional stains for light microscopy in histology because of its relative simplicity and ability to show various structures. **Hematoxylin** is a natural basic dye, extracted from the logwood tree *Haematoxylum campechianum*, that binds to acidic components that are thus called basophilic. Oxidation converts it to hematein, a compound with a rich blue-purple color. Nuclei, which contain acidic substances such as DNA and RNA, stain blue. **Eosin**—an acidic, anionic orange-pink dye extracted from coal tar—is used as a counterstain to hematoxylin. Its name derives from Eos, the Greek goddess of the dawn, because of its color. It imparts shades of pink, red, and orange to the cytoplasm of most cells and to connective tissue fibers, which are acidophilic.

Wright's and Giemsa stains, used in hematology for blood and bone marrow smears, contain eosin and methylene blue, so protein stains pink and nuclei, bluish purple. Granules of granular leukocytes stain characteristic colors because of metachromasia, whereby materials such as basophilic granules alter the color of some stains, such as methylene blue.

Luxol fast blue plus cresyl violet (LFB/CV) is a combination used for neural tissues. It stains myelin blue and nuclei and Nissl substances of nerve cell bodies violet to purple.

Osmic acid—both a fixative and a stain—is used in light microscopy to preserve fats (lipid), which stain black. It is also used in electron microscopy to preserve and stain ultrastructural components of cells, especially membranes. Other stains for fats in paraffin or frozen sections are **oil red O** and **Sudan black.**

Gomori aldehyde fuchsin (GAF) contains basic fuchsin, which is used to stain elastic fibers and mucins dark purple. Counterstaining with **orange G** and **phloxine** shows collagen as yellow to orange and muscle as bright pink to red. Other stains used for elastin and elastic fibers are **Verhoeff's, Weigert's resorcin-fuchsin,** and **van Gieson's.**

Trichrome stains are a class of stains made from a mixture of three or more chromophores or coloring agents, which allows one method to stain several tissue components differently. It can differentiate connective tissue from muscle and detect other tissue constituents. **Masson's trichrome** commonly stains collagen blue or green, nuclei blue-black, and muscle fibers red. With the trichrome stain **hematoxylin plus phloxine plus orange G (HPO),** hematoxylin stains RNA and DNA blue, phloxine stains muscle red, and orange G stains collagen yellow to orange.

Periodic acid-Schiff (PAS) is a histochemical stain for carbohydrates that detects aldehyde groups, such as those in glycogen in cells. Carbohydrate components of some glycosaminoglycans (such as those in mucins, basement membranes, and brush [striated] borders) normally stain purple to magenta. Hematoxylin may be used to counterstain cell nuclei purple. **Alcian blue,** which mainly shows acidic mucins at low pH, is often used with PAS, which detects neutral mucins.

Chromaffin is a fixative that contains chromic acid or potassium dichromate salt. After chromate oxidation, a brown color, from the **chromaffin reaction,** develops in fresh tissues (such as adrenal medulla and paraganglia). Chromaffin cells of the adrenal medulla stain yellow-brown, which indicates the presence of epinephrine and related compounds.

Silver stains are used to reveal fine reticular fibers of connective tissue, which appear black. Stroma of many lymphoid organs is best shown with these stains. Metallic impregnation techniques using silver also demonstrate nerve fibers and axon terminals (following methods developed and modified by **Golgi, Cajal,** and **Bielschowsky**).

Toluidine blue is a bluish-violet metachromatic stain for mast cell granules and extracellular components such as cartilage matrix. It is also commonly used to stain semithin plastic sections for light microscopic study before electron microscopy.

Immunocytochemistry utilizes antibodies to antigens (proteins), which are attached to a color reagent via a series of steps. First, a primary antibody is attached to the antigen (e.g., insulin in beta cells of the pancreas); then a secondary antibody, which is covalently linked to a coloring agent, is attached to the primary antibody. Compared with conventional optical microscopy, **fluorescence microscopy** and **confocal microscopy** offer advantages when combined with immunocytochemistry. Coupled to immunofluorescence agents—e.g., **fluorescein isothiocyanate** (FITC), **Alexa Fluor, Texas red**—that are conjugated to antibodies, they selectively probe subcellular structures.

Electron microscopy is a technique that utilizes electrons rather than light (photons) to produce images. Two types are **transmission electron microscopy** (whereby thin sections of tissues are collected on small grids and electrons are projected through specimens) and **scanning electron microscopy** (whereby electrons are used to scan specimen surfaces to produce three-dimensional images of the topography). Preparation of tissue samples for electron microscopy typically requires more time than that for paraffin sections. Staining starts before sectioning of the material: small pieces of tissue are immersed in heavy metal-containing solutions, such as osmium tetroxide and uranyl acetate. These agents accumulate in tissue and make tissue and cell structures electron dense. After immersion staining of samples, they are dehydrated in ethanol and infiltrated with a resin that can be polymerized to form a hardened block. Samples are then sectioned with an ultramicrotome to be 70-100 nm thick and are floated on water. Small copper grids are immersed under the sections and are drawn upward to collect the sections. Additional staining of sections on grids with uranyl acetate and lead citrate solutions enhances contrast in tissues. For scanning electron microscopy, biologic samples are fixed with aldehydes and then stained with osmium tetroxide to impregnate tissues with heavy metal and make them conductive. Samples must be completely dehydrated and dried to avoid surface tension drying artifacts. Samples are adhered to an aluminum stub and sputter coated with a thin layer of gold to create a conductive layer of metal on the surface. **High-resolution scanning electron microscopy** allows fractured internal surfaces of cells to be studied in three dimensions.

471

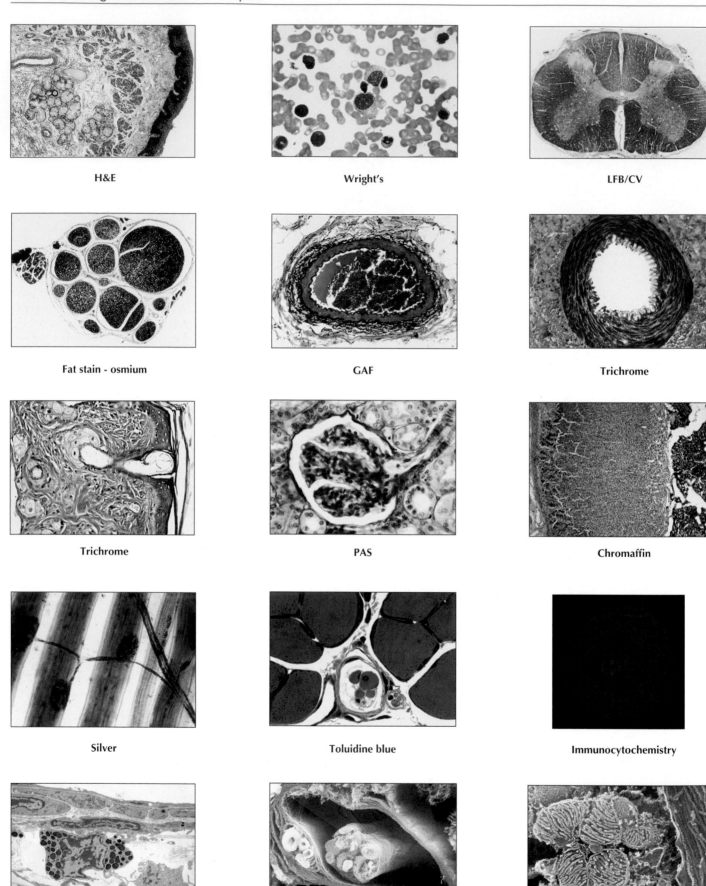

H&E

Wright's

LFB/CV

Fat stain - osmium

GAF

Trichrome

Trichrome

PAS

Chromaffin

Silver

Toluidine blue

Immunocytochemistry

TEM

SEM

HRSEM

Index

Page numbers followed by f indicates figures; t, tables

A

A band, 75
  H zone of, 76
  thick filaments and, 76, 79, 80
Abdominal cavity, 296
Acetylcholine, exocytosis and release of, 88
Acid phosphatase, lysosome, 19
Acidophils, adenohypophysis, 222
Acini, 33, 43
  mucous, 274, 276
  mucus-producing, 45
  pancreatic, 330, 330f
  seromucous, 276
  serous, 275, 276
Acne vulgaris, 256
Acquired immune deficiency syndrome (AIDS), 207
  neutropenia and, 161
Acrosomal granule, 383
Acrosome, 383, 384
Actin filaments, 6, 25, 28, 40, 79
  muscle fiber, 72
  myosin interaction with, in contraction, 79f
  thin, 97
  zonulae anchored by, 7
α-Actinin, 79, 85, 97
Acute otitis externa, 450
Addison disease, 234
Adenocarcinoma, 49, 279, 291
  cervical, 417
  prostate, 394
Adenohypophysis, 216, 220
  acidophils in, 222
  anterior lobe, 217
  basophils in, 222
  functions, 222, 222f, 222t
  pars intermedia, 217
  pars tuberalis, 217
Adenomas, pituitary, 216
ADH. *See* Antidiuretic hormone
Adipocytes, 22, 67, 167
  connective tissue, 52
  multilocular, in brown fat, 69, 69f
  peripheral nerve, 67f
  unilocular, in white fat, 68
  white, 68, 68f
  white adipose tissue, 67f
Adipose connective tissue, 53
Adipose tissue, 46, 49
  adventitia, 183
  brown, 67
    adipocytes in, 69f
  epicardium, 175
  fat droplet, 67
  histology, 67
  multilocular, 67

Adipose tissue (cont'd)
  unilocular, 67
  white, 67, 67f
    adipocytes in, 67f, 68f
Adnexa, 412, 412f, 427-446
  overview, 428
Adrenal glands, 214
  blood supply, 232, 232f
  central vein, 232
  cortex, 232, 235f
    function of, 235
    histology of, 235
    spongiocyte in, 236f
  development, 233, 233f
  histochemistry, 234
  histology, 232f, 234
  medulla, 232, 235f
    chromaffin cells in, ultrastructure of, 237
    function of, 235
    histology of, 235
  overview, 232
Adrenocortical insufficiency, primary, 234
Advanced testicular carcinoma, 27
Adventitia, 183, 187, 281, 281f. *See also* Tunica adventitia
  blood vessel innervation and, 192, 192f
  elastic fiber, 183
  esophageal, 278, 281, 281f
  vaginal, 418
  venae cavae, 181
AIDS. *See* Acquired immune deficiency syndrome
Allergic reactions, mast cells and, 61
Alpha cells, islets of Langerhans and, 240
Alpha chains, 149
Alpha granules, 166
Alpha particles, 21
Alport syndrome, 358
ALS. *See* Amyotrophic lateral sclerosis
Alveolar ducts, bronchioles and, 344
Alveolar macrophages (AM), 348
  ultrastructure, 351
Alveolar sacs, bronchioles and, 344
Alveolar-capillary membrane, 349
Alveoli, 46
  lactation and, 47, 48, 48f
  lumina, 393
  mammary gland
    atrophy and, 49
    function of, 48
    ultrastructure of, 48
Alzheimer disease, 106
AM. *See* Alveolar macrophages
Ameloblasts, 272
Amelogenins, 273
Amino acid sequence, 57

Amniocentesis, 19
Amorphous ground substance, 52
Ampulla, 409
Amylase, 330
Amyotrophic lateral sclerosis (ALS), 123
Anal canal, 308, 308f, 309
  in lower digestive system, 264
  mucosa, 309f
Anaphase, 27
Anaphylaxis, 61
Anastomoses, arteriovenous, 251
Anemia, 63, 160. *See also* Sickle cell anemia
  aplastic, 167
Anencephaly, 103
Aneurysm, 180
Annulus fibrosus, 136
Anorectal junction
  function, 308
  histology, 309, 309f
  structure, 308, 308f
Anosmia, 457
ANP. *See* Atrial natriuretic peptide
Anterograde transport, 109
Antibiotics, acne vulgaris, 256
Antibodies, immunocytochemistry use of, 221
Antidiuretic hormone (ADH), 224
Antigen, binding, 85
α1-Antitrypsin deficiency, 324
Aorta, 180
  rupture of EDS and, 56
  semilunar valve, 177, 177f
  wall, 179f, 180f
Apical blebs, 391
Apical foramina, 271
Aplastic anemia, 167
Apocrine secretion, 48
Apoptosis, 27
  epithelial cell, 49
Appendices epiploicae, 304
Appendicitis, 307
Appendix, 304, 306f
  function, 306
  histology, 307
  plexuses, 307f
  serosa, 307f
  smooth muscle in, 96, 96f
  structure, 306
Aqueous humor, drainage, 436, 436f
Arachidonic acid, mast cells and, 61
Arachnoid, 104, 123
Areolae, 425
Argyrophilia, 60
Arrector pili muscles, 258, 258f
Arteries, 178f. *See also* Coronary artery disease; Pulmonary artery
  arcuate, 355, 413

473